Oat (*Avena sativa*)

This book is a groundbreaking exploration of the multifaceted world of oats, offering a holistic journey from historical roots to cutting-edge applications. Its diverse chapters traverse the genetic and genomic landscape of oats, tracing their origin, domestication, and global spread. From their humble beginnings as animal feed to their evolution into a staple in human diets, this book showcases oats as a pivotal player in sustainable agriculture and nutrition.

The chapters meticulously delve into the bioactive compounds of oats, their health benefits, and the role of oats in disease prevention and management. The book also provides insights into oat processing techniques, storage, and milling, offering a comprehensive understanding of how these processes impact nutritional properties. The international scenario of oat production takes centre stage, emphasizing the vital role of oats in sustainable agriculture and their contribution to soil health and climate-resilient farming systems. The discussion on β-glucans, avenanthramides, and other bioactive compounds underscores the potential of oats in functional foods, catering to the increasing demand for health-focused dietary choices.

Closing with a visionary look into the future, this book explores the development of novel value-added oat-based superfoods, aligning with the global shift towards nutritionally dense, minimally processed options. Readers, including agronomists, farmers, chefs, and health enthusiasts, will find a wealth of knowledge on topics ranging from oat production economics to the nutritional composition that sets oats apart from other cereals.

***Oat* (Avena sativa):** *Production to Plate* is a must-read for anyone seeking a comprehensive and forward-looking guide to the remarkable journey of oats, blending history, agriculture, nutrition, and sustainability into a seamless narrative.

Cereals: Science and Processing Technology

Series Editors: Sneh Punia and Manoj Kumar

Maize
Nutritional Composition, Processing, and Industrial Uses
Edited by Sukhvinder Singh Purewal, Pinderpal Kaur, Sneh Punia, Kawaljit Singh Sandhu, Surender Kumar Singh, and Maninder Kaur

Wheat Science
Nutritional and Anti-Nutritional Properties, Processing, Storage, Bioactivity, and Product Development
Edited by Om Prakash Gupta, Sunil Kumar, Anamika Pandey, Mohd. Kamran Khan, Sanjay Kumar Singh, and Gyanendra Pratap Singh

Oat (*Avena sativa*)
Production to Plate
Edited by Maharishi Tomar and Prabha Singh

For more information about this series, please visit: www.routledge.com/Cereals/book-series/CSPT

Oat (*Avena sativa*)
Production to Plate

Edited by Maharishi Tomar and Prabha Singh

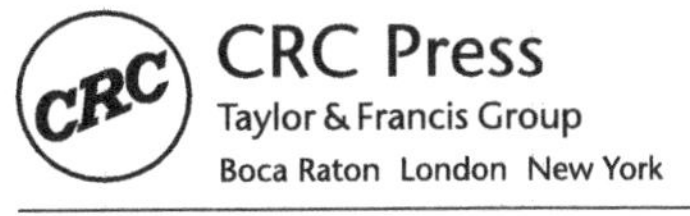

CRC Press
Taylor & Francis Group
Boca Raton London New York

CRC Press is an imprint of the
Taylor & Francis Group, an **informa** business

Cover image: Shutterstock 198199856

First edition published 2025
by CRC Press
2385 NW Executive Center Drive, Suite 320, Boca Raton FL 33431

and by CRC Press
4 Park Square, Milton Park, Abingdon, Oxon, OX14 4RN

CRC Press is an imprint of Taylor & Francis Group, LLC

Library of Congress Cataloging-in-Publication Data
Names: Tomar, Maharishi, editor. | Singh, Prabha, editor.
Title: Oat (avena sativa) : production to plate / edited by Maharishi Tomar and Prabha Singh
Other titles: Cereals: science and processing technology.
Description: First edition | Boca Raton, FL : CRC Press, 2025 | Series: Cereals: science and processing technology | Includes bibliographical references and index
Identifiers: LCCN 2024002999 (print) | LCCN 2024003000 (ebook) | ISBN 9781032199283 (hardback) | ISBN 9781032203522 (paperback) | ISBN 9781003263302 (ebook)
Subjects: LCSH: Oats.
Classification: LCC SB191.O2 O23 2025 (print) | LCC SB191.O2 (ebook) | DDC 633.1/3—dc23/eng/20240515
LC record available at https://lccn.loc.gov/2024002999
LC ebook record available at https://lccn.loc.gov/2024003000

ISBN: 978-1-032-19928-3 (hbk)
ISBN: 978-1-032-20352-2 (pbk)
ISBN: 978-1-003-26330-2 (ebk)

DOI: 10.1201/ 9781003263302

Typeset in Times
by Apex CoVantage, LLC

Contents

About the Editors

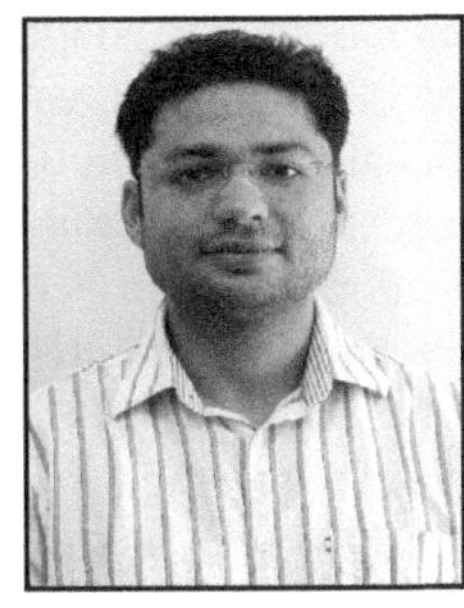

Dr. Maharishi Tomar is a distinguished figure in the field of plant biochemistry, contributing significantly to the realms of nutritional biochemistry, techno-functional analysis, virus-induced gene silencing (VIGS), heat stress, near-infrared spectroscopy (NIRS) prediction modelling, statistical modelling, and chemometrics. With an illustrious career spanning over eight years, Dr. Tomar has emerged as a leading authority in the scientific community. His academic achievements underscore his dedication and excellence. Dr. Tomar secured a commendable all-India rank of 3 in the Agricultural Research Service (ARS) examination, coupled with an all-India rank of 27 in the Council of Scientific and Industrial Research (CSIR) examination. His expertise extends further, having excelled in the Graduate Aptitude Test in Engineering (GATE) and securing a Senior Research Fellowship (SRF). Since July 2015, Dr. Maharishi Tomar has been actively engaged as an ARS scientist specializing in plant biochemistry. In the initial years of his career, from July 2015 to July 2017, he contributed significantly to the field while stationed at the ICAR-Central Potato Research Institute in Shimla, India. Here, his research focused on virus-induced gene silencing (VIGS) in potatoes under heat stress, showcasing his commitment to understanding the molecular intricacies of plant responses to environmental challenges. Subsequently, from 2019 to the present day, Dr. Tomar has been immersed in the study of nutritional biochemistry and NIRS statistical modelling, particularly in the context of pearl millet grains. His research portfolio also includes pivotal contributions to the identification of the berseem stem rot pathogen, employing both morphological and molecular methods. Additionally, he played a crucial role in unravelling the mysteries of ageing-causing enzymes and nutritional quality in various oat genotypes. A prolific author, Dr. Maharishi Tomar has made substantial contributions to scientific literature, with over 40 research papers and several insightful book chapters to his credit. His work reflects a deep understanding of the intricate biochemical processes in plants, contributing significantly to the advancement of knowledge in the field. Dr. Tomar's comprehensive expertise, coupled with his dedication to unravelling complex biochemical phenomena, positions him as a distinguished editor in the field of plant biochemistry.

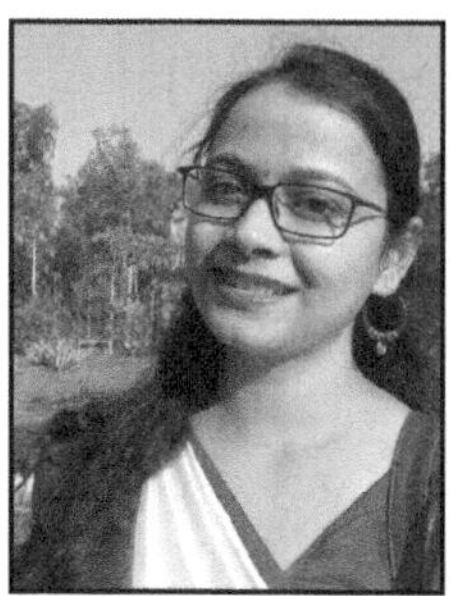**Dr. Prabha Singh** is a distinguished expert in the field of plant physiology, showcasing a remarkable focus on nutrient stress and associated studies. With a specialized emphasis on abiotic stress in cereals such as wheat, maize, and oat, as well as seed physiology and cereal nutritional quality, Dr. Singh brings a wealth of experience spanning approximately four years. Her academic prowess is evident in her outstanding achievements, having secured notable rankings in prestigious examinations. Dr. Singh cleared the Agricultural Research Service (ARS) with an impressive all-India rank of 3, and the Council of Scientific and Industrial Research (CSIR) with an all-India rank of 69. Her academic excellence is further underscored by securing the top position, all-India rank 1, in the Senior Research Fellowship (SRF). Since January 2019, Dr. Prabha Singh has served as an ARS scientist specializing in plant physiology. Her journey in the scientific realm began with focused research on nitrogen and phosphorus stress in maize and wheat, an area she explored prior to joining the Indian Council of Agricultural Research (ICAR). Dr. Singh's significant contributions extend to her role at the ICAR-Indian Grassland and Fodder Research Institute in Jhansi. Here, she is actively engaged in investigating the seed coat dynamics of berseem and studying the impact of karrikinolide (KAR1) on the early establishment of range grasses and legumes. Her diverse research portfolio also encompasses climate change studies and near-infrared spectroscopy (NIRS) statistical modelling, particularly focused on the nutritional aspect of berseem. A prolific author, Dr. Prabha Singh has made substantial contributions to the scientific community through numerous publications. Her body of work includes a collection of international and national research papers, as well as insightful book chapters. Dr. Singh's commitment to advancing knowledge in plant physiology and her multifaceted expertise make her a valuable and respected figure in the field.

Contributors

Dilshad Ahmad
ICAR-Indian Agricultural Research
Institute
New Delhi, India

Meenakshi Arya
Rani Lakshmi Bai Central Agricultural
University
Jhansi, India

Rakesh Bhardwaj
ICAR-National Bureau of Plant Genetic
Resources
New Delhi, India

Sushil S. Changan
ICAR-National Institute of Abiotic Stress
Management
Baramati, India

Prince Choyal
ICAR-Indian Institute of Soybean
Research
Indore, India

Anil Dahuja
ICAR-Indian Agricultural Research
Institute
New Delhi, India

Ajeet Singh Dhaka
ICAR-Indian Agricultural Research
Institute
New Delhi, India

Nitin Kumar Garg
Sri Karan Dev Agriculture University
Jobner, India

Muzaffar Hasan
ICAR-Central Institute of Agricultural
Engineering
Bhopal, India

Deepmala Jain
ICAR-Indian Grassland and Fodder
Research Institute
Jhansi, India

Prashant P. Jambhulkar
Rani Lakshmi Bai Central Agricultural
University
Jhansi, India

Archana T. Janamatti
ICAR-Indian Agricultural Research
Institute
New Delhi, India

Racheal John
ICAR-National Bureau of Plant Genetic
Resources
New Delhi, India

Preetiman Kaur
Punjab Agricultural University (PAU)
Ludhiana, India

Simardeep Kaur
ICAR-Research Complex for North
Eastern Hill (NEH)
Region Umiam, India

Pratapsingh Khapte
ICAR-National Institute of Abiotic Stress
Management
Baramati, India

Veda Krishnan
ICAR-Indian Agricultural Research
   Institute
New Delhi, India

Dharmendra Kumar
ICAR-Central Potato Research Institute
Shimla, India

Kamlesh Kumar
ICAR-Indian Institute of Farming
   Systems Research (IIFSR)
Meerut, India

Manish Kumar
ICAR-Indian Agricultural Research
   Institute
New Delhi, India

Sanjay Kumar
ICAR-Indian Grassland and Fodder
   Research Institute
Jhansi, India

Vinay Kumar
ICAR-Indian Grassland and Fodder
   Research Institute
Jhansi, India

Arti Kumari
ICAR-Indian Agricultural Research
   Institute
New Delhi, India

Milan Kumar Lal
ICAR-Central Potato Research Institute
Shimla, India

Brijesh Lekhak
ICAR-Indian Agricultural Research
   Institute
New Delhi, India

H. S. Mahesha
ICAR-Indian Grassland and Fodder
   Research Institute
Jhansi, India

Chirag Maheshwari
ICAR-Indian Agricultural Research
   Institute
New Delhi, India

Nand Lal Meena
ICAR-National Bureau of Plant Genetic
   Resources
New Delhi, India

Vandana Parmar
ICAR-Central Potato Research Institute
Shimla, India

Arun Prajapati
ICAR-Indian Grassland and Fodder
   Research Institute
Jhansi, India

Prathap V.
ICAR-Indian Institute of Oil Palm Research
Pedavegi, India

Sohel Rahaman
ICAR-Indian Agricultural Research
   Institute
New Delhi, India

Pinky Raigond
ICAR-National Research Centre on
   Pomegranate
Solapur, India

Kanika Rani
Chaudhary Charan Singh Haryana
   Agricultural University
Hisar, India

Archana Sachdev
ICAR-Indian Agricultural Research
   Institute
New Delhi, India

Ravi Prakash Saini
ICAR-Indian Grassland and Fodder
   Research Institute
Jhansi, India

Karishma Seem
ICAR-Indian Agricultural Research
  Institute (IARI)
New Delhi, India

Ajay Kumar Singh
ICAR-Indian Grassland and Fodder
  Research Institute
Jhansi, India

Awnindra Kumar Singh
ICAR-Indian Grassland and Fodder
  Research Institute
Jhansi, India

Binay Kumar Singh
ICAR-Research Complex for North
  Eastern Hill (NEH) Region
Umiam, India

Brajesh Kumar Singh
ICAR-Central Potato Research Institute
Shimla, India

Ishwar Singh
(FFC)-ICAR Krishi Bhawan
New Delhi, India

Naseeb Singh
ICAR-Research Complex for North
  Eastern Hill (NEH) Region
Umiam, India

Tejveer Singh
ICAR-Indian Grassland and Fodder
  Research Institute
Jhansi, India

Sunil Ramling Swami
ICAR-Indian Grassland and Fodder
  Research Institute
Jhansi, India

Kailashpati Tripathi
ICAR-National Research Centre on
  Seed Spices
Ajmer, India

Aruna Tyagi
ICAR-Indian Agricultural Research
  Institute
New Delhi, India

Vijay Kumar Yadav
ICAR-Indian Grassland and Fodder
  Research Institute
Jhansi, India

Preface

In the intricate tapestry of agriculture, nutrition, and sustainability, oats emerge as a resilient and versatile protagonist. This book embarks on a captivating journey through the chapters, each unfolding a distinct facet of oats – *Avena sativa*, a cereal that has weathered the winds of time, evolving from a humble weed to a global player in the realms of nutrition, agriculture, and health. Chapter 1 initiates the exploration, unravelling the historical narrative of oats' cultivation that spans over four millennia. From Central Europe to China, and eventually finding their way to the Americas and Australia, oats have not only adapted to diverse climates but also transformed from fodder to a vital component of human diets. The chapter extends beyond history to delve into the genetic intricacies of oats, emphasizing their indispensable role in crop improvement and achieving Sustainable Development Goals. As we navigate through global challenges, the urgency of diversifying food sources takes centre stage, with oats poised as a key player in this quest. Chapter 2 broadens the horizon, providing a panoramic view of oats on the global stage. Russia, Canada, Poland, Australia, and Finland take the lead in oat production, highlighting the cereal's significance in livestock feed and human consumption. The chapter underscores the pivotal role of oats in sustainable agriculture, weaving a narrative that connects oats to soil health, erosion mitigation, and climate-resilient farming systems. As we delve deeper into the nutritional realm in Chapter 3, oats shine as a beacon of hope amid global challenges of food insecurity and malnutrition. The nutritional composition of oats stands out, offering a rich tapestry of proteins, fats, dietary fibre, vitamins, and minerals. The chapter advocates for plant-based diets and positions oats as a solution to address malnutrition, showcasing their potential to improve public health. Chapter 4 unravels the bioactive compounds and phytochemicals in oats, portraying them not just as a staple but as a potential therapeutic agent. From avenanthramides to flavonoids and antioxidants, oats showcase a rich portfolio that extends beyond their fibre content, contributing to heart health, cancer prevention, and more. The chapter ignites the curiosity for future research to explore and enhance the health benefits of these compounds. The journey through the chapters continues with Chapter 5, where the focus shifts to the journey of oats from the field to our tables. A historical survey of grain milling, processing techniques, and storage strategies unfolds, revealing the evolution of oats from rudimentary methods to sophisticated technologies. The chapter offers insights into preserving grain quality during storage and presents a diverse array of oat mill products. Chapter 6 takes a detour into the realm of health benefits and medicinal properties of oats. Oats, with their diverse bioactive compounds, become not just a dietary choice but a potential ally in disease prevention and treatment. From diabetes management to cancer prevention, oats showcase a spectrum of health-promoting properties, transcending their role as a mere staple. The spotlight then shifts to the star player, β-glucan, in Chapter 7. This soluble oat fibre takes centre stage, demonstrating its prowess in mitigating glycaemic responses, reducing cholesterol levels, and enhancing immune responses. The chapter provides a comprehensive overview of the physiological functions of β-glucans and their potential applications across biomedical, pharmaceutical, food, and cosmetic industries. In Chapter 8, oats step onto the culinary stage, becoming integral components of diverse functional food products. Despite challenges in integrating oats into food production, innovative oat ingredients enriched with β-glucan emerge, catering to the preferences of health-conscious consumers. Oat proteins, starch, and β-glucan play pivotal roles in addressing dietary and nutritional needs, spanning from gluten-free alternatives to plant-based protein sources. Chapter 9 delves into the biotechnological, molecular, and processing strategies for improving the nutritional and functional properties of oats. The complex genetic landscape of cultivated oats takes centre stage, with advancements in molecular genetics, genomics, and biotechnology contributing to a deeper understanding of oat genetics. These advancements empower plant breeders to continually enhance oat quality, offering potential solutions to global food security challenges. As we reach the concluding chapter, Chapter 10, the spotlight turns to the future prospects and the development of novel value-added oat-based superfoods. Oats, exemplified as superfoods, play a pivotal role in the pursuit of healthier and more sustainable nutrition sources. The chapter explores the nutraceutical and superfood potential of oats, emphasizing their impact on gut microbiota, consumer acceptability, and future research prospects. This book is an odyssey through the diverse dimensions of oats, intertwining history, agriculture, nutrition, and health. Each chapter contributes a unique thread to the narrative, weaving a tapestry that illuminates the significance of oats in our global journey towards sustainable, nutritious, and wholesome living.

Oat, a Distinct Cereal

Origin, History, Production Practices, and Production Economics

Deepmala Jain, Prabha Singh, Kanika Rani, Sanjay Kumar, Vinay Kumar, and Arun Prajapati

1.1 INTRODUCTION

Oats (*Avena sativa*) belong to the Poaceae grass family, characterized by a genomic composition of AACCDD ($2n = 6x = 42$) and have been cultivated for over 2000 years globally. Particularly popular in the northwestern regions of India due to their favourable growth habits and high nutritional value for animals, oats have recently gained traction as a fodder crop [1]. With an average annual global production of approximately 20,565 (1000 MT), leading oat-producing nations include the European Union (EU), Russia, Canada, Brazil, Australia, the United Kingdom, the United States, Argentina, China, and Chile (USDA 2023) [2]. In India, oats are predominantly used for winter fodder, although certain regions cultivate them for grain used in infant food and animal feed [3]. Key oat-producing regions in India include Uttar Pradesh, Himachal Pradesh, Haryana, Punjab, Madhya Pradesh, Bihar, Gujarat, Andhra Pradesh, Rajasthan, and Tamil Nadu, with hilly areas in southern India also participating in oat farming [4].

DOI: 10.1201/ 9781003263302-1

Although oats are often underutilized on a global scale, they boast a wealth of diverse nutrients. Notably, 100 grams of oats typically contain 379 kcal of energy, 67.7 grams of carbohydrates, 10.84 grams of water, 13.15 grams of protein, 10.1 grams of fibre, and 6.52 grams of lipids [5]. Studies have revealed that oats possess cholesterol-lowering properties, attributed to their β-glucan content, offering benefits such as improved obesity management, postprandial glycaemic control, and reduced risks of cardiovascular diseases and colon cancer [6].

Although oats were domesticated later than wheat and barley, their cultivation dates back no earlier than 4000 years ago. Initially perceived as a weed in wheat and barley fields, oats gained prominence due to their superior adaptation to cooler and more humid climates [7]. While the domestication of oats likely occurred outside the centre of origin during the Neolithic revolution, the exact time and place remain undetermined. However, evidence suggests that oat domestication occurred independently from the domestication of other grains [8]. Archaeological findings place the beginnings of oat cultivation in Central Europe at the dawn of the modern era, with oat cultivation also taking root in China around the same time. Over time, oats gained recognition as both animal feed and human food, particularly in regions with poor soil conditions [3], [9], [10]. Oats were introduced to the Americas in the 16th and 17th centuries, with red oats arriving via Spanish settlers and common oats following suit with English and German settlers. Oats also found their way to Australia through English settlers [11]. Traditionally utilized as feed for horses, calves, young stock, poultry, and sheep, oats have recently gained popularity among human consumers, especially in developed countries, owing to their content of β-glucan, known for its cholesterol-reducing properties [12]. Oats serve as a valuable source of proteins, lipids, vitamins, minerals, and antioxidants, leading to increased interest from the food, pharmaceutical, and cosmetic industries [13]. While primarily cultivated for grain, pastures, and forage, oats have also gained traction in diverse areas, including sustainable agriculture and biofuel production. This chapter will extensively review the genetic and genomic resources of oats, emphasizing their origin, domestication, diversity, and taxonomy, alongside discussions on conservation, characterization, evaluation, and the current status of oat germplasm and its role in crop improvement.

Significant advancements have been made in improving global survival rates, nutritional standards, and educational opportunities over recent decades. However, despite these strides, global efforts to accomplish the Sustainable Development Goals, aimed at eradicating malnutrition and poverty by 2030, have significantly veered off track [14]. The prevalence of severe food insecurity has escalated, impacting a staggering 11.7% of the global population. This rise is evidenced by a surge of 112 million individuals unable to afford a nutritious diet, bringing the total affected population to approximately 3.1 billion, highlighting the growing issue of inadequate access to safe and nourishing food [3], [9], [10], [15]. Child malnutrition continues to persist as a critical public health concern, with only a quarter of countries demonstrating progress towards meeting targets for addressing stunting, wasting, and childhood obesity. Presently, children are confronted with the dual challenge of malnutrition, where undernutrition coincides with issues such as overweight, obesity, and other diet-related non-communicable diseases [16]. Beyond the burden of malnutrition, today's children confront an uncertain future marked by environmental changes, conflicts, the COVID-19 pandemic, and entrenched inequalities that jeopardize their health and well-being. As the global population continues to grow at a rapid pace, it poses increasingly complex challenges to both food security and environmental sustainability [3]. These challenges underscore the urgent need to diversify food sources, particularly through the incorporation of more plant-based materials [17]. A plant-based diet primarily comprises or is entirely composed of foods derived from plants. It encompasses various eating patterns that limit the consumption of animal products while emphasizing the intake of plant-based foods such as vegetables, fruits, whole grains, legumes, nuts, and seeds [18]. Notably, individuals following plant-based diets need not strictly adhere to vegan or vegetarian diets, as the defining characteristic is a reduced consumption of animal-derived foods. The global market for plant-based food materials has witnessed substantial growth in recent years, with the market share of plant-based proteins projected to reach USD 15.6 billion by 2026, demonstrating an annual growth rate of 7.2% [19]–[24].

In this section, we embark on an enlightening exploration of the realm of oats, revealing the origins of this exceptional grain and tracing its historical development. By examining its ancient beginnings and the key milestones that have influenced its journey, our goal is to uncover the intricate history of oats, emphasizing their cultural and agricultural significance across various civilizations. Moreover, this section thoroughly investigates the current landscape of oat cultivation, shedding light on the complexities of modern farming practices. Through a comprehensive analysis of the latest innovations, approaches, and sustainable methods, we aim to provide readers with a thorough grasp of the dynamic procedures involved in nurturing this valuable crop. A significant emphasis of this section is also placed on dissecting the intricate economics of oat production. By analysing the diverse factors that impact production, including market trends, pricing mechanisms, and cost-efficient strategies, we seek to offer readers valuable insights into the economic dynamics that underlie the oat industry. Additionally, we strive to underscore the crucial role of oats in promoting agricultural sustainability and their potential contribution to the broader economic sphere.

1.2 EVOLUTION AND GLOBAL SIGNIFICANCE OF OAT CULTIVATION

1.2.1 Ancient Roots and Cultural Significance

Oats possess a rich historical background as a fundamental cereal crop for both human and animal sustenance, evidenced by their discovery in various archaeological sites. Notably, explorations of the Grotta Paglicci cave in southeastern Italy, inhabited by Upper Paleolithic hunter-gatherers approximately 32,000 years ago, unveiled substantial oat grain remnants on a stone pestle, pre-dating the era of plant domestication [25]. Likewise, findings from the ancient Neolithic village of Dhra' in the Jordan Valley, dating back to 11,500 to 10,500 BP (Before Present) [26] indicate the gathering of wild oats (*Avena sterilis*) by early humans during that epoch. *A. sterilis*, an Old World wild red oat, distinguishes itself from related species due to its vaguely defined upper florets [27]. This wild oat serves as the precursor of *A. sativa* and its closely associated minor crop, *Avena byzantina*, being naturally hexaploid. Genetic studies propose that the original forms of *A. sterilis* thrived in the Fertile Crescent of the Near East. Notably, the recovery of around 120,000 wild oat seeds at the site implies deliberate cultivation, as the surrounding soil conditions were unsuitable to sustain a significant population of wild cereals [28].

Furthermore, the importance of oats in historical contexts becomes apparent with the recovery of oat grains (presumably *Avena fatua* or *A. sterilis*) associated with archaeological findings, suggesting the development of a substantial oat market alongside favourable climatic changes in the Northern British Isles. Historical records documenting agricultural practices on estates in the British Isles during medieval times affirm the extensive cultivation of oats throughout Britain, underscoring their paramount significance in human diets and as a staple feed for livestock employed in agriculture and other tasks. These changes potentially contributed to the widespread adoption of oat cultivation during the medieval era in Britain [29]. Numerous archaeological surveys from Saxon and medieval sites in England routinely unearth oats, frequently constituting the majority of deposits or found in significant quantities alongside barley deposits, as observed in late Saxon sites in Oxford and Ipswich [30]. This importance is further encapsulated in the writings of the prolific English poet and author Gervase Markham (c. 1568–1637 AD) in his work *A Way to Get Wealth*. Markham accentuates the virtues of oats in the chapter "Of the Excellency of Oats, and the Many Singular Virtues and Use of Them in a Family," emphasizing their adaptability to diverse soil types and their pivotal role in supporting households and agricultural activities.

During the span from the 18th century to the mid-19th century, oats played a pivotal role in the dietary provisions for livestock in Britain. Noteworthy advancements in agricultural practices instigated a considerable surge in yield. However, the ascendancy of wheat and barley as viable substitutes gradually eclipsed oats, predominantly owing to their more lucrative returns. Despite the sustained demand for oats in livestock feed during the mid-17th century, the consumption of oat-based foods by humans experienced a gradual downturn, yielding ground to the prevalence of wheat-based alternatives. Historical evidence suggests the introduction of oats to the New World occurred through two principal routes during the 17th and 18th centuries [3], [21], [23], [31], [32]. The red oat variety, *A. byzantina*, a winter oat, was transported to North and South America by the Spaniards. Conversely, the spring oat variant, *A. sativa*, was introduced to North America by English and German settlers. By the mid-19th century, the eastern regions of the United States were identified as the primary cultivation areas for oats. Subsequently, the upper Mississippi Valley and adjoining prairie provinces in Southern Canada underwent a notable expansion in oat acreage, eventually transforming into the primary oat-growing regions in North America by the turn of the century [33].

Although the exact birthplace of oats remains uncertain, it is widely believed that the greatest genetic diversity is concentrated in the Canary Islands, the Mediterranean, the Middle East, and the Himalayan region. *Avena* species were discovered at various sites in the Near East, dating back to 10,500 to 5750 BC. The expansion of the

Neolithic Revolution from the Near East to regions in Europe, Great Britain, and Asia catalysed the proliferation of farming and trade, leading to the inadvertent introduction of oats and rye as weed contaminants alongside wheat and barley seeds. Limited historical records indicate the existence of cultivated oats in the northern regions of western Europe between 4500 and 400 BC, during a period characterized by cooler and wetter climatic conditions. Oats and rye thrived under these environmental circumstances, exhibiting a comparative advantage over wheat and barley. References by Greek and Roman authors from AD 23 to AD 79 underscored the multifaceted applications of oats, including their uses in fodder, animal feed, human consumption, and medicinal properties [34]. Despite a relatively obscure historical narrative during the Dark Ages, oat cultivation persisted and gained prominence during the Renaissance, securing its place as the fourth most significant crop after wheat, barley, and rye. Scotland, in particular, embraced oats as a dominant crop by the 13th century, owing to its adaptability to regions with lower agricultural productivity. From 1500 to 1700, oats solidified its position as the primary grain crop for human consumption in Scotland, Wales, Ireland, and Britain, while retaining its pivotal role in animal feed for horses, cattle, and sheep [35].

During the dire potato crop failure in Ireland between 1740 and 1741, oats were harnessed in the preparation of soups as a palliative measure against starvation. The migration of British and Spanish immigrants and explorers to North America marked the introduction of oats to the continent. Throughout the 16th and 17th centuries, the English populace brought oats primarily for animal consumption to Canada, New England, and the eastern United States. The assimilation of Scottish settlers in North America further cemented the use of oats in culinary practices and porridge-making. Concurrently, the Spanish influx in the early 1800s disseminated oats along the Pacific coast, as well as the southwestern and southeastern regions of the United States, primarily for equine sustenance. Oats were also embraced by the general public for medicinal purposes, readily procurable from apothecaries during this epoch. The westward migration of oat production gradually transpired, shifting towards the Upper Mississippi River Valley and Canada by the 1880s [36]. The rise in popularity of oatmeal as a breakfast staple burgeoned around 1900 in the United States, as local mills pivoted to processing oats into breakfast cereals, leading to their retail distribution in grocery stores, and displacing their former niche in pharmacies and drugstores. Governor Phillip played a pivotal role in the introduction of oats to New South Wales, Australia, in 1791. Initially, oats were primarily employed as green fodder and hay for horses, dairy cattle, and pigs. However, the late-maturing European oat varieties introduced in Australia limited successful cultivation to Tasmania and the elevated regions of mainland Australia until the advent of the early-maturing Algerian variety, better suited for regions with lower rainfall. The consumption of rolled oats among the Australian populace can be traced back to the influence of British immigrants. Notably, the migration of Leonard and George Parsons from England to Australia in 1861 heralded the establishment of the esteemed John Bull brand of rolled oats by the late 1880s. Similarly, the immigration of Harry Clifford Love from Dublin to Australia in 1854 led to the formation of the Imperial Manufacturing Company, Ltd. The company subsequently initiated the production of Uncle Tobys, a renowned brand of rolled oats, in 1893 [37].

1.2.2 Oat Domestication and Genetic Diversification

Oats, taxonomically categorized within the genus *Avena*, derive their nomenclature from the Latin term *"Avena,"* signifying both "nourishment" and "desire." Linnaeus, in 1735, delineated the initial four species – *sterilis*, *fatua*, *sativa*, and *nuda* – within this genus. The extant *Avena* comprises 27 recognized forms, encompassing 14 biological classifications. *Avena* species are subtypes within the *Avena clauda*, *strigosa*, *barbata*, and *sativa* categories of the Gramineae family, a subdivision of true grasses numbering around 10,000 species across 700 genera [38]. Despite phylogenetic analyses establishing Avena's proximity to cool-season grasses such as brome, wheat, barley, rye, and brachypodium [39], chemical [40] distinctions persist, including elevated β-glucan, oil, and protein content, alongside unique antioxidants. Oats, inherently self-pollinating and cleistogamous under standard environmental conditions, exhibit three levels of polyploidization – ranging from diploid to tetraploid to hexaploidy. Two cultivated species exist: the diploid *A. strigosa*, a significant forage and soil cover crop in Europe, Brazil, Argentina, and Uruguay [41], and the hexaploid *A. sativa*. *A. sativa*, commonly known as cultivated oat, holds paramount economic significance globally, constituting 2% of world grain production with an average of 22.7 million metric tons in 2021–22 [42]. While livestock feed predominantly drives its importance, compounds such as β-glucan and distinctive antioxidants have solidified its place in human diets and cosmetics. Debates surrounding the evolution of cultivated hexaploid oats persist. Early cytological studies suggested progenitor species of the three genomes, with one of the resulting tetraploid genomes duplicating under selection pressure, culminating in the hexaploid state. However, as researchers contend, the historical review supports a departure from the AACCDD genome designations, advocating for a more provisional classification until the genuine progenitors are identified [43] (Figure 1.1) (Table 1.1).

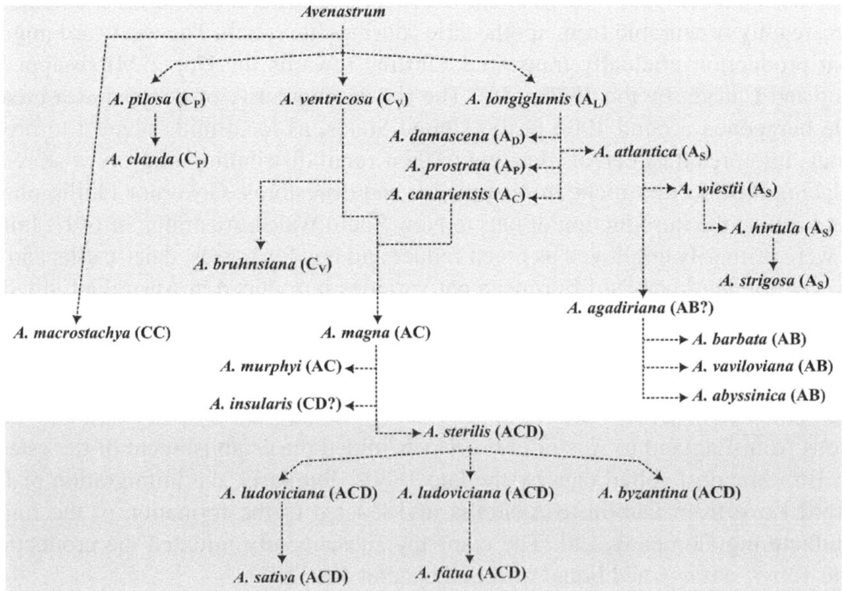

FIGURE 1.1 The origin and historical dissemination of oat species.

TABLE 1.1 Diversity of *Avena* Species: Distribution, Ecological Characteristics, and Conservation Status

AVENA *SPECIES*	*DISTRIBUTION*	*ECOLOGICAL CHARACTERISTICS*	*CONSERVATION STATUS*	*REFERENCES*
Avena sativa	Global distribution, 2% of world grain production	Economically crucial and used in livestock feed, human diets, and cosmetics. High β-glucan, oil, and protein content. Dual domestication events.	Not specified	[42]
Avena strigosa	Europe, Brazil, Argentina, Uruguay	Diploid species and significant forage and soil cover crop. Centre of origin and diversity in Spain and Portugal.	Not specified	[41]
Avena atlantica	Exclusive to Morocco	Endemic to Morocco and found along the Atlantic littoral, with sporadic occurrences in arid habitats.	Not specified	[85]
Avena macro-stachya	Endemic to northeastern Algeria	Abundant in Bellezma region and faces threats from grazing.	Not specified	[76]
Avena insularis	Sicily, Tunisia	Endangered species, observed in Sicily and Tunisia. Grazing poses a significant threat.	Endangered on the European Red List	[74], [85]
Avena canariensis	Canary Islands, possibly Morocco	Endemic to the Canary Islands and categorized as "vulnerable." Divergent views on distribution beyond the Canary Islands.	Vulnerable on the IUCN Red List	[64]
Avena agadiriana	Atlantic Coast of Morocco	Endemic to North Africa and Morocco and resilient in diverse environmental challenges.	Not specified	[86]
Avena magna	Endemic to Morocco	Weedy species with large spikelets and faces threats from agricultural intensification and habitat contraction.	Not specified	[63]

(Continued)

TABLE 1.1 (Continued) Diversity of *Avena* Species: Distribution, Ecological Characteristics, and Conservation Status

AVENA *SPECIES*	*DISTRIBUTION*	*ECOLOGICAL CHARACTERISTICS*	*CONSERVATION STATUS*	*REFERENCES*
Avena murphyi	Southern Spain, northern Morocco	Thrives in the Mediterranean climate and faces threats from intensive agriculture and competition with *A. sterilis*.	Endangered on the Red List of Spanish Flora	[71], [87]
Avena prostrata	Southeast Spain, Morocco	Morphological affinities with *A. hirtula*, *A. wiestii*, and *A. barbata*. Faces threats from agricultural practices in Morocco.	Potentially Red List species (ECPGR)	[61], [63]
Avena vaviloviana	Ethiopia, Eritrea, Yemen	Ubiquitous and often as mixtures with the main crop. Faces threats from changes in agricultural practices and introduction of new crops.	Not specified	[58], [77]
Avena volgensis	Endemic weed associated with a local landrace	Significant decline since the 1950s due to the replacement of landrace by commercial varieties. Suspected high risk of extinction.	High risk of extinction	[63]
Avena longiglumis	Iberian Peninsula, North Africa, Israel	Prevalence in Morocco, two distinct ecotypes with specialization in sandy soils.	Not specified	[63]
Avena damascena	Syria, Morocco	Endemic to Syria, discovered in Morocco with conspecific populations. Extensive distribution in Morocco.	Not specified	[59], [63]
Avena hirtula	Southeast Spain, Morocco	Morphological affinities with *A. prostrata*, *A. wiestii*, and *A. barbata*. Threatened by agricultural practices in Morocco.	ECPGR	[63], [85]

(Continued)

TABLE 1.1   (Continued) Diversity of *Avena* Species: Distribution, Ecological Characteristics, and Conservation Status

AVENA *SPECIES*	*DISTRIBUTION*	*ECOLOGICAL CHARACTERISTICS*	*CONSERVATION STATUS*	*REFERENCES*
Avena wiestii	Southeast Spain, Morocco	Morphological affinities with *A. prostrata*, *A. hirtula*, and *A. barbata*. Threatened by agricultural practices in Morocco.	ECPGR	[63], [85]
Avena barbata	Southeast Spain, Morocco	Coexists with *A. prostrata*, *A. hirtula*, and *A. wiestii*. Threatened by agricultural practices in Morocco.	ECPGR	[63], [85]

Cultivated oat is believed to have undergone dual domestication events – one in the Near East (e.g., Iran, Iraq, Syria, and Turkey) and another in North Africa and the Iberian Peninsula of southern Spain [44]. Modernly, Near East ecotypes are termed common oats, while North African or Iberian ecotypes are designated as byzantina oats. Both ecotypes were introduced to North America between 1500 and 1600 AD [45]. Researchers posit that common oats migrated to North-central Europe around 1200–600 BC, resulting in environmental adaptations favouring colonization of upper latitudes in North America. Byzantina types, sown in autumn, colonized the southern regions. Intriguingly, genetic bottlenecks stemming from different geographic centres of origin endure in North America, presenting substantial opportunities for oat breeders [46].

The western Mediterranean region is acknowledged as a primary centre of diversity for the genus *Avena*, with significant occurrences of wild *Avena* species in this area and the adjoining Middle East. Notably, three biological species of oats – *Avena insularis*, *Avena canariensis*, and *Avena macrostachya* – have yet to be documented in Morocco [47]. Equally intriguing is the exclusivity of *Avena maroccana*, *Avena agadiriana*, and *Avena atlantica* to Morocco, as they have not been found elsewhere. The secondary centre of *Avena* species formation and the origin of cultivated oat (*A. sativa*) is located in the Asia Minor centre of crop origin. Intraspecific diversity analysis of landraces has facilitated the identification of morphogenesis centres for all cultivated oat species [48]. Spain with Portugal serves as the centre of origin and diversity for diploid species (*A. strigosa*), while Great Britain is identified as the centre for naked forms (*A. sativa* subsp. *nudisativa* (Husnot.) Rod. et Sold.) [49]. Ethiopia is designated as the centre for tetraploid species (*Avena abyssinica*); Algeria and Morocco for hexaploid species (*A. byzantina*); Iran, Georgia, and Russia for hulled forms of *A. sativa*; and Mongolia and China for its unhulled forms [27] (Figure 1.1) (Table 1.1).

Vavilov et al.'s assertion that the eastern part of Anterior Asia, characterized by harsher soil and climate conditions than the western Mediterranean areas, harbours the most extensive diversity of polyploids has been substantiated [50]. Allopolyploid species have fostered the development of highly differentiated ecotypes, playing a pivotal role in evolution [50]. Moving from the centre of origin towards the southwestern Asiatic centre, smaller-seeded and more adaptive hexaploid forms of wild species have emerged. Among the 26 oat species, 4 have been domesticated and are cultivated, while 5 are considered weeds. Common oat (*A. sativa*), the most economically crucial species, exhibits a global distribution. Red oat (*A. byzantina*) is cultivated in southern Europe, particularly in Spain and Portugal, as well as in North Africa, Southwest Asia, South America, and Australia [47]. Two other species – *A. strigosa* (cultivated in Europe and Brazil, with landraces on European islands) and *A. abyssinica* (cultivated in Ethiopia) – have regional cultivation significance. Except for common oats, *A. fatua* is the only species found worldwide and is recognized as a noxious weed. Seven wild species within the genus *Avena* are endemic and face imminent threats of genetic erosion or extinction in their natural habitats. The succinct portrayals of the habitats, distributions, and threats of *Avena* species in the Mediterranean, Near East, and Anterior Asia regions are drawn from observations made during expeditions conducted over the past 25 years [51].

Avena ventricosa, indigenous to Algeria, Cyprus, Iraq, Saudi Arabia, and Azerbaijan, manifests a European presence limited to the confines of the Island of Cyprus. An investigation conducted in 2009 on the island revealed the occurrence of *A. ventricosa* in diverse locales, including Kampos and Nicosia, proximal to the Cypriot Agricultural Institute (ARI), Athalass Farm (National Park), Macheras Mt, and Salt Lake (Alykes), in close proximity to Larnaka airport [52]. This species, characterized by its conspicuous rarity and disjunct distribution, likely possesses relic attributes, persisting exclusively within undisturbed habitats. *Avena pilosa* and *A. clauda* exhibit prevalence in steppe mountain passes in the western Transcaucasia, sporadically extending to semidesert and desert zones, as well as mountainous regions of Central Asia, notably Uzbekistan. Both taxa are disseminated throughout Asia Minor, Iran, Turkish and Iraqi Kurdistan, Lebanon, and Syria. While *A. pilosa* and *A. clauda* form substantial populations in Turkish and Iraqi Kurdistan and Iran, their presence in the Mediterranean region is delimited and dispersed [53]. In Turkey, populations have been ascertained in the Chardak and Cheilapinar regions and along the Aegean Sea coast. *A. clauda* maintains an endangered status in Israel, with occurrences documented in Lower Galilee, the hills of Judah, and the Samaria Desert. The species is under protection in the Um Zuka nature reserve in Samaria, currently existing in four stands while extinct in three additional locations [54]. Small populations have been discerned in the Jordanian highlands and in Algeria near Oran and Batna. In Europe, *A. clauda* has been documented in Bulgaria and Greece, spanning Athens, Attica, Macedonia, Thrace, and Crete Island. *A. pilosa* also thrives in various regions of Spain. Moroccan populations of *A. clauda* and *A. pilosa* have been identified in the foothills of the Middle Atlas Mountains near Azrou. *A. clauda* exhibits a proclivity for contaminating wheat and barley fields, as well as irrigated alfalfa fields, often cohabiting with *A. barbata* and *A. pilosa* along roadsides and proximal to structures. *A. clauda* primarily displays segetal and ruderal characteristics. *A. pilosa* is abundant in maquis vegetation, among oaks and pistachio trees, in cenoses of abandoned pastures, on limestone slopes, and in narrow crevices on mountain slopes [55].

Avena longiglumis is sporadically distributed across the Iberian Peninsula, North Africa, and Israel. Observations by researchers indicate its prevalence in Morocco, where two distinct ecotypes have been identified – a coastal variant characterized by robust, towering plants with expansive drooping panicles, and a desert variant featuring shorter, slender plants with diminutive panicles. Both ecotypes specialize in sandy soils, with these populations predominantly inhabiting eucalyptus plantations in Morocco, where grazing activities are restricted [56].

A. atlantica, an autochthonous botanical specimen exclusive to the delimited confines of Morocco, ascertains its unique status within the local flora [57]. The inaugural data collection initiatives, spanning the temporal expanse of 1985–1988 and masterfully orchestrated by Baum and Fedak (1985), fastidiously catalogued its presence along the Atlantic littoral, extending from Essaouira to Tiznit. The species manifests a distributional scope that transcends to the northwestern slopes of the Atlas Mountains, scaling altitudes up to 1000 m above sea level [58]. In a comprehensive investigation, researchers scrutinized *A. atlantica* within its native habitat in the arid precincts of southwestern Morocco, characterized by annual precipitation of approximately 200 mm. Even during comparably pluvial years, its occurrence remains sporadic, materializing as diminutive and disjointed populations. Principally, *A. atlantica* populates sandy substrates, although sporadic instances of its occurrence on brown soil have been documented. Historically circumscribed to a solitary locus in Syria, nearly 60 km from Damascus within the Syrian Desert [59], *Avena damascena* underwent a transformative revelation during a botanical expedition to Morocco, spearheaded by Mike Leggett and Per Hagberg. Seeds were meticulously procured from diverse populations ensconced on the east-facing slopes of the Atlas range, spanning elevations from 700 to 1650 m and characterized by a variably yet predominantly sandy loam soil type. Subsequent hybridization experiments with *A. damascena* from Syria incontrovertibly affirmed the conspecific nature of these populations. This disclosure, signifying the presence of *A. damascena* at both extremities of the Mediterranean basin, precipitates inquiries into the evolutionary chronicle of this oat species [60].

Avena prostrata, delineated by Ladizinsky (1971), shares morphological affinities with concomitant species, namely *Avena hirtula*, *Avena wiestii*, and *A. barbata*, and typically coexists with them in circumscribed regions of Southeast Spain, specifically in the provinces of Murcia and Almeria [61]. Additional occurrences are chronicled in various locales in Morocco [62]. While the topographical impediments and suboptimal soil quality in Spain ostensibly shield its populations from imminent extinction, the Moroccan regions supporting *A. prostrata*, characterized by fertile red-brown soil, confront a palpable threat owing to advancing agricultural practices. Acknowledging the restricted number of documented populations and the encroachment of the greenhouse industry into its primary habitat, the European Cooperative Programme for Plant Genomic Resources (ECPGR) contends that *A. prostrata* should potentially be classified as a Red List species [63].

A. canariensis, meticulously chronicled by Baum et al., stands as an exclusive endemic species confined to the Canary Islands, particularly thriving in Lanzarote and Fuerteventura [64]. Its conservation status, as designated by the International Union for Conservation of Nature (IUCN, 1994) and the "Lista Roja 2008 de la Flora Vascular Española" [65], is categorized as "vulnerable." Although certain subpopulations seek refuge in protected areas of Fuerteventura and Lanzarote, the comprehensive evaluation designates *A. canariensis* as "least concern." Despite confronting grazing pressures in specific locales, its population remains stable and robust, contributing to its prevailing and localized abundance. Divergent accounts persist concerning its distribution beyond the Canary Islands [66].

A. agadiriana, flourishing along the Atlantic Coast of Morocco from Casablanca to Tiznit, distinguishes itself as an endemic species for North Africa and Morocco [67]. The distribution area, intersected by the formidable Haut-Atlas Mountains reaching an altitude of 4165 m, displays considerable variability. The northern segment features dense clay soil, while the southern counterpart, marked by aridity, exhibits sandy soil conditions. The species, a subject of meticulous ecological scrutiny, exhibits resilience despite these diverse environmental challenges [36].

Avena magna, synonymous with *A. maroccana* Gdgr., is acknowledged as an exclusive endemic to Morocco. Initially sampled in 1964 along the Moroccan coast, subsequent revelations unveiled numerous populations to the south of Rabat (altitude: 1000–1300 m above sea level), southeast of Casablanca (altitude: 500 m above sea level), and northwest of Fes on the slopes of the Atlas Mountains (altitude: up to 600 m above sea level) [68]. Characterized as a weedy species, *A. magna*, distinguished by its large spikelet, thrives in cereal fields on heavy alluvial soil. Notably, its occurrence is intertwined with the less frequent weeding of cultivated crops compared to its counterpart, *A. sterilis*. The jeopardy to its existence becomes apparent in regions with rich alluvial soils intensely utilized for farming, where it contends with the more aggressive *A. sterilis* [69]. Predominantly located at the peripheries of cultivation, the species confronts potential eradication or displacement due to evolving agricultural practices and the contraction of its primary habitat, attributed to overgrazing and alterations in farming methods. Diligent soil plant management strategies are imperative for the sustained survival of this oat species [70].

Avena murphyi, identified in the southern reaches of Spain, specifically spanning from Tarifa to Vejer de la Frontera, thrives within the parameters of a distinctly Mediterranean climate. Frequently encountered in conjunction with the hexaploid oat species *A. sterilis*, it shares morphological affinities with the latter. Initial samplings were extended to the coastal zone of southwestern Spain, revealing a proliferation of *A. murphyi* specimens. However, recent observations in the Cadiz province indicate a conspicuous reduction in the population, suggestive of a potential decline or partial disappearance from Spanish territories [71]. Subsequent field surveys in 2010 identified new sites near Atlanterra, Barbate, and north of Alcala de los Gazules, where diminutive *A. murphyi* populations persisted [52]. Additionally, the species has been sighted in the northern region of Morocco near Tangier. The Moroccan population faces threats stemming from intensive agricultural activities on fertile alluvial soils, which may lead to its extirpation or displacement by the more assertive hexaploid *A. sterilis*, posing challenges to cultivated crops [72]. In acknowledgement of these conservation concerns, the Andalusian government has included *A. murphyi* on the Red List, securing positions on the Red List of Spanish Vascular Flora in the vulnerable category [73]. *A. insularis*, initially documented in Sicily in 1996, boasts four populations flourishing in the region between Gela and Butera, situated in southern Sicily. These populations inhabit undisturbed cenoses on hills at elevations ranging from 50 to 150 m above sea level, featuring alluvial clay soils with sand–clay and conglomerate–stony subsoils [74]. *A. insularis* holds an endangered status on the European Red List of Vascular Plants [75]. *A. macrostachya* has been exclusively documented in the elevated regions of two mountain chains in northeastern Algeria, namely the Aures and Djurdjura Mountains. Acknowledged as an endemic species of Algeria, *A. macrostachya*'s presence extends across the Aures and Bellezma Mountains, with additional encounters in the Djebel Chenntgouma area west of Kenchala [76].

A. macrostachya exhibits a notable variability in distribution across northeastern Algeria. While not particularly common in the Aures area, it thrives in large populations in the Bellezma region. In Djurdjura, the species is abundant throughout the *Festuca* sp. grassland areas above approximately 1500 m, a consequence of cedar woodland degradation. The distribution in Djurdjura appears more continuous than in the Aures and Bellezma. Although the situation in Djurdjura is relatively secure due to the species' commonness and abundance, grazing pressure poses a significant challenge, despite the area's partial protection status. The national park in Djurdjura, established in 1925 under French colonial rule and reestablished after Algeria gained independence, plays a crucial role in preserving this unique ecosystem. *A. macrostachya*, once established, forms robust tussocks, making complete dislodgment challenging. However, livestock grazing, particularly in heavily grazed areas, poses a threat, with flowering culms often restricted to unpalatable or spiny shrubs [76].

The primary threats faced by wild *Avena* species include the destruction of natural habitats, grazing, alterations in agricultural practices, and, in some instances, afforestation. For endemic species with narrow or disjunctive distributions, climate changes may impact their existence. A more complex situation arises with semicultivated and cultivated species, where diversity could rapidly diminish due to cultivation abandonment unless survival through a soil seed bank is ensured, necessitating annual replanting. Among the species listed in the Red List of Plants of Ethiopia and Eritrea, *A. abyssinica* and *Avena vaviloviana* stand out. These species, endemic to Ethiopia, Eritrea, and Yemen, grow ubiquitously and often as mixtures with the main crop. *A. vaviloviana* typically occurs as a weed in crops, preferring cultivated fertile soils and is recorded on the Ethiopian plateau at altitudes of 2200–2800 m. *A. abyssinica*, found in more humid areas of northern Ethiopia, has displaced other crops and become a cultivated plant. In the south, it serves as a segetal weed of emmer and barley. While *A. abyssinica* is widespread as a weed in Ethiopia and not currently considered threatened, changes in agricultural practices and the introduction of new crops or varieties may impact its existence, given its association with landraces of common oats [58], [77].

Avena strigosa, commonly known as bristle oat, traces its origins to the Mediterranean region and has been utilized in European nations since the Bronze Age for both cereal and fodder purposes [78]. Throughout history, bristle oats held a significant role as the predominant oat crop in Europe, especially in regions characterized by impoverished or marginal soils. However, its prominence in Europe experienced a marked decline following the introduction of the more productive common oat species (*A. sativa*). Remnant populations of bristle oats persist in regions where common oats fail to yield seeds without substantial inputs [79]. The native range and distribution of *A. strigosa* (sensu stricto) encompass a substantial portion of West and Central Europe, historically extending into the Nordic countries. Until the 17th century, a majority of oats cultivated in Great Britain and Ireland comprised *A. strigosa*. *A. strigosa* maintained popularity, particularly in mountainous regions, persisting in the Karpaty until 1980 as a feed crop for horses and pigs [80]. Despite its historical significance, several authors have classified bristle oats as a species on the brink of extinction. Podyma highlighted the diminishing presence of this synanthropic species in Poland, attributing it to evolving agricultural practices. Conversely, Korniak et al. reported renewed occurrences in northeastern Poland, suggesting a resurgence in specific areas. Simultaneously, the status of *A. strigosa* in other parts of Northern Europe underwent rapid deterioration [81].

Recent discoveries unveil new populations of *A. strigosa* in the eastern part of Lithuania, particularly within the Aukštaitija National Park. Given that these locations are situated in villages practising extensive agriculture, there is a reasonable expectation that these populations will endure. However, previously identified populations in the southern regions of the country (Alytus District) seemingly vanished, following a change in seed by the landowner. This underscores the extreme sensitivity of *A. strigosa* to alterations in agricultural practices, indicating that its survival does not rely on a seed reserve but necessitates annual replanting alongside the associated crops. Moreover, unfavourable agroeconomic policies and disputes over land properties have left extensive areas fallow [82].

The transition from cultivating traditional and genetically and morphologically heterogeneous landraces to more standardized "line" cultivars marked a significant shift in the characteristics of common oat cultivars. Grau Nersting et al. conducted a comprehensive study examining genetic diversity using microsatellites and agronomic traits in Nordic oat cultivars (*A. sativa*) spanning the 20th century, encompassing both landraces and contemporary cultivars [83]. A discernible evolution in agronomic traits was observed over this period. However, when comparing cultivars released post-1940 with landraces, the reduction in diversity evident in agronomic traits was corroborated by molecular data. The study highlighted a clear diminishing trend in the number of alleles from landraces to modern cultivars, a phenomenon previously noted in Canadian oats by Fu et al. [84]. It is noteworthy to mention the alterations in the diversity of weedy forms of hexaploid oats. The IUCN Red List of Threatened Species documents the history of *Avena volgensis* (Vavilov) Nevski syn. *A. fatua* subspecies *nodopilosa* var. *subglabra* subvar. *speltiformis Vavilov* ex Malzev, a specialized weed associated with a local landrace of *Triticum dicoccum*. Since the 1950s, the landrace has been supplanted by commercial varieties, resulting in a precipitous decline in the population of this weed, estimated at approximately 80%. This taxon is suspected to be at a high risk of extinction.

1.2.3 Classification

Historical endeavours to classify oats have a rich lineage, with Linnaeus in 1753 offering an initial taxonomy comprising four species: *A. sterilis*, *A. fatua*, *A. sativa*, and *A. nuda*. Linnaeus later bifurcated oats into wild and cultivated categories, further subdividing cultivated oats into covered and naked variants. Subsequent attempts by scholars and scientists sought to refine these classifications based on the morphology of the panicle, size and the number of kernels, grain shape and size, panicle shape, grain colour, spikelet grain count, maturation period length, and grain shape. Despite these efforts, many classifications were either speculative or relied on non-definitive plant parameters, impeding their widespread acceptance. Notably, the cytological classification by O'Mara (1961) based on chromosome number has emerged as the most pertinent [88]. This classification categorizes oats into three groups:

Group I comprises diploid oat species with a chromosome count of $2n = 14$ ($n = 7$), including *Avena brevis*, *A. strigosa*, and *A. nudibrevis*.

Group II encompasses tetraploid oat species with a chromosome count of $2n = 28$ ($n = 14$), exemplified by *A. barbata* and *A. abyssinica*.

Group III encompasses hexaploid oat species with a chromosome count of $2n = 42$ ($n = 21$). Prominent members of this group include *A. sativa*, *A. fatua*, *A. sterilis*, *A. byzantina*, and *A. nuda* – representative of common cultivated oats, wild oats, wild red oats, cultivated red oats, and hull-less oats, respectively.

1.3 PRODUCTION PRACTICES AND MANAGEMENT STRATEGIES

1.3.1 Botanical Description, Morphology, and Climatic Requirement

Within the taxonomic expanse of the Plantae kingdom, the oat plant, scientifically classified under the Order Poales, Family Poaceae (also known as Gramineae), finds its niche in the esteemed Genus *Avena*. Specifically, the most commonly cultivated species is *A. sativa*, accompanied by several other variants. Oat, a resolute winter annual grass, unveils a morphological semblance akin to its winter grass counterparts, notably wheat and barley. Its root system, distinguished by adventitious roots, originates from the initial node and, subsequently, from nodes proximate to the earth's surface along the primary culm [89]. The stem, or culm, comprises a sequence of nodes and internodes, characterized by their solid nature. During the nascent vegetative phase, internodes exhibit solidity or subtle indications of pith disintegration, whereas the elongated internodes in the mature stem manifest a hollow core. Nodes that bear the inflorescence, termed peduncles, branch elegantly. The leaves, possessing a linear, alternate, and acuminate structure, extend between 15 and 40 cm in length and 0.6 and 1.5 cm in breadth. Enveloping the leaf is a sheath, and in juvenile plants, the old leaf sheath conceals the emerging shoot [90]. Noteworthy is the presence of ligule on the leaves. The inflorescence, a terminal, loose, curving panicle, branches gracefully and houses singular, pendulous spikelets. These spikelets, oft adorned with two overlapping glumes (husks), precede the development of the fruit. The fruit, a caryopsis measuring 0.6 to 0.8 cm in length, boasts a hairy, cylindrical structure with slight ridges, ensconced in hulls presenting a formidable challenge for removal. In concert, these botanical characteristics paint a vivid portrait of the *Avena* genus, particularly the *A. sativa* species, elucidating its place within the intricate tapestry of plant taxonomy [85] (Figure 1.2).

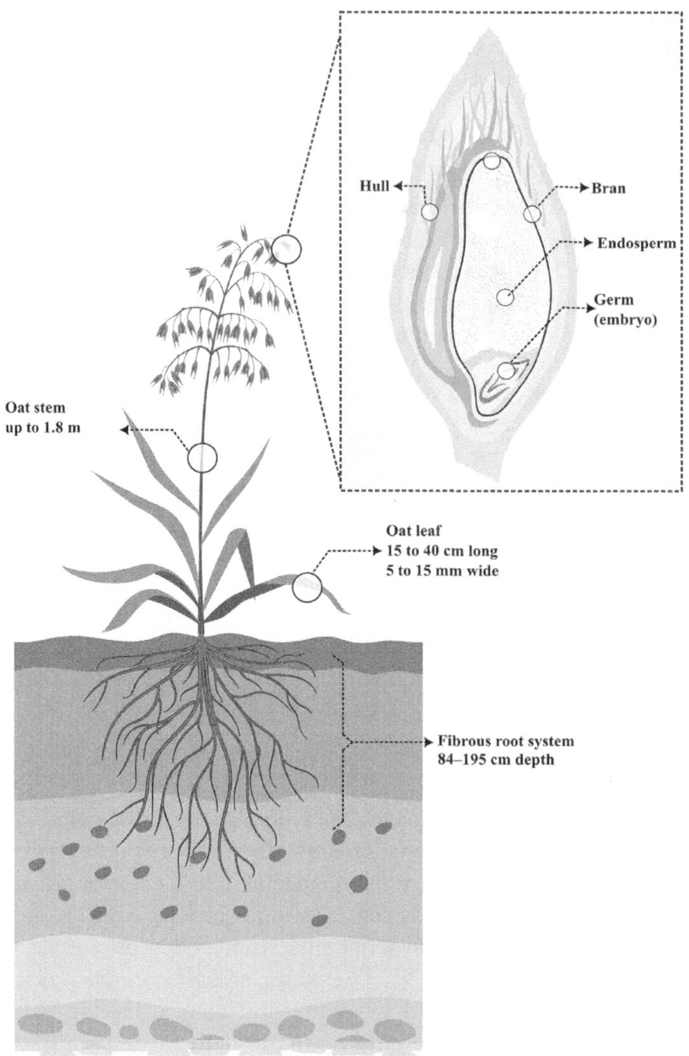

FIGURE 1.2   Botanical description of the oat plant and seed.

The oat, a venerable staple crop flourishing in temperate and sub-tropical climes, exhibits a discerning nature in its climatic predilections, demanding a cooler temperature regime for optimal growth. In the northern reaches of India, oats assert their presence as a winter annual crop, cultivated primarily for both green fodder and seed due to their affinity for cooler climates [91]. The pivotal phases of oat growth, spanning germination, tillering, booting, and heading unfold most favourably within a cool temperature milieu, ideally oscillating between 10°C and 15°C. This foundational temperature requirement, crucial during the vegetative stages, transitions to an optimal range of 20°C to 25°C for the crop's overall flourishing [92]. Notably, exceeding this temperature range, especially during the later stages of reproductive development and maturity, proves deleterious. Elevated temperatures at this juncture impede fertilization, resulting in an increased proportion of empty spikelets and subsequent diminution in seed yield. The crop's vulnerability extends beyond temperature considerations; adverse conditions such as waterlogging and frost inflict considerable harm. While oats do exhibit a degree of resilience to frost, circumstances characterized by high temperatures and aridity exert an adverse influence on both feed output and quality. For optimal thriving, oats exhibit a penchant for regions where the mean annual rainfall spans from 38 to 114 cm, encapsulating an ecological niche that complements their growth requirements [93] (Figure 1.2).

In this intricate interplay between climatic variables, oats emerge as a crop with nuanced preferences, their cultivation intricately intertwined with the tapestry of temperature, precipitation, and environmental conditions. The most substantial climatic factors influencing oat productivity are temperature and moisture. Oats flourish in cool, moist environments, requiring more moisture to produce a unit of dry matter than other cereals. Oat-producing regions in North America, Europe, and Asia are primarily situated between 40°N and 60°N latitudes [47]. Maritime climates in northern Europe also serve as prime oat-producing regions. The length of the growing season in the northern hemisphere varies from 90 to 110 days, with decreasing day length as the growing season progresses. In the southern hemisphere, prime oat-growing regions occur within latitudes 20°S and 45°S. Oats are cultivated between 30°S and 40°S latitudes in Australia, between 25°S and 45°S latitudes in New Zealand, and between 20°S and 30°S latitude in South America [94]. The growing season in Australia and South America can vary from 150 to 180 days, with increasing day length as the growing season progresses. While oats exhibit cold tolerance during seedling and tillering stages, yield loss may occur once the panicle emerges. However, oats tolerate frost better than wheat and barley. Conversely, hot dry weather can reduce grain yield and quality, especially from anthesis to grain filling. The intricate dance between climatic conditions and agronomic considerations underscores the delicate balance required for the successful cultivation of oats [95].

The global cultivation of oats, a resilient grain, is underscored by its impressive adaptability to a spectrum of soil types. While the scholarly scrutiny of oat soil requirements remains relatively modest, a discernible consensus emerges, drawing parallels with the soil preferences of wheat and barley, oats exhibit a notable sensitivity to salinity, acidity, and waterlogging, discouraging cultivation in soils characterized by these adverse conditions. In-depth investigations by Keilling et al. shed light on the deleterious impact of salinity on oats, attributing diminished crop performance to osmotic influences induced by salt, resulting in imbalances of specific ion nutrition or toxicity from certain ions [96]. The aversion of oats to acidic soil conditions is accentuated by presumed poor performance due to the toxicity of aluminium ions. Hence, the imperative arises to eschew soils marked by salinity, alkalinity, acidity, or waterlogging, fostering an environment conducive to oat cultivation [97]. Optimal soil conditions for oats materialize in well-drained, porous loam to sandy loam soils. This particular soil profile strikes a harmonious balance between water retention and drainage, creating an optimal medium for robust oat growth. In navigating the intricate relationship between oats and their soil milieu, the judicious selection of suitable soil types emerges as a pivotal factor in nurturing high-quality oat yields [98]. Oats exhibit a commendable tolerance for a diverse range of soil types, accommodating acidity down to a pH of 4.5 and alkalinity up to a pH of 8.5. While oats can endure acidic soils, the crop's productivity peaks within a pH range of 5 to 6. Acidic soils, associated with aluminium toxicity, are recognized as potential hindrances to oat success. Oats, although not as salt-tolerant as wheat, barley, and rye, surpass sorghum in this regard [99]. Australian oat varieties demonstrate heightened tolerance to boron compared to barley, albeit slightly less tolerant than wheat. Furthermore, oats exhibit general resilience to elevated manganese levels in the soil, further contributing to the crop's adaptability across diverse agricultural landscapes [100].

To ensure the efficacious germination and optimal proliferation of plants, meticulous preparation of a fine and compact seedbed is imperative. Typically, the preparatory groundwork involves an initial deep ploughing, executed with either a country plough or a disc plough. This preliminary step serves the dual purpose of eliminating any residual stubble from the antecedent crop and priming the soil for subsequent processes. Following the initial ploughing, a crisscross pattern of harrowing is employed, meticulously orchestrated to instil porosity in the soil matrix [101]. This method serves the dual function of breaking down clods that may impede seedling emergence and ensuring a homogenously textured substrate. The resultant effect is a harmoniously refined canvas, receptive to the imminent botanical life that will unfold. The landscape, having undergone this preparatory ballet, is then meticulously levelled through the assiduous application of planking [102]. This nuanced intervention not only facilitates an even and uniform topography but also fosters an environment conducive to the uniform distribution of seeds. The choreography of planking, akin to a skilled artisan refining their masterpiece, contributes to the creation of an optimal milieu for the germination and subsequent growth of the nascent flora. Integral to this sylvan orchestration is the establishment of a judicious drainage system. A requisite complement to the preparatory measures, this drainage infrastructure mitigates the risk of waterlogging and ensures the judicious disposition of excess moisture. Such prescient water management aligns with the overarching objective of cultivating an environment where seeds can burgeon and plants can establish robust roots [103].

1.3.2 Seeding and Sowing Practices within Diverse Cropping Systems

In the agricultural context of the southern hemisphere, where winter months prevail, the predominant practice involves sowing spring varieties during the winter months. Meanwhile, in the northern hemisphere, both spring and winter oat varieties find cultivation, and the optimal time for sowing varies in accordance with latitude [104]. This latitude-dependent variability underscores the need for region-specific considerations in oat cultivation practices. Sowing rates, a critical determinant of successful oat cultivation, are intricately linked to climate, soil conditions, and the intended purpose of the crop. Notably, sowing rates are higher for fodder production when compared to grain production, reflecting the diverse applications of oats in agriculture [105]. Moreover, owing to the extensive variation in oat seed sizes, a departure from conventional weight-based calculations is recommended. Instead, sowing rates should be meticulously calculated as the number of seeds per square meter (seeds/m²), ensuring an optimal plant density that accounts for the inherent variability in seed size [106] (Figure 1.3).

In the Indian context, the pinnacle period for oat sowing spans from mid-October to mid-November. Researchers pinpointed November 15 as the zenith, emphasizing its role

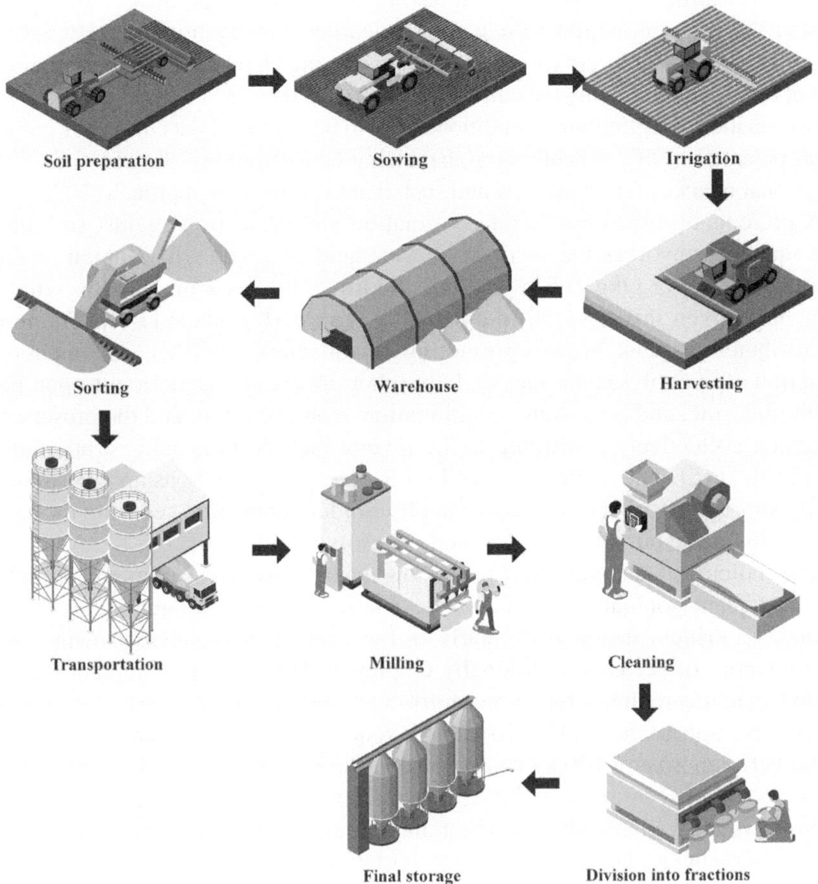

FIGURE 1.3 The sequential steps involved in oat cultivation, encompassing essential agronomic practices. (1) Soil Preparation: Depicting activities such as ploughing and cultivation to create a suitable soil environment for oat growth. (2) Sorting: Illustrating the process of selecting high-quality oat seeds for sowing, ensuring uniformity and optimal crop performance. (3) Transportation: Representing the movement of sorted seeds from the sorting facility to the sowing area. (4) Sowing: Showing the distribution of oat seeds in prepared soil, a crucial step in initiating the growth cycle. (5) Warehouse: Highlighting the storage facility for harvested oats, ensuring proper conditions for maintaining seed quality. (6) Milling: Depicting the processing of harvested oats into various oat-based products, contributing to the food industry. (7) Final Storage: Representing the long-term storage of milled oats, maintaining quality for subsequent use. (8) Irrigation: Illustrating the application of water to the oat fields, a critical practice for ensuring optimal growth and yield. (9) Harvesting: Showing the mechanical or manual harvesting of mature oat crops for further processing. (10) Cleaning: Depicting the removal of impurities and debris from harvested oats before storage or processing. (11) Division into Fractions: Highlighting the separation of different oat components or fractions based on size or quality during processing. This comprehensive figure provides a visual guide to the diverse agronomic practices involved in cultivating oats, from soil preparation to the final stages of processing and storage.

in not only ensuring maximal yield but also guaranteeing the production of high-quality fodder [107]. Aligning with the findings of an earlier investigation, it is advised to commence sowing for a multi-cut forage crop of oats during October, underscoring the significance of timing in optimizing oat cultivation practices. By tailoring sowing practices to the unique climatic and agricultural conditions of each hemisphere, oat cultivators can harness the full potential of this versatile crop, balancing considerations of yield, fodder quality, and regional nuances for an optimal and sustainable cultivation approach [108].

A prerequisite for robust seed germination and protection against soil and seed-borne maladies involves the meticulous treatment of seeds with Captan or Agrosan GN at a rate of 2.5 g/kg before sowing. Additionally, seed inoculation with *Azotobacter* has proven instrumental in enhancing crop performance [109]. The multifaceted attributes of plant growth-promoting rhizobacteria (PGPR), encompassing the production of exopolysaccharides and phytohormones, atmospheric nitrogen fixation, phosphorus, zinc, and potassium solubilization, iron chelation, and the preservation of soil health, collectively contribute to the pivotal factors influencing crop quality and yield [110]–[115]. The deployment of PGPR emerges not only as an environmentally friendly strategy but also as an economically prudent approach, securing its status as a stalwart ally in the pursuit of heightened oat crop output [116].

The judicious selection and proper sowing of seeds are paramount in achieving an optimal plant population for any crop. The seed rate, contingent upon the sowing method, is a critical factor, particularly in the context of broadcast sowing, where a higher quantity of seeds is traditionally employed. However, the inherent flaw of this method lies in its proclivity for a non-uniform plant stand, underscoring the significance of alternative approaches [117]. To attain a requisite plant stand, an optimal seed rate ranging between 80 and 100 kg has been identified as efficacious. The strategic placement of seeds between rows, set 20–25 cm apart, is pivotal to this process. The depth of sowing, a critical variable akin to wheat and barley cultivation, should range from 2 to 3 cm. Maintaining a plant-to-plant distance of 10 cm further reinforces the importance of meticulous spacing for optimal plant distribution [118].

Cereal crops, known for their nutrient-extractive nature, pose a risk of depleting soil fertility, a concern acutely applicable to oats, a member of the Poaceae family [110], [111], [113], [115]. The recurrent monoculture of oats can precipitate a decline in soil fertility, potentially leading to barrenness. Mitigating this risk necessitates the adoption of alternative cropping systems, as delineated in the next subsections.

1.3.2.1 Intercropping

Introducing oats into a symbiotic relationship with leguminous crops from the Leguminaceae family, such as peas, berseem, senji, chickpeas, and lucerne, proves advantageous. The atmospheric nitrogen-fixing ability of these leguminous companions enhances soil fertility and confers economic benefits [110]–[112], [115], [119].

1.3.2.2 Mixed Cropping

In rainfed areas where traditional broadcasting methods prevail, mixed cropping offers a viable alternative. Oats can be broadcasted alongside compatible crops such as peas, lucerne, and mustard, diversifying the crop composition and optimizing resource utilization [120].

1.3.2.3 Crop Rotation/Sequencing

The adoption of a judicious crop rotation or sequencing strategy becomes imperative in the context of oat monoculture. Integrating oats into a rotational cycle with leguminous crops serves as a prudent approach to sustaining soil fertility and texture [121]. A suggested rotation includes pulses, followed by oats for one year, Sudan grass coupled with oats and maize with cowpea for one year, and sorghum with cowpea preceding oats with lucerne. This systematic rotation ensures the replenishment of nutrients and prevents the detrimental consequences of continuous oat monocropping [122].

In conclusion, the implementation of diversified cropping systems, encompassing intercropping, mixed cropping, and strategic crop rotation, emerges as a panacea for mitigating the potential soil fertility decline associated with oat cultivation. These practices not only contribute to enhanced agricultural productivity but also embody a sustainable ethos, safeguarding the long-term health and viability of the soil.

1.3.3 Nutrient Management

The conventional reliance on residual soil fertility from previous crops for oat cultivation is a practice fraught with drawbacks, diminishing both yield quantity and grain quality. The nuanced requirement for specific nutrients is contingent upon various factors, including regional climate, soil type, and fertility, as well as the physical and chemical properties of the soil [110], [112], [115], [123]–[125]. Relying solely on inorganic sources for nutrient supplementation not only compromises crop quality but also poses environmental hazards and contributes to soil erosion. A more judicious approach involves the integration of organic sources, such as Farm Yard Manure and Vermicompost, into the soil [126]. These organic manures not only furnish essential NPK nutrients but also supply micronutrients critical for plant development. Moreover, they play a pivotal role in enhancing soil physical properties, including water-holding capacity and soil structure. To address potential zinc deficiency in the soil, a prudent measure is the application of 10 kg of zinc sulphate per hectare during land preparation. This comprehensive approach to nutrient management not only optimizes oat crop productivity but also aligns with sustainable agricultural practices, mitigating the adverse environmental impacts associated with exclusive reliance on inorganic fertilizers [110]–[112], [114], [115] (Figure 1.3).

1.3.4 Irrigation Scheduling and Weed Management

In rainfed cultivation, where the crop is entirely reliant on winter rains, prudent measures should be instituted in regions where rainfall surpasses the crop's tolerance levels [114], [125], [127]. Specifically, surplus water should be efficiently drained to mitigate potential adverse effects. Under irrigated conditions, strategic pre-sowing irrigation is recommended, particularly if residual soil moisture is insufficient or if the soil composition is skewed towards a higher proportion of sand relative to silt and clay [110], [111], [113], [123], [125], [128]. This initial irrigation catalyses proper germination, laying the groundwork for a robust start to the oat cultivation cycle. It is imperative to align irrigation schedules with rainfall patterns; if sufficient rainfall coincides with the planned irrigation, the latter should be omitted. A general guideline for irrigation comprises four to five sessions, commencing with the first irrigation at 20–25 days after sowing (DAS). Subsequent irrigations for loamy soils should be administered at monthly intervals, while sandy soils necessitate more frequent irrigation at 10-day intervals [129].

In summary, the establishment of a judicious water management strategy, involving careful consideration of critical stages, irrigation frequency, and the integration of rainfall patterns, is essential for optimizing oat cultivation outcomes. This approach, grounded in the synthesis of scientific insights, promotes both water-use efficiency and crop resilience, thereby contributing to sustainable agricultural practices. The meticulous management of intercultivation practices is an inherent necessity, albeit one reluctantly acknowledged. For oats cultivated for fodder, the density of the sown seeds typically obviates the need for extensive weeding. However, a single manual weeding or hoeing session is deemed essential 20–25 DAS. This operation serves to maintain the desired crop geometry and optimize plant population (Figure 1.3).

1.3.5 Plant Protection Measures

In the realm of cereals, oats distinguish themselves as notably resilient, showcasing a heightened resistance to a majority of pests and diseases in comparison to their counterparts. However, it is imperative to note that oats, albeit robust, are not impervious to certain diseases, primarily fungal [111]–[113], [123], [125], [127]. These infections have the potential to detrimentally impact both the quality and yield of the oat crop. This nuanced susceptibility underscores the importance of vigilance and targeted management strategies to safeguard against specific fungal pathogens that may pose a threat to oats. Implementing preventive measures, such as disease-resistant oat varieties and judicious agricultural practices, becomes paramount in ensuring the longevity and productivity of oat cultivation. As with any crop, a comprehensive understanding of the specific diseases affecting oats and the deployment of effective control measures are integral to maintaining the resilience and viability of oat crops in agricultural ecosystems.

1.3.5.1 Disease Management

The predilection for affliction by various maladies is an inherent vulnerability of oats, with several prevalent diseases demanding meticulous consideration (Table 1.2). Foremost among these is *Fusarium head blight*, orchestrated by an array of *Fusarium* species, including *Fusarium graminearum*, *Fusarium culmorum*, *Fusarium poae*, *Fusarium avenaceum*, and *Fusarium langsethiae*. The insidious nature of this pathogenic intrusion is exacerbated by the imperceptibility of symptoms due to the oat's formidable hull, concealing the kernel with an elusive subtlety. This pestilence extends its influence beyond oats, encroaching upon wheat and barley. Prudent measures such as rigorous field sanitation through deep ploughing, solarization, and judicious crop rotation are imperative to disrupt the pathogen's life cycle. Preemptive seed treatment assumes paramount significance, and should this vigilant defence falter, recourse to fungicides such as propiconazole, prothioconazole, and tebuconazole becomes an imperative last line of defence [130].

TABLE 1.2   A Comprehensive Table for Oat Disease Management

DISEASE	PATHOGEN	SYMPTOMS	CONTROL AND MANAGEMENT STRATEGIES
Fusarium Head Blight	*Fusarium* species	Imperceptible symptoms due to oat's hull	Field sanitation, deep ploughing, solarization, crop rotation, seed treatment, fungicides (propiconazole, prothioconazole, tebuconazole)
Crown rust	*Puccinia coronata*	Yellow and brown streaks, chlorotic specks, and orange pustules	Seed treatment with Oxycarboxin and sprays of Zineb
Stem rust	*Puccinia graminis f. sp. Avenae*	Brown to dark brown pustules on stems	Similar strategies to crown rust
Loose smut	*Ustilago avenae*	Complete transformation of floret, smut sori	Use of certified seeds and seed treatments with hot water or fungicides
Covered smut	*Ustilago kolleri*	Kernels shrouded with sori and membrane	Resistant varieties and seed treatment with systemic fungicides
Septoria leaf blotch	*Stagonospora avenae*	Minor disease with a substantial impact on yields	Worldwide occurrence, impacts Western Australia, management strategies needed
Pyrenophora leaf blotch	*Pyrenophora avenae Ito* and *Kuribayashi*	Global presence with economic impact	Third most important disease in Germany, significant in Brazil and Scandinavia
Red leather leaf	*Spermospora avenae Sprague* and A.G. Johnson	Minor disease in specific regions	Vigilance and localized management strategies
Powdery mildew	*Erysiphe graminis*	Greyish-white powder, brown hue, chlorotic patches	Resistant varieties, removal of pathogenic hosts, seed treatments with thiram or captan

Crown rust, orchestrated by *Puccinia coronata*, manifests through a spectrum of symptoms – yellow streaks, brown necrotic streaks, chlorotic specks on leaves or stems, and conspicuous orange pustules adorning lesions [131].

Stem rust, wrought by *Puccinia graminis f.* sp. *Avenae*, instigates a similar assault on the plant's stem, engendering the emergence of brown to dark brown pustules that metamorphose into an ominous black hue. Remedial strategies mirror those of crown rust [132].

Loose smut, induced by *Ustilago avenae*, orchestrates a complete transformation of the floret, enveloping every part in smut sori concealed by a delicate membrane. The dissemination of this seed-borne scourge is abated through the conscientious use of certified seeds and meticulous seed treatments with either hot water or systemic fungicides during sowing [133].

Covered smut, attributable to *Ustilago kolleri*, enshrouds kernels with sori, enveloped in an extended membrane composed of intact floral bracts and pericarp. Resilience against this malady is fostered through the deployment of resistant varieties and judicious seed treatment with systemic fungicides [134].

Septoria leaf blotch, attributed to the pathogen *Stagonospora avenae*, is often categorized as a minor disease in comparison to more prominent afflictions such as stem and leaf rust. However, its impact on crop yields can be substantial when it does manifest. This disease has been reported in diverse regions worldwide, including eastern Canada, the United States, Australia, Europe, Great Britain, and Israel. Notably, it emerges as a significant production constraint in Western Australia, underscoring its regional importance [135].

Pyrenophora leaf blotch, caused by *Pyrenophora avenae* Ito & Kuribayashi apud Ito, exhibits a global presence with varying economic implications. In Germany, it ranks as the third most important disease, holds significance in Brazil, and is prevalent in Scandinavia. The ubiquity of Pyrenophora leaf blotch underscores its adaptability and diverse economic impact in different agricultural landscapes [136].

The malady known as red leather leaf, induced by *Spermospora avenae* Sprague & A.G. Johnson, is regarded as a minor disease and has been identified in regions such as the northwestern United States, Turkey, and Australia. Although it may not command the same level of attention as some major diseases, its localized occurrence in these regions highlights the need for vigilance and management strategies [137].

Powdery mildew, orchestrated by *Blumeria graminis*, paints the upper leaf surface with a greyish-white powder that evolves into a disconcerting brown hue. On the reverse side, chlorotic patches burgeon, eventually giving rise to discernible black dots – fungal fruiting bodies. Control strategies encompass the utilization of resistant varieties, the removal of potential pathogenic hosts in the form of crop debris, and seed treatments employing thiram or captan [138].

The tandem afflictions of *halo*, attributed to *Pseudomonas syringae pv. coronafaciens*, and *stripe blight*, caused by *P. syringae pv. striafaciens*, collectively constitute *bacterial blight*. This malady tends to manifest prominently under conditions characterized by coolness and moisture. The prevalence of bacterial blight is particularly notable during periods of cool, moist weather. It is under these environmental conditions that the disease gains traction and exerts its impact on oat crops [139].

Barley yellow dwarf virus (BYDV) stands out as the most economically significant viral disease afflicting oats, exerting a substantial impact on crop yields globally. This viral threat poses a pervasive challenge to oat cultivation, with repercussions that extend across diverse regions. The primary mode of transmission for BYDV involves a range of aphid species, marking a critical link in the virus's life cycle and its spread [140].

Despite their varying degrees of prominence, each of these oat diseases presents unique challenges to oat cultivation in different parts of the world. The recognition of their global presence emphasizes the importance of vigilance, research, and targeted management strategies to mitigate the impact of these diseases on oat yields and ensure sustainable oat production worldwide.

1.3.5.2 Pest Management

Oats, a fundamental cereal crop, face challenges from a spectrum of insect pests that can significantly impact productivity [112], [114], [123], [124], [127]. Among these pests, the Russian wheat aphid (*Diuraphis noxia*), greenbug (*Schizaphis graminum*), bird cherry-oat aphid (*Rhopalosiphum padi*), grain aphid (*Macrosiphum avenae*), and rosegrain aphid (*Metopolophium dirhodum*) collectively exert their influence on oat crops with varying effects [141] (Table 1.3).

TABLE 1.3 A Comprehensive Table for Oat Pest Management

PEST	SCIENTIFIC NAME	IMPACT ON OATS	CONTROL AND MANAGEMENT STRATEGIES
Russian wheat aphid	*Diuraphis noxia*	Detrimental effects on crop yields	Integrated approach with cultural practices, biological control, insecticides
Greenbug	*Schizaphis graminum*	Influences oat crops with varying effects	Similar integrated approach to the Russian wheat aphid
Bird cherry-oat aphid	*Rhopalosiphum padi*	Impacts oats with varying effects	Similar integrated approach to the Russian wheat aphid
Grain aphid	*Macrosiphum avenae*	Affects oats with distinct influences	Similar integrated approach to the Russian wheat aphid
Rosegrain aphid	*Metopolophium dirhodum*	Contributes to insect-related challenges faced by oat growers	Similar integrated approach to the Russian wheat aphid
Armyworms, fruit flies	*Phalaenidae spp., Oscinella*	Distinct adversaries with different modus operandi and impact	Nuanced and integrated approach with cultural practices, biological control, insecticides
Cereal cyst nematode (CCN)	*Heterodera avenae Wollenweber*	Formidable economic threat with an impact on yields globally	Genetic resistance, genetic tolerance, and resistant oat varieties
Stem nematode	*Ditylenchus dipsaci (Kuhn)*	Challenges in cool and moist conditions, more closely associated	Genetic factors influencing resistance and tolerance
Root lesion nematode	*Pratylenchus neglectus*	Affects oat crops globally with significant yield losses	Genetic resistance, genetic tolerance, and resistant oat varieties
Root knot nematode	*Meloidogyne sp.*	Distinctive galls, spindle-like formations	Crop rotation to disrupt nematode life cycle, strategic control measures

The Russian wheat aphid, known scientifically as *Diuraphis noxia*, represents a formidable threat to oat production, capable of inducing detrimental effects on crop yields. Similarly, the greenbug (*Schizaphis graminum*), bird cherry-oat aphid (*R. padi*), grain aphid (*M. avenae*), and rosegrain aphid (*Metopolophium dirhodum*) can all impact oats, with their respective influences contributing to the complex tapestry of insect-related challenges faced by oat growers [142].

Beyond aphids, other insect pests, such as armyworms (*Phalaenidae* spp.), fruit flies (*Oscinella frit* (L.)), and wireworms (*Agriotes* spp.), further compound the challenges in oat production. The armyworm, fruit fly, and wireworms operate as distinct adversaries, each with its own modus operandi and capacity to affect oats in various ways. The management and mitigation of these insect pests demand a nuanced and integrated approach, combining cultural practices, biological control methods, and, when necessary, judicious use of insecticides. By understanding the ecology and behaviour of these pests, oat producers can tailor their strategies to effectively combat and minimize the impact of insect infestations, thereby safeguarding oat productivity on a global scale.

The *cereal cyst nematode (CCN)*, specifically *Heterodera avenae* Wollenweber, emerges as a formidable economic threat to oat production on a global scale. In regions where CCN is prevalent, the implementation of genetic resistance becomes instrumental in mitigating its impact, effectively reducing CCN population sizes. Additionally, oat varieties endowed with genetic tolerance play a crucial role in optimizing productivity under the persistent threat of CCN. It is noteworthy that genetic resistance and tolerance are independently inherited traits, each contributing independently to the oat plant's defence mechanisms [143].

The *stem nematode, Ditylenchus dipsaci* (Kuhn) *Filipjev*, poses challenges to oat production in cool and moist climatic conditions. This nematode manifests its impact on winter oats in regions characterized by mild winters and on spring oats sown during the winter, particularly in Mediterranean climates. Unlike CCN, resistance and tolerance for the stem nematode appear to be more closely associated, suggesting a nuanced interplay of genetic factors influencing the oat plant's response to this specific nematode [144].

Root lesion nematode, Pratylenchus neglectus, is implicated in affecting oat crops in diverse regions, including Europe, Iran, the United States, and Australia. Recent trials in South Australia have demonstrated yield losses of up to 37% in areas with high nematode populations. Similar to CCN, resistance and tolerance mechanisms for the root lesion nematode are inherited traits, reinforcing the importance of genetic factors in oat plant defences against nematode infestations [145].

Delving beneath the soil's surface, the *root knot nematode (Meloidogyne* sp.) manifests its presence through distinctive galls and spindle-like formations on uprooted plants. The strategic response to this nematode involves judicious crop rotation, a tactical manoeuvre designed to disrupt the nefarious life cycle of the pest. By implementing these control measures, agricultural practitioners seek to manage and mitigate the impact of nematode infestations on oat production, safeguarding the economic viability of this essential cereal crop [146].

1.4 INTERPLAY OF AGRONOMICS AND PRODUCTION ECONOMICS

1.4.1 Optimizing Yield and Quality

Oat yield and quality are intricately linked to agronomic and environmental factors throughout the growth cycle. Researchers have found that plump kernels, groat percentage, and test weight suffer adverse impacts from interactions between seeding dates, cultivars, and delayed seeding. Similarly, protein and β-glucan concentrations respond positively to varying nitrogen levels and seed doses [147]. The influence of agronomic parameters is evident in the impact of seeding rate and nitrogen rates on pivotal yield components, such as the number of panicles and the weight and quantity of grains responsive to nitrogen application [110]–[114], [114], [115], [123]–[125], [127], [128]. This highlights the complex interplay of cultivation strategies in shaping oat productivity and quality. Sowing high-quality oat grain begins with planting premium seeds, crucial for ensuring superior yield [148]. These seeds must give rise to disease-resistant plants, as diseases commonly lead to a decline in grain quality. Additionally, the environment plays a pivotal role, affecting crucial parameters such as groat starch, ash concentrations, and overall grain output. Optimal oat yields and premium grain quality are achieved under warm, sunny conditions during spring, coupled with lower summer temperatures and minimal precipitation during grain loading. The physical attributes of oat grain and the mechanistic facets of the dehulling process intricately intertwine to impact groat percentage, underscoring the multifaceted nature of factors influencing oat grain quality [149].

Leaf removal during panicle emergence significantly reduces grain yield, emphasizing the pivotal role of the penultimate leaf in oats. Removal of the flag and penultimate leaves or systematic defoliation results in a substantial decrease in grain yield, attributed to a reduction in the number of developed grains [150]. Defoliation during anthesis induces a 20% reduction in yield, primarily due to diminished single-grain weights. Studies on source-sink adjustments during the grain-filling phase highlight the resilience of temperate cereals, demonstrating compensatory mechanisms for factors affecting grain yield, including spikes per plant, spikelets per spike, and grains per spikelet. This resilience underscores the intricate adaptability of temperate cereals in navigating challenges to reproductive success, ultimately influencing grain yield dynamics [151].

1.4.2 Economic Viability and Market Dynamics

The lower total energy yield of oats compared to other cereals is attributed to the presence of hulls, akin to straw in energy yield [114], [124], [128]. Despite oats' favourable fat and amino acid composition for animal feed, their utilization lags behind crops with higher energy content. Economic outcomes in oat cultivation are linked to key variables: feed value, yield level, and market prices. Oat production costs hinge on inputs influenced by cultivation circumstances, crop type, methods, machinery, work efficiency, farm size, and related factors [152]. Insights into Finnish farm models reveal that 57% of production costs are fixed, encompassing labour costs for family-run enterprises. Variable costs include items like fuel, fertilizer, pesticides, and herbicides. Given oats' minimal input requirements on less fertile land, the financial feasibility of chemical pesticide management becomes questionable. Oats, adaptable to diverse soils, enable cost reduction in calcification and fertilization compared to other cereals, with gross margins akin to wheat and barley. Naked and conventional oats exhibit no discernible cost differences in various aspects [153]. The ultimate cost of oat cultivation is influenced by multiple factors, detailed below.

1.4.2.1 Sowing

Optimal seeding rate determination is nuanced due to oats' capacity to adjust development and tillering in response to plant density, addressing lodging concerns economically [110], [111], [115], [125]. Seed rates vary globally, impacting seed expenses within total variable production costs. The pursuit of an optimal seeding rate requires nuanced consideration of agronomic factors and economic considerations [154].

1.4.2.2 Plant Protection

Oat farming's reduced reliance on pesticides and herbicides underscores the crop's resilience to pests and weeds, offering economic benefits aligned with sustainable practices [155].

1.4.2.3 Threshing

Infrequent threshing issues in oats cultivation require prudence to prevent mature oat dispersion. A standard combine harvester is predominant for mechanized threshing, reflecting contemporary trends where machinery replaces manual labour. Labour costs become pivotal in manual threshing scenarios, impacting economic considerations [156].

1.4.2.4 Drying and Storage

Safe oat grain storage requires airtight storage or moisture reduction to 14% or below. Chemical preservation methods may be employed, with drying processes impacting costs based on factors like end moisture level, drying oven size, initial moisture content, and external air temperature. Drying is critical, demanding a balance between effective preservation and associated energy expenditures [157].

1.4.2.5 Global Market Trends and Consumer Preferences Driving the Demand for Oats and Oat-Based Products

Oat-based cereals, the epitome of wholesome breakfast options, derive their essence from the nutritional powerhouse, that is, oats. Renowned for their abundance of fibre, vitamins, and minerals, oats contribute significantly to the nutritional profile of these cereals. Typically savoured in conjunction with milk or yoghurt, these cereals have garnered favour among the health-conscious demographic. The current landscape of the oat-based cereal market paints a promising picture. A burgeoning awareness of the health dividends associated with oats is propelling a surge in demand for these products [158]. The contemporary consumer, driven by a quest for both nutrition and convenience, finds the perfect amalgamation of these attributes in oat-based cereals. Furthermore, the escalating incidence of chronic diseases and the burgeoning ageing demographic have substantively fuelled the quest for healthier breakfast alternatives [159]. On a global scale, the oats market exhibits substantial growth, with an estimated valuation of USD 6.1 billion in 2022. Projections augur even more impressive figures, anticipating a rise to USD 10.8 billion by 2032, signifying a commendable compound annual growth rate (CAGR) of 5.9% from 2022 to 2032. Beyond the numerical growth, the market is poised to manifest an absolute financial opportunity of approximately USD 4.7 billion by 2032. The inherent quality of oats to offer a comprehensive meal without necessitating supplementary ingredients positions it as the premier grain of choice, elucidating its escalating popularity across diverse regions, notably the Asia Pacific region. The trajectory of the oats market is inexorably linked to its intrinsic value as a self-sufficient and nutritionally robust cereal option, making it an indispensable player in the global dietary landscape [160].

Oats stand as paragons of satiety and nutritional excellence in the realm of breakfast choices, owed to their remarkably high soluble fibre content. In comparison to cereals such as rice and wheat, oats distinguish themselves by providing an elevated sense of fullness, a phenomenon attributed to the abundant presence of β-glucan and the inherent viscosity of oatmeal. Notably, the oats market constitutes approximately 8% of the broader cereal market, underscoring its significance in the dietary landscape [161]. The viscosity inherent in oats imparts a distinctive quality to the digestive process, instigating a heightened sensation of fullness coupled with a commensurate reduction in feelings of hunger. Furthermore, the caloric content of oats is notably lower than that of other cereals, rendering them a superior option for individuals pursuing weight loss goals. This confluence of attributes positions oats as a front-runner in the quest for a filling and health-conscious breakfast [162]. Anticipating an upsurge in demand in the foreseeable future, this market is poised for substantial growth. The factors driving this demand are manifold, primarily rooted in the demographic landscape and innovative considerations, all under the subjective sway of macro and industry-specific influences. As the consummate choice for those seeking a satisfying and healthful breakfast option, oats are set to emerge as a pivotal player in the evolving narrative of dietary preferences. Some recent developments underscore a strategic and nutritional repositioning of oats within the broader food industry. From enhanced market presence in breakfast cereals to serving as a beacon of health-conscious choices, oats are carving a niche as a versatile and convenient ingredient in contemporary culinary landscapes:

(i) Market Integration of Oats in Breakfast Cereal Products:
    Oats are increasingly finding their way into the food industry, primarily driven by a surge in the market penetration of breakfast cereal products. This strategic integration is a response to the growing recognition of oats as a versatile and nutrient-rich ingredient.

(ii) Nutritional Abundance and Health Consciousness:
The global oats market is propelled by the richness of nutrients, with a particular emphasis on the high dietary fibre content found in oats. As health consciousness becomes more pervasive among consumers, oats emerge as a key player in meeting the demand for wholesome and nutritionally dense food options.

(iii) Impact of Convenience Food Consumption:
The rising consumption of convenience and on-the-go food products positively influences the oats market. Oats, with their adaptability to modern, fast-paced lifestyles, serve as an ideal component in convenient food options, aligning seamlessly with evolving consumer preferences [163].

1.4.2.5.1 Temporal Dynamics: Assessing the Oats Market Landscape from 2017 to 2021 and Anticipating Growth Patterns in the Forecasted Period of 2022–2032

In the realm of future market projections, as elucidated by Future Market Insights, the oats market is poised to retain its allure, manifesting a robust growth trajectory at a CAGR of 5.9% between the temporal expanse of 2022 and 2032. This signifies a notable uptick from the CAGR of 4.3% documented during the antecedent period spanning from 2017 to 2021. Oats, venerable for their profound nutritional richness, are notably distinguished by their propensity to mitigate blood cholesterol levels when incorporated into the regular dietary regimen. The consummate versatility of oats is evident in their various consumable forms, ranging from the esteemed rolled and steel-cut oats to the more diminutive yet equally consequential crushed variants such as oatmeal and refined oat flour. The culinary landscape is graced by the pre-eminence of oatmeal, finding its paramount application in the quintessential morning porridge [164]. However, the ubiquity of oats transcends the confines of the breakfast table, permeating the realm of bakery products with an omnipresence that extends to the crafting of delectable oatcakes, oatmeal cookies, and hearty oat bread. This diversification of applications underscores the resilience and adaptability of oats in the culinary domain, elucidating a nuanced facet of their commercial significance. Beyond the purview of human consumption, oats have emerged as a stalwart component in the formulation of livestock feed, thereby expanding their sphere of influence into the agricultural domain. The multifaceted utility of oats across disparate domains augurs well for the anticipated remarkable growth trajectory poised to unfold in the impending decade [165].

In summation, the oats market, propelled by its intrinsic nutritional benefits and diverse applications spanning both human and animal consumption, is poised for a commendable ascent in the ensuing decade. The projected growth at a CAGR of 5.9% underscores the resilience and adaptability of oats, cementing their status as a pivotal player in the dynamic landscape of culinary and agricultural markets.

In the United States, oats play a prominent role in a variety of food products, including hot breakfast cereals, cold cereals, bakery items, baby food, and granola bars. Additionally, oats are a significant component of breakfast traditions, often consumed with fruits. This prevalence in diverse food categories is expected to drive an increase in demand for oats in the North American oats market throughout the forecast period from 2022 to 2031. A notable trend contributing to the growth of the oats market is the evolving breakfast preferences observed among consumers in emerging countries, such as India and China [166]. As breakfast routines undergo transformations, there is a discernible shift in consumer preference towards healthier eating habits, with an emphasis on promoting weight loss. This changing dietary inclination is anticipated to lead to increased consumption of oats in these regions, thereby influencing market growth positively during the assessment period from 2022 to 2031. The expanding popularity of oats in various forms, coupled with their association with health-conscious choices, positions oats as a versatile and sought-after ingredient in the evolving global food market. The anticipation of heightened demand in both North America and emerging markets underscores oats' integral role in catering to evolving consumer preferences and dietary trends [167].

1.4.2.5.2 Revolutionizing Oats Distribution: The Ascendance of Modern Trade and Online Retail Formats

Within the product type segment, oat flour is anticipated to exhibit a noteworthy growth rate of 6.4% in terms of revenue in the global oats market. This growth can be attributed to the increasing consumer inclination towards ready-to-cook food products. Oats, in particular, have emerged as the most favoured ready-to-cook food item owing to their myriad health benefits. This preference is further accentuated by the contemporary trend of busier lifestyles and the rise in income levels among consumers. The versatility and health-conscious appeal of oat flour position it as a sought-after ingredient in the realm of ready-to-cook food products. The convenience it offers aligns seamlessly with the demands of modern lifestyles, contributing to its popularity among consumers. As a result, the projected growth in revenue for oat flour underscores its significance in meeting the evolving preferences and lifestyle choices of consumers in the global oats market [168].

The rising prevalence of mobile phones and the widespread use of social media platforms have empowered consumers with unparalleled access to information about various products. Furthermore, this connectivity allows consumers to share insights and information regarding the benefits of the products they encounter. The dissemination of information through digital channels has created a dynamic environment where consumer awareness and engagement play pivotal roles in shaping purchasing decisions. In tandem with the digital landscape, offline channels, notably hypermarkets/supermarkets, and online retail services contribute significantly to the sales of food products globally [169]. The convenience and diversity offered by these channels cater to a broad spectrum of consumer preferences. Additionally, the advent of modern retail formats has given rise to innovative operational models, such as food courts and speciality stores within malls [3], [21], [22], [24], [32]. These formats provide consumers with unique and curated food experiences, further diversifying the retail landscape. This evolving ecosystem, encompassing both digital and physical channels, reflects the changing dynamics of consumer behaviour and the retail industry at large. The synergy between mobile connectivity, social media influence, and diverse retail formats underscores the multifaceted ways in which consumers discover, share, and engage with food products in the contemporary marketplace [170].

1.4.3 Policy Implications and Farmer Empowerment

In major oat markets, the influential currents are shaped by pivotal government policies, notably EU export subsidies, the reform initiatives within the EU Common Agricultural Policy (CAP), and the determinative U.S. loan rate. Central to the dynamics of oat market evolution are the EU export subsidies, a forceful impetus that propels the trajectory of trade. These subsidies, wielded by the EU, exert a discernible influence on the ebb and flow of oat commerce, steering market dynamics through financial incentives and economic levers. The nuanced interplay between these subsidies and market forces demands astute observation to unravel the intricacies of their impact on the global oat landscape. Simultaneously, the reformations underway within the EU CAP constitute a formidable current shaping the contours of oat markets [171]. As this policy framework transforms, its repercussions are felt across the agricultural expanse, instigating shifts in production, distribution, and consumption patterns. The discerning gaze of market participants must navigate this complex terrain to fathom the nuanced repercussions of these reforms on the oat market's equilibrium. Across the Atlantic, the U.S. loan rate emerges as a linchpin in the economic machinery steering oat trade dynamics. This rate, hailing from the corridors of U.S. agricultural policy, casts a defining shadow on the pricing mechanisms and commercial strategies that underpin the oat market. Its role as a determinant in shaping market behaviour necessitates a comprehensive understanding of its implications for producers, traders, and consumers. In synthesizing these policy currents, the kaleidoscope of government interventions converges to shape the collective destiny of major oat markets. The nuanced interplay of EU export subsidies, the evolving landscape of the EU CAP, and the influential U.S. loan rate collectively serve as the orchestrators of change in this dynamic arena. As we scrutinize the intricacies of their impact, we unravel the tapestry of forces guiding the course of oat market evolution on the global stage [172].

1.4.3.1 Examining EU Export Subsidies: A Closer Look at Economic Impacts

The sustenance of Scandinavia's prominence in the global oat export market hinges significantly on the strategic utilization of subsidies by the EU, particularly for oat exports to the United States. This deliberate policy has been a linchpin in preserving the market share of Sweden and Finland, acknowledging the pivotal role oat trade plays in their respective economies. A crucial milestone in this trajectory occurred in 1995 when, upon their accession to the EU, special provisions for subsidies on oat exports were tailored to accommodate the unique economic significance of oats for Sweden and Finland. Operationalized through a meticulous weekly tendering process, these subsidies exclusively target oats originating from Sweden and Finland. It is essential to underscore that participation in the open tender does not guarantee the allocation of export subsidies. Rather, each bid undergoes scrutiny on an individual basis, with the potential for acceptance or rejection based on nuanced considerations. A notable facet of this policy landscape is the flexibility afforded by the EU's commitments under the Uruguay Round of the World Trade Organization (WTO). Unlike constraints specific to oats, the

WTO commitments pertain to export subsidies for all coarse grains. As of the present writing, the EU has adhered to these commitments, thereby possessing the latitude to augment expenditures on oats should such a course of action align with its objectives. The convergence of interests between Canada and the United States is palpable in their joint pursuit of eliminating export subsidies, a shared objective slated for discussion in the upcoming WTO negotiations. Meanwhile, both nations are actively engaged in exploring avenues to incentivize the EU to cease export subsidies on oat sales to North America. Crucially, the absence of support payments for oats, be it for production or exports, poses a palpable threat to the sustainability of oat production and exports from Sweden and Finland. The interplay of economic forces underscores the indispensability of subsidies in maintaining current levels of oat production and ensuring the continued viability of exports to the United States. In navigating this complex terrain, the imperatives of international trade dynamics, WTO commitments, and bilateral negotiations underscore the delicate balance that shapes the fate of Scandinavian oats on the global stage [173].

1.4.3.2 Transformative Changes: Analysing the Reforms in the EU CAP

The financial underpinning for agriculture in Finland and Sweden derives its sustenance from the support measures delineated within the CAP of the EU. A significant watershed moment unfolded in 2003 when the EU member countries collectively sanctioned a comprehensive reform of the CAP. This reform ushered in transformative changes, foremost among them being the introduction of a single farm payment disentangled from production, a reduction in direct payments, and a bolstering of the rural development policy. The implementation of the single farm payment, representing a paradigm shift in agricultural subsidy structures, was realized on January 1, 2005. Particularly noteworthy in this CAP reform is the incorporation of special provisions tailored to accommodate the distinctive agricultural challenges faced by Finland and Sweden. These provisions take cognizance of the exigencies imposed by a colder climate, offering additional compensation to mitigate the drying costs associated with cereal production in these regions. The conceptual cornerstone of the reform lies in the decoupling of the single farm payment from production levels. This departure from traditional models of agricultural support reflects a strategic shift towards a more nuanced and diversified approach. Simultaneously, the reduction in direct payments underscores a recalibration of financial incentives within the agricultural sector, urging greater efficiency and adaptability. The amplification of the rural development policy stands out as another hallmark of the CAP reform. This augmentation underscores an expanded focus on holistic rural development, acknowledging the multifaceted dimensions of agriculture beyond mere production. The intent is to foster a resilient and sustainable agricultural landscape, attuned to the socioeconomic fabric of the regions it serves.

In essence, the CAP reform not only reshapes the financial architecture supporting agriculture in Finland and Sweden but also signals a broader philosophical shift towards sustainability and adaptability. The tailored provisions for addressing the unique challenges posed by a colder climate demonstrate the nuanced approach taken to accommodate the diverse needs of EU member countries. As these policies unfold, they represent a dynamic response to the evolving landscape of European agriculture, with Finland and Sweden positioned to navigate their distinct agricultural terrains within the broader framework of EU policies [174].

1.4.3.3 Navigating U.S. Loan Landscape: Understanding Current Interest Rates and Trends

Non-recourse loans constitute a pivotal financial instrument enabling producers to secure loans at predetermined levels to offset the expenses incurred during production. Central to this mechanism is the establishment of a loan rate that effectively functions as the minimum threshold for the market price of major commodities. In instances where the prevailing market price falls below this predetermined loan rate, farmers are afforded a distinctive recourse: rather than repaying the loan, they have the option to annul it by relinquishing their grain to the Commodity Credit Corporation. The profound impact of commodity loan rates on producers' decisions regarding acreage cannot be overstated. The support provided through marketing loans is contingent upon prevailing production and market prices. Consequently, these rates assume a role of paramount significance in shaping the economic landscape of agricultural operations. Within the historical context, the loan rate assigned to oats has, regrettably, found itself at a disadvantage when juxtaposed with rates allocated to other crops such as corn, soybeans, and wheat. This asymmetry has proven to be a consequential factor contributing significantly to the dwindling acreage and production of oats in the United States. The historical discrepancy in loan rates has precipitated a tangible and adverse effect on the economic viability of oat cultivation, hastening its decline. The potential revitalization of U.S. oat acreage and production hinges upon rectifying this historical disadvantage. Elevating the loan rate for oats relative to that of other crops emerges as a plausible strategy to ameliorate the production outlook. However, the extent of such gains would inherently be circumscribed by the intrinsic factors of yield limitations and varietal considerations. In contemplating the recalibration of loan rates, policymakers must reckon with the nuanced interplay of economic factors, agricultural dynamics, and the imperative to cultivate a resilient and diverse agricultural landscape. A judicious adjustment in loan rates, particularly favouring oats, holds promise for mitigating the historical decline in oat cultivation, potentially fostering a more balanced and sustainable agricultural portfolio in the United States [175].

1.5 CONCLUSION AND FUTURE PROSPECTS

The exploration of "Oat, a Distinct Cereal: Origin, History, Production Practices, and Production Economics" has provided a comprehensive understanding of the multifaceted aspects of oat cultivation. From its origins and historical significance to the intricacies of modern production practices and economic considerations, this chapter has delved into the unique characteristics that set oats apart as a cereal crop. Throughout the chapter, it became evident that oats have a rich historical legacy and have evolved into a distinct cereal with unique attributes. The examination of production practices highlighted the significance of factors such as optimal sowing times, disease management, and the role of genetic resistance in ensuring successful oat cultivation. Additionally, the economic considerations underscored the importance of balancing production costs with market demands, emphasizing the need for sustainable and economically viable approaches. The implications of this research extend beyond the agronomic realm. Oats, with their versatility and nutritional benefits, play a vital role in global food security. Moreover, sustainable oat cultivation practices can contribute to environmental conservation through soil health maintenance and reduced chemical inputs. Looking forward, future research initiatives should focus on advancing sustainable oat cultivation practices. Exploring innovative technologies, such as precision agriculture and genomic advancements, can enhance disease resistance, improve crop yields, and optimize resource utilization. Collaborative efforts between researchers, farmers, and policymakers will be essential in developing and disseminating best practices globally. Addressing challenges related to pests, diseases, and changing climatic conditions will require ongoing research and adaptive management strategies. By investing in education and extension services, farmers can be empowered to implement the latest advancements in oat production. Furthermore, exploring value-added products and market diversification can contribute to maximizing economic returns for oat farmers, fostering resilience in the face of market fluctuations.

In conclusion, the chapter has unravelled the intricacies of oat cultivation, emphasizing its historical significance, production nuances, and economic dimensions. Sustainable oat cultivation is not just a choice but a necessity for a resilient and environmentally conscious agriculture sector. By fostering collaboration, embracing innovative practices, and continually advancing our understanding of oats, we can contribute to global food security, environmental sustainability, and the prosperity of oat farmers worldwide.

REFERENCES

[1] M. Rh et al., "Effect of sowing windows and cutting management on growth and seed yield of oat (Avena sativa L.)," *Pharma Innov. J.*, vol. 12, no. 2, pp. 968–972, 2023. Accessed: Oct. 31, 2023. [Online]. Available: www.thepharmajournal.com/archives/?year=2023&vol=12&issue=2&ArticleId=18563

[2] USDA 2023, "Oats explorer, 2023." Accessed: Oct. 31, 2023. [Online]. Available: https://ipad.fas.usda.gov/cropexplorer/cropview/commodityView.aspx?cropid=0452000

[3] M. Tomar et al., "Interactome of millet-based food matrices: A review," *Food Chem.*, vol. 385, p. 132636, Aug. 2022, doi: 10.1016/j.foodchem.2022.132636.

[4] A. Kujur and T. Abra, "Effect of different organic sources of nitrogen and different planting pattern on growth, yield and quality of oats (avena sativa l.)," *Progress. Res.*, vol. 12, pp. 2471–2475, Jan. 2017, doi: 10.1007/978-94-011-0015-1.

[5] N. Ben Halima, R. Ben Saad, B. Khemakhem, I. Fendri and S. Abdelkafi, "Oat (avena sativa L.): Oil and nutriment compounds valorization for potential use in industrial applications," *J. Oleo Sci.*, vol. 64, no. 9, pp. 915–932, 2015, doi: 10.5650/jos.ess15074.

[6] S. A. Joyce, A. Kamil, L. Fleige and C. G. M. Gahan, "The cholesterol-lowering effect of oats and oat beta glucan: Modes of action and potential role of bile acids and the microbiome," *Front. Nutr.*, vol. 6, p. 171, Nov. 2019, doi: 10.3389/fnut.2019.00171.

[7] D. Zohary and M. Hopf, "Domestication of plants in the old world: The origin and spread of cultivated plants in West Asia, Europe and the Nile Valley," *Domest. Plants Old World Orig. Spread Cultiv. Plants West Asia Eur. Nile Val.*, no. Ed.3, 2000, Accessed: Oct. 31, 2023. [Online]. Available: www.cabdirect.org/cabdirect/abstract/20013014838

[8] J. R. Harlan, "The origins of cereal agriculture in the old world," in *The Origins of Cereal Agriculture in the Old World*, De Gruyter Mouton, 2011, pp. 357–384, doi: 10.1515/9783110813487.357.

[9] M. Tomar et al., "Nutritional composition patterns and application of multivariate analysis to evaluate indigenous Pearl millet ((*Pennisetum glaucum* (L.) R. Br.) germplasm," *J. Food Compos. Anal.*, vol. 103, p. 104086, Oct. 2021, doi: 10.1016/j.jfca.2021.104086.

[10] V. Krishnan, M. Tomar, L. N. Malunga and S. J. Thandapilly, "Food matrix: Implications for nutritional quality," in *Conceptualizing Plant-Based Nutrition: Bioresources, Nutrients Repertoire and Bioavailability*, Ramesh S. V. and S. Praveen, Eds. Singapore, Singapore: Springer Nature, 2022, pp. 43–60, doi: 10.1007/978-981-19-4590-8_3.

[11] J. P. Murphy and T. D. Phillips, "Isozyme variation in cultivated oat and its progenitor species," *Crop Sci.*, vol. 33, no. 6, pp. 1366–1372, Nov. 1993, doi: 10.2135/cropsci1993 .0011183X003300060048x.

[12] D. Ryan, M. Kendall and K. Robards, "Bioactivity of oats as it relates to cardiovascular disease," *Nutr. Res. Rev.*, vol. 20, no. 2, pp. 147–162, Dec. 2007, doi: 10.1017/ S0954422407782884.

[13] A. Marshall et al., "Crops that feed the world 9. Oats- a cereal crop for human and livestock feed with industrial applications," *Food Secur.*, vol. 5, no. 1, pp. 13–33, Feb. 2013, doi: 10.1007/s12571-012-0232-x.

[14] C. Agostoni, M. Baglioni, A. La Vecchia, G. Molari and C. Berti, "Interlinkages between climate change and food systems: The impact on child malnutrition – Narrative review," *Nutrients*, vol. 15, no. 2, Art. no. 2, Jan. 2023, doi: 10.3390/nu15020416.

[15] E. Muñoz-Redondo et al., "New perspectives on frailty in light of the global leadership initiative on malnutrition, the global leadership initiative on sarcopenia, and the WHO's concept of intrinsic capacity: A narrative review," *Maturitas*, vol. 177, p. 107799, Nov. 2023, doi: 10.1016/j.maturitas.2023.107799.

[16] S. A. O. Adeyeye, T. J. Ashaolu, O. T. Bolaji, T. A. Abegunde and A. O. Omoyajowo, "Africa and the nexus of poverty, malnutrition and diseases," *Crit. Rev. Food Sci. Nutr.*, vol. 63, no. 5, pp. 641–656, Feb. 2023, doi: 10.1080/10408398.2021.1952160.

[17] M. Springmann et al., "Options for keeping the food system within environmental limits," *Nature*, vol. 562, no. 7728, Art. no. 7728, Oct. 2018, doi: 10.1038/s41586-018-0594-0.

[18] A. Manzoor, B. Yousuf, J. A. Pandith and S. Ahmad, "Plant-derived active substances incorporated as antioxidant, antibacterial or antifungal components in coatings/films for food packaging applications," *Food Biosci.*, vol. 53, p. 102717, Jun. 2023, doi: 10.1016/j.fbio.2023.102717.

[19] Y. Wang et al., "Flavor challenges in extruded plant-based meat alternatives: A review," *Compr. Rev. Food Sci. Food Saf.*, vol. 21, no. 3, pp. 2898–2929, 2022, doi: 10.1111/1541-4337.12964.

[20] M. Tomar et al., "Development of NIR spectroscopy based prediction models for nutritional profiling of pearl millet (*Pennisetum glaucum* (L.)) R.Br: A chemometrics approach," *LWT*, vol. 149, p. 111813, Sep. 2021, doi: 10.1016/j.lwt.2021.111813.

[21] M. Kumar et al., "Advances in the plant protein extraction: Mechanism and recommendations," *Food Hydrocoll.*, vol. 115, p. 106595, Jun. 2021, doi: 10.1016/j.foodhyd.2021.106595.

[22] M. Kumar et al., "Cottonseed feedstock as a source of plant-based protein and bioactive peptides: Evidence based on biofunctionalities and industrial applications," *Food Hydrocoll.*, vol. 131, p. 107776, May 2022, doi: 10.1016/j.foodhyd.2022.107776.

[23] M. Kumar et al., "Cottonseed: A sustainable contributor to global protein requirements," *Trends Food Sci. Technol.*, vol. 111, pp. 100–113, May 2021, doi: 10.1016/j.tifs.2021.02.058.

[24] M. Kumar et al., "Plant-based proteins and their multifaceted industrial applications," *LWT*, vol. 154, p. 112620, Jan. 2022, doi: 10.1016/j.lwt.2021.112620.

[25] M. Mariotti Lippi, B. Foggi, B. Aranguren, A. Ronchitelli and A. Revedin, "Multistep food plant processing at Grotta Paglicci (Southern Italy) around 32,600 cal B.P.," *Proc. Natl. Acad. Sci.*, vol. 112, no. 39, pp. 12075–12080, Sep. 2015, doi: 10.1073/pnas.1505213112.

[26] I. Kuijt and B. Finlayson, "Evidence for food storage and predomestication granaries 11,000 years ago in the Jordan Valley," *Proc. Natl. Acad. Sci.*, vol. 106, no. 27, pp. 10966–10970, Jul. 2009, doi: 10.1073/pnas.0812764106.

[27] D. R. Sampson, "On the origin of oats," *Bot. Mus. Leafl. Harv. Univ.*, vol. 16, no. 10, pp. 265–303, 1954, Accessed: Nov. 13, 2023. [Online]. Available: www.jstor.org/stable/41762157

[28] E. Weiss, M. E. Kislev and A. Hartmann, "Autonomous cultivation before domestication," *Science*, vol. 312, no. 5780, pp. 1608–1610, Jun. 2006, doi: 10.1126/science.1127235.

[29] R. J. Moore-Colyer, "Oats and oat production in history and pre-history," in *The Oat Crop: Production and Utilization* (World Crop Series), R. W. Welch, Ed. Dordrecht, The Netherlands: Springer Netherlands, 1995, pp. 1–33, doi: 10.1007/978-94-011-0015-1_1.

[30] J. Kenney and L. W. Parry, "Excavations at Ysgol yr Hendre, Llanbeblig, Caernarfon: An early medieval cemetery and possible construction camp for Segontium fort," *Archaeol. Cambrensis.*, vol. 161, pp. 249–284, Jan. 2012.

[31] M. Kumar et al., "Delineating the inherent functional descriptors and biofunctionalities of pectic polysaccharides," *Carbohydr. Polym.*, vol. 269, p. 118319, Oct. 2021, doi: 10.1016/j.carbpol.2021.118319.

[32] M. Kumar et al., "Functional characterization of plant-based protein to determine its quality for food applications," *Food Hydrocoll.*, p. 106986, Jun. 2021, doi: 10.1016/j.foodhyd.2021.106986.

[33] F. A. Coffman, "Oat history: Identification and classification," *Tech. Bull.*, Art. no. 158127, Feb. 1977, Accessed: Nov. 13, 2023. [Online]. Available: https://ideas.repec.org//p/ags/uerstb/158127.html

[34] A. W. Read, "The history of Dr. Johnson's definition of 'oats,' " *Agric. Hist.*, vol. 8, no. 3, pp. 81–94, 1934, Accessed: Nov. 13, 2023. [Online]. Available: www.jstor.org/stable/3739459

[35] A. Koroluk, E. Paczos-Grzęda, S. Sowa, M. Boczkowska and J. Toporowska, "Diversity of polish oat cultivars with a glance at breeding history and perspectives," *Agronomy.*, vol. 12, no. 10, Art. No. 10, Oct. 2022, doi: 10.3390/agronomy12102423.

[36] Y.-B. Fu, "Oat evolution revealed in the maternal lineages of 25 Avena species," *Sci. Rep.*, vol. 8, no. 1, Art. No. 1, Mar. 2018, doi: 10.1038/s41598-018-22478-4.

[37] P. K. Zwer, "Oat: Overview," in *Reference Module in Food Science*, Elsevier, 2016, doi: 10.1016/B978-0-08-100596-5.00013-5.

[38] B. R. Baum, "Classification of the oat species (Avena, Poaceae) using various taximetric methods and an information–theoretic model," *Can. J. Bot.*, vol. 52, no. 11, pp. 2241–2262, Nov. 1974, doi: 10.1139/b74-292.

[39] E. A. Kellogg, "Evolutionary history of the grasses1," *Plant Physiol.*, vol. 125, no. 3, pp. 1198–1205, Mar. 2001, doi: 10.1104/pp.125.3.1198.

[40] J. Valentine, A. (Sandy) A. Cowan and A. H. Marshall, "Oat breeding," in *Oats (Second Edition)* (American Associate of Cereal Chemists International), F. H. Webster and P. J. Wood, Eds. AACC International Press, 2011, pp. 11–30, doi: 10.1016/B978-1-891127-64-9.50007-5.

[41] L. C. Federizzi and C. M. Mundstock, "Fodder oats: An overview for South America," *Fodd. Oats World Overv.*, pp. 37–51, 2004, Accessed: Nov. 13, 2023. [Online]. Available: www.cabdirect.org/cabdirect/abstract/20056705031

[42] M. Shahbandeh, "Leading oats producers worldwide 2022," *Statista.* Accessed: Nov. 13, 2023. [Online]. Available: www.statista.com/statistics/1073550/global-leading-oats-producers/

[43] P. Chew et al., "A study on the genetic relationships of Avena taxa and the origins of hexaploid oat," *Theor. Appl. Genet.*, vol. 129, no. 7, pp. 1405–1415, Jul. 2016, doi: 10.1007/s00122-016-2712-4.

[44] B. Trevaskis et al., "Advancing understanding of oat phenology for crop adaptation," *Front. Plant Sci.*, vol. 13, 2022, Accessed: Nov. 13, 2023. [Online]. Available: www.frontiersin.org/articles/10.3389/fpls.2022.955623

[45] L. Leišová-Svobodová, S. Michel, I. Tamm, M. Chourová, D. Janovska and H. Grausgruber, "Diversity and pre-breeding prospects for local adaptation in oat genetic resources," *Sustainability*, vol. 11, no. 24, Art. No. 24, Jan. 2019, doi: 10.3390/su11246950.

[46] I. G. Loskutov, A. A. Gnutikov, E. V. Blinova and A. V. Rodionov, "The origin and resource potential of wild and cultivated species of the genus of oats (avena L.)," *Russ. J. Genet.*, vol. 57, no. 6, pp. 642–661, Jun. 2021, doi: 10.1134/S1022795421060065.

[47] H. Buerstmayr, N. Krenn, U. Stephan, H. Grausgruber and E. Zechner, "Agronomic performance and quality of oat (Avena sativa L.) genotypes of worldwide origin produced under Central European growing conditions," *Field Crops Res.*, vol. 101, no. 3, pp. 343–351, Mar. 2007, doi: 10.1016/j.fcr.2006.12.011.

[48] A. Achleitner, N. A. Tinker, E. Zechner and H. Buerstmayr, "Genetic diversity among oat varieties of worldwide origin and associations of AFLP markers with quantitative traits," *Theor. Appl. Genet.*, vol. 117, no. 7, pp. 1041–1053, Nov. 2008, doi: 10.1007/s00122-008-0843-y.

[49] M. A. Newell, F. G. Asoro, M. P. Scott, P. J. White, W. D. Beavis and J.-L. Jannink, "Genome-wide association study for oat (Avena sativa L.) beta-glucan concentration using germplasm of worldwide origin," *Theor. Appl. Genet.*, vol. 125, no. 8, pp. 1687–1696, Dec. 2012, doi: 10.1007/s00122-012-1945-0.

[50] N. Vavilov, "Centers of origin of cultivated plants," *N Vavilov Orig. Geogr. Cultiv. Plants*, 1926, Accessed: Nov. 13, 2023. [Online]. Available: https://cir.nii.ac.jp/crid/1573950400013464832

[51] C. Polanco and M. P. De La Vega, "Intergenic ribosomal spacer variability in hexaploid oat cultivars and landraces," *Heredity*, vol. 78, no. 2, Art. No. 2, Feb. 1997, doi: 10.1038/hdy.1997.19.

[52] A. Katsiotis and G. Ladizinsky, "Surveying and conserving European Avena species diversity," 2011. Accessed: Nov. 13, 2023. [Online]. Available: https://ktisis.cut.ac.cy/handle/20.500.14279/14635

[53] B. R. Baum, G. Fleischmann, J. W. Martens, T. Rajhathy and H. Thomas, "Notes on the habitat and distribution of Avena species in the Mediterranean and Middle East," *Can. J. Bot.*, vol. 50, no. 6, pp. 1385–1397, Jun. 1972, doi: 10.1139/b72-167.

[54] A. Shmida, O. Fragman-Sapir, R. Nathan, Z. Shamir and Y. Sapir, "The red plants of Israel: A proposal of updated and revised list of plant species protected by the law," *Ecol. Mediterr.*, vol. 28, Jan. 2002, doi: 10.3406/ecmed.2002.1918.

[55] O. Yu. Shelukhina, E. D. Badaeva, T. A. Brezhneva, I. G. Loskutov and V. A. Pukhalsky, "Comparative analysis of diploid species of Avena L. using cytogenetic and biochemical markers: Avena pilosa M. B. and A. clauda Dur.," *Russ. J. Genet.*, vol. 44, no. 9, pp. 1087–1091, Sep. 2008, doi: 10.1134/S1022795408090111.

[56] J. M. Leggett and H. Thomas, "Oat evolution and cytogenetics," in *The Oat Crop: Production and Utilization* (World Crop Series), R. W. Welch, Ed. Dordrecht, The Netherlands: Springer Netherlands, 1995, pp. 120–149, doi: 10.1007/978-94-011-0015-1_5.

[57] B. R. Baum and G. Fedak, "Avena atlantica, a new diploid species of the oat genus from Morocco," *Can. J. Bot.*, vol. 63, no. 6, pp. 1057–1060, Jun. 1985, doi: 10.1139/b85-144.

[58] I. G. Loskutov, "On evolutionary pathways of Avena species," *Genet. Resour. Crop Evol.*, vol. 55, no. 2, pp. 211–220, Mar. 2008, doi: 10.1007/s10722-007-9229-2.

[59] T. Rajhathy and B. Baum, "Avena damascena: A new diploid oat species," *Can. J. Genet. Cytol.*, vol. 14, pp. 645–654, Jan. 2011, doi: 10.1139/g72-079.

[60] E. D. Badaeva, O. Y. Shelukhina, S. V. Goryunova, I. G. Loskutov and V. A. Pukhalskiy, "Phylogenetic relationships of tetraploid AB-genome *Avena* species evaluated by means of cytogenetic (C-banding and FISH) and RAPD analyses," *J. Bot.*, vol. 2010, p. e742307, Jun. 2010, doi: 10.1155/2010/742307.

[61] G. Ladizinsky and D. Zohary, "Notes on species delimination, species relationships and polyploidy in Avena L.," *Euphytica*, vol. 20, no. 3, pp. 380–395, Aug. 1971, doi: 10.1007/BF00035663.

[62] J. Valentine, "Studies in oat evolution: A man's life with *Avena*. By G. Ladizinsky. Heidelberg, Germany: Springer (2012), pp. 87, £44.99 (pb). ISBN 978-3-642-30546-7," *Exp. Agric.*, vol. 49, no. 1, pp. 159–160, Jan. 2013, doi: 10.1017/S0014479712000956.

[63] J. M. Leggett, G. Ladizinsky, P. Hagberg and M. Obanni, "The distribution of nine Avena species in Spain and Morocco," *Can. J. Bot.*, vol. 70, no. 2, pp. 240–244, Feb. 1992, doi: 10.1139/b92-033.

[64] B. R. Baum, T. Rajhathy and D. R. Sampson, "An important new diploid Avena species discovered on the Canary Islands," *Can. J. Bot.*, vol. 51, no. 4, pp. 759–762, Apr. 1973, doi: 10.1139/b73-095.

[65] S. Moreno, J. P. Martín and J. M. Ortiz, "Inter-simple sequence repeats PCR for characterization of closely related grapevine germplasm," *Euphytica*, vol. 101, no. 1, pp. 117–125, May 1998, doi: 10.1023/A:1018379805873.

[66] T. Morikawa and J. M. Leggett, "Isozyme polymorphism in natural populations of Avena canariensis from the Canary Islands," *Heredity*, vol. 64, no. 3, Art. No. 3, Jun. 1990, doi: 10.1038/hdy.1990.51.

[67] T. Morikawa, Y. Gushiken and N. Tsurukawa, "Chromosomal diversity and morphological dimorphism in Moroccan wild oat, Avena agadiriana," *Plant Syst. Evol.*, vol. 281, no. 1, pp. 107–113, Aug. 2009, doi: 10.1007/s00606-009-0192-6.

[68] G. Ladizinsky, "The taxonomic status of Avena magna-reappraisal," *Lagascalia*, vol. 17, no. 2, pp. 325–328, 1994, Accessed: Nov. 13, 2023. [Online]. Available: https://dialnet.unirioja.es/servlet/articulo?codigo=291864

[69] T. Rajhathy and R. S. Sadasivaiah, "The chromosomes of avena magna," *Can. J. Genet. Cytol.*, vol. 10, no. 2, pp. 385–389, Jun. 1968, doi: 10.1139/g68-051.

[70] G. Ladizinsky, "Domestication via hybridization of the wild tetraploid oats Avena magna and A. murphyi," *Theor. Appl. Genet.*, vol. 91, no. 4, pp. 639–646, Sep. 1995, doi: 10.1007/BF00223291.

[71] O. Yu. Shelukhina, E. D. Badaeva, I. G. Loskutov and V. A. Pukhal'sky, "A comparative cytogenetic study of the tetraploid oat species with the A and C genomes: Avena insularis, A. magna, and A. murphyi," *Russ. J. Genet.*, vol. 43, no. 6, pp. 613–626, Jun. 2007, doi: 10.1134/S102279540706004X.

[72] I. L. Craig, B. E. Murray and T. Rajhathy, "Avena canariensis: Morphological and electrophoretic polymorphism and relationship to the a. magna–a. murphyi complex and a. sterilis," *Can. J. Genet. Cytol.*, vol. 16, no. 3, pp. 677–689, Sep. 1974, doi: 10.1139/g74-074.

[73] P. García, L. Sáenz de Miera, F. J. Vences, M. Benchacho and M. De La Vega, "Conservation of spanish wild oats: Avena canariensis, a. prostrata and a. murphyi," *Crop Wild Relat. Conserv. Use*, pp. 413–428, Dec. 2007.

[74] G. Ladizinsky, "A new species of Avena from Sicily, possibly the tetraploid progenitor of hexaploid oats," *Genet. Resour. Crop Evol.*, vol. 45, no. 3, pp. 263–269, Jun. 1998, doi: 10.1023/A:1008657530466.

[75] M. Bilz, S. Kell, N. Maxted and R. Lansdown, *European Red List of Vascular Plants.* 2011, doi: 10.2779/8515.

[76] L. Guarino, H. Chadja and A. Mokkadem, "Collection of Avena macrostachya Bal. ex Coss. Et Dur. (Poaceae) Germplasm in Algeria," *Econ. Bot.*, vol. 45, no. 4, pp. 460–466, 1991, Accessed: Nov. 13, 2023. [Online]. Available: www.jstor.org/stable/4255388

[77] J. Vivero, E. Kelbessa and S. Demissew, "Progress on the red list of plants of Ethiopia and Eritrea: Conservation and biogeography of endemic flowering taxa," 2006, pp. 761–778, doi: 10.13140/2.1.1746.9767.

[78] K. Kubiak, "Genetic diversity of Avena strigosa Schreb. Ecotypes on the basis of isoenzyme markers," *Biodivers. Res. Conserv.*, vol. 15, pp. 23–28, Jan. 2009, doi: 10.2478/v10119-009-0013-3.

[79] M. Scholten, B. Spoor and N. Green, "Machair corn: Management and conservation of a historical machair component," *Glasg. Nat.*, vol. 25, no. Supplement-Machair Conservation: Successes and Challenges, pp. 63–71, 2009.

[80] W. Podyma et al., "A multilevel exploration of Avena strigosa diversity as a prelude to promote alternative crop," *BMC Plant Biol.*, vol. 19, p. 291, Jul. 2019, doi: 10.1186/s12870-019-1819-6.

[81] T. Korniak, "Avena strigosa [Poaceae] in north-eastern Poland," *Fragm. Florist. Geobot.*, vol. 2, no. 42, 1997, Accessed: Nov. 13, 2023. [Online]. Available: www.infona.pl//resource/bwmeta1.element.agro-article-94a8aea2-18e0-4ac1-9a30-8964eb078d9d

[82] H. A. Waterson and G. J. Davies, "The Distribution of Avena Fatua L., Avena Strigosa Schreb. And Agropyron Repens (l.) Beauv. In Barley Crops in the West of Scotland," *Weed Res.*, vol. 13, no. 2, pp. 192–199, 1973, doi: 10.1111/j.1365-3180.1973.tb01263.x.

[83] L. Grau Nersting, S. Bode Andersen, R. von Bothmer, M. Gullord and R. Bagger Jørgensen, "Morphological and molecular diversity of Nordic oat through one hundred years of breeding," *Euphytica*, vol. 150, no. 3, pp. 327–337, Aug. 2006, doi: 10.1007/s10681-006-9116-5.

[84] Y.-B. Fu, G. W. Peterson, G. Scoles, B. Rossnagel, D. J. Schoen and K. W. Richards, "Allelic diversity changes in 96 Canadian oat cultivars released from 1886 to 2001," *Crop Sci.*, vol. 43, no. 6, pp. 1989–1995, 2003, doi: 10.2135/cropsci2003.1989.

[85] G. Ladizinsky, "Oat morphology and taxonomy," in *Studies in Oat Evolution*, Berlin and Heidelberg, Germany: Springer, 2012, pp. 1–18, doi: 10.1007/978-3-642-30547-4_1.

[86] M. Boczkowska, W. Podyma and B. Łapiński, "Oat," in *Genetic and Genomic Resources for Grain Cereals Improvement*, M. Singh and H. D. Upadhyaya, Eds. San Diego, CA, USA: Academic Press, 2016, pp. 159–225, doi: 10.1016/B978-0-12-802000-5.00004-6.

[87] A. Katsiotis and G. Ladizinsky, "Surveying and conserving European Avena species diversity," *Agrobiodiversity Conserv. Secur. Divers. Crop Wild Relat. Landrac.*, pp. 65–71, Jan. 2012, doi: 10.1079/9781845938512.0065.

[88] J. C. O'Mara, "Cytogenetics," in *Oats and Oat Improvement*, F. A. Coffman, Ed. Madison, WI, USA: American Society of Agronomy, 1961, pp. 112–124.

[89] M. Portillo, T. Ball and J. Manwaring, "Morphometric analysis of inflorescence phytoliths produced by Avena sativa L. andAvena strigos schreb," *Econ. Bot.*, vol. 60, no. 2, pp. 121–129, Jun. 2006, doi: 10.1663/0013-0001(2006)60[121:MAOIPP]2.0.CO;2.

[90] H. J. Ougham, G. Latipova and J. Valentine, "Morphological and biochemical characterization of spikelet development in naked oats (Avena sativa)," *New Phytol.*, vol. 134, no. 1, pp. 5–12, 1996, doi: 10.1111/j.1469-8137.1996.tb01141.x.

[91] B. Sera, P. Špatenka, M. Šerý, N. Vrchotova and I. Hrušková, "Influence of plasma treatment on wheat and oat germination and early growth," *IEEE Trans. Plasma Sci.*, vol. 38, no. 10, pp. 2963–2968, Oct. 2010, doi: 10.1109/TPS.2010.2060728.

[92] L. Elsgaard et al., "Shifts in comparative advantages for maize, oat and wheat cropping under climate change in Europe," *Food Addit. Contam. Part A*, vol. 29, no. 10, pp. 1514–1526, Oct. 2012, doi: 10.1080/19440049.2012.700953.

[93] D. Stewart and G. McDougall, "Oat agriculture, cultivation and breeding targets: Implications for human nutrition and health," *Br. J. Nutr.*, vol. 112, no. S2, pp. S50–S57, Oct. 2014, doi: 10.1017/S0007114514002736.

[94] M. Djanaguiraman et al., "Agroclimatology of oats, barley, and minor millets," in *Agroclimatology*, John Wiley & Sons, Ltd, 2020, pp. 243–277, doi: 10.2134/agronmonogr60.2018.0020.

[95] P. Peltonen-Sainio, L. Jauhiainen and K. Hakala, "Crop responses to temperature and precipitation according to long-term multi-location trials at high-latitude conditions," *J. Agric. Sci.*, vol. 149, no. 1, pp. 49–62, Feb. 2011, doi: 10.1017/S0021859610000791.

[96] K. A. Kelling and P. E. Fixen, "Soil and nutrient requirements for oat production," in *Oat Science and Technology*, John Wiley & Sons, Ltd., 1992, pp. 165–190, doi: 10.2134/agronmonogr33.c6.

[97] E. George, W. J. Horst and E. Neumann, "Adaptation of plants to adverse chemical soil conditions," in *Marschner's Mineral Nutrition of Higher Plants (Third Edition)*, P. Marschner, Ed. San Diego, CA, USA: Academic Press, 2012, pp. 409–472, doi: 10.1016/B978-0-12-384905-2.00017-0.

[98] S. P. Hoad, G. Russell, M. E. Lucas and I. J. Bingham, "The management of wheat, barley, and oat root systems," in *Advances in Agronomy*, vol. 74, Academic Press, 2001, pp. 193–246, doi: 10.1016/S0065-2113(01)74034-5.

[99] P. H. Oliveira, L. C. Federizzi, S. C. K. Milach, C. Gotuzzo and J. T. Sawasato, "Inheritance in oat (Avena sativa L.) of tolerance to soil aluminum toxicity," *Cropp Breed. Appl. Biotechnol.*, vol. 5, no. 3, pp. 302–309, Sep. 2005, doi: 10.12702/1984-7033.v05n03a07.

[100] D. G. Westfall, D. A. Whitney and D. M. Brandon, "Plant analysis as an aid in fertilizing small grains," in *Soil Testing and Plant Analysis*, John Wiley & Sons, Ltd, 1990, pp. 495–519, doi: 10.2136/sssabookser3.3ed.c19.

[101] A. Wasaya, T. A. Yasir, M. Ijaz and S. Ahmad, "Tillage effects on agronomic crop production," in *Agronomic Crops*, Singapore, Singapore: Springer, 2019, pp. 73–99, doi: 10.1007/978-981-32-9783-8_5.

[102] A. Gronle et al., "Effect of ploughing depth and mechanical soil loading on soil physical properties, weed infestation, yield performance and grain quality in sole and intercrops of pea and oat in organic farming," *Soil Tillage Res.*, vol. 148, pp. 59–73, May 2015, doi: 10.1016/j.still.2014.12.004.

[103] Yu. I. Mitrofanov, L. V. Pugacheva, N. A. Smirnova and V. N. Lapushkina, "Oat-sowing methods on drained lands," *Russ. Agric. Sci.*, vol. 44, no. 6, pp. 493–498, Nov. 2018, doi: 10.3103/S1068367418060101.

[104] S. S. Kadam, N. S. Solanki, M. Arif, L. N. Dashora, S. L. Mundra and B. Upadhyay, "Productivity and quality of fodder oats (Avena sativa L.) as influenced by sowing time, cutting schedules and nitrogen levels," *Indian J. Anim. Nutr.*, vol. 36, no. 2, pp. 179–186, 2019, Accessed: Dec. 07, 2023. [Online]. Available: www.cabdirect.org/cabdirect/abstract/20193366664

[105] G. Mahajan and B. S. Chauhan, "Biological traits of six sterile oat biotypes in response to planting time," *Agron. J.*, vol. 113, no. 1, pp. 42–51, 2021, doi: 10.1002/agj2.20507.

[106] M. V. Romitti et al., "The sowing density on oat productivity indicators," *Afr. J. Agric. Res.*, vol. 12, no. 11, pp. 905–915, Mar. 2017, doi: 10.5897/AJAR2016.12095.

[107] P. Sharma and K. Choudhary, "Effect of sowing methods and nitrogen levels on growth, yield and economics of oats (Avena sativa L.) under mid-hills of Himachal Pradesh, India," *Int. J. Environ. Clim. Change*, vol. 13, no. 11, Art. No. 11, Oct. 2023, doi: 10.9734/ijecc/2023/v13i113321.

[108] A. Singh, D. S. K. Jha and D. V. K. Samadhiya, "Effect of different varieties, date of sowing and cutting management on yield attributes and yield for seed productivity of oat (Avena sativa L.)," *Pharma Innov. J.*, vol. 11, no. 12, pp. 1076–1086, 2022, Accessed: Dec. 07, 2023. [Online]. Available: www.thepharmajournal.com/archives/?year=2022&vol=11&issue=12&ArticleId=17363

[109] N. Aggarwal, S. K. Thind and S. Sharma, "Role of secondary metabolites of actinomycetes in crop protection," in *Plant Growth Promoting Actinobacteria: A New Avenue for Enhancing the Productivity and Soil Fertility of Grain Legumes*, G. Subramaniam, S. Arumugam and V. Rajendran, Eds. Singapore, Singapore: Springer, 2016, pp. 99–121, doi: 10.1007/978-981-10-0707-1_7.

[110] R. K. Singhal et al., "Beneficial elements: New players in improving nutrient use efficiency and abiotic stress tolerance," *Plant Growth Regul.*, vol. 100, no. 2, pp. 237–265, Jun. 2023, doi: 10.1007/s10725-022-00843-8.

[111] P. Singh et al., "Global gene expression profiling under nitrogen stress identifies key genes involved in nitrogen stress adaptation in maize (Zea mays L.)," *Sci. Rep.*, vol. 12, no. 1, Art. No. 1, Mar. 2022, doi: 10.1038/s41598-022-07709-z.

[112] P. Singh, R. S. Tomar, K. Kumar, B. Kumar, S. Rakshit and I. Singh, "Morpho-physiological and biochemical characterization of maize genotypes under nitrogen stress conditions," *Indian J. Genet. Plant Breed.*, vol. 81, no. 2, Art. No. 2, May 2021, doi: 10.31742/IJGPB.81.2.8.

[113] P. Singh, S. Jaiswal, S. Sheokand and S. Duhan, "Morpho-physiological and oxidative responses of nitrogen and phosphorus deficiency in wheat (Triticum aestivum L.)," *Indian J. Agric. Res.*, vol. 52, no. 1, pp. 40–45, 2018, doi: 10.18805/IJARe.A-4905.

[114] I. Singh, K. Kumar, P. Singh, P. Yadava and S. Rakshit, "Physiological and molecular interventions for improving nitrogen-use efficiency in maize," in *Molecular Breeding in Wheat, Maize and Sorghum: Strategies for Improving Abiotic Stress Tolerance and Yield*, M. A. Hossain, M. Alam, S. Seneweera, S. Rakshit, R. Henry, Eds. Wallingford: CABI, 2021, pp. 325–339.

[115] P. Singh et al., "Role of range grasses in conservation and restoration of biodiversity," in *Agro-biodiversity and Agri-ecosystem Management*, P. Kumar, R. S. Tomar, J. A. Bhat, M. Dobriyal and M. Rani, Eds. Singapore, Singapore: Springer Nature, 2022, pp. 53–69, doi: 10.1007/978-981-19-0928-3_4.

[116] Y. Zhang, C. Li, T. Yao, M. Li, X. Lan and Z. Wang, "Plant growth–promoting rhizobacteria enhance salt tolerance in oat by upregulating the antioxidant system and promoting root growth," *J. Plant Growth Regul.*, vol. 42, no. 6, pp. 3568–3581, Jun. 2023, doi: 10.1007/s00344-022-10821-z.

[117] J. M. Finnan, L. Hyland and B. Burke, "The effect of seeding rate on radiation interception, grain yield and grain quality of autumn sown oats," *Eur. J. Agron.*, vol. 101, pp. 239–247, Nov. 2018, doi: 10.1016/j.eja.2018.09.008.

[118] A. K. Obour, J. D. Holman and A. J. Schlegel, "Seeding rate and nitrogen application effects on oat forage yield and nutritive value," *J. Plant Nutr.*, vol. 42, no. 13, pp. 1452–1460, Aug. 2019, doi: 10.1080/01904167.2019.1617311.

[119] V. Gecaitė, A. Arlauskienė and J. Ceseviciene, "Competition effects and productivity in oat–forage legume relay intercropping systems under organic farming conditions," *Agriculture.*, vol. 11, no. 2, Art. No. 2, Feb. 2021, doi: 10.3390/agriculture11020099.

[120] M. Li, J. Zhang, S. Liu, U. Ashraf, B. Zhao and S. Qiu, "Mixed-cropping systems of different rice cultivars have grain yield and quality advantages over mono-cropping systems," *J. Sci. Food Agric.*, vol. 99, no. 7, pp. 3326–3334, 2019, doi: 10.1002/jsfa.9547.

[121] K. N. Harker et al., "Diverse rotations and optimal cultural practices control wild oat (Avena fatua)," *Weed Sci.*, vol. 64, no. 1, pp. 170–180, Mar. 2016, doi: 10.1614/WS-D-15-00133.1.

[122] E. G. Smith et al., "The profitability of diverse crop rotations and other cultural methods that reduce wild oat (Avena fatua)," *Can. J. Plant Sci.*, vol. 98, no. 5, pp. 1094–1101, Oct. 2018, doi: 10.1139/cjps-2018-0019.

[123] R. S. Tomar et al., "Genomics approaches for restoration and conservation of agro-biodiversity," in *Agro-biodiversity and Agri-ecosystem Management*, P. Kumar, R. S. Tomar, J. A. Bhat, M. Dobriyal and M. Rani, Eds. Singapore, Singapore: Springer Nature, 2022, pp. 273–283, doi: 10.1007/978-981-19-0928-3_14.

[124] A. Kumar et al., "Genomics-assisted improvement of grain quality and nutraceutical properties in millets," in *Millets and Millet Technology*, A. Kumar, M. K. Tripathi, D. Joshi and V. Kumar, Eds. Singapore, Singapore: Springer, 2021, pp. 333–343, doi: 10.1007/978-981-16-0676-2_17.

[125] S. Singh, P. Singh, R. S. Tomar, R. A. Sharma and S. K. Singh, "Proline: A key player to regulate biotic and abiotic stress in plants," in *Towards Sustainable Natural Resources: Monitoring and Managing Ecosystem Biodiversity*, M. Rani, B. S. Chaudhary, S. Jamal and P. Kumar, Eds. Cham, Germany: Springer International Publishing, 2022, pp. 333–346, doi: 10.1007/978-3-031-06443-2_18.

[126] S. Biswas and R. Das, "Role of integrated nutrient management on oat: A review," *Int. J. Environ. Clim. Change*, vol. 12, pp. 66–79, Mar. 2022, doi: 10.9734/IJECC/2022/v12i530675.

[127] S. N. Dheeravathu et al., "Open top chamber: An innovative screening technique for temperature stress tolerance of morpho-physiological and fodder yield traits in forage cowpea varieties," *Range Manag. Agrofor.*, vol. 44, no. 1, pp. 58–65, Sep. 2023, doi: 10.59515/rma.2023.v44.i1.07.

[128] R. S. Singh Tomar, S. Tiwari, P. Singh, K. B. Naik and A. Kumar, "Genome editing for improvement of wheat and millets," in *Genome Editing in Plants (First Edition)*, Boca Raton, Florida: CRC Press, 2021, pp. 1–12.

[129] K. Djaman, M. O'Neill, C. Owen, K. Koudahe and K. Lombard, "Evapotranspiration, grain yield, and water productivity of spring oat (Avena sativa L.) under semiarid climate," *Agric. Sci.*, vol. 9, no. 9, Art. No. 9, Sep. 2018, doi: 10.4236/as.2018.99083.

[130] A. G. Xue et al., "Timing of inoculation and fusarium species affect the severity of Fusarium head blight on oat," *Can. J. Plant Sci.*, vol. 95, no. 3, pp. 517–524, May 2015, doi: 10.4141/cjps-2014-300.

[131] J. G. Menzies et al., "Virulence of puccinia coronata var avenae f. sp. Avenae (oat crown rust) in Canada during 2010 to 2015," *Can. J. Plant Pathol.*, vol. 41, no. 3, pp. 379–391, Jul. 2019, doi: 10.1080/07060661.2019.1577300.

[132] Y. Li, P. Lv, J. Mi, B. Zhao and J. Liu, "Integrative transcriptome and metabolome analyses of the interaction of oat–oat stem rust," *Agronomy.*, vol. 12, no. 10, Art. no. 10, Oct. 2022, doi: 10.3390/agronomy12102353.

[133] L. Necheporenko and S. Vorozhko, "Perspective resources of resistance of spring oats to loose smut," *Quar. Plant Prot.*, no. 5–6, Art. no. 5–6, May 2019, doi: 10.36495/2312-0614.2019.5-6.20-23.

[134] L. R. Winkler, J. Michael Bonman, S. Chao, B. Admassu Yimer, H. Bockelman and K. Esvelt Klos, "Population structure and genotype–phenotype associations in a collection of oat landraces and historic cultivars," *Front. Plant Sci.*, vol. 7, 2016, Accessed: Dec. 7, 2023. [Online]. Available: www.frontiersin.org/articles/10.3389/fpls.2016.01077

[135] R. Kapoor and T. P. Singh, "Breeding oats for biotic and abiotic stresses," *Int. J. Curr. Microbiol. Appl. Sci.*, vol. 9, no. 1, pp. 274–283, Jan. 2020, doi: 10.20546/ijcmas.2020.901.032.

[136] H. Chen, L. Xue, J. F. White, M. Kamran and C. Li, "Identification and characterization of Pyrenophora species causing leaf spot on oat (Avena sativa) in western China," *Plant Pathol.*, vol. 71, no. 3, pp. 566–577, 2022, doi: 10.1111/ppa.13491.

[137]   A. Zaveri et al., "Phylogenetic placement of Spermospora avenae, causal agent of red leather leaf disease of oats," *Australas. Plant Pathol.*, vol. 49, no. 5, pp. 551–559, Sep. 2020, doi: 10.1007/s13313-020-00730-8.

[138]   A. Reilly, S. Okoń, M. Cieplak, J. Finnan, S. Kildea and A. Feechan, "Breadth of resistance to powdery mildew in commercial oat cultivars available in Ireland," *Crop Prot.*, vol. 176, p. 106517, Feb. 2024, doi: 10.1016/j.cropro.2023.106517.

[139]   C. J. Pretorius, P. A. Steenkamp, F. Tugizimana, L. A. Piater and I. A. Dubery, "Metabolomic characterisation of discriminatory metabolites involved in halo blight disease in oat cultivars caused by pseudomonas syringae pv. coronafaciens," *Metabolites*, vol. 12, no. 3, Art. no. 3, Mar. 2022, doi: 10.3390/metabo12030248.

[140]   S. F. Jan, M. R. Khan, A. Iqbal, F. U. Khan and S. Ali, "Genetic diversity in exotic oat germplasm & resistance against barley yellow dwarf virus," *Saudi J. Biol. Sci.*, vol. 27, no. 10, pp. 2622–2631, Oct. 2020, doi: 10.1016/j.sjbs.2020.05.042.

[141]   A. Wenda-Piesik and D. Piesik, "Diversity of species and the occurrence and development of a specialized pest population – A review article," *Agriculture.*, vol. 11, no. 1, Art. no. 1, Jan. 2021, doi: 10.3390/agriculture11010016.

[142]   S. Ward, M. van Helden, T. Heddle, P. M. Ridland, E. Pirtle and P. A. Umina, "Biology, ecology and management of Diuraphis noxia (Hemiptera: Aphididae) in Australia," *Austral Entomol.*, vol. 59, no. 2, pp. 238–252, 2020, doi: 10.1111/aen.12453.

[143]   N. Wen, Y. Manning-Thompson, K. Garland-Campbell and T. Paulitz, "Distribution of cereal cyst nematodes (heterodera avenae and H. filipjevi) in Eastern Washington State," *Plant Dis.*, vol. 103, no. 9, pp. 2171–2178, Sep. 2019, doi: 10.1094/PDIS-10-18-1881-SR.

[144]   E. Yavuzaslanoglu and G. Aksay, "Susceptibility of different plant species to two populations of Ditylenchus dipsaci Kühn, 1857 (Tylenchida: Anguinidae) from Turkey," *Turk. J. Entomol.*, vol. 45, no. 1, Art. no. 1, Mar. 2021, doi: 10.16970/entoted.795993.

[145]   F. Mokrini, N. Viaene, L. Waeyenberge, A. A. Dababat and M. Moens, "Root-lesion nematodes in cereal fields: Importance, distribution, identification, and management strategies," *J. Plant Dis. Prot.*, vol. 126, no. 1, pp. 1–11, Feb. 2019, doi: 10.1007/s41348-018-0195-z.

[146]   N. Hamidi and A. Hajihassani, "Differences in parasitism of root-knot nematodes (spp.) on oilseed radish and oat," *J. Nematol.*, vol. 52, no. 1, pp. 1–10, Jan. 2020, doi: 10.21307/jofnem-2020-043.

[147]   C. J. Howarth et al., "Genotype and environment affect the grain quality and yield of winter oats (avena sativa L.)," *Foods*, vol. 10, no. 10, Art. no. 10, Oct. 2021, doi: 10.3390/foods10102356.

[148]   V. Ugrenović et al., "Black oat (avena strigosa schreb.) ontogenesis and agronomic performance in organic cropping system and pannonian environments," *Agriculture.*, vol. 11, no. 1, Art. no. 1, Jan. 2021, doi: 10.3390/agriculture11010055.

[149]   C. P. McCabe and J. I. Burke, "Oat (Avena sativa) yield and grain fill responses to varying agronomic and weather factors," *J. Agric. Sci.*, vol. 159, no. 1–2, pp. 90–105, Jan. 2021, doi: 10.1017/S0021859621000320.

[150]   B. Bytyqi and E. Kutasy, "Leaf reflectance characteristics and yield of spring oat varieties as influenced by varietal divergences and nutritional supply," *Acta Agrar. Debreceniensis.*, no. 1, Art. no. 1, Jun. 2023, doi: 10.34101/actaagrar/1/12144.

[151]   E. A. Tambussi, M. L. Maydup, C. A. Carrión, J. J. Guiamet and J. L. Araus, "Ear photosynthesis in C3 cereals and its contribution to grain yield: Methodologies, controversies, and perspectives," *J. Exp. Bot.*, vol. 72, no. 11, pp. 3956–3970, May 2021, doi: 10.1093/jxb/erab125.

[152]   R. Tobiasz-Salach, B. Stadnik and M. Bajcar, "Oat as a potential source of energy," *Energies*, vol. 16, no. 16, Art. no. 16, Jan. 2023, doi: 10.3390/en16166019.

[153] T. R. Sarker, R. Azargohar, A. K. Dalai and M. Venkatesh, "Physicochemical and fuel characteristics of torrefied agricultural residues for sustainable fuel production," *Energy Fuels*, vol. 34, no. 11, pp. 14169–14181, Nov. 2020, doi: 10.1021/acs.energyfuels.0c02121.

[154] E. R. da S. Santos et al., "Seeding rate affects the performance of oat and black oat," *Crop Forage Turfgrass Manag.*, vol. 8, no. 2, p. e20192, 2022, doi: 10.1002/cft2.20192.

[155] J. M. Luna and G. J. House, "Pest management in sustainable agricultural systems," in *Sustainable Agricultural Systems (First Edition)*, Boca Raton, Florida: CRC Press, 1990, pp. 1–17.

[156] A. Juostas, E. Jotautiene and G. Juodisius, "Evaluation of combine harvester performance telemetry data," presented at the 21st International Scientific Conference Engineering for Rural Development, May 2022, pp. 267–271, doi: 10.22616/ERDev.2022.21.TF079

[157] V. Ziegler, R. T. Paraginski and C. D. Ferreira, "Grain storage systems and effects of moisture, temperature and time on grain quality – A review," *J. Stored Prod. Res.*, vol. 91, p. 101770, Mar. 2021, doi: 10.1016/j.jspr.2021.101770.

[158] O. Laaksonen, X. Ma, E. Pasanen, P. Zhou, B. Yang and K. M. Linderborg, "Sensory characteristics contributing to pleasantness of oat product concepts by Finnish and Chinese consumers," *Foods*, vol. 9, no. 9, Art. no. 9, Sep. 2020, doi: 10.3390/foods9091234.

[159] D. V. Byrne, "Current trends in food health and safety in cross-cultural sensory and consumer science," *Foods*, vol. 10, no. 5, Art. no. 5, May 2021, doi: 10.3390/foods10050965.

[160] M. G. Mumolo et al., "Is gluten the only culprit for non-celiac gluten/wheat sensitivity?," *Nutrients*, vol. 12, no. 12, Art. no. 12, Dec. 2020, doi: 10.3390/nu12123785.

[161] S. C. Paterson, T. C. Mulholland, A. Mehta and L. Serventi, "Carbohydrates for fibre," in *Sustainable Food Innovation* (Sustainable Development Goals Series), L. Serventi, Ed. Cham, Germany: Springer International Publishing, 2023, pp. 29–43, doi: 10.1007/978-3-031-12358-0_3.

[162] A. Xie et al., "A review of plant-based drinks addressing nutrients, flavor, and processing technologies," *Foods*, vol. 12, no. 21, Art. no. 21, Jan. 2023, doi: 10.3390/foods12213952.

[163] N. Bocken, L. S. Morales and M. Lehner, "Sufficiency business strategies in the food industry – The case of oatly," *Sustainability*, vol. 12, no. 3, Art. no. 3, Jan. 2020, doi: 10.3390/su12030824.

[164] Z. Şahin, M. H. Aydoğdu, G. Sevinç and N. Küçük, "The analysis of the recent periods of oat market in Turkey," *ITEGAM-JETIA*, vol. 7, no. 28, Art. no. 28, Apr. 2021, doi: 10.5935/jetia.v7i28.741.

[165] K. Hakala, L. Jauhiainen, A. A. Rajala, M. Jalli, M. Kujala and A. Laine, "Different responses to weather events may change the cultivation balance of spring barley and oats in the future," *Field Crops Res.*, vol. 259, p. 107956, Dec. 2020, doi: 10.1016/j.fcr.2020.107956.

[166] E. Dohlman, J. Hansen and D. Boussios, Eds., *USDA Agricultural Projections to 2031*. OCE-2022-01. 2022, doi: 10.22004/ag.econ.323859.

[167] Z. Yang, C. Xie, Y. Bao, F. Liu, H. Wang and Y. Wang, "Oat: Current state and challenges in plant-based food applications," *Trends Food Sci. Technol.*, vol. 134, pp. 56–71, Apr. 2023, doi: 10.1016/j.tifs.2023.02.017.

[168] X. Xu and Y. Zhang, "Commodity price forecasting via neural networks for coffee, corn, cotton, oats, soybeans, soybean oil, sugar, and wheat," *Intell. Syst. Account. Finance Manag.*, vol. 29, no. 3, pp. 169–181, 2022, doi: 10.1002/isaf.1519.

[169] D. Panagiotou and A. Tseriki, "Directional predictability between trading volume and price returns in the agricultural futures markets: Risk implications for traders," *J. Risk Finance*, vol. 23, no. 3, pp. 264–288, Jan. 2022, doi: 10.1108/JRF-04-2021-0063.

[170] D. Panagiotou and K. Karamanis, "Testing for monotonicity, linearity and symmetry between trading volume and price returns in the futures markets of agricultural commodities: A discussion on the financial implications," *Stud. Econ. Finance*, vol. 40, no. 5, pp. 996–1020, Jan. 2023, doi: 10.1108/SEF-03-2023-0138.

[171] G. Graddy-Lovelace et al., "Parity as radical pragmatism: Centering farm justice and agrarian expertise in agricultural policy," *Front. Sustain. Food Syst.*, vol. 7, 2023, Accessed: Dec. 10, 2023. [Online]. Available: www.frontiersin.org/articles/10.3389/fsufs.2023.1066465

[172] K. Anderson, "Agriculture's globalization: Endowments, technologies, tastes and policies," *J. Econ. Surv.*, vol. 37, no. 4, pp. 1314–1352, 2023, doi: 10.1111/joes.12529.

[173] N. Andrusenko, L. Martynova, V. Sharko, K. Garbazhii, S. Hyrych and O. Vasylyshyna, "Changes in the organic products market as a result of the 2022 events in eastern Europe." Rochester, NY, Oct. 31, 2022. Accessed: Dec. 10, 2023. [Online]. Available: https://papers.ssrn.com/abstract=4262798

[174] I. Rac, K. Erjavec and E. Erjavec, "Agriculture and environment: Friends or foes? Conceptualising agri-environmental discourses under the European Union's Common Agricultural Policy," *Agric. Hum. Values.*, Jun. 2023, doi: 10.1007/s10460-023-10474-y.

[175] E. Mulligan, E. Bassey, D. De Widt, M. Greggi, D. Kiesewetter and L. Oats, "Regulation of intermediaries, including tax advisers, in the EU/member states and best practices from inside and outside the EU." Accessed: Dec. 10, 2023, doi: 10.2861/13951.

International Scenario of Oat Production and Its Potential Role in Sustainable Agriculture

2

Prabha Singh, Maharishi Tomar,
Awnindra Kumar Singh, Vijay Kumar Yadav,
Ravi Prakash Saini, Sunil Ramling Swami,
H. S. Mahesha, Ajay Kumar Singh,
and Tejveer Singh

2.1 INTRODUCTION

Oats (*Avena sativa* L.) occupy a pivotal position as a consequential global livestock feed, serving as both a nutrient-rich grain and a vital forage. Renowned for their protein, fibre, and mineral content, oats historically reigned as the foremost protein source in livestock feed until eclipsed by soybeans [1]. Despite a significant decline in global oat production over the past seven decades due to increased farm mechanization from 1930 to 1950, oats persist as a vital grain crop. This enduring relevance is particularly pronounced in

DOI: 10.1201/ 9781003263302-2

developing regions and advanced economies, where oats find application in diverse agricultural niches [2]. Globally, oats are cultivated for various purposes, including grain, forage, fodder, straw, bedding, hay, haylage, silage, and chaff. Approximately 25% of the oat-seeded area is dedicated to green feed across numerous regions. Data from the U.S. Department of Agriculture (USDA) spanning from 1995 to 2005 reveals that livestock feed constitutes the primary use of oats, accounting for an average of 74% of the world's oat utilization. However, the versatility of oats extends beyond animal consumption into human food products and industrial applications. Oatmeal, oat flour, oat bran, and oat flakes, integral components of breakfast cereals and various food products, exemplify the diverse applications of oats in human consumption [3].

Russia leads global oat production, harvesting over 22 million tons, with Canada, Poland, Australia, and Finland following suit [4]. The United States, Brazil, Spain, the United Kingdom, and Argentina round out the top-ten oat-producing nations [5]. Presently cultivated in over 70 countries worldwide, oats contributed to global production of 20,425,000 metric tons in 2023. The peak of worldwide oat production was observed in 1960, reaching an impressive 55.9 million metric tons. Canada ranked as the second-largest global oat producer in 2022, following the European Union (EU), with an output of approximately 4.6 million metric tons. The global oats market, valued at US$5.4 billion in 2022, is poised for further expansion. Projections from the international market analysis research and consulting group (IMARC) Group anticipate the market reaching US$6.10 billion by 2028, reflecting a compound annual growth rate (CAGR) of 2.10% during 2023–2028. This growth is fuelled by increasing health consciousness, a rising preference for gluten-free and plant-based diets, and a growing demand for breakfast cereals, granola bars, muesli, and healthy snacks. Against the backdrop of the burgeoning oats market, the imperative of sustainable agriculture has gained ascendancy since the Brundtland Report's inception in 1987. However, the conceptual ambiguity surrounding sustainable agriculture has hindered its effective use and implementation. This systematic review aims to enhance the understanding of sustainable agriculture from a social science and governance perspective, identifying areas of complementarity and concern among emerging definitions.

The seemingly humble oats, often overshadowed in breakfast bowls, emerge as silent architects of sustainability within agriculture. Their role transcends culinary delight, encompassing pivotal functions crucial for fostering resilient and environmentally conscious farming systems [6]. Deployed as cover crops and green manure, oats act as protective shields for the soil, mitigating erosion and suppressing weeds. Integration into diversified crop rotations aids in breaking pest and disease cycles, promoting soil health, and reducing reliance on chemical inputs [7]. As a low-input crop, oats align with sustainable agriculture principles, requiring fewer fertilizers and pesticides while offering robust nutritional value. Beyond the farm gate, oats support livestock by providing a nutritious and energy-rich feed source [8].

Moreover, the use of oats contributes to nitrogen management within agroecosystems, especially when strategically paired with nitrogen-fixing legumes in cover crop rotations. While oats themselves do not fix nitrogen, their synergy with legumes allows for a comprehensive approach to soil fertility, reducing reliance on synthetic nitrogen fertilizers and minimizing associated environmental impacts [9]–[16]. With a relatively shallow root system, oats play a pivotal role in water management, preventing soil erosion and enhancing water infiltration, thereby contributing to overall sustainability in the agricultural landscape.

In the context of climate change, the cold-hardy nature of oats becomes a valuable asset in regions with shorter growing seasons. Their adaptability to cooler climates not only expands the geographic scope for sustainable agriculture but also positions oats as a climate-resilient crop choice [17]. The incorporation of oats into agroecological practices presents an opportunity to build climate-smart farming systems capable of withstanding the unpredictable challenges posed by a changing climate. In essence, the potential role of oats in sustainable agriculture extends far beyond the confines of a popular breakfast grain [18]. It encompasses a holistic approach to farming that addresses soil health, biodiversity, water conservation, and climate resilience. As we delve into the nuanced contributions of oats within the agricultural landscape, a compelling narrative unfolds – one where this unassuming cereal takes centre stage in the ongoing pursuit of a more sustainable and harmonious coexistence between humanity and the earth we cultivate [19]. In this chapter, we will delve into the contemporary global landscape of oat cultivation, shedding light on its pivotal role in fostering sustainable agricultural practices. We'll explore the current state of international oat production and underscore its significance in promoting environmentally conscious and resource-efficient farming methods.

2.2 PRODUCTION

The global landscape of oat production reveals a conspicuous lull in comparison to its grain counterparts. According to the USDA Foreign Agricultural Service, the worldwide output of oats hovers between 22 and 25 million tons. This figure, while dwarfed by other cereals, signifies a minute fraction within the expansive realm of global grain production. The Food and Agriculture Organization, in its latest prognostications for 2023, maintains an anticipated world cereal production of 2819 million tons. This projection signals a modest uptick of 0.9%, equivalent to a 26 million ton increase from the preceding year. Notably, the sector of coarse grains is estimated to hold steady at 1510 million tons, constituting a 2.7% (38.8 million tons) surge from the prior year's yield.

In the hierarchical echelons of grain production, oats find themselves occupying the sixth position globally. This ranking places oats in the company of more prolific cereal crops such as corn, wheat, barley, sorghum, and millets (Figure 2.1). However, oats contribute a mere fraction, accounting for less than 2% of the total grain production, with the lion's share employed for on-farm fodder. Examining the dynamics of oat production from 2012 to 2022 reveals a striking growth trajectory, particularly in Brazil, where a commendable CAGR of +8.7% was achieved. In contrast, other leading oat-producing nations experienced more restrained rates of expansion during the same period. In the year 2022, the global average oat yield exhibited a modest ascent to 2.36 metric tons per hectare, registering a 4.4% increase from the previous year. The upward trend in yield has been a consistent feature, advancing at an average annual rate of +1.0% over the 2012–2022 period, punctuated by notable fluctuations. The most remarkable surge occurred in 2013, marked by a conspicuous 9.3% increase. The USDA's "Grain: World Markets and Trade Report," published in October 2021, underscores the evolution

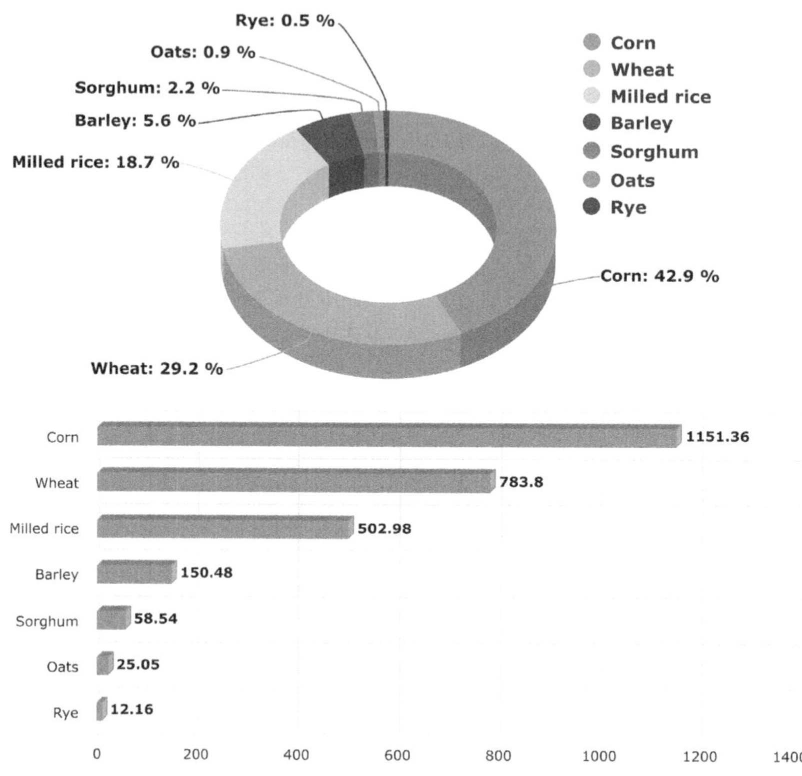

FIGURE 2.1   Global grain production for the 2022/23 crop year. This figure illustrates the worldwide production of grain for the agricultural season 2022/23, categorized by grain type and measured in million metric tons. The data provides a comprehensive overview of the distribution of major grain varieties, offering insights into the global dynamics of food production and agricultural trends during this specific crop year.

of world oat production, escalating from 22.1 million tons in the 2018/19 season to 23.2 million tons in 2019/20, and further to 25.5 million tons in 2020/21. However, a noteworthy downturn is observed in the ongoing 2021/22 season, with global oat production poised to contract by 3 million tons, reaching a projected 22.7 million tons. This decline is attributed significantly to drought conditions prevailing in numerous regions worldwide (Table 2.1) (Figure 2.2).

Considering the distribution of oat production among nations, the EU emerged as the preeminent contributor. According to USDA's 2020/21 data, the EU leads the world in oat production, yielding 8.4 million tons, trailed by Canada with 4.5 million tons, Russia with 4.1 million tons, Australia with 1.6 million tons, and the United Kingdom with 1 million tons. Forecasts for the 2021/22 season anticipate a marginal dip in EU production to 8.2 million tons. Concurrently, while Russia's production remains relatively stable, Canada is poised to experience the most significant contraction, with an expected decrease of approximately 2.2 million tons, plummeting to 2.3 million tons.

TABLE 2.1 Oats Area, Yield, and Production

	AREA (MILLION HECTARES)				YIELD (METRIC TONS PER HECTARE)				PRODUCTION (MILLION METRIC TONS)			
REGION	2021/22	2022/23	2023/24 OCTOBER	2023/24 NOVEMBER	2021/22	2022/23	2023/24 OCTOBER	2023/24 NOVEMBER	2021/22	2022/23	2023/24 OCTOBER	2023/24 NOVEMBER
World	9.63	9.33	8.41	8.39	2.36	2.69	2.43	2.43	22.69	25.13	20.45	20.43
United States	0.26	0.36	0.34	0.34	2.20	2.33	2.46	2.46	0.58	0.84	0.83	0.83
Total foreign	9.36	8.97	8.07	8.06	2.36	2.71	2.43	2.43	22.11	24.29	19.62	19.60
European Union	2.54	2.34	2.31	2.31	2.94	3.17	2.92	2.95	7.47	7.41	6.75	6.81
Former Soviet Union – 12												
Russia	2.17	2.13	1.80	1.80	1.72	2.11	1.94	1.94	3.73	4.50	3.50	3.50
Ukraine	0.18	0.15	0.15	0.15	2.61	2.47	2.33	2.33	0.48	0.38	0.35	0.35
Belarus	0.15	0.16	0.16	0.16	2.33	2.42	2.26	2.26	0.35	0.38	0.35	0.35
Kazakhstan	0.20	0.20	0.19	0.19	0.90	1.16	1.16	1.16	0.18	0.23	0.22	0.22
Canada	1.21	1.40	0.85	0.85	2.39	3.73	2.94	2.94	2.90	5.23	2.50	2.50
South America												
Argentina	0.35	0.26	0.29	0.29	2.07	1.67	2.14	2.14	0.73	0.43	0.61	0.61
Brazil	0.50	0.50	0.51	0.51	2.27	2.38	2.39	2.39	1.14	1.19	1.22	1.22
Chile	0.12	0.07	0.10	0.10	4.70	4.38	4.74	4.74	0.58	0.32	0.45	0.45
Uruguay	0.01	0.02	0.01	0.01	2.21	2.40	2.20	2.20	0.03	0.04	0.02	0.02
Oceania												
Australia	0.84	0.75	0.70	0.70	2.06	2.13	1.57	1.57	1.74	1.59	1.10	1.10
New Zealand	0.00	0.01	0.01	0.01	6.25	5.67	5.67	5.67	0.03	0.03	0.03	0.03

(Continued)

TABLE 2.1 (Continued) Oats Area, Yield, and Production

REGION	AREA (MILLION HECTARES)				YIELD (METRIC TONS PER HECTARE)				PRODUCTION (MILLION METRIC TONS)			
	2021/22	2022/23	2023/24 OCTOBER	2023/24 NOVEMBER	2021/22	2022/23	2023/24 OCTOBER	2023/24 NOVEMBER	2021/22	2022/23	2023/24 OCTOBER	2023/24 NOVEMBER
China	0.41	0.41	0.41	0.41	1.48	1.48	1.48	1.48	0.60	0.60	0.60	0.60
Africa												
Algeria	0.08	0.08	0.08	0.08	1.31	1.31	1.31	1.31	0.11	0.11	0.11	0.11
Morocco	0.02	0.02	0.01	0.01	0.33	0.40	0.31	0.31	0.01	0.01	0.00	0.00
South Africa	0.04	0.03	0.03	0.03	1.64	1.04	1.79	1.79	0.06	0.03	0.05	0.05
Other Europe												
United Kingdom	0.20	0.17	0.17	0.17	5.62	5.79	5.45	5.15	1.12	1.01	0.90	0.85
Norway	0.07	0.07	0.07	0.07	4.29	4.29	4.29	4.29	0.30	0.30	0.30	0.30
Serbia	0.02	0.02	0.02	0.02	3.11	2.80	3.00	3.00	0.06	0.04	0.06	0.06
Albania	0.02	0.02	0.02	0.02	2.20	2.20	2.27	2.27	0.03	0.03	0.03	0.03
Bosnia and Herzegovina	0.01	0.01	0.01	0.01	2.82	4.00	3.43	3.43	0.03	0.04	0.02	0.02
Turkey	0.11	0.11	0.11	0.11	2.38	2.38	2.38	2.38	0.25	0.25	0.25	0.25
Mexico	0.05	0.05	0.05	0.03	2.02	2.22	2.00	2.00	0.09	0.11	0.09	0.06
Others	0.06	0.03	0.06	0.06	1.66	1.63	1.68	1.68	0.10	0.05	0.09	0.09

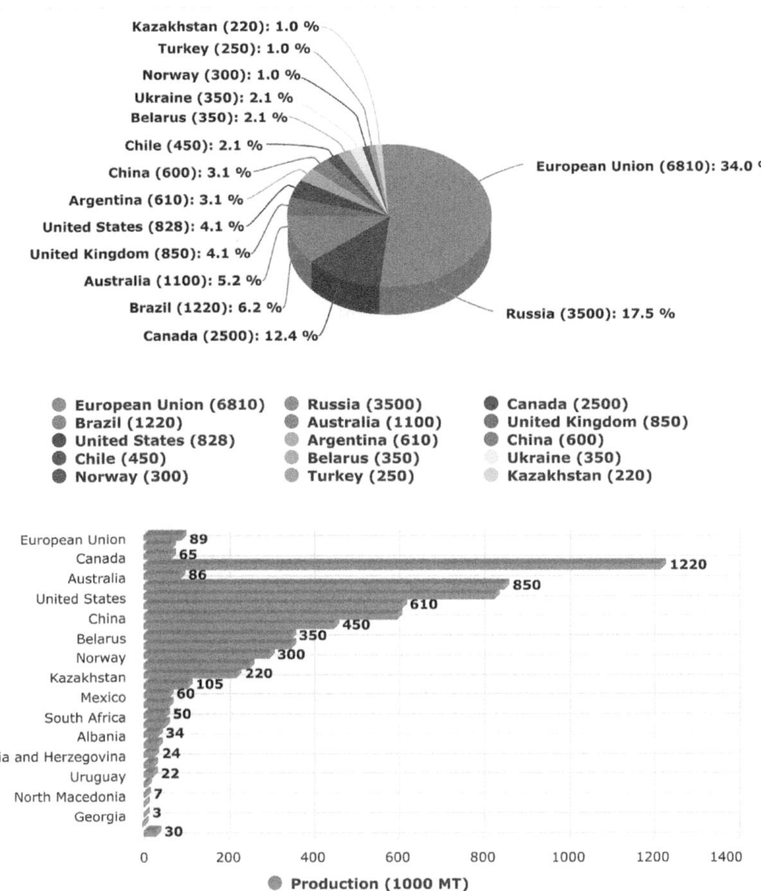

FIGURE 2.2   Oat production by place 1000 MT during 2023. Number in brackets indicates production (1000 MT)

The global trajectory of oat production has undergone a discernible descent, attributed in part to the mechanization of farms and a substantial decline in the demand for oats in horse feed. Remarkably, this decline, spanning over four decades, culminated in a precipitous 60% reduction; however, recent years have witnessed a stabilization, with global oat production hovering slightly above 25 million tons. Oat cultivation, constituting less than 5% of total cropping in numerous countries (and dipping to less than 2% in some instances), has also found equilibrium at its current levels. This stabilization can be attributed to several factors. Oats, serving as a cover crop in crop rotations, contribute to soil health. Additionally, oats present an economically viable and nutritionally rich feedstock for young cattle, albeit constrained by their modest energy content. Furthermore, augmented demand for human consumption has buoyed commercial utilization of oats, a surge initially fuelled by the promotion of oats for heart health in the United States during the 1980s. However, this surge has plateaued and, in certain regions, experienced a decline. Human consumption typically constitutes around 25% of total domestic oat use in most countries.

Forecasts for the future paint a picture of specialized oat production, with commercial entities increasingly engaging in contracted milling-quality oat acreage with growers to ensure both consistent quantity and quality. The global outlook, however, does not augur a substantial increase in oat production beyond Canada. The allure of biofuel-related crops, such as corn, soybeans, and canola/rapeseed, coupled with the modest feed value of oats, poses challenges to significant growth. Even in Canada, a global oat export leader with one of the largest oat-milling industries, competition from other crops looms large. Despite the commendable nutritional profile of oats, their limited energy content restrains their commercial viability as a feed grain, restricting their utility to specific niches like hobby horses and young calves. Consequently, the expansion of oat production remains constrained in most regions, as reflected in the steady or declining trend in oat production as a percentage of total cropping in oat-producing countries.

The decline in oat production presents a predicament for the oat-milling industry, as the selection base for milling-quality oats continues to shrink. Nevertheless, the overall trade in oats and oat products remains relatively stable. A notable proportion of the decline in raw oat production is offset by increased global trade in oat products such as flakes, groats, and flour. However, the rising costs of freight, both container and vessel, pose challenges for net oat and oat-product importers, potentially limiting trade for feed use. Oats, resilient in adapting to variable soil types, particularly excel in cool, moist climates, showcasing adaptability to acid soils. Geographically, their cultivation is concentrated between latitudes 35 and 65°N (including Finland and Sweden) and between 20 and 46°S (encompassing Argentina, Brazil, and Chile). The versatility of oats in crop rotations and their adaptability to different climates make them a preferred choice for many producers.

While spring-sown cultivars dominate global oat production, autumn sowing is practised in regions such as Australia and southern U.S. states, where hot and dry summers prevail. Severe winters in Scandinavia, northern U.S. states, Canada, and higher-altitude regions in the tropics prompt the use of short-season to mid-maturing oat cultivars. In the United States, fall-sown oats find favour among livestock producers in Texas, Gulf states, and southeastern seaboard states, serving as a nutritious pasture. Noteworthy oat production occurs in Russia, Canada, the United States, the EU, and Australia, collectively accounting for approximately 77% of the world's supply of grain oats, seed, and industrial-grade oats. Although Russia leads as the largest global producer of oats, a substantial portion of its production is consumed domestically on farms, mirroring the global trend of decline in oat production for feed and human consumption.

Canada solidifies its status as the pre-eminent global commercial producer and exporter of oats, wielding considerable influence with a commanding 15% share of total global production and a staggering 60% of global exports. Remarkably, exports constitute one-third of Canada's total oat production, a figure that stands in stark contrast to the global average export rate of 7% of production. The sustained ascendancy of Canada's oat production is attributed to a confluence of strategic factors. Proximity to the U.S. oat-milling market emerges as a pivotal advantage, facilitating efficient trade dynamics. Unlike other major oat-producing nations, Canada abstains from providing production or trade subsidies, determining seeding decisions based on return per acre. This economic approach has favoured oat cultivation in Canada, positioning it as a stalwart oat-producing nation for the past 15 years. Additionally, Canada's higher production trend is fortified by a robust forward-contracting programme, empowering growers to secure prices for nearly 90% of the milling-quality crop they cultivate. In some instances, production contracts are sealed a year before the actual seeding, underscoring the strategic foresight embedded in the Canadian oat industry.

In stark contrast, Sweden and Finland, the two other major commercial oat-producing countries, grapple with the necessity for subsidies to support production and exports. These subsidies, typically granted annually post-harvest, introduce an element of uncertainty for growers and grain marketers. The loss of subsidized rail rates in 1995 prompted a substantial shift in oat production within Canada, redirecting it eastward from western Canada. The provinces of Manitoba and Saskatchewan witnessed a surge in production, driven by their closer proximity to the midwestern U.S. milling market. Simultaneously, a significant alteration in grade standards, coinciding with the loss of subsidized rates, catalysed the production increase. This change narrowed the permissible percentage of other grains and foreign material for each grade, enabling growers to command higher premiums for superior-quality oats.

The EU-27 collectively contributes 34% to the total world oat production. Predominantly consumed internally for feed, particularly cattle and hog feed, approximately 80% of the EU-27's total oat usage is met through domestic production. Despite an overall decline in acreage since 1991, steadily increasing yields have kept production robust at 8–9 million tons over an extended period. Among the major oat-producing EU-27 countries, Sweden and Finland emerge as the primary exporting nations. Finland has maintained steady or slightly increased production over a decade, whereas Sweden has experienced a decline. Spain and Denmark exhibit upward production trends, while the United Kingdom has sustained steady to somewhat higher production since 1991. Some decline is noticeable in other major oat-producing EU-27 countries, such as Germany, France, and Poland. Smaller-production countries in Europe show no discernible major trends. Australia, another key player, witnesses a somewhat lower production trend, primarily attributable to declines in major cash-grain-growing regions in eastern and southern Australia. Consequently, the harvested area has experienced a downward trend since 1991, with occasional years of elevated production due to exceptional yields. The bulk of Australian oat production is utilized on farms, with just over 11% earmarked for exports. Overall, the global production trend in smaller-producing countries remains largely stable and is anticipated to persist into the foreseeable future.

In recent decades, the trajectory of oat yields has experienced a commendable ascent, a testament to the progress achieved in oat varieties and agronomic practices. Since 1960, oat yields have steadily increased, witnessing a noteworthy rise of nearly 0.75 kg/ha. This impressive surge represents a substantial 139% improvement, highlighting significant strides in advancing oat cultivation. It is crucial to note, however, that this increase in oat yields, while noteworthy, stands as the most modest among major cereal grains, rivalled only by sorghum. A comparative analysis reveals that corn yields, for instance, soared by approximately 240% during the same period. This discrepancy emphasizes a distinct emphasis on hybrid crops such as corn, wheat, and soybeans by various stakeholders, including governments, private industry, and researchers.

The disproportionate focus on hybrid crops has played a pivotal role in harnessing molecular biology techniques to significantly augment yield potential. Both corn and soybeans have reaped the benefits of these techniques, experiencing dramatic increases in yield and capitalizing on technology that allows for specific trait enhancements.

This multifaceted approach, encompassing genetic improvements and technological innovations, has propelled hybrid crops to the forefront of agricultural productivity. The contrast in yield improvements across different cereal grains underscores the dynamic landscape of agricultural research and development. While oat yields have made considerable strides, the relatively lower enhancement signals a variance in priorities and investments within the realm of crop improvement efforts. As advancements in molecular biology continue to shape the trajectory of crop yields, it remains imperative to strike a balance between traditional crops like oats and high-yielding hybrid varieties to meet the diverse demands of global agriculture.

2.3 OAT CONSUMPTION

Analysing USDA data provides a comprehensive perspective on the global dynamics of oat consumption and production. In the 2018/19 season, world oat consumption stood at 23 million tons, slightly surpassing the production figure of 22 million tons. This resulted in a marginal decrease in stocks for that season. The following season, 2019/20, witnessed global oat consumption rise to approximately 24.8 million tons, still trailing production. A slight increase in production during these two seasons mitigated the impact on stocks. Projections for the 2021/22 season indicate a decrease in both production and consumption. However, the anticipated decline in production, totalling 2.8 million tons, significantly outweighs the projected decrease in consumption, amounting to 1.3 million tons. Consequently, it is forecasted that approximately 1.5 million tons of existing stocks will be utilized in the current season. A closer examination of oat consumption on a national scale reveals that prominent oat-producing nations such as the EU, Russia, the United States, Canada, Australia, and the United Kingdom consistently rank among the top ten countries in both consumption and production. As per USDA data, oat consumption in the 2020/21 season was 8.2 million tons in the EU, 4 million tons in Russia, 2.3 million tons in the United States, 2.3 million tons in Canada, 1.1 million tons in Australia, and approximately 1 million tons in the United Kingdom. Projections for the 2021/22 season suggest that these countries are expected to maintain similar consumption rates, with perhaps slight declines. This intricate interplay between production and consumption underscores the delicate balance in the oat market. The nuanced variations in these figures across different seasons and countries highlight the need for careful monitoring and analysis to navigate the intricacies of the global oat landscape.

2.4 TRADE

The oats market, valued at US$7483.84 million in the year 2020, is anticipated to exhibit robust growth at a CAGR of 3.6% during the forecast period from 2021 to 2028. By the end of the forecast period, it is projected to attain a valuation of approximately

IJS\$9939.82 million in the year 2028. This forecast indicates a positive trajectory for the oats market, suggesting sustained expansion and an increasing market valuation over the specified timeframe. Various factors, including changing consumer preferences, nutritional awareness, and potentially expanding applications of oats in the food industry, could contribute to this growth. However, it's essential to consider that market forecasts are subject to dynamic factors, and actual outcomes may vary based on evolving market dynamics and external influences [20]. The global oat trade, which has fluctuated between 2 and 2.5 million tons over the past decade, has experienced a noteworthy evolution in recent years.

The geopolitical conflict between Russia and Ukraine has adversely affected the immediate prospects of a global economic rebound following the COVID-19 pandemic. The ongoing war has precipitated the imposition of economic sanctions on multiple nations, precipitated a notable uptick in commodity prices, and induced disruptions within global supply chains [21]. Consequently, inflationary pressures have manifested across various sectors, influencing markets on a global scale. Despite these challenges, the oatmeal market is projected to witness growth, reaching a valuation of US\$7.68 billion by 2027, with a CAGR of 4.2%.

From a 45-year low of 1.250 million tons in the 1982/83 crop year, oat exports have consistently trended higher, reflecting changing dynamics in international trade. According to USDA data, world oat trade stood at 2.3 million tons in the 2018/19 season, increasing to 2.6 million tons in 2019/20 and reaching an estimated 2.7 million tons in the 2020/21 season. However, forecasts for the 2021/22 season anticipate a decline, predicting that the volume of oats subject to world trade will decrease to 2.1 million tons, marking a reduction of 560,000 tons.

The leading countries in international oat trade have remained relatively stable in recent seasons. Canada, Australia, the EU, the United Kingdom, and Russia consistently lead in exports. Canada, estimated to have exported 2 million tons in the 2020/21 season, is expected to witness a decline in exports in the current season, exporting 1.1 million tons in line with expectations of reduced production. Simultaneously, Australia is forecasted to export 600,000 tons, the EU 200,000 tons, the United Kingdom 115,000 tons, and Russia 100,000 tons of oats in the same period.

On the imports side, the United States emerges as the largest commercial importer of oats globally, contributing to about two-thirds of all annual imports. Other countries, such as China and Mexico, import smaller amounts, each representing less than 2% of the annual total. The United States plays a pivotal role in driving the global oat trade, with Canadian production predominantly oriented towards exporting to this market. Canadian exports, ranging from 1.4 to 2.4 million tons annually, are primarily destined for the United States, which contrasts with an annual domestic mill use of 0.600 million tons. The high-quality and high-priced U.S. market significantly influences Canadian production, which would likely trend lower without access to this market.

The pervasive adoption of enduring solutions and products has experienced a surge, driven by the dynamic shifts in consumer preferences and lifestyles. This trend, considered a pivotal factor, is exerting a profound influence on the expansive growth trajectory of the global oats market. Foreseen as a key driver, the market is poised to ascend, propelled by the nourishing attributes and health benefits inherently associated with oat consumption, complemented by an escalating global consciousness regarding the imperative for enhanced food utilization. In response to the escalating demand for oats, a prominent market participant has strategically positioned itself by offering innovative products rooted in these wholesome ingredients. This strategic move not only satiates the burgeoning demand for oats but also emerges as a substantive growth driver, fortifying the market share of oats within the broader landscape.

The landscape, however, is not devoid of challenges. As dietary preferences undergo perpetual evolution, a critical juncture looms for the market's growth, anticipated to manifest between 2022 and 2030. A formidable impediment is posed by the premium pricing associated with these ingredients, serving as a potential deterrent to market growth when juxtaposed with analogous offerings. These limitations, in turn, manifest as formidable challenges, casting shadows on the unfettered expansion and development of the oats market during the forecasted period. Despite these challenges, a promising vista beckons the global oats market, characterized by an escalating appetite for refined dining experiences and the discernible shift in consumer dietary inclinations. The enduring demand for comfort food, coupled with the inherent high nutritional value of cereals, serves as a bulwark, sustaining the vitality of the oats market. Noteworthy growth opportunities abound, propelled by the diversification of oats and their integration into the cosmetics industry.

The market, however, has weathered the turbulent tides of the COVID-19 pandemic. Consumer goods, food, and beverage enterprises grappled with a drastic downturn in demand and supply chain disruptions. Notably, in contrast to the surge in at-home consumption, out-of-home consumption witnessed minimal fluctuations. The disrupted production and supply chain dynamics, coupled with a contraction in the retail sector, led to a paradigm shift in the consumption of oats – traditionally a home-bound affair. Notwithstanding these challenges, oats emerged as a resilient nutritional snack, fortifying immune systems. Consequently, a post-COVID-19 resurgence in oats demand is anticipated, driven by a renewed emphasis on maintaining healthy diets.

The geographical analysis of the oats market encompasses North America, Europe, South America, Asia Pacific, the Middle East, and Africa. In 2021, North America emerged as the preeminent market, commanding a formidable 37.04% share of the market revenue. This regional dominance was underpinned by the widespread and substantial consumption of oats, particularly in the form of porridge. The prevalence of such consumption habits solidified North America's position as the leading market player. Notwithstanding North America's dominance, the Asia Pacific region is poised for robust development, buoyed by an increased demand for diet foods offering nutritional advantages. The Middle East and South Africa also present growth opportunities, driven by a similar surge in demand for diet foods. The dynamics of these regional markets are thus intricately interwoven with evolving dietary preferences and health-conscious consumption patterns.

The market's type segment is stratified into whole oats, steel cuts, instant oats, and others. Remarkably, in 2021, the whole oats segment commanded the lion's share, accounting for 32.85% of the market. Whole oats, derived from the meticulous processes of collecting, washing, and hull removal, are commonly found in health food stores. Their preparation is more intricate compared to other types, as they retain the entire grain, including the germ and bran. The endosperm, rich in easily digestible energy, contributes to the nutritional appeal of whole oats.

Further delving into the market's segments, the application facet includes breakfast cereals, bakery and confectionery, animal feed, and others. Strikingly, the animal feed segment claimed a substantial market share of 35.58% in 2021. Oats, being a versatile cereal item, find utility in animal diets, catering to pets such as cats, dogs, and game animals. The fat content in oats enhances their energy levels, particularly vital in horse meals. Moreover, oats exhibit allergen-reducing properties in cat meals and contribute to gastrointestinal tract soothing. The high hull and fibre content positions oats as an excellent grain for initiating calves onto feed, a preference often exercised by knowledgeable cattlemen for weaned calves. Oats prove to be an optimal diet for youngstock and breeding animals, reflecting the diverse applications of this nutritious grain in the animal feed sector.

2.5 ROLE OF OATS IN SUSTAINABLE AGRICULTURE

The imperative for sustainability in agricultural systems pivots on the imperative to cultivate technologies and practices that steer clear of deleterious impacts on environmental goods and services, ensuring accessibility and efficacy for farmers while concurrently fostering advancements in food productivity [8]. Despite the considerable strides made in agricultural productivity over the past half-century – marked by heightened crop and livestock yields propelled by increased utilization of fertilizers, irrigation water, agricultural machinery, pesticides, and land – it is overly optimistic to presume that these relationships will perpetually follow linear trajectories. Anticipating a future characterized by non-linearity necessitates innovative approaches, entailing the integration of biological and ecological processes into food production. The quest for sustainability compels a strategic shift towards minimizing the reliance on non-renewable inputs that pose threats to the environment and the well-being of farmers and consumers [22]. This transformative trajectory calls for harnessing the knowledge and skills embedded in the farming community, thereby substituting human capital for resource-intensive external inputs. Simultaneously, it advocates leveraging collective capacities to collaboratively address shared agricultural and natural resource challenges, ranging from pest and watershed management to irrigation, forest conservation, and credit systems [23].

These foundational principles not only guide the trajectory towards agricultural sustainability but also contribute to the cultivation of essential capital assets for agricultural systems, encompassing natural, social, human, physical, and financial capital. Central to this pursuit is the enhancement of natural capital, with dividends accruing from optimizing the genotypes of crops and animals within the ecological conditions of cultivation or husbandry [8]. The paradigm of agricultural sustainability underscores the need for a simultaneous focus on genotype enhancements through contemporary biological methodologies and an enriched understanding of the advantages inherent in ecological and agronomic management, manipulation, and redesign [24].

The ecological management of agroecosystems, addressing energy flows, nutrient cycling, population-regulating mechanisms, and system resilience, holds the promise of transforming agriculture on a landscape scale. Positive outcomes of sustainable agriculture manifest in improved food productivity, reduced reliance on pesticides, and favourable carbon balances [25]. Nevertheless, formidable challenges persist, necessitating the formulation of comprehensive national and international policies that champion the widespread adoption of sustainable agricultural practices, spanning both industrialized and developing nations [26]. In essence, these cardinal principles form a coherent framework for fostering sustainable agricultural practices, delineating a pathway that integrates ecological processes, minimizes environmental impact, leverages the expertise of farmers, and fosters collective action for addressing common challenges in agriculture and natural resource management [27].

The pivotal tenets underpinning sustainability can be succinctly delineated as follows:

(i) Integration of biological and ecological processes, encompassing nutrient cycling, nitrogen fixation, soil regeneration, allelopathy, competition, predation, and parasitism, within the ambit of food production processes.

(ii) Minimization of the utilization of non-renewable inputs that inflict harm upon the environment or compromise the well-being of farmers and consumers.

(iii) Effective harnessing of the knowledge and skills inherent in farmers, thereby enhancing their self-reliance and substituting human capital for expensive external inputs.

(iv) Strategic mobilization of collective capacities, fostering collaborative endeavours to address shared agricultural and natural resource challenges. This collaborative approach extends to problem-solving in areas such as pest management, watershed conservation, irrigation practices, forest management, and credit systems.

Oats stand as an exemplary low-input crop, and when strategically integrated into crop rotations, they foster a diversified agricultural landscape, yielding benefits that extend beyond the direct value of the crop, encompassing both grain and straw. The inclusion of oats in a three-year rotation cycle, such as corn/oats/soybeans, emerges as an effective strategy to mitigate challenges associated with corn rootworm eggs. This rotation disrupts extended dormancy, substantially reducing the necessity for chemical insecticides targeted at rootworms.

2.6 AS COVER CROPS AND GREEN MANURES

Oats serve as a commendable winter cover crop, offering soil protection with minimal springtime management demands due to their susceptibility to frost-induced termination. While their shallow incorporation into the soil may be required before subsequent crop planting, oats obviate the need for intensive management efforts in the spring [28]. To ensure adequate soil protection, it is advisable to plant oats by late August at a rate of approximately 100 lb/acre. This strategic timing allows for sufficient growth before the first frost sets in. The residues of oats, whether incorporated into the soil or left on the surface, exhibit dual functionality. They not only act as a physical barrier but also possess the capacity to chemically suppress weed growth. This inherent weed suppression ability adds to the appeal of oats as a cover crop, offering an eco-friendly means of curtailing weed proliferation. Oats further distinguish themselves as a versatile cover crop that can be sown at any time during the spring or summer when land is temporarily out of production. In contrast to winter rye, oats exhibit robust and upright growth when seeded in the spring or summer, effectively outcompeting weeds in the process. This adaptability contributes to their efficacy as a cover crop throughout various seasons, augmenting their utility in diverse agricultural contexts. Notably, oats demonstrate resilience by thriving in soils with low pH levels, as low as 5.5. This adaptability underscores their suitability for deployment in a wide array of soil conditions, enhancing their versatility as a cover crop. Overall, oats emerge as a pragmatic choice for farmers seeking an effective and low-maintenance winter cover crop that confers multiple agronomic benefits.

2.7 NITROGEN METABOLISM

The impact of living plants on net nitrogen mineralization in soil exhibits a complex spectrum, with reported instances of stimulation, inhibition, or no discernible effect. In the pursuit of understanding this phenomenon, a series of experiments were meticulously undertaken to assess the influence of living oat plants on net nitrogen mineralization [9]–[16], [29]. These experiments involved cultivating oat plants in plastic cylinders containing soil, and the assessment of net nitrogen mineralization was achieved by scrutinizing the nitrogen balance within these controlled microcosms. The measured nitrogen inputs encompassed nitrogen content inherent in oat seeds and nitrogen fixation, while nitrogen losses were quantified through NH_3 volatilization and denitrification measurements [13], [30]. The findings yielded intriguing insights, revealing a significant stimulation of net nitrogen mineralization in certain soils, reaching an augmentation of up to 81%. However, it is noteworthy that, in other soils, the presence of living oat plants exhibited no discernible effect on net nitrogen mineralization. This variability in responses is not arbitrary but is intricately linked to the historical cropping patterns of the respective soils [31]. The observed diversity in net nitrogen mineralization responses underscores the nuanced interplay between living oat plants and soil nitrogen dynamics [10]–[16]. The multifaceted nature of these interactions suggests that the influence of living plants on net nitrogen mineralization is contingent upon intricate soil-specific factors, including but not limited to past cropping histories [32]. These findings contribute valuable insights into the complex dynamics governing nitrogen cycling in soil–plant systems and underscore the need for a nuanced understanding of the interdependencies at play in agroecosystems [13], [14], [29].

2.8 AS ANIMAL FEED

Oats have a rich history as a traditional feed grain, enduring centuries of use. Despite the recent decline in oat production for feed, owing to advances in other feed grains such as corn, wheat, barley, soybean, and canola, oats persist as a primary feed grain. In the bygone era, oats held a pivotal role as the primary feed for horses powering farm equipment before the advent of mechanization [33]. Oats find application in feeding both ruminant and monogastric animals. Their versatility extends to various animals, including dairy and beef cattle, sheep, horses, cats, dogs, birds, rabbits, bison, deer, and fish. The unique attributes of naked oats position them as an ideal feed for weaner and grower pigs, poultry, racehorses, and birds [34], [35]. The fat content in oats enhances their energy content, a crucial aspect in horse feeds, contributing to improved fur shine and reduced incidence of diarrhoea. Oats in pet foods play a role in preventing allergies and intestinal irritation, making them a preferred choice [36]. Oat fodder boasts nutrient values, including 10.0–11.5% crude proteins, 55–63% NDF, 30–32% ADF, 22.0–23.5% cellulose, and 17–20% hemicellulose [37].

The nutrient value for animal feed is contingent upon the groat-to-hull ratio, influenced by variety and growing conditions. The high oil content in oats, primarily comprising unsaturated fatty acids, can impact the fatty-acid composition of animal fat positively. Additionally, oats are characterized by high protein content, with a greater proportion of lysine compared to other cereals, offering nutritional benefits to animals [38]–[43]. The hull, a major component in feed, serves a dual role by reducing digestive problems like acidosis and acting as a constraint for non-ruminants, such as poultry and pigs, due to their inability to digest cellulose, hemicellulose, and lignin [44]. In contrast, naked oats, lacking hulls, emerge as a favourable energy source for grower and weaner pigs, broilers, laying hens, and turkeys.

Beyond their role as feed grains, oats contribute to increased milk production in cattle, owing to their high-fat and nutrition-rich content. The demand for oats in the cattle feed industry is on the rise, further accelerated by their use as a substitute for high-energy content cereals like barley and corn [45]. This growth in demand underscores the multifaceted utility of oats as a feed ingredient. Moreover, oats exhibit environmental benefits, such as reduced methane emissions when consumed by animals. This attribute, coupled with their increasing use as a substitute for high-energy cereals, contributes to the high growth rate observed in the oats feed ingredients market. In the Asia Pacific region, the demand for oats as a feed ingredient is particularly pronounced, fuelled by factors such as population growth, rising disposable incomes, and an increased preference for protein-rich meat diets [39], [40], [42], [43], [46]. The poultry industry in countries like India and China is poised for expansion, further driving the demand for oats in starter feed formulations. The heterogeneity in the Asia Pacific region, encompassing diverse income levels, technology adoption, and consumer demands, presents ample opportunities for future growth in the oats feed ingredients market.

2.9 OTHER ROLES

The deployment of oats at elevated densities during early planting establishes a robust cover that effectively curtails weed competition. Incorporating oats into crop rotation programmes extends the weed suppression effects to subsequent row crops, presenting an eco-friendly alternative to chemical herbicides [47]. Collaborating with legumes such as hairy vetch and peas, oats function as a nurse crop, curbing the risk of surface and groundwater contamination resulting from excessive herbicide use [48]. Moreover, oats exhibit a frugal nutrient uptake, particularly in nitrogen, contributing to a potential reduction in the need for excessive fertilizer applications. This not only holds promise for mitigating surface and groundwater nitrate contamination but aligns with sustainable agricultural practices [13], [14], [29], [49]. Furthermore, the water-efficient nature of oats, requiring less irrigation compared to crops like corn, proves advantageous in safeguarding underground aquifers, particularly in geographically vulnerable regions [50].

The dense cover provided by oats, coupled with their low water requirements, serves as a formidable bulwark against soil erosion caused by wind and water. Oat stubble, left in the ground after harvest, emerges as an ideal candidate for no-till or minimum-till programmes. Its presence enhances soil moisture retention, facilitating the establishment of seedlings for subsequent crops. This holistic approach not only fortifies soil health but also contributes to sustainable land management practices [51]. Beyond the agronomic benefits, oats yield hulls, a by-product with the potential for clean and renewable energy generation. Notably, oat hulls have been successfully employed to replace coal in generating electricity, powering large institutions and homes in the Midwest [52]. Additionally, they play a role in steam generation, facilitating the processing of cleaned oats into various food products. This dual functionality positions oats not only as a valuable agricultural commodity but also as a contributor to environmentally conscious energy practices [53]. Oats are known for their ability to grow in cooler climates and are often used in regions with shorter growing seasons. This can contribute to climate-resilient agriculture by providing a viable crop option in areas where other crops may struggle [54]. Oats, when used in diverse crop rotations, contribute to overall biodiversity on the farm. This diversity can support a range of beneficial insects, microbes, and other organisms that contribute to a healthy and balanced ecosystem. Oats have a relatively shallow root system, which can help with water management in the soil [55]. Their roots can help prevent soil erosion and improve water infiltration, reducing the risk of runoff and enhancing water conservation [56].

2.10 CONCLUSION

The enduring trajectory of oat production and utilization hinges upon several pivotal factors, with a paramount emphasis on the augmentation of feed value, the exploration of non-food applications, and the expansive integration of oats within the food sector. Although the area allocated for oat cultivation has achieved a degree of stabilization, the prospect of significant acreage expansion remains contingent upon substantial enhancements in the feed characteristics inherent to oats. The impetus driving future oat cultivation is intricately tied to the pursuit of heightened feed value. To catalyse an increase in acreage, a discernible enhancement in the nutritional profile and qualities that render oats an enticing feed grain is imperative. This enhancement has the potential to catalyse growth in oat production, positioning it as a pivotal and cost-effective feed source for livestock. Moreover, the diversification of oat applications beyond traditional food products holds promise for the future. The development of non-food products derived from oats could unlock novel avenues and markets, furnishing additional incentives for growers and industries engaged in oat production. The inherent versatility of oats lends itself adeptly to various industrial applications, spanning cosmetics, pharmaceuticals, and other non-food sectors, thereby contributing substantively to the overall sustainability and economic viability of oat cultivation. Expanding the footprint of oats within the food sector represents another dimension of long-term growth. This entails exploring innovative culinary applications, advocating for the nutritional merits of oats, and creating inventive oat-based products attuned to evolving consumer preferences. As awareness of the health benefits associated with oat consumption burgeons, there lies a prospect for an augmented demand for oat-based food products. While substantial acreage expansion may pose challenges in the absence of feed characteristic improvements, it is unlikely that oat production will witness a precipitous decline from current levels. Oats, characterized by ease of cultivation and compatibility with crop rotations, coupled with relatively modest input costs, present a compelling proposition for producers. The economic advantages linked to oats as a feed grain are poised to sustain continued cultivation, solidifying oats as a cost-effective and invaluable feed source for livestock. Furthermore, gains in yields, facilitated by advancements in agricultural practices and technology, have the potential to offset any modest declines in acreage. These strides in efficiency can contribute substantially to maintaining oat production at sustainable levels, ensuring a consistent supply for both established and emerging markets. In summation, the long-term outlook for oat production is intricately interwoven with progress in feed characteristics, exploration of non-food applications, and strategic expansion within the food sector. Despite prevailing challenges and constraints, the inherent merits of oats in agriculture, coupled with ongoing endeavours to augment their appeal and adaptability, position oats as a resilient and potentially burgeoning component of the agricultural landscape.

REFERENCES

[1] S. Chand, Indu, R. K. Singhal and P. Govindasamy, "Agronomical and breeding approaches to improve the nutritional status of forage crops for better livestock productivity," *Grass Forage Sci.*, vol. 77, pp. 11–32, 2022, doi: 10.1111/gfs.12557.

[2] M. Ahmad, Gul-Zaffar, Z. A. Dar and M. Habib, "A review on Oat (Avena sativa L.) as a dual-purpose crop," *SRE.*, vol. 9, pp. 52–59, 2014, doi: 10.5897/SRE2014.5820.

[3] P. Rasane, A. Jha, L. Sabikhi, A. Kumar and V. S. Unnikrishnan, "Nutritional advantages of oats and opportunities for its processing as value added foods – A review," *J. Food Sci. Technol.*, vol. 52, pp. 662–675, 2015, doi: 10.1007/s13197-013-1072-1.

[4]   A. M. Agapkin and I. A. Makhotina, "The grain market of Russia," *IOP Conf. Ser. Earth Environ. Sci.*, vol. 839, p. 022023, 2021, doi: 10.1088/1755-1315/839/2/022023.

[5]   M. Pinheiro et al., "Survey of freshly harvested oat grains from Southern Brazil reveals high incidence of type B trichothecenes and associated fusarium species," *Toxins.*, vol. 13, p. 855, 2021, doi: 10.3390/toxins13120855.

[6]   N. Nemeth, I. Rudnak, P. Ymeri and C. Fogarassy, "The role of cultural factors in sustainable food consumption – an investigation of the consumption habits among international students in Hungary," *Sustainability*, vol. 11, p. 3052, 2019, doi: 10.3390/su11113052.

[7]   N. Kumar, K. K. Hazra, C. P. Nath, C. S. Praharaj and U. Singh, "Grain legumes for resource conservation and agricultural sustainability in South Asia," in *Legumes for Soil Health and Sustainable Management*, R. S. Meena, A. Das, G. S. Yadav and R. Lal, Eds. Singapore, Singapore: Springer, 2018, pp. 77–107, doi: 10.1007/978-981-13-0253-4_3.

[8]   J. Pretty, "Agricultural sustainability: Concepts, principles and evidence," *Philos. Trans. R. Soc. B: Biol. Sci.*, vol. 363, pp. 447–465, 2007, doi: 10.1098/rstb.2007.2163.

[9]   R. K. Singhal et al., "Beneficial elements: New players in improving nutrient use efficiency and abiotic stress tolerance," *Plant Growth Regul.*, vol. 100, pp. 237–265, 2023, doi: 10.1007/s10725-022-00843-8.

[10] R. S. Singh Tomar, S. Tiwari, P. Singh, K. B. Naik and A. Kumar, "Genome editing for improvement of wheat and millets," in *Genome Editing in Plants (First Edition)*, Boca Raton, Florida: CRC Press, 2021, pp. 1–12.

[11] R. S. Tomar et al., "Genomics approaches for restoration and conservation of agro-biodiversity," in *Agro-Biodiversity and Agri-Ecosystem Management*, P. Kumar, R. S. Tomar, J. A. Bhat, M. Dobriyal and M. Rani, Eds. Singapore, Singapore: Springer Nature, 2022, pp. 273–283, doi: 10.1007/978-981-19-0928-3_14.

[12] A. Kumar et al., "Genomics-assisted improvement of grain quality and nutraceutical properties in millets," in *Millets and Millet Technology*, A. Kumar, M. K. Tripathi, D. Joshi and V. Kumar, Eds. Singapore, Singapore: Springer, 2021, pp. 333–343, doi: 10.1007/978-981-16-0676-2_17.

[13] P. Singh et al., "Global gene expression profiling under nitrogen stress identifies key genes involved in nitrogen stress adaptation in maize (Zea mays L.)," *Sci. Rep.* vol. 12, p. 4211, 2022, doi: 10.1038/s41598-022-07709-z.

[14] P. Singh, R. S. Tomar, K. Kumar, B. Kumar, S. Rakshit and I. Singh, "Morpho-physiological and biochemical characterization of maize genotypes under nitrogen stress conditions," *Indian J. Genet. Plant Breed.*, vol. 81, pp. 255–265, 2021, doi: 10.31742/IJGPB.81.2.8.

[15] I. Singh, K. Kumar, P. Singh, P. Yadava and S. Rakshit, "Physiological and molecular interventions for improving nitrogen-use efficiency in maize," in *Molecular Breeding in Wheat, Maize and Sorghum: Strategies for Improving Abiotic Stress Tolerance and Yield*, M. A. Hossain, M. Alam, S. Seneweera, S. Rakshit, R. Henry, Eds. Wallingford: CABI, 2021, pp. 325–339.

[16] P. Singh et al., "Role of range grasses in conservation and restoration of biodiversity," in *Agro-Biodiversity and Agri-Ecosystem Management*, P. Kumar, R. S. Tomar, J. A. Bhat, M. Dobriyal and M. Rani, Eds. Singapore, Singapore: Springer Nature, 2022, pp. 53–69, doi: 10.1007/978-981-19-0928-3_4.

[17] M. Heinz, V. Galetti and A. Holzkämper, "How to find alternative crops for climate-resilient regional food production," *Agric. Syst.*, vol. 213, p. 103793, 2024, doi: 10.1016/j.agsy.2023.103793.

[18] R. Singh and G. S. Singh, "Traditional agriculture: A climate-smart approach for sustainable food production," *Energ. Ecol. Environ.*, vol. 2, pp. 296–316, 2017, doi: 10.1007/s40974-017-0074-7.

[19] K. Akpoti, A. T. Kabo-Bah and S. J. Zwart, "Review – agricultural land suitability analysis: State-of-the-art and outlooks for integration of climate change analysis," *Agric. Syst.*, vol. 173, pp. 172–208, 2019, doi: 10.1016/j.agsy.2019.02.013.

[20] M. J. M. Smulders et al., "Oats in healthy gluten-free and regular diets: A perspective," *Food Res. Int.*, vol. 110, pp. 3–10, 2018, doi: 10.1016/j.foodres.2017.11.031.

[21] E. Hatipoglu, M. A. Soytas and F. Belaïd, "Environmental consequences of geopolitical crises: The case of economic sanctions and emissions," *Resour. Policy*, vol. 85, p. 104011, 2023, doi: 10.1016/j.resourpol.2023.104011.

[22] K. Zhang, Z. Rengel, F. Zhang, P. J. White and J. Shen, "Rhizosphere engineering for sustainable crop production: Entropy-based insights," *Trends Plant Sci.*, vol. 28, pp. 390–398, 2023, doi: 10.1016/j.tplants.2022.11.008.

[23] H. Gosnell, N. Gill and M. Voyer, "Transformational adaptation on the farm: Processes of change and persistence in transitions to 'climate-smart' regenerative agriculture," *Glob. Environ. Change.*, vol. 59, p. 101965, 2019, doi: 10.1016/j.gloenvcha.2019.101965.

[24] P. Schröder et al., "Discussion paper: Sustainable increase of crop production through improved technical strategies, breeding and adapted management – A European perspective," *Sci. Total Environ.*, vol. 678, pp. 146–161, 2019, doi: 10.1016/j.scitotenv.2019.04.212.

[25] A. Wezel, M. Casagrande, F. Celette, J.-F. Vian, A. Ferrer, J. Peigné, "Agroecological practices for sustainable agriculture. A review, Agron." *Sustain. Dev.*, vol. 34, pp. 1–20, 2014, doi: 10.1007/s13593-013-0180-7.

[26] R. Bali Swain and F. Yang-Wallentin, "Achieving sustainable development goals: Predicaments and strategies," *Int. J. Sustain. Dev. World Ecol.*, vol. 27, pp. 96–106, 2020, doi: 10.1080/13504509.2019.1692316.

[27] S. D. Sarasvathy and A. Ramesh, "An effectual model of collective action for addressing sustainability challenges," *AMP.*, vol. 33, pp. 405–424, 2019, doi: 10.5465/amp.2017.0090.

[28] E. B. Brennan and R. F. Smith, "Winter cover crop growth and weed suppression on the Central Coast of California," *Weed Technology.*, vol. 19, pp. 1017–1024, 2005, doi: 10.1614/WT-04-246R1.1.

[29] P. Singh, S. Jaiswal, S. Sheokand and S. Duhan, "Morpho-physiological and oxidative responses of nitrogen and phosphorus deficiency in wheat (Triticum aestivum L.).," *Indian J. Agric. Res.*, vol. 52, pp. 40–45, 2018, doi: 10.18805/IJARe.A-4905.

[30] T. B. Parkin, T. C. Kaspar and C. Cambardella, "Oat plant effects on net nitrogen mineralization," *Plant Soil.*, vol. 243, pp. 187–195, 2002. Accessed Dec. 6, 2023. Available: www.jstor.org/stable/24122504

[31] D. Ebersberger, P. A. Niklaus and E. Kandeler, "Long term CO_2 enrichment stimulates N-mineralisation and enzyme activities in calcareous grassland," *Soil Biol. Biochem.*, vol. 35, pp. 965–972, 2003, doi: 10.1016/S0038-0717(03)00156-1.

[32] L. Barton et al., "Soil nitrogen supply and N fertilizer losses from Australian dryland grain cropping systems," in *Advances in Agronomy*, D. L. Sparks, Ed. Academic Press, 2022, pp. 1–52, doi: 10.1016/bs.agron.2022.03.001.

[33] A. Marshall et al., "Crops that feed the world 9. Oats- a cereal crop for human and livestock feed with industrial applications," *Food Sec.*, vol. 5, pp. 13–33, 2013, doi: 10.1007/s12571-012-0232-x.

[34] P. Bikker and A. J. M. Jansman, "Review: Composition and utilisation of feed by monogastric animals in the context of circular food production systems," *Animal.*, vol. 17, p. 100892, 2023, doi: 10.1016/j.animal.2023.100892.

[35] W.-Y. Chuang, L.-J. Lin, H.-D. Shih, Y.-M. Shy, S.-C. Chang and T.-T. Lee, "The potential utilization of high-fiber agricultural by-products as monogastric animal feed and feed additives: A review," *Animals.*, vol. 11, p. 2098, 2021, doi: 10.3390/ani11072098.

[36] M. R. C. De Godoy, K. R. Kerr and J. Fahey, "Alternative dietary fiber sources in companion animal nutrition," *Nutrients*, vol. 5, pp. 3099–3117, 2013, doi: 10.3390/nu5083099.

[37] A. Chahal et al., "Impact of different nutrient sources on forage yield, nutritive value and economics of sorghum Sudan grass hybrid-oat cropping system," *J. Plant Nutr.*, vol. 44, pp. 1223–1240, 2020, doi: 10.1080/01904167.2020.1866603.

[38] N. Ames, C. Rhymer and J. Storsley, "Food oat quality throughout the value chain," in *Oats Nutrition and Technology*, John Wiley & Sons, Ltd, 2013, pp. 33–70, doi: 10.1002/9781118354100.ch3.

[39] M. Kumar et al., "Advances in the plant protein extraction: Mechanism and recommendations," *Food Hydrocoll.*, vol. 115, p. 106595, 2021, doi: 10.1016/j.foodhyd.2021.106595.

[40] M. Kumar et al., "Cottonseed feedstock as a source of plant-based protein and bioactive peptides: Evidence based on biofunctionalities and industrial applications," *Food Hydrocoll.*, vol. 131, p. 107776, 2022, doi: 10.1016/j.foodhyd.2022.107776.

[41] V. Krishnan, M. Tomar, L. N. Malunga and S. J. Thandapilly, "Food matrix: Implications for nutritional quality," in *Conceptualizing Plant-Based Nutrition: Bioresources, Nutrients Repertoire and Bioavailability*, Ramesh S. V. and S. Praveen, Eds. Singapore, Singapore: Springer Nature, 2022, pp. 43–60, doi: 10.1007/978-981-19-4590-8_3.

[42] M. Kumar et al., "Functional characterization of plant-based protein to determine its quality for food applications," *Food Hydrocoll.*, p. 106986, 2021, doi: 10.1016/j.foodhyd.2021.106986.

[43] M. Kumar et al., "Plant-based proteins and their multifaceted industrial applications," *LWT.*, vol. 154, p. 112620, 2022, doi: 10.1016/j.lwt.2021.112620.

[44] P. Zwer, "Oats: Characteristics and quality requirements," in *Cereal Grains*, C. W. Wrigley and I. L. Batey, Eds. Woodhead Publishing, 2010, pp. 163–182, doi: 10.1533/9781845699529.2.163.

[45] L. M. S. Magaña, L. L. López, E. O. C. Rodríguez and D. M. D. Arispuro, "Cereal based functional products," in *Cereal-Based Food Products*, M. A. Shah, K. Valiyapeediyekkal Sunooj and S. A. Mir, Eds. Cham, Germany: Springer International Publishing, 2023, pp. 273–311, doi: 10.1007/978-3-031-40308-8_13.

[46] M. Kumar et al., "Cottonseed: A sustainable contributor to global protein requirements," *Trends Food Sci. Technol.*, vol. 111, pp. 100–113, 2021, doi: 10.1016/j.tifs.2021.02.058.

[47] A. Zohry and S. Ouda, "Crop rotation defeats pests and weeds," in *Crop Rotation: An Approach to Secure Future Food*, S. Ouda, A. E.-H. Zohry and T. Noreldin, Eds. Cham, Germany: Springer International Publishing, 2018, pp. 77–88, doi: 10.1007/978-3-030-05351-2_5.

[48] R. K. Shrestha, L. R. Cooperband and A. E. MacGuidwin, "Strategies to reduce nitrate leaching into groundwater in potato grown in sandy soils: Case study from North Central USA," *Am. J. Pot Res.*, vol. 87, pp. 229–244, 2010, doi: 10.1007/s12230-010-9131-x.

[49] M. J. Adegbeye et al., "Sustainable agriculture options for production, greenhouse gasses and pollution alleviation, and nutrient recycling in emerging and transitional nations – an overview," *J. Clean. Prod.*, vol. 242, p. 118319, 2020, doi: 10.1016/j.jclepro.2019.118319.

[50] M. S. Kukal and S. Irmak, "Impact of irrigation on interannual variability in United States agricultural productivity," *Agric. Water Manag.*, vol. 234, p. 106141, 2020, doi: 10.1016/j.agwat.2020.106141.

[51] L. Carretta, P. Tarolli, A. Cardinali, P. Nasta, N. Romano and R. Masin, "Evaluation of runoff and soil erosion under conventional tillage and no-till management: A case study in northeast Italy," *CATENA.*, vol. 197, p. 104972, 2021, doi: 10.1016/j.catena.2020.104972.

[52] A. Abedi and A. K. Dalai, "Study on the quality of oat hull fuel pellets using bio-additives," *Biomass. Bioenerg.*, vol. 106, pp. 166–175, 2017, doi: 10.1016/j.biombioe.2017.08.024.

[53] I. S. Arvanitoyannis and P. Tserkezou, "Wheat, barley and oat waste: A comparative and critical presentation of methods and potential uses of treated waste," *Int. J. Food Sci. Technol.*, vol. 43, pp. 694–725, 2008, doi: 10.1111/j.1365-2621.2006.01510.x.

[54] T. Roitsch, K. Himanen, A. Chawade, L. Jaakola, A. Nehe and E. Alexandersson, "Functional phenomics for improved climate resilience in Nordic agriculture," *J. Exp. Bot.*, vol. 73, pp. 5111–5127, 2022, doi: 10.1093/jxb/erac246.

[55] C. Liu et al., "Diversifying crop rotations enhances agroecosystem services and resilience," in *Advances in Agronomy*, D. L. Sparks, Ed. Academic Press, 2022, pp. 299–335, doi: 10.1016/bs.agron.2022.02.007.

[56] T. C. Kaspar, J. K. Radke and J. M. Laflen, "Small grain cover crops and wheel traffic effects on infiltration, runoff, and erosion," *J. Soil Water Conserv.*, vol. 56, pp. 160–164, 2001. Accessed Dec. 6, 2023. Available: www.jswconline.org/content/56/2/160.

Nutritional Composition of Oats and Its Comparison with Other Major Cereal Crops

Arti Kumari, Manish Kumar, Aruna Tyagi, Chirag Maheshwari, and Nand Lal Meena

3.1 INTRODUCTION

Progress has been made in enhancing survival rates, nutritional standards, and educational opportunities over recent decades. Nevertheless, global efforts towards achieving the Sustainable Development Goals, which aim to eradicate malnutrition and poverty by 2030, remain significantly off track [1]. Severe food insecurity has become more widespread, affecting 11.7% of the world's population at alarming levels. The number of individuals unable to afford a nutritious diet has increased by 112 million, reaching nearly 3.1 billion, underscoring the growing problem of inadequate access to safe and nourishing food [2]. Child malnutrition remains a significant public health issue, with only one-quarter of countries making progress towards meeting targets for addressing stunting, wasting, and overweight in children. Children now face the dual challenge

DOI: 10.1201/ 9781003263302-3

of malnutrition, where undernutrition coexists with issues such as overweight, obesity, and other diet-related non-communicable diseases [3]. Beyond the burden of malnutrition, today's children confront an uncertain future characterized by environmental changes, conflicts, the COVID-19 pandemic, and deep-seated inequalities that threaten their health and well-being. As the global population continues to grow rapidly, it poses increasingly complex challenges to both food security and environmental sustainability. These challenges underscore the urgent need to diversify our food sources, particularly by incorporating more plant-based materials [4].

A plant-based diet primarily consists of or is entirely composed of foods derived from plants. Plant-based diets encompass various eating patterns that limit the consumption of animal products while emphasizing the intake of plant-based foods like vegetables, fruits, whole grains, legumes, nuts, and seeds [5]. It's important to note that individuals following plant-based diets need not be strictly vegan or vegetarian, as the defining characteristic is a reduced consumption of animal-derived foods. The global market for plant-based food materials has seen significant growth in recent years. For example, the market share of plant-based proteins is projected to reach \$15.6 billion by 2026, with an annual growth rate of 7.2% [6]–[12].

Cereals, including wheat, rice, maize, rye, barley, and oats, are widely consumed for human nutrition and animal feed. In many developing countries, approximately 60% of calorie intake comes from cereal-based foods. Oats have been cultivated for over two millennia in various regions worldwide and are one of the oldest known crops in human history. They entered cultivation several thousand years after other grains like wheat and barley. Historically, Oats were seen as a poor version of wheat by the ancient Romans, who utilized them as inexpensive horse feed. The elite looked down on communities that ate oats in their meals. Over the period oat gained popularity due to a variety of health benefits [13]. Oats rank sixth in world cereal production, following wheat, maize, rice, barley, and sorghum. Notably, Russia leads in oat production, producing 4.4 million tons, closely followed by Canada, which produces 4.2 million tons [14]. Oats stand out among cereal crops due to their rich nutritional value, which is valuable for human food, animal feed, healthcare, and cosmetics [15]. Oats are a significant source of carbohydrates, dietary soluble fibre, well-balanced proteins, lipids, various phenolic compounds, vitamins, and minerals [16]. Given the growing public awareness of healthy eating habits, oats have garnered increased attention from both scientific researchers and industries. Oats are a member of the Gramineae family, and two significant hexaploid oat varieties that are frequently grown are *Avena sativa* L. (commonly known as husked oat) and *Avena nuda* L. (known as naked oats). Among these, *A. sativa* L. is the most widely cultivated species.

The nutritional composition of oats significantly differs from that of other cereals. Oats are distinctively rich in protein content and contain ample essential amino acids. Moreover, oats have a higher fat content (ranging from 6% to 10%) compared to wheat and most other cereals, which typically have a fat content of 2% to 3% [17]. Oats have the highest fat content among all cereals, and a substantial portion of this fat is composed of unsaturated fats. The nutritional value of oats is further enhanced by their high β-glucan content. β-Glucan is a crucial functional component used in various food industries. Additionally, oats contain over 20 unique polyphenolic compounds known as avenanthramides (AVNs), which exhibit antioxidant activity that is 10 to 30 times

higher than that of other cereals. These polyphenolic compounds include ferulic acid, gentisic acid, *p*-hydroxybenzoic acid, protocatechuic acid, syringic acid, vanillic acid, and vanillin [18].

Oat grains consist of four parts: the husk, bran, endosperm, and germ. In the oat grain, the husk represents about 20–30% of the dry mass and contains hemicellulose (24–33%), lignin (12–25%), cellulose (12–25%), starch (2–17%), proteins (1–8%), lipids (0.3–2%), and ash (5–7%). Oat groats, which are used for human consumption, are produced by mechanically removing the husk. They are spindle-shaped and elongated, with lengths of up to 0.5 inches and widths of up to 0.125 inches [19]. The bran, the outermost layer of the oat groat, contains carbohydrates (67.9%), protein (17.1%), fat (8.6%), dietary fibre (15–22%), and various minerals (iron 6.4 mg, magnesium 171 mg, copper 0.17 mg, potassium 441 mg) and vitamins (niacin 1.3 mg, α-tocopherol <0.5 mg). Oat bran is also a rich source of minerals, vitamins, and phytochemicals [20]. The endosperm, which makes up the bulk of the oat grain, consists of starch (70–80%), protein (9–12%), fat (6–8%), and dietary fibres (4–6%). Lastly, the germ is the embryo of the oat grain, which has the potential to develop into a complete plant. It is rich in proteins, lipids, vitamins, vitamin E, and other antioxidants [21], [22].

Oats do not contain gluten, making them unsuitable for bread making. However, they are rich in lipids and dietary fibres; oats have garnered attention in the food industry and are used as ingredients in a wide range of food products, including infant foods, bread, biscuits, cookies, thickeners, muesli, porridge, breakfast meals, and flakes, among others [23], [24]. Oat flour, with its antioxidants, oat gum containing β-glucan, and oat proteins, is employed to stabilize milk and meat products, enhance ice cream texture, and even contribute to the production of heat-resistant chocolate [19]. The popularity of oats can be attributed to their remarkable attributes, including a high protein content (approximately 12–20%), excellent digestibility (around 90–94%), and a substantial amount of dietary fibre, particularly β-glucan (typically 4–8%) [25]. Key factors that define the quality of oat grains encompass the percentage of grains, test weight, levels of protein and fat, and the concentration of β-glucan. Additionally, considerations such as ease of dehulling, uniform kernel size, minimal groat breakage during dehulling, and consistency in colour and taste hold significance in the milling of oats [26].

The consumption of whole grains like oats is associated with a reduced risk of developing certain diet-related disorders such as type 2 diabetes, obesity, cancer, and cardiovascular disease. Oats are commonly consumed in their whole-grain form, providing essential nutrients like proteins, unsaturated fatty acids, vitamins, and minerals [27]. Numerous laboratory and clinical studies have demonstrated that the inclusion of oat-based products in one's diet can lead to lower serum cholesterol levels, reduced glucose absorption, and decreased plasma insulin response [28], [29]. These beneficial properties of oats are attributed to their functional components, including lipids, starch components, and dietary fibres like β-glucan [30]. Oats are also a rich source of micronutrients such as zinc, iron, selenium, copper, manganese, chromium, molybdenum, iodine, and various vitamins, both fat-soluble and from the B complex. The bran, found in the outer layer of the oat kernel, is particularly abundant in antioxidants. Oats' antioxidant properties are linked to substances like vitamin E, phytic acid, phenolic compounds, AVNs, flavonoids, and sterols [31].

This chapter embarks on a thorough examination of the nutritional makeup of oats. Its goal is to offer a deep insight into the diverse elements that render oats a valuable dietary resource. The primary emphasis will be on pivotal nutritional elements including protein, oil, carbohydrates, dietary fibre, minerals, and vitamins. Additionally, this chapter will explore the physiological and nutritional characteristics that distinguish oats, underscoring the importance of β-glucans, tocopherols, and innate antioxidants in the realm of human nutrition.

3.2 NUTRITIONAL COMPOSITION OF OATS

Oats contain a wealth of nutritional elements. The entire oat grain can be categorized into three components: the germ, endosperm, and bran, which serve as storage for essential nutrients. A diverse array of chemical constituents, including carbohydrates, proteins, AVNs, tocols, lipids, alkaloids, flavonoids, saponins, vitamins, minerals, phytochemicals, and sterols, have been documented in oat [32]. It is worth mentioning that the quantity and makeup of these nutrients are influenced by genetic factors and the conditions in which the oats are cultivated.

3.2.1 Carbohydrate

Carbohydrates play a fundamental role in the functioning of all living organisms. Primary metabolic processes rely on the conversion of carbon and energy, regardless of whether an organism follows autotrophic or heterotrophic nutrition, and, thus, carbohydrates are at the core of these processes [12], [33]. Consequently, it is not surprising that polysaccharides are the most prevalent polymers in the biosphere. Oats are classified as a high-carbohydrate food, containing approximately 70.7 g of carbohydrates per 100 g of oats. It's worth emphasizing that the carbohydrates found in oats fall into the category of "complex" carbohydrates, serving as a primary source of energy for our bodies (Table 3.1). Oats earn this distinction as complex carbohydrates due to their substantial dietary fibre content, encompassing both soluble and insoluble fibres, along with a notable presence of β-glucan [34] (Figure 3.1).

3.2.1.1 Starch

Starch holds the distinction of being the most abundant storage carbohydrate on Earth, primarily synthesized by plants and some cyanobacteria. Unlike many other organisms that produce water-soluble glycogen for carbohydrate storage, starch is stored in the form of water-insoluble particles known as starch granules. Despite this difference, both starch and glycogen share similar biological functions and chemical compositions, consisting of glucose units connected through α-1,4 and α-1,6 glycosidic bonds (Figure 3.1). What sets starch apart is its distinct physical properties, which greatly differ from those of glycogen. These unique characteristics contribute to the high value of starch across various applications. Starch is a versatile biomaterial that garners special interest due

TABLE 3.1 Proximate Constituents and Energy Values (Representative Values per 100 g) for Oats and Other Whole Grains

PARTICULARS	OATMEAL	CORNMEAL	WHOLE-GRAIN RYE	SORGHUM	WHOLE-GRAIN WHEAT	BROWN RICE	PEARLED BARLEY
Carbohydrate, g	58.7	70.6	58.7	65.6	60.2	73.9	69.7
Dietary fibre, g	9.0	4.8	12.8	6.9	10.6	2.3	8.0
Ash, g	1.8	1.1	2.0	1.6	1.6	1.4	1.2
Fat, g	8.0	3.5	2.3	3.3	2.1	2.8	1.6
Protein, g	14.0	8.8	11.2	11.0	13.5	7.4	9.2
Water, g	8.5	11.2	13.0	11.6	12.0	12.2	10.3
Energy, kcal	363	349	300	336	314	350	330
Energy, kJ	1,473	1,409	1,215	1,359	1,270	1,412	1,331

Source: Compiled from data from the U.S. Department of Agriculture, Agricultural Research Service (2008) and Welch (2006).

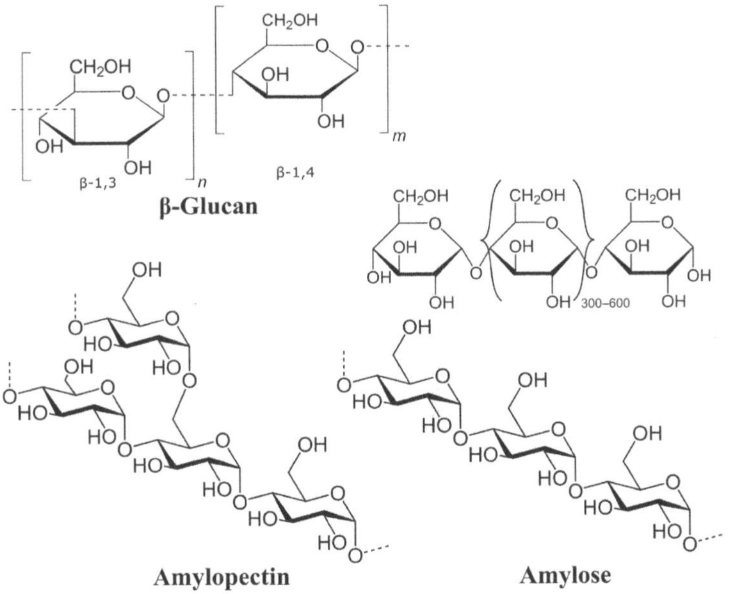

FIGURE 3.1 Chemical structures of starch (amylose and amylopectin) and β-glucan in oats. This figure presents the molecular structures of key components in oats, specifically focusing on starch (comprising amylose and amylopectin) and β-glucan. The chemical structure of amylose is depicted as a linear chain of glucose units linked by α(1→4) glycosidic bonds, showcasing its characteristic helical arrangement. Amylopectin, characterized by a branched structure, is illustrated with both linear and branching segments connected by α(1→6) glycosidic bonds. Additionally, the figure includes the chemical structure of β-glucan, emphasizing its beta (1→3,1→4) glycosidic linkages, which contribute to its unique functional and nutritional properties.

to its widespread availability, affordability, non-toxic nature, and ability to biodegrade [35]. As a result, starch finds utility in a multitude of industries, encompassing both food and non-food sectors.

Starch makes up approximately 51–65% of the composition of oat grains. The specific chemical makeup of oat starch can vary depending on the oat variety and the method used for its extraction. It is primarily found in the endosperm of the oat grain and serves as a prominent ingredient in oat-based food applications. Oat starch granules are distinctive, existing in A- and B-types with polyhedral shapes. These granules consist predominantly of amylose and amylopectin, making up roughly 98–99% of the carbohydrate content. Notably, the physicochemical properties of oat starch set it apart from many other cereal starches. For example, oat starch exhibits a higher affinity for binding lipids, increased relative crystallinity, and more pronounced coiling of amylose and amylopectin [36]. However, it has shorter amylose chains and smaller granule sizes compared to regular cereal starches. Variations in physicochemical properties can also be observed among different oat cultivars. These distinctions likely arise from differences in the interactions among starch chains within both the amorphous and crystalline regions of the native granules, as well as variations in the chain lengths of amylose and amylopectin fractions within oat starch. Oat starch exhibits unique characteristics, including small granule size, a well-developed granule surface, and a higher lipid content compared to other starches [37]. Studies have indicated that oat starches possess distinctive traits such as reduced amylose leaching, higher peak viscosity, heightened susceptibility to acid hydrolysis, low gel rigidity, increased swelling capacity, increased setback, co-leaching of a branched starch component, and greater resistance to α-amylase activity, amylose during the pasting process, and enhanced freeze–thaw stability [38]. However, it's important to note that these properties can vary significantly among different oat cultivars [39].

Oats contain approximately 7% of rapidly digestible starch (RDS), 22% of slowly digestible starch (SDS), and 25% of resistant starch (RS). This composition allows oats to be classified as a low-glycaemic index food, making them a favourable choice for individuals seeking foods with slower and more controlled carbohydrate digestion [40]. The gradual digestion of starch plays a crucial role in maintaining stable blood glucose levels, which is vital for human health. Among these fractions, SDS holds particular significance as it helps moderate the body's glycaemic response and enhances the nutritional quality of food [41]. RS has been acknowledged as a functional fibre that contributes significantly to digestive physiology. Unlike other starches, it avoids complete digestion and serves as fermentable carbohydrates for colonic bacteria, similar to substances like fructo-oligosaccharides. Additionally, it offers various benefits, such as the production of beneficial metabolites like short-chain fatty acids in the colon. Beyond its therapeutic effects, RS also improves the appearance, texture, and mouthfeel of food compared to conventional fibres. RS occurs naturally in cereal grains and heated starch or starch-containing foods, although it is often lost during processing [42]. To experience the physiological benefits of consuming RS, one typically needs to intake doses ranging from 20 to 30 g per day. However, this level is significantly higher (about three to four times) than what is commonly found in the typical human diet, where estimated RS intake among the U.S. population typically ranges from 5 to 10 g per day. Most foods contain less than 3 g of RS per serving. Oats stand out as a notable source of RS and other starch fractions, with approximately 7% consisting of RDS, 22% of SDS, and 25% of RS in the total starch content of oats. Regular consumption of oats can serve as a valuable dietary supplement to increase the intake of these beneficial starches [43].

In the oat grain, starch is primarily found in the endosperm, which is encased by the bran layers rich in β-glucan and protein. In contrast to other cereals, isolating starch from oats is a relatively complex process. This complexity arises from the strong association between starch and protein, as well as the presence of β-glucan. The removal of proteins is a crucial step that significantly enhances the yield of starch extraction from oats [36], [38].

If we talk about the morphological characteristics, in the majority of cereal starches, granules are typically discrete, solid, and appear optically clear. In contrast, oat starch displays a distinct granule structure [44]. Oat starch granules tend to aggregate into clusters, resulting in irregular or polygonal shapes for the majority of these granules. Some granules, particularly those situated on the outer layer of these clusters, exhibit polygonal shapes on one side and an ovoid shape on the other. These clusters generally vary in diameter from 20 to 150 μm, with an average size of approximately 60 μm. When oat starch is extracted, the resulting granules typically have diameters that span from 2 to 12 μm [45]. In a comparative study conducted by Zwer et al., the analysis of granule sizes in various cereal starches revealed distinctive characteristics of oat starch [46]. Oat starch granules were observed to form clusters comprised of irregularly shaped granules, which included a mixture of both A- and B-type granules. In terms of size, oat starch granules were found to be similar in dimension to rice starch but smaller than those found in wheat, maize, and potato starches. Specifically, the typical length range, width range, and mean granule width of native starches fell within the ranges of 5.85–6.9 μm, 3.0–7.5 μm, and 1.5–9.7165 μm, respectively [47]. These oat starch granules presented smooth surfaces without any noticeable fissures. Unlike some other starches, oat starch granules exhibited weak birefringence, indicating a lack of strong optical properties. They displayed irregular shapes, tended to cluster together, and did not conform to the discrete size distributions commonly observed in wheat and barley starches, which typically feature distinct A- and B-type granules [48].

Oat starch can be found in a wide range of both food and non-food products. Starch is composed of soluble macromolecules that offer valuable properties such as adhesion, high viscosity, and the ability to coat surfaces, all of which are highly beneficial in the food industry. Starches are employed for various purposes in food applications, including stabilizing, thickening, fat replacement, bulking, texturizing, and gelling [42]. Oat starch has garnered less attention in industrial applications when compared to other cereals due to its relatively higher cost and limited availability. However, despite these challenges, oat starch possesses unique characteristics that render it particularly suitable for specific and specialized uses [49]. The soluble macromolecules present in oat starch provide desirable attributes like adhesion, surface coating capabilities, and high viscosity, which are sought after in food products. Beyond the food industry, oat starch finds utility in the paper and pulp sector, where it is used for sizing and coating papers. This is due to its small granule size and elevated lipid content, which are advantageous in this context. Oat starch is widely incorporated into the processing of oat-based foods, including snacks, sauces, dairy products, noodles, baked goods, and even non-food items [50].

Oat starch finds valuable applications in the medical sectors and cosmetics. It can serve as a substitute for talcum powder and is utilized as a dusting powder for medical gloves. Alpine Gloves Inc. has even patented latex gloves that are powdered with oat starch, claiming that this choice reduces the risk of latex allergies [51]. Unlike corn starch, oat starch does not bind to latex protein. Furthermore, oat starch has been explored as a fat replacer in various culinary applications [52]. In a study, both annealed and native oat starches were employed to replace fat in mayonnaise. This substitution was carried out at levels of 0%, 50%, and 75%, and the results demonstrated that, as the quantity of starch increased, the stability of the mayonnaise also increased [53]. Oatrim, a notable fat substitute developed by the U.S. Department of Agriculture, is a significant industrial application of oat starch [54]. It offers a healthier alternative by replacing the fat content in various food products. The RS found in oats has been harnessed to create nutritious meals, such as granola cereals and bars, which are low in fat and calories while being rich in dietary fibre. This highlights the versatility and beneficial properties of oat starch in both cosmetic and food industries [55].

Oat starch has gained popularity in both food and non-food products due to its content of soluble macromolecules, which impart favourable properties like high viscosity and adhesion to various foods. The interest in utilizing oat starch for nutritional and technological purposes has been steadily increasing. However, its application has been somewhat limited by the challenges associated with separating starch from other components, such as fibre and protein, as well as its relatively low availability and higher cost compared to other starch sources [7], [56]. While the advantages of using oat starch may not surpass those of more commonly used starches like maize, wheat, and potato starch, it is still employed as an ingredient in a variety of food products. These include soups, baked goods, noodles, snack bars, and certain health-conscious foods, often after undergoing modification to enhance their properties. Nonetheless, there is a notable absence of comprehensive comparative studies pitting oat starch against other starch sources in terms of their applications [21]. Further research is necessary to determine whether oat starch can indeed serve as a viable alternative to traditional starch sources and to expand its potential applications within the food industry. The quality of food products is significantly influenced by the pasting and rheological properties of oat starch. However, natural oat starch may come with certain limitations. For instance, it tends to have a higher lipid content in comparison to other cereal starches. Additionally, it is characterized by a high pasting temperature and viscosity, relatively low resistance, low paste clarity to shear stress, and a low degree of crystallinity. These characteristics make natural oat starch unsuitable for direct use in food applications. As a result, the modification of oat starch to imbue it with more desirable properties becomes crucial for its broader and more effective utilization in the food industry [57].

3.2.1.1.1 Amylose

Oats primarily consist of starch, making up about 50–60% or more of their composition. This starch contains various components, including lipids (approximately 5–7.5%), proteins (about 0.3–1%), minerals, and carbohydrate constituents known as amylose and amylopectin (making up 90–95%). Oat starch possesses distinctive characteristics, such as having a short amylose chain, relatively high crystallinity, and small granule surface structure. These unique properties distinguish oat starch from starches found in other cereal grains [58].

Amylose, a polysaccharide composed of α-d-glucose units, is a significant component of oat starch. It is formed by α(1→4) glycosidic bonds between glucose units, resulting in a relatively low degree of polymerization (DP) of around 3,000 and a low frequency of branching with α-1,6 linkages (Figure 3.1). Amylose molecules are predominantly linear, with a few long-chain branches and a smaller molecular weight (around 105–106) [59]. Amylose molecules have a natural helical structure and exhibit interactions with substances like iodine, organic alcohols, and fatty acids. When these interactions occur, they form helical inclusion complexes. In the presence of fatty acids, these complexes are known as amylose–lipid complexes. Amylose can be relatively easily extracted using hot water. The amylose content in oat starch varies, ranging from 25.2% to 29.4%, depending on factors such as the oat genotype, environmental conditions, and the analytical methods employed [60]. The apparent amylose content, considering lipid complexing, falls in the range of 16.7% to 22%, while the amylose content without lipid complexing can range from 19.4% to 33.6%. Various research studies have presented divergent findings. For instance, the total amylose content in oat starch ranges from 27.5% to 29.5%. In Canadian oats, it falls within the range of 19.4% to 22.7%, while for hulless and hulled oat cultivars, the amylose content is approximately 22.5% and 22.2%, respectively [61]–[63].

3.2.1.1.2 Amylopectin

Amylopectin tends to have a high DP (N 5,000) and higher α-1, 6 linkage frequency (3–4%). Amylopectin is highly branched with many short chains and has a high molecular weight (107–8) [44]. The side chain branches of amylopectin are made up of about 30 glucose units attached with 1α→6 linkages approximately every 20 to 30 glucose units along the chain. Starch digestion behaviour is also influenced by chemical structure, including molecular weight, amylose content, and degree of branching. The digestion rate is associated with the branch chain size of amylopectin, and shorter chains can result in higher digestion rates [45]. Other factors contributing to the slower digestion of oat starch were fewer short branch chains (DP < 13) and less branching of amylopectin, causing reduced enzyme accessibility. In contrast, a relatively lower proportion of the longest branch chains was also observed, which may increase digestibility to some extent [64].

The structure of starch can be broken down into several hierarchical levels of organization. At the first level, individual branches are connected by α-(1→4) glycosidic linkages, which determine the chain length distribution (CLD) [60] (Figure 3.1). These chains are then linked together at the reducing end by α-(1→6) glycosidic linkages, forming amylose and amylopectin. This represents the second level of structure, encompassing whole starch molecules. The third level of structure involves the formation of a lamellar structure, created by the entwining of branches of amylopectin into double helices and then into clusters. These clusters give rise to alternating amorphous and crystalline lamellae with an average repeat distance of approximately 9 nm within granules. These lamellae form semi-crystalline growth rings alternated with amorphous growth rings, which are constructed from amylose and portions of amylopectin. This constitutes the fourth level of structure, defining starch granules. The fifth level of structure involves the starch granules and their interactions with non-starch components, such as proteins and lipids [65].

The intricate structure of starch is formed through the coordinated efforts of three classes of enzymes: starch synthases (SSs), starch branching enzymes (SBEs), and starch debranching enzymes (DBEs). SSs can be further divided into soluble starch synthases (SSSs), which are primarily responsible for building amylopectin by transferring glucose from ADP-glucose to the non-reducing end of growing chains, and granule-bound starch synthases (GBSSs), which oversee the synthesis of amylose. SBEs function by cleaving linear glucose chains and then attaching the cleaved portion to an adjacent glucan chain through α-(1→6) glycosidic linkages [66]. On the other hand, DBEs play a role in removing branches that are in "improper positions" during the formation of amylopectin. The ratios of specific enzymatic activities of SSs, GBSSs, SBEs, and DBEs exert control over the CLDs of both amylose and amylopectin [67].

3.2.1.2 Dietary Fibre

In the realm of human nutrition, the term "dietary fibre" was initially introduced by Hipsley during the 1950s to refer to the indigestible components found in plant cell walls [68]. The characteristics of dietary fibre, including its chemical composition, physiological functions, and the specific food context in which it is found, can vary significantly. The American Association of Cereal Chemists International defines dietary fibre as follows: "The edible portions of plants and similar carbohydrates that resist digestion and absorption within the human small intestine, undergoing either complete or partial fermentation in the large intestine. Dietary fibre encompasses polysaccharides, oligosaccharides, lignin, and related plant substances." This definition also recognizes the beneficial physiological effects of dietary fibre [69]. It is important to differentiate dietary fibre from functional fibre, which comprises isolated, indigestible carbohydrates that confer positive physiological effects in humans. The sum of dietary fibre and functional fibre is collectively referred to as total fibre. It's worth noting that dietary fibre, primarily composed of carbohydrate polymers that remain undigested by human enzymes, has not been formally designated as an essential dietary component. Oats, typically processed as whole grains, are notably rich in a specific type of dietary fibre. Both soluble and insoluble fibres are present in oats, with a significant content of soluble fibre in the form of β-glucan, alongside insoluble fibres such as arabinoxylans and cellulose [70].

Dietary fibre includes a significant component known as β-d-glucan. Purified oat β-glucan is a linear, unbranched polysaccharide consisting of 1–4-O-linked (70%) and 1–3-O-linked (30%) β-d-glucopyranosyl units. The 1–3 linkages occur individually, while most of the 1–4 linkages occur in clusters of two or three, predominantly resulting in a structure of β-(1–3)-linked cellotriosyl and cellotetraosyl units [71]. Linkage analysis reveals that oat β-glucan and non-cereal β-glucan seem identical, but differences emerge when examining oligosaccharide fragments released through enzymatic hydrolysis. The physiological effects of dietary fibre are determined by its physical and chemical properties, which include hydration, solubility, viscosity, and its ability to absorb organic molecules [72]. While some β-glucan is found in the aleurone cell wall, it is in smaller amounts compared to the starchy endosperm beneath, which serves as the primary storage site for starch, protein, lipid, and β-glucan. Oat groats contain varying amounts of β-glucan, ranging from 2.3 to 8.5 g/100 g. β-Glucan consists primarily of β-1–3 linked cellotriosyl and cellotetraosyl units, but it also contains cellulose-like β-1–4 linked glucose units [73]. The water solubility of β-glucan is influenced by its structure, with the soluble form having a higher ratio of (1–4) linkages and cellotriosyl units compared to the insoluble form. Oats typically contain 3% to 5% β-glucan on a dry weight basis. The native chain length of oat β-glucan is approximately 20,000 glucosidyl units, with a molecular weight of up to 3 million Da. β-Glucan is also present in other cereals such as sorghum, rye, maize, triticale, wheat, and rice, as well as in specific seaweed and mushroom species. However, the β-glucan content in these sources is significantly lower than that found in oats or barley. For instance, wheat contains approximately 1% β-glucan, whereas oats typically range from 3% to 7% in β-glucan content [74].

Dietary fibres resist digestion in the small intestine, and soluble β-glucan is thought to elevate the viscosity of the food mass. This results in a delay in gastric emptying, an increased sensation of fullness in the gut, and a slower absorption of nutrients [75]. The potential impact of dietary fibre has been discussed in its ability to potentially prevent conditions such as coronary heart disease, colorectal and other cancers, type 2 diabetes, and obesity. Furthermore, β-glucan can serve as a thickening agent in the food industry and may affect the sensory characteristics of beverages, making it particularly significant in the field of human nutrition [76], [77] (Table 3.2).

3.2.2 Protein

Oats, represent a cereal crop characterized by a notably higher protein content (ranging from 12.4% to 24.5% in oat groats) compared to other commonly cultivated cereal crops such as wheat or rye [79]. Furthermore, oats exhibit a protein quality of significant nutritional value and possess a unique protein composition. The embryonic axis and the scutellum within the oat kernel contain more abundant quantities of amino acids compared to other kernel sections. Enzymes play a pivotal role in metabolic activity. The distribution of proteins within the oat grain is not uniform, showing an increasing gradient from the inner to the outer regions. Proteins are predominantly located in the germ and bran but are less abundant in the endosperm [21]. Additionally, oats are

TABLE 3.2 Comparative Dietary Fibre Content in Different Crops [78]

FOOD	DIETARY FIBRE (G/100 G)
Oat	10.3
Nuts	4.0–12.0
Wheat	9.5
Rice	2.8
Corn	7.3
Pulses	5.0–18.0
Fruit and vegetables	0.5–5.0
Barley	9.2

TABLE 3.3 Total Protein Content, Molecular Weights, and Isoelectric Points of Protein Fractions from Oats Isolated by Osborne Fractionation [78]

PROTEIN FRACTION	% OF TOTAL PROTEIN OATS	ISOELECTRIC POINTS
Albumin	1–12	pH 4.0–7.0
Globulin	50–80	pH 5.5 and pH 8.0–10.0
Prolamin	4–15	pH 5.0–9.0
Glutelin	< 10	—

generally gluten-free, making them a suitable dietary option for individuals with celiac disease. Oats represent a potential source of cost-effective protein due to their elevated protein content (ranging from 9% to 20%) when compared to other commercially cultivated cereal grains such as corn, barley, wheat, and sorghum. The structural properties and distribution of protein fractions in oat protein differ from those observed in other cereal grains [25] (Table 3.3).

The nutritional quality of proteins is commonly assessed using the protein digestibility-corrected amino acid score (PDCAAS). Research on oat proteins has indicated a PDCAAS range of 0.41 to 0.60, with lysine being the amino acid in the shortest supply [80], [81]. Consequently, oat proteins have a lower PDCAAS compared to certain other plant protein sources like soy proteins (0.90–0.93) and pea proteins (0.73–0.89), but they fare better in comparison to almond proteins (0.32–0.34) and wheat proteins (0.37–0.54) [82]. In contrast, pulse proteins like lentil and pea proteins are rich in lysine but limited in sulphur-containing amino acids, making them complementary when combined with oat proteins. These combinations of plant proteins offer an opportunity to create plant-based dairy alternatives with PDCAAS values like cow's milk (PDCAAS = 1) [82]. Oats are commonly utilized in commercial liquid and semi-solid applications, such as milk substitutes and plant-based yoghurt-like products. However, in cases where oat is the sole source of protein, the total protein content in such products is low (typically ranging from 0% to 1%). This is primarily due to the relatively low protein content in oat flours and flakes (typically around 10% to 15%), combined with the unintentional removal of a significant amount of oat protein during the processing of these products [83].

Oats can be categorized into four distinct protein groups based on the Osborne classification: globulins (comprising 70–80% of the total protein), prolamins (constituting 4–15%), albumins (making up 1–12%), and glutelins (comprising less than 10%) [84]. Most cereals like wheat, barley, and rye predominantly contain prolamins, which are alcohol-soluble proteins and typically house most storage proteins. However, oats and rice stand out as exceptions, as their primary storage proteins belong to the globulin fraction. In oats, the prolamins are known to have a low presence, with estimates ranging from approximately 4% to 15% of the total protein content [85]. The significance of oats having a high proportion of globulins and a low proportion of prolamins is that their protein composition offers a more balanced profile of essential amino acids for humans and other monogastric animals compared to other cereal proteins. Another protein fraction in oats is albumins, which are primarily composed of enzymes and represent a minor component, with levels ranging from 1% to 12% of the total protein content. Regarding globulins, there has been some variation in reported proportions (saltwater-soluble proteins) in oats. Quantitative data on the proportion of globulins can vary widely, with estimates ranging from 40% to 50% up to 70% to 80%. Nevertheless, it is universally agreed that the globulin fraction accounts for most oat grain storage proteins. In total, water-soluble proteins and glutelins typically make up about 30% of the total protein in oats, with globulins and prolamins being distributed roughly in a 2:1 ratio [86].

Most of the protein in oat grains can be dissolved in a buffered salt solution, classifying it as globulin. These globulins generally have isoelectric points around pH 5.5, though some proteins exhibit higher pH values in the range of 8–10 [87]. Oat globulin displays significant heterogeneity, a characteristic shared with the seed storage proteins of other cereal grains. This diversity is attributed to the expression of multigene families. Unlike wheat, barley, and rye, where different components dominate, oats are primarily composed of the 12 S globulin [88]. This 12 S globulin is an oligomeric protein with a quaternary structure like that of legumins. The first comprehensive characterization of this protein was carried out by Peterson in 1978, revealing a molecular weight of 322,000 for the 12 S fraction. Oats also contain smaller quantities of 3S and 7S globulins, which are thought to resemble vicilin-like proteins [86]. Oat globulin (12S) is an oligomeric protein composed of six quaternary monomer subunits, each weighing in at 54–60 kDa, reminiscent of the structure of soy 11S globulin (glycinin). Within the 12S globulin, there are two major subunits: the A-subunit (32 kDa), an acidic polypeptide, and the B-subunit (22 kDa), a basic polypeptide, linked by a disulphide bond. In contrast, the 7S globulins are comprised of polypeptides ranging from 55 to 65 kDa, while the 3S fraction consists of two polypeptides with molecular weights of approximately 15 and 21 kDa. Oat globulins possess a high denaturation temperature of around 110°C, attributed to strong hydrophobic interactions between the subunits that become more pronounced at higher temperatures [89].

Oats stand out among cereals in terms of their amino acid composition, primarily due to their higher levels of essential amino acids like lysine and threonine, which are often considered limiting in other cereal grains. During germination, there is an observed increase in essential amino acids such as lysine and tryptophan, enhancing the nutritional value of germinated oats. Avenins play a vital role in protein storage in oats, accounting for approximately 10 to 13% of the total protein content [90]. Oat proteins contain a higher proportion of limiting amino acids like glutamine, lysine, and threonine, and comparatively less proline when compared to other cereal grains (Table 3.4) (Figure 3.2). This results in oats being particularly rich in lysine content, thanks to the albumin and globulin fractions, which have a higher concentration of lysine, while the content of glutamic acid is lower. Among the various protein fractions in oats, globulins have the highest levels of most essential amino acids (e.g., phenylalanine, lysine, histidine, and valine) as well as non-essential amino acids (e.g., glutamic acid and arginine) [91]. When evaluating the ratio of essential amino acid content to the total amino acid content, both albumin (39%) and globulin (36%) exhibit values higher than 36%, thus meeting the criteria for high-quality proteins as recommended by the FAO for adults. This distinguishes them from the prolamin and glutelin fractions. Notably, oats are

TABLE 3.4   Amino Acid Content of Oat Proteins

	OAT	FAO STANDARD (ADULT)	WHEAT	SOY	RICE	PEA
Protein content[1]	64		81	91	79	80
Essential amino acids[2]						
Leucine	3.8	1.9	5	5	5.8	5.7
Phenylalanine	2.7	1.9	3.7	3.2	3.7	3.7
Histidine	0.9	1.6	1.4	1.5	1.5	1.6
Methionine	0.1	1.7	0.7	0.3	2	0.3
Threonine	1.5	0.9	1.8	2.3	2	2.5
Lysine	1.3	1.6	1.1	3.4	1.9	4.7
Valine	2	1.3	2.3	2.2	2.8	2.7
Isoleucine	1.3	1.3	2	1.9	2	2.3
ΣEAA	13.7	—	18	19.9	22.1	23.6
Non-essential amino acids						
Alanine	2.2	—	1.8	2.8	4.3	3.2
Glutamic acid	11	—	26.9	12.4	12.7	12.9
Glycine	1.7	—	2.4	2.7	3.4	2.8
Cysteine	0.4	—	0.7	0.2	0.6	0.2
Serine	2.2	—	3.5	3.4	3.4	3.6
Tyrosine	1.5	—	2.4	2.2	3.5	2.6
Proline	2.5	—	8.8	3.3	3.4	3.1
Arginine	3.1	—	2.4	4.8	5.4	5.9
ΣNEAA	24.7	—	48.9	31.9	36.8	34.4
ΣAA	38.4	—	66.9	51.8	58.9	58
ΣEAA/ΣAA	36	36	27	38	37	41

Source: Compiled from data from the U.S. Department of Agriculture, Agricultural Research Service (2008) and Welch (2006).
Values are presented in g/100 g of commercially available isolated protein powder. ΣEAA, sum of all essential amino acids; ΣNEAA, sum of all non-essential amino acids; ΣAA, sum of all amino acids; ΣEAA/ΣAA, the essential amino acid content to the total amino acid content ratio.
Notes:
[1] Determined using the Dumas combustion method.
[2] Determined using ultra-performance liquid chromatography tandem mass spectrometry.

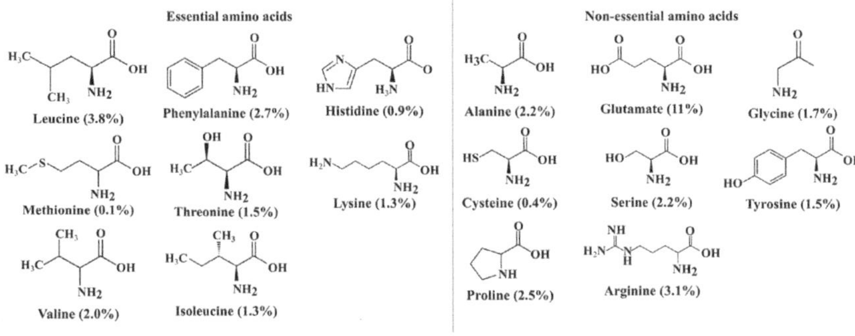

FIGURE 3.2   Chemical structures of essential and non-essential amino acids in oats.

unique among cereals in that they contain a globulin or legume-like protein called avenalin, which makes up the majority (around 80%) of their storage protein. Globulins are water-soluble proteins, whereas other cereal proteins are categorized as gluten and zein, belonging to the prolamin or prolamin category [92].

Albumins, typically having molecular weights in the range of 19 to 21 kDa, primarily serve as enzymes that contribute to the overall protein quality and play a role in plant defence mechanisms. These proteins, which are soluble in water, are predominantly composed of enzymes. On the other hand, glutelins are polypeptides with a wider range of molecular weights, spanning from 10 to 90 kDa [93]. Oats, in comparison to legumes, contain higher levels of sulfur-containing amino acids such as cysteine and methionine. A minor portion of proteins in oats, referred to as glutelins, can be dissolved either under acidic or alkaline conditions. Oat prolamins belong to the category of prolamins rich in sulphur and have low levels of basic amino acids while exhibiting high levels of glutamic acid and proline. Prolamins are highly soluble in aqueous alcohol solutions. Within the prolamin fraction, oats display valuable and consistent polymorphism among different genotypes, which, together with the glutelins, are collectively known as avenins. The diversity of avenin patterns is greater compared to the globulin fraction. Avenins in oats form a group of alcohol-soluble proteins with sizes ranging from 17 to 34,000 kDa and typically have isoelectric points falling within the range of 5.0 to 9.0 [94]. The alcohol-soluble prolamin fraction, avenins, consists of four subfractions: α, β, γ, and ω-avenins. These proteins have relatively low molecular weights (20–40 kDa) and exhibit structural similarities to the sulfur-rich subgroups α-gliadins and γ-gliadins in wheat, B-hordeins in barley, and γ-secalins in rye. They serve a storage function like wheat gluten but have a different amino acid composition, particularly lower levels of proline and glutamine. Seed storage proteins, including avenins and globulins in oats, are typically encoded by multigene families. The number of potential avenin coding sequences can vary, ranging from as few as 6–8 in *A. hirtula* and *A. magna* to as many as 25 in A. sativa. Avenins are primarily located within protein bodies in the endosperm and are absent from the aleurone layer [95].

3.2.3 Lipid

The energy content of oat grains is significantly determined by their lipid component, which in turn plays a vital role in shaping their nutritional quality due to the specific fatty acid composition. These lipids are thought to have an impact on the pasting properties of oat starch, thus influencing its functional properties. Furthermore, lipids are involved in shaping the flavour profile of oats and any potential off-flavour attributes. *A. sativa* L. grains are renowned for their high oil content, ranging from 3% to 18%, in contrast to the approximately 2–3% found in wheat and most other cereals (around 17% in maize) [96]. This lipid content is primarily concentrated in the endosperm tissues of the grain and exhibits variations among different oat cultivars. In 1979, Sahasrabudhe provided a detailed breakdown of typical oat lipid composition, reporting the following components: 51% triacylglycerols, 7% free fatty acids, 3% sterols, 3% sterol esters, 8% glycolipids, and 20% phospholipids [97] (Table 3.5). Oat lipids can be categorized into polar and non-polar fractions, with polar lipids mainly comprising glycolipids and phospholipids. Non-polar lipids constitute approximately 80% of all lipids in oats and contain valuable fatty acids, primarily palmitic acid (20%), oleic acid (35%), and linoleic acid (40%), along with fat-soluble antioxidants [98].

Several studies have suggested that the content of free fatty acids is influenced by the sample preparation process, as grinding the grain can increase lipase activity, resulting in a higher concentration of free fatty acids. Significant factors affecting lipid and fatty acid content in oats include soil and climatic conditions, as well as genetic characteristics during the plant's growth and development.

3.2.3.1 Polar Lipids

The oil derived from *A. sativa* seeds is noteworthy for its substantial concentration of polar lipids, specifically glycolipids and phospholipids, which can make up a substantial portion, up to 34%, of the total lipid content. These polar lipids possess an amphiphilic

TABLE 3.5 Lipid (%) Content of Grains [18]

CROPS	LIPID (%)
Oat	4.41 ± 0.20%
Wheat	1.7–2.39 ± 0.44%
Maize	4.36 ± 0.36%
Millet	4.8 ± 0.70%
Barley	2.45–2.75%
Buckwheat	1.62%
Quinoa	7.48%
Amaranth	7.00%

structure, rendering them valuable candidates for use as emulsifiers in oil-in-water emulsions. Phospholipids, often referred to as phosphatides, are essential structural components in both food products and cellular membranes. They are primarily composed of phosphatidic acids, esters consisting of 1,2-diacylated 3-glycerophosphoric acid, associated with organic bases or other functional groups [99]. A study conducted by Price and Parsons in 1975 identified the prevalent phospholipids in oat grains as 1-α-phosphatidylcholine (PC), 1-α-phosphatidylethanolamine (PE), and 1-α-lysophosphatidylcholine (Lyso-PC). Furthermore, phospholipids play a critical role in maintaining cellular structure and are renowned for their antioxidant properties [100]. Oat grains typically contain a phospholipid fraction estimated to range from 5% to 26% of the total lipids. Among these, phosphatidylcholine is the primary constituent, comprising 45–51% of all phospholipids, with phosphatidylethanolamine and phosphatidylglycerol also present. Oat grains are distinguished by their remarkable capacity to accumulate a significant amount of oil within the endosperm, especially in comparison to other cereal grains. It is worth noting that maize is the sole cereal exhibiting a similarly high grain oil content as oats, although in maize, the oil is predominantly stored in the embryo [101].

The polar lipid fraction of oat oil is noteworthy for its high content of glycolipids, including specific compounds such as monogalactosyldiacylglycerols (MGDG), digalactosyldiacylglycerols (DGDG), and sulpholipids. DGDGs, in particular, are of great significance as they contribute to membrane formation in chloroplasts found in higher plants and various cell organelles. These compounds are present in tissues involved in photosynthesis, including higher plants, algae, and certain bacteria. The glycolipid content in oat oil typically falls within the range of 7% to 12%. Oat oil, obtained through extraction with hexane or ethanol from oat flour, is notably characterized by a high concentration of DGDG, a feature commonly observed in oat seeds. Researchers suggest that oat glycolipids possess viscosity-reducing properties, making them valuable emulsifiers in chocolate products [102] (Figure 3.3).

3.2.3.2 Non-Polar Lipids

Inert lipids predominantly include free fatty acids, triacylglycerols, segments of glycerides, sterol esters, and free sterols. Roughly 50–60% of oat fats are composed of this lipid component, with triacylglycerols being the most prevalent [103]. Scientific investigations have established significant disparities in the quantities of both free and bound lipids, as well as variations in the composition of free fatty acids, contingent on the specific oat variety. Palmitic, oleic, and linoleic acids are the prevailing constituents found in all segments of oat fat (Table 3.6).

Oat lecithin, when used as an additive, is an oil extracted from oat grains using ethanol as the solvent. This oil is subsequently fractionated to obtain lipids with higher polarity. The resulting lecithin has a yellow-brown colour and a flavour reminiscent of oat flakes. Oat lecithin primarily consists of non-polar lipids (about 58% by weight) and polar lipids (about 35% by weight) [104]. The non-polar fraction is mainly composed of triglycerides, while the polar lipids include approximately 20–25% glycolipids such as MGDG and DGDG and 15–20% phospholipids, including phosphatidylcholine and N-acylphosphatidylethanolamine. This lecithin also contains saturated fatty acids

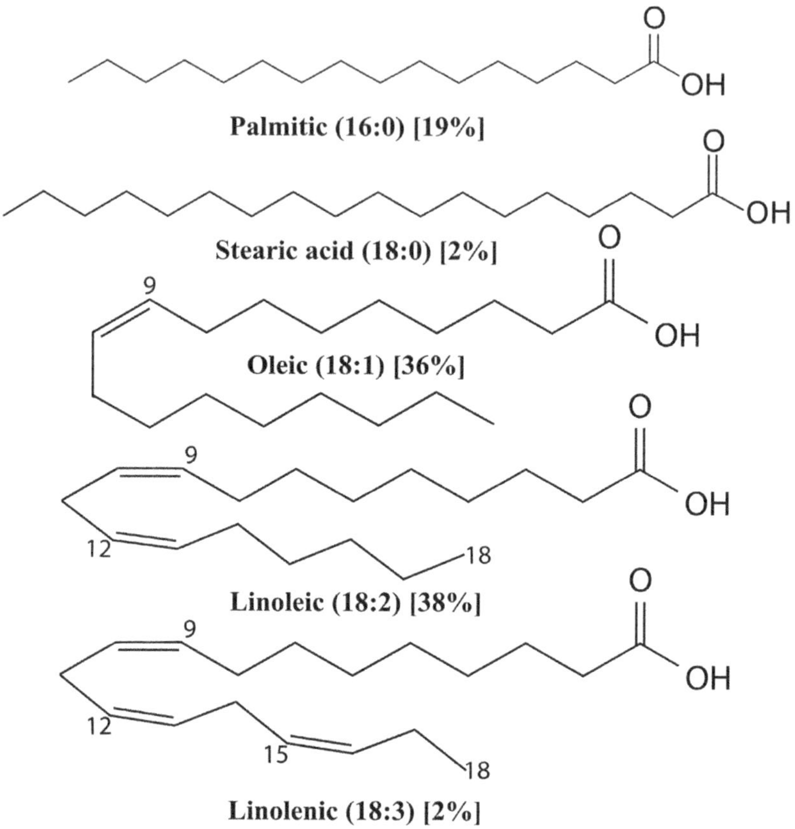

Palmitic (16:0) [19%]

Stearic acid (18:0) [2%]

Oleic (18:1) [36%]

Linoleic (18:2) [38%]

Linolenic (18:3) [2%]

FIGURE 3.3 Various predominant fatty acids in oat.

TABLE 3.6 Fatty Acid Composition (Representative Values, g/100 g of Total Fatty Acids) of Oats and Other Whole Grains

FATTY ACID	OATMEAL	CORNMEAL	WHOLE-GRAIN RYE	SORGHUM	BROWN RICE	WHOLE-GRAIN WHEAT	PEARLED BARLEY
Palmitic (16:0)	19	12	15	13	22	18	22
Stearic (18:0)	2	2	1	2	2	2	1
Oleic (18:1)	36	32	17	34	34	18	13
Linoleic (18:2)	38	50	58	46	38	56	56
Linolenic (18:3)	2	2	7	2	2	3	5

Source: Compiled from data from the U.S. Department of Agriculture, Agricultural Research Service (2008) and Welch (2006).

(primarily palmitic and stearic), monounsaturated fatty acids (oleic), and polyunsaturated fatty acids (linoleic and alpha-linolenic). As a result, grains with a high fat content are typically preferred for animal feeds rather than human consumption, as they lack flavour and tend to brown excessively during cooking. Lipids are categorized into free or bound lipids based on their solubility properties [105]. Studies found that approximately 80% of the total groat lipids were free lipids, which could be extracted using non-polar solvents like n-hexane, while the remaining 20%, referred to as bound lipids, required polar solvents such as water-saturated n-butanol (WSB) for extraction [106]. Freshly harvested oats have a mild taste. An essential function of lipids in oats is to develop the desirable flavour profile, characterized by a nutty, sweet, and cereal-like aroma. This unique oat flavour is the outcome of lipid oxidation products and N-heterocyclic compounds that emerge during the heat processing of oat groats. However, the utilization of oat lipids is often hindered by various lipid-related challenges. The quality of oat lipids significantly deteriorates through hydrolytic and oxidative processes, resulting in the development of a bitter, acrid taste or the formation of a rancid flavour. This deterioration primarily occurs because polyunsaturated fatty acids (especially linoleic and linolenic acids) are prone to oxidation due to the actions of lipid-degrading enzymes or chemical reactions [107]. During oat storage and processing, undesirable off-flavours may arise, typically originating from chemical reactions such as lipid autoxidation and the Maillard reaction, as well as enzymatic reactions catalysed by lipid-degrading enzymes. Autoxidation is a process involving free radicals, triplet oxygen ($3O_2$), and unsaturated lipids, typically progressing through three phases: chain initiation, propagation, and termination. This reaction tends to generate off-flavour compounds over extended oat storage periods. Conversely, the Maillard reaction takes place between reducing sugars and amino acids, resulting in desirable flavours, browning, and the production of certain antioxidants that can enhance lipid stability. Given the vital role of oats in daily dietary and nutritional consumption, it is imperative to comprehend the mechanisms behind the formation of off-flavour compounds, their sensory characteristics in oat-based foods, and potential strategies to mitigate them [108] (Figure 3.3).

3.2.4 Minerals and Vitamins

Minerals and vitamins, collectively known as micronutrients, are vital dietary components required in significantly smaller quantities compared to macronutrients like carbohydrates, proteins, and fats. Minerals constitute the inorganic or ash component, while vitamins are minor organic constituents [109].

Oats, in particular, boast a wealth of vitamins and minerals, each contributing to various aspects of health. They are notably abundant in B vitamins, encompassing B1, B2, B3, and B6, and contain vitamin E, which possesses the capacity to dilate peripheral blood vessels, thereby improving blood circulation and mitigating menopausal symptoms [110]. Furthermore, oat bran harbours trace elements and minerals such as calcium, phosphorus, iron, zinc, manganese, and chromium, all of which can be effectively assimilated by the body. These elements and compounds hold substantial potential in the prevention of conditions like osteoporosis and anaemia, while simultaneously promoting the healing of wounds. Among various grains, such as rice, wheat, and corn, oats reign supreme in selenium content, a mineral renowned for enhancing immune function and playing a pivotal role in safeguarding against cancer and the ageing process [111].

3.2.4.1 Minerals

Minerals can be classified into two main categories: major minerals and minor (or trace) minerals. Major minerals are typically found in larger quantities and are required in greater amounts for proper nutrition, whereas minor minerals are necessary in smaller quantities [112].

The major minerals encompass potassium, phosphorus, magnesium, calcium, and sodium. In physiological terms, potassium and sodium serve critical roles as electrolytes within both intercellular and intracellular fluids. Calcium, phosphorus, and magnesium are integral components of bones and teeth. Additionally, major minerals function as essential enzyme cofactors, contributing to various biochemical processes. Phosphorus, for instance, is also found in phospholipids like lecithin, which are minor lipid components with vital physiological functions [113]. Oats, in comparison to other cereals, boast relatively high concentrations of these major minerals. Although naturally low in sodium, it is often added in excess during processing, either in the form of sodium chloride (salt) or as a component of leavening agents like sodium bicarbonate. The category of minor minerals includes iron, zinc, manganese, and copper. Iron is a pivotal component of haemoglobin and, along with zinc, manganese, and copper, acts as an essential enzyme cofactor [114]. There are other minor minerals like selenium, chromium, and cobalt, which may hold dietary significance. Conversely, cadmium, arsenic, and lead are generally considered toxic and are found at significant levels only in crops grown on land contaminated with mining or industrial waste. Oats typically contain higher levels of minor minerals like iron, zinc, and manganese compared to other cereals. The amounts of these minor minerals in oats can be strongly influenced by the availability of these minerals in the soil in which they are grown [115] (Table 3.7).

3.2.4.2 Vitamins

Vitamins exhibit considerable variability in their chemical structures and physiological functions. They assume a diverse array of essential roles in various metabolic processes. Due to their inability to be synthesized by the body or being synthesizable only in limited quantities, vitamins are indispensable constituents of a well-rounded and healthful diet. Insufficient intake of vitamins can give rise to a spectrum of deficiency diseases. Moreover, emerging evidence is establishing a connection between inadequate vitamin intake, particularly in the cases of folic acid and vitamin E, and the incidence of chronic ailments like heart disease and various forms of cancer. Vitamins can be categorized based on their solubility characteristics into two primary groups: fat-soluble and water-soluble vitamins [116].

Vitamins A, D, E, and K belong to the category of fat-soluble vitamins. Vitamin A, or retinol, is not inherently present in plant-based foods but can be synthesized from

TABLE 3.7 Mineral Content (Representative Values, mg/100 g of Fresh Weight) of Oats and Other Whole Grains

	OATMEAL	SORGHUM	BROWN RICE	PEARLED BARLEY	CORNMEAL	WHOLE-GRAIN WHEAT	WHOLE-GRAIN RYE
Calcium	54	28	22	24	12	36	32
Magnesium	145	156	127	80	134	129	107
Phosphorus	459	289	302	242	266	333	367
Sodium	9	15	4	5	38	4	3
Potassium	389	318	247	286	319	373	337
Zinc	3.4	2.2	1.9	2.1	1.9	2.9	3.4
Copper	0.44	0.98	0.56	0.39	0.30	0.42	0.44
Manganese	4.1	1.8	3.0	1.2	0.6	3.5	1.7
Iron	4.3	4.8	1.6	2.7	3.2	3.9	2.7

Source: Compiled from data from the U.S. Department of Agriculture, Agricultural Research Service (2008) and Welch (2006).

carotenoids, such as β-carotene, referred to as "provitamin A." It's worth noting that β-carotene is not found in oats, although it occurs in modest quantities (<100 μg/kg) in wheat and rye, and is more prevalent in certain varieties of corn and genetically modified "golden rice." Vitamin D is not naturally present in cereals, while most cereals do contain small amounts of phylloquinone, which is the plant form of vitamin K. Vitamin E, represented by tocols including tocopherols and tocotrienols, is present in all cereal grains [117]. Its primary role is as a fat-soluble antioxidant, guarding against lipid oxidation and mitigating damage caused by free radicals. Vitamin E is renowned for protecting the body against free radical-induced harm and is significant in the prevention of conditions such as cancer, arthritis, atherosclerosis, and cataracts. Oat germ is particularly rich in tocopherols, encompassing both α and γ isomers, whereas tocotrienols are mainly concentrated in the endosperm but are absent in the germ. The primary tocol in oats is α-tocotrienol, but small quantities of tocopherols and their β homologs are also present. Conversely, water-soluble vitamins, such as vitamin C (ascorbic acid), act as antioxidants within the aqueous phase of physiological systems [118]. They also function as enzyme cofactors and enhance the absorption of dietary iron. However, vitamin C is not naturally occurring in cereal grains. Similarly, vitamin B12, crucial in the prevention of megaloblastic anaemia, is not found naturally in cereals. Nevertheless, all other water-soluble vitamins, including thiamin (B1), riboflavin (B2), niacin, vitamin B6 (comprising pyridoxine, pyridoxal, and pyridoxamine), pantothenic acid, folic acid, and biotin, are present in significant quantities in cereals. These vitamins serve as cofactors for enzymes engaged in various metabolic processes, including amino acid metabolism, energy production and methyl group metabolism [119] (Figure 3.4).

While humans possess the capability to synthesize choline in limited amounts, it is imperative to obtain dietary sources of choline to maintain overall health. Choline has gained recognition as an essential nutrient in recent years [120]. Though not categorized

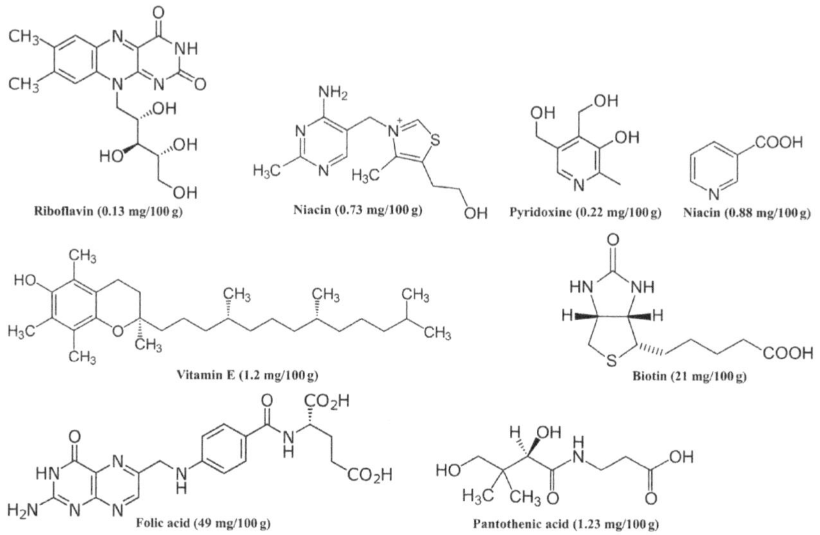

FIGURE 3.4 Vitamins in oat.

as a vitamin, recommended dietary intakes have been established. Choline plays a crucial role in methyl metabolism, ensuring cell membrane integrity, and contributing to various neurological functions [121]. Dietary niacin is another vital component. Nevertheless, niacin can be produced in the liver through the conversion of the amino acid tryptophan. It is estimated that 1 mg of niacin equivalents can be synthesized from every 60 mg of tryptophan ingested. Therefore, the total niacin equivalents are determined as the sum of niacin and (tryptophan/60). In comparison to other cereal grains, oats stand out for their elevated levels of thiamin, biotin, and choline [122]. They also exhibit relatively higher quantities of vitamin E, pantothenic acid, riboflavin, and folic acid. However, oats are relatively lower in niacin, niacin equivalents, and vitamin B6. It is important to emphasize that when assessing analytical data for vitamins, one must consider the context of nutritional requirements and availability [123] (Table 3.8).

3.2.5 Antioxidants

Antioxidants are compounds that can neutralize harmful oxidation reactions without interfering with essential oxidation processes in the body. The definition of an antioxidant is context-dependent and associated with oxidative stress in a biological setting. Scientifically, an antioxidant is described as a redox-active compound that mitigates oxidative stress by reacting non-enzymatically with a reactive oxidant [124]. In contrast, an antioxidant enzyme is defined as a protein that restricts oxidative stress by catalysing a redox reaction with a reactive oxidant. In human and animal biology, an antioxidant refers to any compound or mechanism that mitigates or counters oxidative stress either by lessening its cause or its effects [125].

TABLE 3.8 Vitamin Content (Representative Values per 100 g of Fresh Weight) of Oats and Other Whole Grains

	OATMEAL	CORNMEAL	WHOLE-GRAIN RYE	SORGHUM	WHOLE-GRAIN WHEAT	BROWN RICE	PEARLED BARLEY
Niacin (vitamin B_3) eq., mg	3.93	3.93	4.65	5.42	9.38	6.50	6.95
Niacin, mg	0.88	2.9	2.6	3.4	6.0	4.9	4.5
Thiamin (vitamin B_1), mg	0.73	0.39	0.36	0.29	0.47	0.47	0.23
Vitamin E, mg	1.2	0.50	1.4	1.13	1.1	1.0	0.33
Riboflavin (vitamin B_2), mg	0.13	0.16	0.24	0.15	0.15	0.07	0.08
Pyridoxine (vitamin B_6), mg	0.22	0.42	0.32	0.50	0.42	0.60	0.29
Biotin (vitamin B_7), mg	21	10	6	42	7	7	ND
Folic acid (vitamin B_9), mg	49	33	69	19	51	30	17
Pantothenic acid (vitamin B_5), mg	1.23	0.51	1.23	1.20	0.90	1.35	0.31
Choline, mg	40	22	30	ND	31	31	38

Source: Compiled from data from the U.S. Department of Agriculture, Agricultural Research Service (2008) and Welch (2006).
ND, no data available.
Niacin equivalents = niacin + (tryptophan/60).

A. sativa (Duke, 1992) has yielded an indole alkaloid, gramine, from its fruit, believed to be responsible for a mild sedative effect. Oats contain various polyphenolic compounds, including simple phenols like various phenolic acids, flavonoids, and anthranilamide compounds [126]. Among these, anthranilamide compounds serve as antioxidant components. Ferulic acid is the most abundant anthranilamide in oats, followed by *p*-coumaric acid, coffee phenol, and other simple phenols connected with 5-hydroxyanthranilic acid via amide bonds. Oats are also rich in physiologically active ingredients like polyphenols and gamma-aminobutyric acid [127]. These polyphenols have diverse physiological effects, encompassing anti-oxidative, anti-ageing, and anti-cancer properties, as well as cardiovascular and cerebrovascular protective effects. The contents of polyphenols and gamma-aminobutyric acid significantly increase during oat germination [128]. Although these compounds are primarily bound to cell wall cellulose or hemicellulose via ester bonds, they can be released upon germination. Moreover, oats contain unique antioxidants known as AVNs, which exhibit demonstrable beneficial effects in cardiovascular diseases [129].

Avenanthramides are phenolic compounds comprising anthranilic and hydroanthranilic acids linked to various hydroxycinnamic acids through amide bonds. The primary AVNs found in oats are A, B, and C [130]. These compounds have been reported to have beneficial effects, including antioxidant, antiproliferative, anti-atherogenic, and anti-inflammatory properties. Furthermore, oats contain tocols (tocopherols and tocotrienols), which are natural antioxidants existing as lipid-soluble compounds. Oats also harbour various organic acids such as maleic, citric, malonic, aconitic, and oxalic acid, along with antioxidant hydrolysed products like caffeic and ferulic acids and aliphatic alcohol [131]. Additionally, avenic acid A and B have been identified from the green herb of *A. sativa*, and avenalumic acids have been found in oat groats and hulls. Moreover, oats contain a range of flavonoids, triterpenoid saponins, and sterols. These various bioactive molecules of oats have demonstrated significant positive health outcomes [132]. They have been shown to possess anti-oxidative, anti-inflammatory, and bioactive properties, all of which contribute to reducing the risk of various diseases associated with oxidative stress. Furthermore, AVNs have been recognized for their heat stability under commercial processing conditions. The beneficial effects of oats' phenolic compounds have attracted considerable attention in both the scientific and health communities [133]. These compounds, especially AVNs, flavonoids, and sterols, have demonstrated potent antioxidant properties. Studies have revealed a strong correlation between antioxidant-rich oat-based foods and a reduced risk of diseases related to oxidative stress, including cancer, cardiovascular issues, and neurodegenerative diseases. Further research on oats and their bioactive components is ongoing, emphasizing the potential health benefits associated with their consumption [134].

3.2.6 Antinutritional Compounds

Antinutrients, compounds found in certain foods, can hinder the absorption of essential nutrients. Typically identified in plant-based foods, these antinutrients, such as phytate, tannins, lectins, and oxalates, may counteract the beneficial effects of the nutrient-rich whole grain, oats. Despite oats being recognized for their abundant reserves of vitamins, minerals, and dietary fibre, the presence of these interfering compounds can potentially exert unfavourable impacts on the body [114]. Also referred to as antinutritional factors, these substances, found ubiquitously in many food sources, can restrict the body's access to crucial nutrients. Antinutrients can be categorized into two primary groups based on their response to temperature changes. The first group comprises heat-stable antinutrients like phytic acid, condensed tannins, alkaloids, and saponins, which remain resistant even under high-temperature conditions. Conversely, the second group includes heat-labile antinutrients such as lectins, cyanogenic glycosides, protease inhibitors, and toxic amino acids, which are sensitive to standard temperatures and tend to degrade at higher temperatures [32]. Notably, some of the prominent antinutritional compounds identified in oats are described in the following subsections.

3.2.6.1 Phytic Acid

Oats, akin to several other grains, contain phytic acid, which can bind to crucial minerals like iron, zinc, and calcium, thereby impeding their absorption within the body. Notably, phytate stands out as one of the most prevalent antinutrients in oats [135]. Serving as a primary storage form of phosphorous and minerals in plants, phytate constitutes a significant proportion, ranging from 60% to 97%, of the total phosphorous in legumes and cereals. This compound undergoes hydrolysis by endogenous phytases during seed germination, facilitating the release of phosphates and minerals for the nourishment of the seedlings [136].

While oats possess a notable phytate content, their endogenous phytase activity is relatively lower compared to other cereals. Besides its recognized high antioxidant capacity, phytate is classified as an antinutrient owing to its tendency to bind with trace elements and minerals like zinc, iron, calcium, copper, and magnesium, consequently hindering their absorption in the human digestive system [114]. Moreover, phytate can also form complexes with protein and starch, thereby modifying their functionality and reducing their bioavailability. The salts of phytic acid, commonly referred to as phytates or phytin, are prevalent in various seed crops, where they restrict the bioavailability of essential minerals such as calcium, magnesium, iron, zinc, and manganese [137]. Consequently, accurate evaluations of grain crops necessitate cautious consideration of total phosphorus analyses, as a substantial portion of it may remain nutritionally inaccessible.

Despite its role as a storage compound within oats, phytic acid content diminishes significantly during germination, releasing inorganic phosphorus. Notably, in mature oat grains, the proportion of total phosphorus present as phytic acid remains consistently between 61% and 63%. Analyses of oat cultivars indicate the predominance of phosphorus, calcium, and magnesium in oat phytate, with smaller yet significant amounts of manganese [138]. Measurements across various oat cultivars highlight the total phosphorus content ranging from 0.37% to 0.45% on a dry weight basis, while phytic acid levels range from 0.82% to 1.01% in the same context. Naturally occurring in grains such as cereals, legumes, nuts, and oilseeds, phytic acid content in grains intensifies with maturity, constituting a substantial percentage, approximately 60% to 90%, of the dormant grain's total phosphorus [139]. Its characteristic negative charge allows it to bind with positively charged metal ions, forming complexes that diminish the bioavailability of these ions by impeding absorption rates [140]. Renowned for its role as a potent natural chelating agent due to the presence of six reactive phosphate groups, phytic acid represents the most significant antinutrient in food, contributing to mineral ion deficiencies in human and animal nutrition primarily through its chelating effects [141].

3.2.6.2 Avenin and Saponins

Oats, containing the protein avenin, might trigger allergic reactions in some, leading to digestive discomfort, skin rashes, or respiratory issues. Nonetheless, owing to the absence of gluten, oats are a favourable inclusion in gluten-free diets for individuals with celiac disease, as avenins are less prone to causing allergies [19]. Despite this advantage, the lack of gluten restricts their use in bakery products. Saponins, identified as secondary, non-volatile, active surface metabolites, occur in various plants and can either be steroids or triterpenes, with triterpenoid saponins commonly found in legumes, spinach leaves, quinoa grain, and other sources [142]. On the other hand, steroid saponins are present in oats, tomato seeds, fenugreek seeds, and yams. Adverse effects of saponins on human health include reduced iron absorption and impaired growth. Additionally, these compounds affect protein digestibility by altering protein structure and obstructing the action of digestive enzymes. Saponins are also recognized for their ability to cause hemolysis by interacting with the cholesterol group in the erythrocyte membrane [30].

Saponins, characterized as amphiphilic compounds with a lipophilic sapogenin part and a hydrophilic sugar part, are linked by a glycosidic bond. The carbohydrate component may consist of various oligosaccharide chains such as glucose, galactose, or pentose, while the sapogenin part can either be a steroid or triterpenoid [91]. There are two classes of saponins: steroidal saponins, featuring the characteristic four-ringed steroid nucleus, and triterpenoid saponins, lacking these extra rings. Although saponins are not commonly found in cereals and grasses, oats, switchgrass, and klein grass are exceptions, with oats synthesizing two distinct families of saponins, namely steroids avenacosides and triterpenoid avenacin, present in both their leaves and roots, with a concentration of 1.3 g/kg of dry weight [99].

While polyphenols are acknowledged for their antioxidant properties, they can hinder the absorption of certain nutrients, although their impact on nutrient absorption is relatively minor compared to other antinutritional factors [143]. Oats contain enzyme inhibitors that can disrupt the digestion and utilization of specific proteins, potentially leading to digestive disturbances and decreased nutrient absorption. Adequate processing techniques, such as soaking, fermenting, or cooking, can alleviate these antinutritional compounds in oats, enhancing their digestibility and overall nutritional quality. Individuals with specific allergies or sensitivities should consider moderating their intake or exploring alternative grains [144].

3.2.7 Conclusion

Oats, known for their rich nutrient content and drought-resistant nature, are valued sources of crucial nutrients, particularly protein and fat. They contain a notable concentration of beneficial mono and polyunsaturated fatty acids, along with a well-balanced amino acid composition. Notably, oats are also abundant in essential minerals vital for our overall well-being. Serving as an essential source of natural antioxidants, oat grains contribute significantly to human health, mitigating the risk of various diseases. This has led to their widespread use in functional food formulations, cementing their position as a pivotal component of a healthy diet and a promising plant-based food for the future, aligning with the goal of global health improvement. In the context of nutritional security, oats present a viable solution, especially for populations with limited access to diverse dietary sources. However, the unique challenges posed by coarse cereal grains, including issues related to grain quality and shelf life, call for innovative processing technologies to produce stable, readily consumable products. Considering the potential of coarse cereal grains for the food processing industry, it is imperative to explore their commercialization for alternative and healthy food purposes, taking into account the associated challenges and opportunities. Given the escalating prevalence of chronic diseases globally, preventative measures, including dietary and lifestyle modifications, are critical. Cereal grains, such as oats, play a pivotal role in a healthy diet, offering a comprehensive range of macronutrients, micronutrients, phytonutrients, and fibre, each contributing unique health benefits. Extensive research on oats has highlighted their potential to lower the risk of coronary heart disease and regulate glycaemia, with emerging evidence suggesting additional benefits for immunity, digestive health, and satiety.

In conclusion, the high nutritional and health value of oats, primarily attributed to their soluble dietary fibre β-glucan content, solidifies their significance as a global cereal crop. To unlock their full potential, further research is imperative to unravel the intricate interactions of oat compounds in the digestive tract, offering valuable insights for the development of healthier food products. Robust advertising and promotion of oat-based foods, alongside ongoing research and development in food systems, are pivotal for the continuous advancement and utilization of oats in diverse food products.

REFERENCES

[1] C. Agostoni, M. Baglioni, A. La Vecchia, G. Molari and C. Berti, "Interlinkages between climate change and food systems: The impact on child malnutrition – Narrative review," *Nutrients.*, vol. 15, p. 416, 2023, doi: 10.3390/nu15020416.

[2] E. Muñoz-Redondo et al., "New perspectives on frailty in light of the global leadership initiative on malnutrition, the global leadership initiative on sarcopenia, and the WHO's concept of intrinsic capacity: A narrative review," *Maturitas.*, vol. 177, p. 107799, 2023, doi: 10.1016/j.maturitas.2023.107799.

[3] S. A. O. Adeyeye, T. J. Ashaolu, O. T. Bolaji, T. A. Abegunde and A. O. Omoyajowo, "Africa and the Nexus of poverty, malnutrition and diseases," *Crit. Rev. Food Sci. Nutr.*, vol. 63, pp. 641–656, 2023, doi: 10.1080/10408398.2021.1952160.

[4] M. Springmann et al., "Options for keeping the food system within environmental limits," *Nature.*, vol. 562, pp. 519–525, 2018, doi: 10.1038/s41586-018-0594-0.

[5] A. Manzoor, B. Yousuf, J. A. Pandith and S. Ahmad, "Plant-derived active substances incorporated as antioxidant, antibacterial or antifungal components in coatings/films for food packaging applications," *Food Biosci.*, vol. 53, p. 102717, 2023, doi: 10.1016/j.fbio.2023.102717.

[6] Y. Wang et al., "Flavor challenges in extruded plant-based meat alternatives: A review," *Compr. Rev. Food Sci. Food Saf.*, vol. 21, pp. 2898–2929, 2022, doi: 10.1111/1541-4337.12964.

[7] M. Kumar et al., "Advances in the plant protein extraction: Mechanism and recommendations," *Food Hydrocoll.*, vol. 115, p. 106595, 2021, doi: 10.1016/j.foodhyd.2021.106595.

[8] M. Kumar et al., "Cottonseed feedstock as a source of plant-based protein and bioactive peptides: Evidence based on biofunctionalities and industrial applications," *Food Hydrocoll.*, vol. 131, p. 107776, 2022, doi: 10.1016/j.foodhyd.2022.107776.

[9] M. Kumar et al., "Cottonseed: A sustainable contributor to global protein requirements," *Trends Food Sci. Technol.*, vol. 111, pp. 100–113, 2021, doi: 10.1016/j.tifs.2021.02.058.

[10] M. Kumar et al., "Functional characterization of plant-based protein to determine its quality for food applications," *Food Hydrocoll.*, p. 106986, 2021, doi: 10.1016/j.foodhyd.2021.106986.

[11] M. Kumar et al., "Plant-based proteins and their multifaceted industrial applications," *LWT.*, vol. 154, p. 112620, 2022, doi: 10.1016/j.lwt.2021.112620.

[12] M. Tomar et al., "Interactome of millet-based food matrices: A review," *Food Chem.*, vol. 385, p. 132636, 2022, doi: 10.1016/j.foodchem.2022.132636.

[13] H. Choi and S. W. Kim, "Characterization of β-glucans from cereal and microbial sources and their roles in feeds for intestinal health and growth of nursery pigs," *Animals.*, vol. 13, p. 2236, 2023, doi: 10.3390/ani13132236.

[14] R. F. Park et al., "Breeding oat for resistance to the crown rust pathogen Puccinia coronata f. sp. avenae: Achievements and prospects," *Theor. Appl. Genet.*, vol. 135, pp. 3709–3734, 2022, doi: 10.1007/s00122-022-04121-z.

[15] N. Kamal et al., "The mosaic oat genome gives insights into a uniquely healthy cereal crop," *Nature.*, vol. 606, pp. 113–119, 2022, doi: 10.1038/s41586-022-04732-y.

[16] N. U. Sruthi and P. S. Rao, "Effect of processing on storage stability of millet flour: A review," *Trends Food Sci. Technol.*, vol. 112, pp. 58–74, 2021, doi: 10.1016/j.tifs.2021.03.043.

[17] G. F. Alemayehu, S. F. Forsido, Y. B. Tola and E. Amare, "Nutritional and phytochemical composition and associated health benefits of oat (*Avena sativa*) grains and oat-based fermented food products," *Sci. World J.*, vol. 2023, p. e2730175, 2023, doi: 10.1155/2023/2730175.

[18] B. Nemzer and F. Al-Taher, "Analysis of fatty acid composition in sprouted grains," *Foods.*, vol. 12, p. 1853, 2023, doi: 10.3390/foods12091853.

[19] D. Paudel, B. Dhungana, M. Caffe and P. Krishnan, "A review of health-beneficial properties of oats," *Foods.*, vol. 10, p. 2591, 2021, doi: 10.3390/foods10112591.

[20] I. G. Loskutov and E. K. Khlestkina, "Wheat, barley, and oat breeding for health benefit components in grain," *Plants.*, vol. 10, p. 86, 2021, doi: 10.3390/plants10010086.

[21] J. Spaen and J. V. C. Silva, "Oat proteins: Review of extraction methods and techno-functionality for liquid and semi-solid applications," *LWT.*, vol. 147, p. 111478, 2021, doi: 10.1016/j.lwt.2021.111478.

[22] M. Tomar, Reetu and S. S. Changan, "Potato vitamins," in *Potatoes for Food and Nutritional Security*, P. Raigond, B. Singh, S. Dutt and S. K. Chakrabarti, Eds. Singapore, Singapore: Springer, 2020, pp. 113–132, doi: 10.1007/978-981-15-7662-1_7.

[23] R. J. McGorrin, "Key aroma compounds in oats and oat cereals," *J. Agric. Food Chem.*, vol. 67, pp. 13778–13789, 2019, doi: 10.1021/acs.jafc.9b00994.

[24] C.-N. Popa, R.-M. Tamba-Berehoiu, "Chapter 10 – Oat flour in bread manufacturing," in *Trends in Wheat and Bread Making*, C. M. Galanakis, Ed. Academic Press, 2021, pp. 279–309, doi: 10.1016/B978-0-12-821048-2.00010-6.

[25] L. Kumar, R. Sehrawat and Y. Kong, "Oat proteins: A perspective on functional properties," *LWT.*, vol. 152, p. 112307, 2021, doi: 10.1016/j.lwt.2021.112307.

[26] Y.-F. Chu et al., "In vitro antioxidant capacity and anti-inflammatory activity of seven common oats," *Food Chem.*, vol. 139, pp. 426–431, 2013, doi: 10.1016/j.foodchem.2013.01.104.

[27] S. S. Cho, L. Qi, G. C. Fahey Jr and D. M. Klurfeld, "Consumption of cereal fiber, mixtures of whole grains and bran, and whole grains and risk reduction in type 2 diabetes, obesity, and cardiovascular disease1234," *Am. J. Clin. Nutr.*, vol. 98, pp. 594–619, 2013, doi: 10.3945/ajcn.113.067629.

[28] D. Aune et al., "Dietary fibre, whole grains, and risk of colorectal cancer: Systematic review and dose-response meta-analysis of prospective studies," *BMJ.*, vol. 343, p. d6617, 2011, doi: 10.1136/bmj.d6617.

[29] R. Singh, S. De and A. Belkheir, "Avena sativa (oat), a potential neutraceutical and therapeutic agent: An overview," *Crit. Rev. Food Sci. Nutr.*, vol. 53, pp. 126–144, 2013, doi: 10.1080/10408398.2010.526725.

[30] Y. Tang et al., "Bioactive components and health functions of oat," *Food Rev. Int.*, vol. 39, pp. 4545–4564, 2023, doi: 10.1080/87559129.2022.2029477.

[31] H. Rafique et al., "Dietary-nutraceutical properties of oat protein and peptides," *Front. Nutr.*, vol. 9, 2022. Accessed: Sept. 23, 2023. [Online]. Available: www.frontiersin.org/articles/10.3389/fnut.2022.950400.

[32] Q. Yu, J. Qian, Y. Guo, H. Qian, W. Yao and Y. Cheng, "Applicable strains, processing techniques and health benefits of fermented oat beverages: A review," *Foods.*, vol. 12, p. 1708, 2023, doi: 10.3390/foods12081708.

[33] M. Tomar et al., "Nutritional composition patterns and application of multivariate analysis to evaluate indigenous Pearl millet ((*Pennisetum glaucum* (L.) R. Br.) germplasm," *J. Food Compos. Anal.*, vol. 103, p. 104086, 2021, doi: 10.1016/j.jfca.2021.104086.

[34] A. Naderi et al., "Carbohydrates and endurance exercise: A narrative review of a food first approach," *Nutrients.*, vol. 15, p. 1367, 2023, doi: 10.3390/nu15061367.

[35] A. Apriyanto, J. Compart and J. Fettke, "A review of starch, a unique biopolymer – Structure, metabolism and in planta modifications," *Plant Sci.*, vol. 318, p. 111223, 2022, doi: 10.1016/j.plantsci.2022.111223.

[36] S. L. M. El Halal, D. H. Kringel, E. D. R. Zavareze and A. R. G. Dias, "Methods for extracting cereal starches from different sources: A review," *Starch – Stärke.*, vol. 71, p. 1900128, 2019, doi: 10.1002/star.201900128.

[37] C. Yi, N. Qiang, H. Zhu, Q. Xiao and Z. Li, "Extrusion processing: A strategy for improving the functional components, physicochemical properties, and health benefits of whole grains," *Food Res. Int.*, vol. 160, p. 111681, 2022, doi: 10.1016/j.foodres.2022.111681.

[38] R. Hoover and T. Vasanthan, "Studies on isolation and characterization of starch from oat (Avena nuda) grains," *Carbohydr. Polym.*, vol. 19, pp. 285–297, 1992, doi: 10.1016/0144-8617(92)90082-2.

[39] H. Rostamabadi et al., "Oat starch – How physical and chemical modifications affect the physicochemical attributes and digestibility?," *Carbohydr. Polym.*, vol. 296, p. 119931, 2022, doi: 10.1016/j.carbpol.2022.119931.

[40] K. Zhang, R. Dong, X. Hu, C. Ren and Y. Li, "Oat-based foods: Chemical constituents, glycemic index, and the effect of processing," *Foods.*, vol. 10, p. 1304, 2021, doi: 10.3390/foods10061304.

[41] M. Ovando-Martínez, K. Whitney, B. L. Reuhs, D. C. Doehlert and S. Simsek, "Effect of hydrothermal treatment on physicochemical and digestibility properties of oat starch," *Food Res. Int.*, vol. 52, pp. 17–25, 2013, doi: 10.1016/j.foodres.2013.02.035.

[42] P. Kaur, K. Kaur, S. J. Basha and J. F. Kennedy, "Current trends in the preparation, characterization and applications of oat starch – A review," *Int. J. Biol. Macromol.*, vol. 212, pp. 172–181, 2022, doi: 10.1016/j.ijbiomac.2022.05.117.

[43] N. M. Thani, M. M. Mazlan, N. I. N. Haris and M. H. Wondi, "Oat thermoplastic starch nanocomposite films reinforced with nanocellulose," *Phys. Sci. Rev.*, 2023, doi: 10.1515/psr-2022-0036.

[44] M. Papageorgiou and A. Skendi, "Introduction to cereal processing and by-products," in *Sustainable Recovery and Reutilization of Cereal Processing by-Products*, C. M. Galanakis, Ed. Woodhead Publishing, 2018, pp. 1–25, doi: 10.1016/B978-0-08-102162-0.00001-0.

[45] A. Shah, F. A. Masoodi, A. Gani and B. Ashwar, "Dual enzyme modified oat starch: Structural characterisation, rheological properties, and digestibility in simulated GI tract," *Int. J. Biol. Macromol.*, vol. 106, pp. 140–147, 2018, doi: 10.1016/j.ijbiomac.2017.08.013.

[46] P. Zwer, "Oats: Characteristics and quality requirements," in *Cereal Grains*, C. W. Wrigley and I. L. Batey, Eds. Woodhead Publishing, 2010, pp. 163–182, doi: 10.1533/9781845699529.2.163.

[47] D. Cozzolino, "The use of the rapid visco analyser (RVA) in breeding and selection of cereals," *J. Cereal Sci.*, vol. 70, pp. 282–290, 2016, doi: 10.1016/j.jcs.2016.07.003.

[48] R. Mukhtar et al., "γ-Irradiation of oat grain – Effect on physico-chemical, structural, thermal, and antioxidant properties of extracted starch," *Int. J. Biol. Macromol.*, vol. 104, pp. 1313–1320, 2017, doi: 10.1016/j.ijbiomac.2017.05.092.

[49] A. Aigster, S. E. Duncan, F. D. Conforti and W. E. Barbeau, "Physicochemical properties and sensory attributes of resistant starch-supplemented granola bars and cereals," *LWT Food Sci. Technol.*, vol. 44, pp. 2159–2165, 2011, doi: 10.1016/j.lwt.2011.07.018.

[50] J. H. Jeong, S. Y. Hong, J.-S. Cho, D.-H. Cho and E. Y. Park, "Impact of enzyme modification on physicochemical properties of oat flake and starch," *Starch – Stärke.*, vol. 74, p. 2100292, 2022, doi: 10.1002/star.202100292.

[51] W. Truscott, "Glove powder reduction and alternative approaches," *Methods.*, vol. 27, pp. 69–76, 2002, doi: 10.1016/S1046-2023(02)00054-3.

[52] N. Ren, Z. Ma, J. Xu and X. Hu, "Insights into the supramolecular structure and techno-functional properties of starch isolated from oat rice kernels subjected to different processing treatments," *Food Chem.*, vol. 317, p. 126464, 2020, doi: 10.1016/j.foodchem.2020.126464.

[53] Y. I. Cornejo-Ramírez, O. Martínez-Cruz, C. L. Del Toro-Sánchez, F. J. Wong-Corral, J. Borboa-Flores and F. J. Cinco-Moroyoqui, "The structural characteristics of starches and their functional properties," *CyTA J. Food.*, vol. 16, pp. 1003–1017, 2018, doi: 10.1080/19476337.2018.1518343.

[54] P. Kasturi and N. Bordenave, "Oat starch," in *Oats Nutrition and Technology*, John Wiley & Sons, Ltd, 2013, pp. 95–121, doi: 10.1002/9781118354100.ch5.

[55] A. Bojarczuk, S. Skąpska, A. Mousavi Khaneghah and K. Marszałek, "Health benefits of resistant starch: A review of the literature," *J. Funct. Foods.*, vol. 93, p. 105094, 2022, doi: 10.1016/j.jff.2022.105094.

[56] E. Ünlü and Ç. Aykaç, "Effect of ultrasound on isolation and properties of oat starch," *Czech J. Food Sci.*, vol. 41, 2023, doi: 10.17221/94/2022-CJFS.

[57] L. Sushytskyi et al., "Perspectives in the application of high, medium, and low molecular weight oat β-d-glucans in dietary nutrition and food technology – A short overview," *Foods.*, vol. 12, p. 1121, 2023, doi: 10.3390/foods12061121.

[58] Y. Li, M. Obadi, J. Shi, B. Xu and Y.-C. Shi, "Rheological and thermal properties of oat flours and starch affected by oat lipids," *J. Cereal Sci.*, vol. 102, p. 103337, 2021, doi: 10.1016/j.jcs.2021.103337.

[59] Y. Wen, T. Yao, Y. Xu, H. Corke and Z. Sui, "Pasting, thermal and rheological properties of octenylsuccinylate modified starches from diverse small granule starches differing in amylose content," *J. Cereal Sci.*, vol. 95, p. 103030, 2020, doi: 10.1016/j.jcs.2020.103030.

[60] R. F. Tester, J. Karkalas and X. Qi, "Starch – Composition, fine structure and architecture," *J. Cereal Sci.*, vol. 39, pp. 151–165, 2004, doi: 10.1016/j.jcs.2003.12.001.

[61] M. Gallo et al., "Lactic fermentation of cereal flour: Feasibility tests on rice, oat and wheat," *Appl. Food Biotechnol.*, vol. 6, pp. 165–172, 2019, doi: 10.22037/afb. v6i3.24299.

[62] Y. Gu, X. Qian, B. Sun, S. Ma, X. Tian and X. Wang, "Nutritional composition and physicochemical properties of oat flour sieving fractions with different particle size," *LWT.*, vol. 154, p. 112757, 2022, doi: 10.1016/j.lwt.2021.112757.

[63] X. Qian, B. Sun, C. Zhu, Z. Zhang, X. Tian and X. Wang, "Effect of stir-frying on oat milling and pasting properties and rheological properties of oat flour," *J. Cereal Sci.*, vol. 92, p. 102908, 2020, doi: 10.1016/j.jcs.2020.102908.

[64] H. Li, S. Prakash, T. M. Nicholson, M. A. Fitzgerald and R. G. Gilbert, "The importance of amylose and amylopectin fine structure for textural properties of cooked rice grains," *Food Chem.*, vol. 196, pp. 702–711, 2016, doi: 10.1016/j.foodchem.2015.09.112.

[65] T. T. L. Nguyen, S. Mitra, R. G. Gilbert, M. J. Gidley and G. P. Fox, "Influence of heat treatment on starch structure and physicochemical properties of oats," *J. Cereal Sci.*, vol. 89, p. 102805, 2019, doi: 10.1016/j.jcs.2019.102805.

[66] K. Wang, R. J. Henry and R. G. Gilbert, "Causal relations among starch biosynthesis, structure, and properties," *Springer Sci. Rev.*, vol. 2, pp. 15–33, 2014, doi: 10.1007/s40362-014-0016-0.

[67] B. Pfister and S. C. Zeeman, "Formation of starch in plant cells," *Cell. Mol. Life Sci.*, vol. 73, pp. 2781–2807, 2016, doi: 10.1007/s00018-016-2250-x.

[68] E. H. Hipsley and K. O. A. Vickery, "Dietary fat and dietary sugar," *Lancet.*, vol. 284, pp. 759–760, 1964, doi: 10.1016/S0140-6736(64)92590-5.

[69] T. M. Barber, S. Kabisch, A. F. H. Pfeiffer and M. O. Weickert, "The health benefits of dietary fibre," *Nutrients.*, vol. 12, p. 3209, 2020, doi: 10.3390/nu12103209.

[70] S. K. Gill, M. Rossi, B. Bajka and K. Whelan, "Dietary fibre in gastrointestinal health and disease," *Nat. Rev. Gastroenterol. Hepatol.*, vol. 18, pp. 101–116, 2021, doi: 10.1038/s41575-020-00375-4.

[71] P. Cronin, S. A. Joyce, P. W. O'Toole and E. M. O'Connor, "Dietary fibre modulates the gut microbiota," *Nutrients.*, vol. 13, p. 1655, 2021, doi: 10.3390/nu13051655.

[72] H. Zhou et al., "Regulation of poultry lipid metabolism by dietary fibre: A review," *Worlds Poult. Sci. J.*, vol. 79, pp. 485–496, 2023, doi: 10.1080/00439339.2023.2234337.

[73] N. Prasad and I. Joye, "Dietary fibre from whole grains and their benefits on metabolic health," *Nutrients.*, vol. 12, p. 3045, 2020, doi: 10.3390/nu12103045.

[74] A. N. Reynolds, A. Akerman, S. Kumar, H. T. Diep Pham, S. Coffey and J. Mann, "Dietary fibre in hypertension and cardiovascular disease management: Systematic review and meta-analyses," *BMC Med.*, vol. 20, p. 139, 2022, doi: 10.1186/s12916-022-02328-x.

[75] P. Wróblewska, T. Hikawczuk, K. Sierżant, A. Wiliczkiewicz and A. Szuba-Trznadel, "Effect of oat hull as a source of insoluble dietary fibre on changes in the microbial status of gastrointestinal tract in broiler chickens," *Animals.*, vol. 12, p. 2721, 2022, doi: 10.3390/ani12192721.

[76] M. Nikinmaa, O. Zehnder-Wyss, L. Nyström and N. Sozer, "Effect of extrusion processing parameters on structure, texture and dietary fibre composition of directly expanded wholegrain oat-based matrices," *LWT.*, vol. 184, p. 114972, 2023, doi: 10.1016/j.lwt.2023.114972.

[77] A. Torbica, M. Radosavljević, M. Belović, T. Tamilselvan and P. Prabhasankar, "Biotechnological tools for cereal and pseudocereal dietary fibre modification in the bakery products creation – Advantages, disadvantages and challenges," *Trends Food Sci. Technol.*, vol. 129, pp. 194–209, 2022, doi: 10.1016/j.tifs.2022.09.018.

[78] L. Saturni, G. Ferretti and T. Bacchetti, "The gluten-free diet: Safety and nutritional quality," *Nutrients.*, vol. 2, pp. 16–34, 2010, doi: 10.3390/nu2010016.

[79] F. Boukid, "Oat proteins as emerging ingredients for food formulation: Where we stand?," *Eur. Food Res. Technol.*, vol. 247, pp. 535–544, 2021, doi: 10.1007/s00217-020-03661-2.

[80] L. L'Hocine et al., "Assessment of protein nutritional quality of novel hairless canary seed in comparison to wheat and oat using in vitro static digestion models," *Nutrients.*, vol. 15, p. 1347, 2023, doi: 10.3390/nu15061347.

[81] M. Yaman, H. S. SargÄ±n, Ã. F. MÄ±zrak, H. UÄŸur, J. Ãatak and E. Duman, "Amino acid profile and in vitro protein digestibility-corrected amino acid score (PDCAAS) of ready-to-eat breakfast cereals: An assessment of protein quality: Protein quality of ready-to-eat breakfast cereals," *Lat. Am. Appl. Res. Int. J.*, vol. 51, pp. 203–210, 2021, doi: 10.52292/j.laar.2021.739.

[82] D. Anwar and G. El-Chaghaby, "Nutritional quality, amino acid profiles, protein digestibility corrected amino acid scores and antioxidant properties of fried tofu and seitan," *Food Environ. Saf.*, vol. 18, pp. 176–190, 2019. Accessed: Oct. 13, 2023. Available: www.cabdirect.org/globalhealth/abstract/20193475132

[83] A. K. Stone, M. G. Nosworthy, C. Chiremba, J. D. House and M. T. Nickerson, "A comparative study of the functionality and protein quality of a variety of legume and cereal flours," *Cereal Chem.*, vol. 96, pp. 1159–1169, 2019, doi: 10.1002/cche.10226.

[84] Y. Zheng et al., "Isolation of novel ACE-inhibitory peptide from naked oat globulin hydrolysates in silico approach: Molecular docking, in vivo antihypertension and effects on renin and intracellular endothelin-1," *J. Food Sci.*, vol. 85, pp. 1328–1337, 2020, doi: 10.1111/1750-3841.15115.

[85] S. Ma, M. Zhang, X. Bao and Y. Fu, "Preparation of antioxidant peptides from oat globulin," *CyTA J. Food.*, vol. 18, pp. 108–115, 2020, doi: 10.1080/19476337.2020.1716076.

[86] B. Korpela, L. Pitkänen and M. Heinonen, "Enzymatic modification of oat globulin enables covalent interaction with procyanidin B2," *Food Chem.*, vol. 395, p. 133568, 2022, doi: 10.1016/j.foodchem.2022.133568.

[87] T. He, J. Wang and X. Hu, "Effect of heat treatment on the structure and digestion properties of oat globulin," *Cereal Chem.*, vol. 98, pp. 740–748, 2021, doi: 10.1002/cche.10417.

[88] R. Mel and M. Malalgoda, "Oat protein as a novel protein ingredient: Structure, functionality, and factors impacting utilization," *Cereal Chem.*, vol. 99, pp. 21–36, 2022, doi: 10.1002/cche.10488.

[89] J. Zhou et al., "Oat plant amyloids for sustainable functional materials," *Adv. Sci.*, vol. 9, p. 2104445, 2022, doi: 10.1002/advs.202104445.

[90] B. A. Sunilkumar and E. Tareke, "Review of analytical methods for measurement of oat proteins: The need for standardized methods," *Crit. Rev. Food Sci. Nutr.*, vol. 59, pp. 1467–1485, 2019, doi: 10.1080/10408398.2017.1414029.

[91] D. J. Liska, E. Dioum, Y. Chu and E. Mah, "Narrative review on the effects of oat and sprouted oat components on blood pressure," *Nutrients.*, vol. 14, p. 4772, 2022, doi: 10.3390/nu14224772.

[92] F. Islam et al., "Vegetable proteins as encapsulating agents: Recent updates and future perspectives," *Food Sci. Nutr.*, vol. 11, pp. 1705–1717, 2023, doi: 10.1002/fsn3.3234.

[93] K. Kosová, L. Leišová-Svobodová and V. Dvořáček, "Oats as a safe alternative to triticeae cereals for people suffering from celiac disease? A review," *Plant Foods Hum. Nutr.*, vol. 75, pp. 131–141, 2020, doi: 10.1007/s11130-020-00800-8.

[94] D. Dhakal, T. Younas, R. P. Bhusal, L. Devkota, C. J. Henry and S. Dhital, "Design rules of plant-based yoghurt-mimic: Formulation, functionality, sensory profile and nutritional value," *Food Hydrocoll.*, vol. 142, p. 108786, 2023, doi: 10.1016/j.foodhyd.2023.108786.

[95] I. Cohen, A. S. Day and R. Shaoul, "To be oats or not to be? An update on the ongoing debate on oats for patients with celiac disease," *Front. Pediatr.*, vol. 7, 2019. Accessed: Oct. 6, 2023. [Online] Available: www.frontiersin.org/articles/10.3389/fped.2019.00384.

[96] A. F. G. Cicero et al., "A randomized placebo-controlled clinical trial to evaluate the medium-term effects of oat fibers on human health: The beta-glucan effects on lipid profile, glycemia and intestinal health (BELT) study," *Nutrients.*, vol. 12, p. 686, 2020, doi: 10.3390/nu12030686.

[97] M. R. Sahasrabudhe, "Lipid composition of oats (Avena sativa L.)," *J. Am. Oil Chem. Soc.*, vol. 56, pp. 80–84, 1979, doi: 10.1007/BF02914274.

[98] M. Havrlentová et al., "The influence of artificial fusarium infection on oat grain quality," *Microorganisms.*, vol. 9, p. 2108, 2021, doi: 10.3390/microorganisms9102108.

[99] J. Bouchard et al., "Impact of oats in the prevention/management of hypertension," *Food Chem.*, vol. 381, p. 132198, 2022, doi: 10.1016/j.foodchem.2022.132198.

[100] P. B. Price and J. G. Parsons, "Lipids of seven cereal grains," *J. Am. Oil Chem. Soc.*, vol. 52, pp. 490–493, 1975, doi: 10.1007/BF02640738.

[101] H. Hu et al., "Heritable temporal gene expression patterns correlate with metabolomic seed content in developing hexaploid oat seed," *Plant Biotechnol. J.*, vol. 18, pp. 1211–1222, 2020, doi: 10.1111/pbi.13286.

[102] M. T. Campbell et al., "Translating insights from the seed metabolome into improved prediction for lipid-composition traits in oat (Avena sativa L.)," *Genetics.*, vol. 217, p. iyaa043, 2021, doi: 10.1093/genetics/iyaa043.

[103] M. Immonen, A. Chandrakusuma, S. Hokkanen, R. Partanen, N. Mäkelä-Salmi and P. Myllärinen, "The effect of deamidation and lipids on the interfacial and foaming properties of ultrafiltered oat protein concentrates," *LWT.*, vol. 169, p. 114016, 2022, doi: 10.1016/j.lwt.2022.114016.

[104] D. Sargautis, T. Kince and I. Gramatina, "Characterisation of the enzymatically extracted oat protein concentrate after defatting and its applicability for wet extrusion," *Foods.*, vol. 12, p. 2333, 2023, doi: 10.3390/foods12122333.

[105] A. Purushothaman, P. Jishnu Gopal and D. Janardanan, "Mechanistic insights on the radical scavenging activity of oat avenanthramides," *J. Phys. Org. Chem.*, vol. 35, p. e4391, 2022, doi: 10.1002/poc.4391.

[106] M. Zhou, K. Robards, M. Glennie-Holmes and S. Helliwell, "Oat lipids," *J. Am. Oil Chem. Soc.*, vol. 76, pp. 159–169, 1999, doi: 10.1007/s11746-999-0213-1

[107] S.-H. Chon, R. Tannahill, X. Yao, M. D. Southall and A. Pappas, "Keratinocyte differentiation and upregulation of ceramide synthesis induced by an oat lipid extract via the activation of PPAR pathways," *Exp. Dermatol.*, vol. 24, pp. 290–295, 2015, doi: 10.1111/exd.12658.

[108] D. C. Doehlert, S. Angelikousis and B. Vick, "Accumulation of oxygenated fatty acids in oat lipids during storage," *Cereal Chem.*, vol. 87, pp. 532–537, 2010, doi: 10.1094/CCHEM-05-10-0074.

[109] I. Marmouzi et al., "Nutritional characteristics, biochemical composition and antioxidant activities of Moroccan Oat varieties," *J. Food Meas. Charact.*, vol. 10, pp. 156–165, 2016, doi: 10.1007/s11694-015-9289-5.

[110] E. Schmitz, E. Nordberg Karlsson and P. Adlercreutz, "Warming weather changes the chemical composition of oat hulls," *Plant Biol.*, vol. 22, pp. 1086–1091, 2020, doi: 10.1111/plb.13171.

[111] A. Chappell et al., "The agronomic performance and nutritional content of oat and barley varieties grown in a northern maritime environment depends on variety and growing conditions," *J. Cereal Sci.*, vol. 74, pp. 1–10, 2017, doi: 10.1016/j.jcs.2017.01.005.

[112] J. V. de Oliveira Maximino et al., "Mineral and fatty acid content variation in white oat genotypes grown in Brazil," *Biol. Trace Elem. Res.*, vol. 199, pp. 1194–1206, 2021, doi: 10.1007/s12011-020-02229-1.

[113] G. E. Inglett, D. Chen and S. X. Liu, "Physical properties of gluten-free sugar cookies made from amaranth–oat composites," *LWT Food Sci. Technol.*, vol. 63, pp. 214–220, 2015, doi: 10.1016/j.lwt.2015.03.056.

[114] S. Kaur, R. D. Bhardwaj, R. Kapoor and S. K. Grewal, "Biochemical characterization of oat (Avena sativa L.) genotypes with high nutritional potential," *LWT.*, vol. 110, pp. 32–39, 2019, doi: 10.1016/j.lwt.2019.04.063.

[115] N. Aparicio-García, C. Martínez-Villaluenga, J. Frias and E. Peñas, "Sprouted oat as a potential gluten-free ingredient with enhanced nutritional and bioactive properties," *Food Chem.*, vol. 338, p. 127972, 2021, doi: 10.1016/j.foodchem.2020.127972.

[116] J. J. Gutierrez-Gonzalez and D. F. Garvin, "Subgenome-specific assembly of vitamin E biosynthesis genes and expression patterns during seed development provide insight into the evolution of oat genome," *Plant Biotechnol. J.*, vol. 14, pp. 2147–2157, 2016, doi: 10.1111/pbi.12571.

[117]   A. Angelov, T. Yaneva-Marinova and V. Gotcheva, "Oats as a matrix of choice for developing fermented functional beverages," *J. Food Sci. Technol.*, vol. 55, pp. 2351–2360, 2018, doi: 10.1007/s13197-018-3186-y.

[118]   P. Russo et al., "Lactobacillus plantarum strains for multifunctional oat-based foods," *LWT Food Sci. Technol.*, vol. 68, pp. 288–294, 2016, doi: 10.1016/j.lwt.2015.12.040.

[119]   M.-Y. Liao et al., "Down-regulation of partial substitution for staple food by oat noodles on blood lipid levels: A randomized, double-blind, clinical trial," *J. Food Drug Anal.*, vol. 27, pp. 93–100, 2019, doi: 10.1016/j.jfda.2018.04.001.

[120]   V. L. Fulgoni, M. Brauchla, L. Fleige and Y. Chu, "Oatmeal-containing breakfast is associated with better diet quality and higher intake of key food groups and nutrients compared to other breakfasts in children," *Nutrients.*, vol. 11, p. 964, 2019, doi: 10.3390/nu11050964.

[121]   V. L. Fulgoni, Y. Chu, M. O'Shea, J. L. Slavin and M. A. DiRienzo, "Oatmeal consumption is associated with better diet quality and lower body mass index in adults: The National Health and Nutrition Examination Survey (NHANES)," *Nutr. Res.*, vol. 35, pp. 1052–1059, 2015, doi: 10.1016/j.nutres.2015.09.015.

[122]   J. W. Allwood et al., "Rapid UHPLC-MS metabolite profiling and phenotypic assays reveal genotypic impacts of nitrogen supplementation in oats," *Metabolomics.*, vol. 15, p. 42, 2019, doi: 10.1007/s11306-019-1501-x.

[123]   T. Steiner, M. Köhrmann, P. D. Schellinger and G. Tsivgoulis, "Non-vitamin K oral anticoagulants associated bleeding and its antidotes," *J. Stroke.*, vol. 20, pp. 292–301, 2018, doi: 10.5853/jos.2018.02250.

[124]   M. Hasanuzzaman et al., "Reactive oxygen species and antioxidant defense in plants under abiotic stress: Revisiting the crucial role of a universal defense regulator," *Antioxidants.*, vol. 9, p. 681, 2020, doi: 10.3390/antiox9080681.

[125]   J. Dumanović, E. Nepovimova, M. Natić, K. Kuča and V. Jaćević, "The significance of reactive oxygen species and antioxidant defense system in plants: A concise overview," *Front. Plant Sci.*, vol. 11, 2021. Accessed: Oct. 27, 2023. [Online]. Available: www.frontiersin.org/articles/10.3389/fpls.2020.552969

[126]   Y. Zhang, Y. Li, X. Ren, X. Zhang, Z. Wu and L. Liu, "The positive correlation of antioxidant activity and prebiotic effect about oat phenolic compounds," *Food Chem.*, vol. 402, p. 134231, 2023, doi: 10.1016/j.foodchem.2022.134231.

[127]   I.-S. Kim, C.-W. Hwang, W.-S. Yang and C.-H. Kim, "Multiple antioxidative and bioactive molecules of oats (Avena sativa L.) in human health," *Antioxidants.*, vol. 10, p. 1454, 2021, doi: 10.3390/antiox10091454.

[128]   S. Singh, M. Kaur, D. S. Sogi and S. S. Purewal, "A comparative study of phytochemicals, antioxidant potential and in-vitro DNA damage protection activity of different oat (Avena sativa) cultivars from India," *J. Food Meas. Charact.*, vol. 13, pp. 347–356, 2019, doi: 10.1007/s11694-018-9950-x.

[129]   E. Turrini, F. Maffei, A. Milelli, C. Calcabrini and C. Fimognari, "Overview of the anticancer profile of avenanthramides from oat," *Int. J. Mol. Sci.*, vol. 20, p. 4536, 2019, doi: 10.3390/ijms20184536.

[130]   N. L. Wankhede et al., "Overview on the polyphenol avenanthramide in oats (Avena sativa Linn.) as regulators of PI3K signaling in the management of neurodegenerative diseases," *Nutrients.*, vol. 15, p. 3751, 2023, doi: 10.3390/nu15173751.

[131]   Z. Li, Y. Chen, D. Meesapyodsuk and X. Qiu, "The biosynthetic pathway of major avenanthramides in oat," *Metabolites.*, vol. 9, p. 163, 2019, doi: 10.3390/metabo9080163.

[132]   G. Soycan et al., "Composition and content of phenolic acids and avenanthramides in commercial oat products: Are oats an important polyphenol source for consumers?," *Food Chem. X.*, vol. 3, p. 100047, 2019, doi: 10.1016/j.fochx.2019.100047.

[133]   Y. Yu et al., "The progress of nomenclature, structure, metabolism, and bioactivities of oat novel phytochemical: Avenanthramides," *J. Agric. Food Chem.*, vol. 70, pp. 446–457, 2022, doi: 10.1021/acs.jafc.1c05704.

[134] D. Wu, Y. Shi, T. Zhang and M. Miao, "The synergistic effect of ascorbic and abscisic acids on enriching AVC-dominated avenanthramides in oat germination process," *Food Biosci.*, vol. 54, p. 102850, 2023, doi: 10.1016/j.fbio.2023.102850.

[135] Y. Li et al., "Fermentation of Lactobacillus fermentum NB02 with feruloyl esterase production increases the phenolic compounds content and antioxidant properties of oat bran," *Food Chem.*, vol. 437, p. 137834, 2024, doi: 10.1016/j.foodchem.2023.137834.

[136] A. Kaleda et al., "Impact of fermentation and phytase treatment of pea-oat protein blend on physicochemical, sensory, and nutritional properties of extruded meat analogs," *Foods.*, vol. 9, p. 1059, 2020, doi: 10.3390/foods9081059.

[137] M. Saka, B. Özkaya and İ. Saka, "The effect of bread-making methods on functional and quality characteristics of oat bran blended bread," *Int. J. Gastron. Food Sci.*, vol. 26, p. 100439, 2021, doi: 10.1016/j.ijgfs.2021.100439.

[138] D. Qin, D. Toyonaga and H. Saneoka, "Characterization of myo-inositol-1-phosphate synthase (MIPS) gene expression and phytic acid accumulation in oat (Avena sativa) during seed development," *Cereal Res. Commun.*, vol. 50, pp. 379–384, 2022, doi: 10.1007/s42976-021-00186-6.

[139] N. Mäkelä, N. Rosa-Sibakov, Y.-J. Wang, O. Mattila, E. Nordlund and T. Sontag-Strohm, "Role of β-glucan content, molecular weight and phytate in the bile acid binding of oat β-glucan," *Food Chem.*, vol. 358, p. 129917, 2021, doi: 10.1016/j.foodchem.2021.129917.

[140] H. Mao et al., "The utilization of oat for the production of wholegrain foods: Processing technology and products," *Food Front.*, vol. 3, pp. 28–45, 2022, doi: 10.1002/fft2.120.

[141] M. S. Ibrahim, A. Ahmad, A. Sohail and M. J. Asad, "Nutritional and functional characterization of different oat (Avena sativa L.) cultivars," *Int. J. Food Prop.*, vol. 23, pp. 1373–1385, 2020, doi: 10.1080/10942912.2020.1806297.

[142] X. Li, L. Zhou, Y. Yu, J. Zhang, J. Wang and B. Sun, "The potential functions and mechanisms of oat on cancer prevention: A review," *J. Agric. Food Chem.*, vol. 70, pp. 14588–14599, 2022, doi: 10.1021/acs.jafc.2c06518.

[143] J. W. Allwood et al., "Assessing the impact of nitrogen supplementation in oats across multiple growth locations and years with targeted phenotyping and high-resolution metabolite profiling approaches," *Food Chem.*, vol. 355, p. 129585, 2021, doi: 10.1016/j.foodchem.2021.129585.

[144] A. V. Sirotkin, "The effect of dietary oat consumption and its constituents on fat storage and obesity," *Physiol. Res.*, vol. 72, pp. S157–S163, 2023.

Novel Bioactive Compounds, Phytochemicals, and Their Characterization in Oats

4

Sushil S. Changan, Vandana Parmar,
Pratapsingh Khapte, Dharmendra Kumar,
Milan Kumar Lal, Pinky Raigond,
and Brajesh Kumar Singh

4.1 INTRODUCTION

Natural compounds have a rich history of global use spanning thousands of years. However, a contemporary worldwide emphasis on health has significantly heightened the quest for natural alternatives to promote well-being. Numerous naturally derived compounds possess bioactive functions and have been extensively studied for diverse applications, particularly in the fields of food and pharmaceuticals [1]. These bioactive compounds encompass both essential and non-essential molecules, such as vitamins and polyphenols, which are found in nature, are integrated into the food chain, and

DOI: 10.1201/ 9781003263302-4

have been demonstrated to exert an impact on human health [2]. These substances are characterized by their unique chemical structures that serve specialized functions at the biological level. Bioactive compounds represent a broad category of naturally occurring essential and non-essential molecules capable of positively influencing human health. This diverse set of molecules exhibits varying chemical structures and distributions in nature and can be broadly categorized into four primary groups: terpenes and terpenoids, glycosides, phenolic compounds, and alkaloids [3].

Terpenes, also referred to as terpenoids, constitute the largest and most diverse group of naturally occurring compounds. They are categorized based on the number of isoprene units they contain, leading to classifications such as mono, di, tri, tetra, and sesquiterpenes. Terpenes play crucial roles in imparting fragrance, taste, and pigmentation to various substances. Terpenes are further categorized according to their structural organization and the number of isoprene units they consist of. An isoprene unit, which serves as the building block of terpenes, is a gaseous hydrocarbon with the molecular formula C_5H_8 [4]. Terpenes are volatile, unsaturated cyclic compounds composed of five carbons and naturally occur in nature. They are known for emitting distinct scents or flavours, which serve as a defence mechanism against organisms that may feed on certain plant types. Terpenoids, on the other hand, represent a modified subset of terpenes. They feature various functional groups and may have undergone oxidation or relocation of methyl groups [5]. While the terms "terpenes" and "terpenoids" are often used interchangeably, there are subtle differences between the two. Terpenes are naturally occurring compounds with volatile, unsaturated 5-carbon cyclic structures, contributing to scents or tastes. In contrast, terpenoids are derived from terpenes but may possess additional functional groups or altered chemical arrangements. Terpenes have multifaceted roles within plants, serving as thermoprotectants, facilitating signalling functions and contributing to attributes such as pigmentation, flavour, and solvency [6]. Additionally, they have various medicinal applications and are utilized in traditional and modern medicine for their therapeutic properties.

Glycosides constitute a substantial group of secondary metabolites originating from plants, and they serve several well-documented functions, including the regulation of growth, allelopathy (inhibition of other plant growth), and acting as defence mechanisms against damage caused by herbivores and pathogens [7]. These glycosides are secondary metabolites that, upon hydrolysis, yield one or more sugar components along with a non-sugar portion. The non-sugar part is referred to as the aglycone or genin, while the sugar portion is known as the glycone. These two components are linked by what is called the glycosidic linkage. The pharmacological action is primarily attributed to the aglycone portion, whereas the sugar portion contributes to solubility, cell permeability, and other pharmacokinetic properties [8]. Glycosides can be categorized based on the type of glycosidic linkage that exists between the carbohydrate and the aglycone. This linkage can occur through oxygen in *O*-glycosides, nitrogen (from an NH group in the aglycone) in *N*-glycosides (which include nucleosides or glycosylamines), sulphur in *S*-glycosides (such as glucosinolates or thioglycosides), and carbon in *C*-glycosides [9]. Among these, *O*-glycosides are the most prevalent in oats. *N*-glycosides encompass nucleosides or glycosylamines, while S-glycosides involve glucosinolates or thioglycosides.

Phenolic compounds constitute a group of small molecules distinguished by their structural feature of containing at least one phenol unit. From a chemical perspective, these compounds possess at least one aromatic ring that carries one or more hydroxyl groups. They can be categorized into two main groups, namely simple phenols and polyphenols, depending on the number of phenol units present within the molecule [10], [11]. Classifying phenolic compounds based on their chemical structures reveals various subgroups, including phenolic acids, flavonoids, tannins, coumarins, lignans, lignins, quinones, stilbenes, and curcuminoids. These subgroups encompass a wide range of chemical diversity [12]. From a biological standpoint, phenolic compounds exhibit numerous activities, with antioxidant activity being one of the most prominent. This antioxidant activity is closely linked to the strong metal-chelating propensity of phenolic compounds and is influenced by factors such as the number and positions of hydroxyl groups and the nature of substitutions on the aromatic rings [10], [11], [13]–[19]. Additionally, phenolic compounds are associated with various other biological activities, including anticarcinogenic, antimutagenic, and anti-inflammatory effects [20]. Many of these activities are interconnected with the antioxidant properties of phenolic compounds, making them of significant importance in the realms of cancer prevention and treatment [10], [17], [19], [21], [22].

An alkaloid is a class of naturally occurring organic compounds characterized by the presence of nitrogen atoms in their structure [23]. Typically, alkaloids contain at least one nitrogen atom in a configuration similar to amines, which are compounds derived from ammonia by replacing hydrogen atoms with hydrocarbon groups. Alkaloids exhibit a wide range of physiological effects on humans and other animals. Some well-known alkaloids include morphine, strychnine, quinine, ephedrine, and nicotine [24]. These alkaloids can have diverse and often significant impacts on the body. Avenanthramides (AVAs), also known as anthranilic acid amides and formerly referred to as "avenalumins," represent a specific group of phenolic alkaloids primarily found in oats [24].

Aside from these primary groups, other molecules have demonstrated some bioactivity, such as polysaccharides, amino acids, and peptides, indicating that the diversity of bioactive compounds is extensive and continues to expand through exploration and research across various sources. Among these compounds, oat terpenoids represent the largest and most diverse category of secondary metabolites in natural products. These bioactive compounds serve as microbiome regulators, including probiotics, prebiotics, symbiotics, and postbiotics [25]. While they may not provide direct nutrition, they are deemed vital ingredients for sustaining human health. Several bioactive compounds, such as flavonoids, curcumin, carotenoids, and ascorbic acid, have undergone extensive research to elucidate their potential to promote human health at various stages. These investigations have progressed to human clinical studies, affirming the effectiveness of these bioactive compounds. In recent years, numerous bioactive compounds have been subjected to rigorous scrutiny for their potential roles as antioxidants, anticancer agents, and anti-inflammatory agents. This exploration has encompassed diverse research settings, including in vitro and in vivo models, as well as clinical trials. It is important to note that among the countless bioactive compounds identified, only a select few have undergone comprehensive testing, transitioning from ancient knowledge to contemporary clinical applications, effectively bridging the gap from traditional plant-based remedies to modern patient-oriented healthcare.

The numerous health advantages of oats are commonly attributed to the presence of a wide variety of phytochemicals within the grain. These phytochemicals encompass phytosterols, phenolics, phytic acid, tocols (such as tocopherols and tocotrienols), dietary fibres (primarily β-glucan), lignans, alkylresorcinols, phytic acid, γ-oryzanols, AVAs, cinamic acid, stanols, ferulic acid, inositols, betaine, AVAs, and saponins [26]. These antioxidants exhibit diverse functions and stability, allowing them to persist throughout the digestive tract for an extended period after consumption [27]. These compounds are secondary metabolites produced by plants as defence mechanisms during growth and serve as antioxidants that mitigate cellular damage caused by oxidative stress by eliminating reactive oxygen species (ROS) in the human body. Additionally, incorporating oat components into food processing aids in suppressing the development of fatty acid plaques due to their antioxidant properties and enhances the preservation of food products.

The biosynthesis of bioactive compounds can occur through various pathways. Terpenes, for instance, are synthesized via the cytosolic mevalonic acid pathway and the methylerythritol phosphate pathway [28]. Phenolic compounds are produced through several pathways, including the shikimic acid pathway, phenylpropanoid pathway, and flavonoid pathway [29]. Conversely, the shikimic acid pathway primarily governs alkaloid biosynthesis. Bioactives have shown their effectiveness in mitigating inflammatory processes by reducing signalling molecules such as pro-inflammatory cytokines, chemokines, interleukins, inducible enzymes like cyclooxygenase-2 and inducible nitric oxide synthase, and inflammatory mediators such as prostaglandins, leukotrienes, and thromboxane. These pathological processes are linked to the onset and progression of numerous chronic diseases, including type 2 diabetes mellitus, obesity, neurodegenerative disorders, cardiovascular diseases, and cancer. Bioactive compounds have also demonstrated antimicrobial activity against various microorganisms, frequently associated with phenolic compounds, where they disrupt microbial cells by employing active redox metals, leading to an imbalance in the cell's redox state and, consequently, cell death. Additionally, bioactive compounds exhibit a range of other effects, including anticancer properties, neuroprotection, hepatoprotection, immunomodulation, and the management of dyslipidemias.

This chapter delves into various bioactive compounds and phytochemicals found in oats, including tocols (namely tocopherols and tocotrienols), phenolic compounds, and sterols. Special attention is given to ferulic acid among the phenolic compounds, and the discussion also covers AVAs (hydroxycinnamoyl anthranilate alkaloids) and steroidal glycosides known as avenacosides A and B. Detailed exploration of their characterization and structure is included.

The major bioactive compounds in oat grains are described in the following sections.

4.2 PHENOLIC COMPOUNDS

Phenolic compounds, also known as polyphenols, constitute a diverse category of chemical compounds encompassing one or more benzene rings with hydroxyl groups. This category includes phenolic acids, flavonoids, stilbenes, coumarins, tannins, and more [17], [19], [21], [22], [30]. These compounds are the byproducts of secondary metabolism in plants and serve vital roles in plant reproduction, growth, defence against pathogens and parasites, and contribution to the plant's coloration. They exhibit a wide range of structural complexity, spanning from simple to highly polymerized phenols. Polyphenolic compounds possess one or more hydroxyl groups within their chemical structure. Given their omnipresence in plants, they inevitably form a part of the human diet.

These compounds can be broadly categorized into two main groups: phenolic acids (primarily hydroxycinnamic, involving carbon atoms from C3 to C6, and hydroxybenzoic acids with carbon atoms from C1 to C6 rings) and flavonoids. Phenolic acids typically consist of a single benzene ring, whereas the fundamental structure of flavonoids comprises 15 carbon atoms arranged in three rings (labelled A, C, and B) in a C6–C3–C6 configuration [31]. Hydroxycinnamic acids, which include *p*-coumaric, caffeic, ferulic, and sinapic acids, are more prevalent than hydroxybenzoic acids. Hydroxybenzoic acid derivatives, such as *p*-hydroxybenzoic, protocatechuic, vanillic, syringic, and gallic acids, are found in the form of esters and glycosides [32] (Figure 4.1). Total phenolics in oat germ, endosperm, and hull range from 180 to 576 mg rutin equivalents (RE)/100. Another study indicated oats contain 6.53 μmol of gallic acid equivalent/g of grain [33].

The term "polyphenol" is used to define plant secondary metabolites exclusively derived from the shikimate-derived phenylpropanoid and/or polyketide pathways. These compounds typically feature multiple phenolic rings and lack nitrogen-based functional groups in their basic structural form. In oats, polyphenolic compounds mainly include simple phenols (such as various phenolic acids), flavonoids, and anthraamide compounds [34]. Notably, anthracamide compounds contribute to the antioxidant properties. In oat flour, one of the predominant phenolic acids is ferulic acid, which is present at a concentration of 66.3 mg/kg. Notably, this ferulic acid is primarily found in a

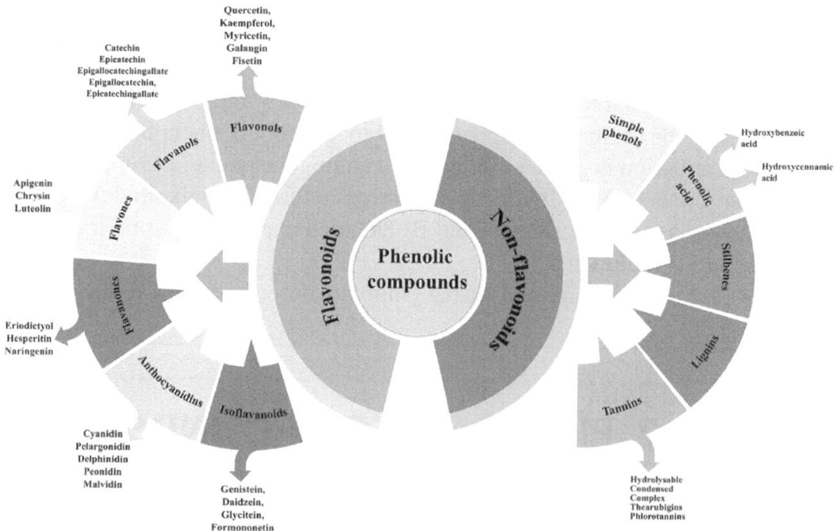

FIGURE 4.1   Comprehensive overview of phenolic compounds.

bound form. Furthermore, within the ferulic acid present, *trans*-ferulic acid constitutes the majority, accounting for more than 96% of the total ferulic acid content, whereas *cis*-ferulic acid is present in a smaller proportion. The hierarchy of phenolic acids found in oat flour is as follows: ferulic acid ranks highest, followed by syringic acid, and then chlorogenic acid and vanillic acid share an equal level of presence. Subsequently, caffeic acid, *p*-coumaric acid, *p*-hydroxybenzoic acid, and protocatechuic acid are found in decreasing order of abundance (Figure 4.2).

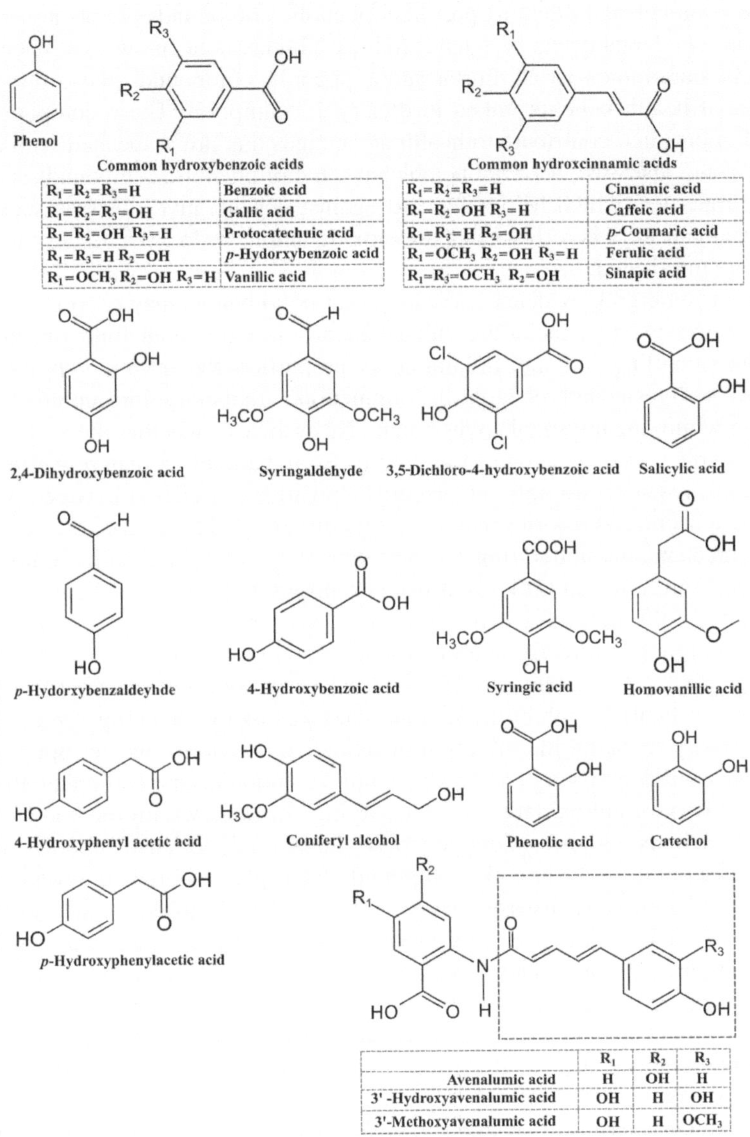

R₁=R₂=R₃=H	Benzoic acid
R₁=R₂=R₃=OH	Gallic acid
R₁=R₂=OH R₃=H	Protocatechuic acid
R₁=R₃=H R₂=OH	*p*-Hydorxybenzoic acid
R₁=OCH₃ R₂=OH R₃=H	Vanillic acid

R₁=R₂=R₃=H	Cinnamic acid
R₁=R₂=OH R₃=H	Caffeic acid
R₁=R₃=H R₂=OH	*p*-Coumaric acid
R₁=OCH₃ R₂=OH R₃=H	Ferulic acid
R₁=R₃=OCH₃ R₂=OH	Sinapic acid

	R₁	R₂	R₃
Avenalumic acid	H	OH	H
3'-Hydroxyavenalumic acid	OH	H	OH
3'-Methoxyavenalumic acid	OH	H	OCH₃

FIGURE 4.2   Various phenolic compounds present in oats.

Polyphenols can be categorized into four primary classes: flavonoids, lignans, stilbenes, and phenolic acids [10], [11], [16], [35]. These classes exhibit a wide range of structural diversity, encompassing both uncomplicated molecules like vanillin, gallic acid, and caffeic acid and more intricate polyphenols like stilbenes and flavonoids, along with polymers derived from these groups. Within their chemical structures, polyphenolic compounds typically contain one or more hydroxyl groups.

The concentration of phenolic compounds in whole-grain cereals varies depending on factors such as grain type, variety, and the specific part of the grain sampled. In whole-grain cereals, the most prevalent phenolic compounds are phenolic acids and flavonoids [11]. Notably, oat bran tends to have a higher concentration of phenolic compounds compared to oat groat. Furthermore, phenolic compounds play a pivotal role in the potential health benefits linked to dietary consumption. These compounds, when included in our diet, contribute to health advantages that are associated with a reduced risk of chronic diseases [36]. One notable attribute of phenolic compounds is their antioxidant properties, which help safeguard against degenerative illnesses such as heart disease and cancer, where ROS like superoxide anion, hydroxyl radicals, and peroxyl radicals are implicated.

There is emerging evidence indicating that polyphenols may exert even more significant effects in vivo, including enhancements in endothelial function, modulation of cellular signalling, and anti-inflammatory properties. Recent research has also suggested that undigested polyphenols, in conjunction with dietary fibre, could offer crucial protection within the intestinal environment. Nevertheless, whether the protective influence of polyphenols on health primarily stems from their antioxidant properties or other mechanisms, research strongly underscores a positive correlation between polyphenol intake and a decreased risk of specific chronic diseases [37].

The mechanisms underlying the antioxidant action of phenolic compounds are intricate and multifaceted [38]. It has been proposed that phenolics manifest their antioxidant effects through three primary actions: (a) direct scavenging of free radicals: phenolic compounds directly neutralize and scavenge free radicals, preventing their damaging effects; (b) prevention of free radical formation: phenolics hinder the formation of free radicals by inhibiting oxidant enzymes or by chelating certain transition metals, thereby reducing the initiation of oxidative reactions; and (c) upregulation of antioxidants and detoxifying enzymes: phenolic compounds may stimulate the production and activity of antioxidants and detoxifying enzymes within the body, enhancing the overall defence against oxidative stress. Substantial evidence supports the notion that the consumption of phenolic compounds from plant sources is inversely related to the risk of numerous diseases triggered by oxidative stress, including cardiovascular diseases and various types of cancer. In oats, phenolic compounds represent a significant source of antioxidants, with phenolic acids and flavonoids being the most prevalent types in oat grains. For instance, flavonoids, which are specific subgroups of polyphenols characterized by their A, B, and C aromatic ring structures, exhibit antioxidant activity that depends on the attached functional groups and the extent of hydroxylation on the rings.

Oats contain a variety of phenolic compounds, primarily consisting of flavonoids and phenolic acids, categorized as either hydroxybenzoic or hydroxycinnamic acids. Some of these phenolic compounds are unique to certain cereal grains (Table 4.1). The biological

TABLE 4.1 Phenolic Compounds in Oat

COMPOUND	PART	REFERENCE
Total phenolics	• Oat (endosperm, germ) (180 mg RE/100 g)	[47]
	• Oat (husk) (265 mg RE/100 g)	
	• Oat (endosperm, germ) (286 mg RE/100 g)	
	• Oat (husk or hull) (576 mg RE/100 g)	
	• Oat (hull, bran, endosperm) (35.1–87.4 mg/100 g)	[48]
	• Oat (hull, bran, endosperm, germ) (23.2 mg/100 g)	[49]
	• Oat (hull) (35.1 mg/100 g)	
	• Oat (hull, bran, endosperm, germ) (0.14–0.16 mg/seed)	[50]
	• Oat (hull, bran, endosperm, germ) (0.4–0.7 µg/seed)	
	• Oat (hull, bran, endosperm, germ) (3.57–14.35 mg/100 g)	[51]
	• Oat (hull, bran, endosperm, germ) (120.1–168.4 mg/100 g)	[52]
	• Oat (bran) (2.52–3.17 mg/100 g)	[53]
	• Oat (seed, bran) (64.5–151.8 mg/100 g)	[42]
	• Oat (113.8 mg GAE/100 g)	[54]
	• Oat (hull, bran, endosperm, germ) (0.62–5.06 mg/100 g)	[48]
	• Oat (bran) (2.2 mg/100 g)	[55]
	• Oat (seeds, hull) (0.54–2.25 mg/100 g)	[56]
2,4-Dihydrobenzoic acid (protocatechuic acid)	• Oat (hull, bran, endosperm, germ) (0.10–1.04 mg/100 g)	[51]
	• Oat (hull, bran, endosperm, germ) (0.50 mg/100 g)	[48]
	• Oat (bran) (5.50–7.62 mg/100 g)	[53]
2-Hydroxycinnamic acid	• Oat (hull, bran, endosperm, germ) (0.05–0.67 mg/100 g)	[48]
o-Coumaric acid	• Oat (hull) (0.69 mg/100 g)	[49]
	• Oat (hull, bran, endosperm, germ) (0.11–0.38 mg/100 g)	[52]
	• Oat (grains) 8.05–210.27 mg/100 g	[57]
p-Coumaric acid	• Oat (hull, bran, endosperm, germ) (0.24–1.19 mg/100 g)	[48]
	• Oat (bran) (1.2 mg/100 g)	[55]
	• Oat (grain) (0.12–0.19 mg/100 g)	[58]
	• Oat (germ, endosperm) (0.57 mg/100 g)	[47]
	• Oat (Hull or husks) (39.9 mg/100 g)	
	• Oat (Germ, endosperm) (1.13 mg/100 g)	
	• Oat (Hull or husks) (26.9 mg/100 g)	

(Continued)

TABLE 4.1 (Continued) Phenolic Compounds in Oat

COMPOUND	PART	REFERENCE
	• Oat (grains) (0.3–29.7 nmol/g)	[59]
	• Oat (hull, bran, endosperm, germ) (4.49 mg/100 g)	[49]
	• Oat (hull) (59.7 mg/100 g)	
	• Oat (hull, bran, endosperm, germ) (0.02–0.04 mg/seed)	[50]
	• Oat (seed, hull) (6.22–368 mg/100 g)	[56]
	• Oat (bran, seed) (0.19–4.94 mg/100 g)	[42]
	• Oat (bran) (0.26–0.30 mg/100 g)	[53]
	• Oat (hull, bran, endosperm, germ) (59.0–82.6 mg/100 g)	[52]
	• Oat (hull) (245 mg/100 g)	[60]
Ferulic acid	• Oat (grains) (0.4–15.4 nmol/l)	[59]
	• Oat (grain) 16.50–149.36 mg/100 g	[57]
	• Oat (hull, bran, endosperm, germ) (0.66–0.84 mg/100 g)	[48]
	• Oat (endosperm, germ) (9.87 mg/100 g)	[47]
	• Oat (grain) (16.50–149.36 mg/100 g)	[57]
	• Oat (husk, hull) (30.9 mg/100 g)	[47]
	• Oat (hull, bran, endosperm, germ) (10.5–45.85 mg/100 g)	
	• Oat (bran) (14 mg/100 g)	[55]
	• Oat (grain) (0.07–0.6 mg/100 g)	[58]
	• Oat (hull, bran, endosperm, germ) (14.2–14.7 mg/100 g)	[49]
	• Oat (hull, bran, endosperm, germ) (0.09–0.13 mg/seed)	[50]
	• Oat (hull, bran, endosperm, germ) (0.14–1.89 mg/100 g)	[51]
	• Oat (hull) (214 mg/100 g)	[60]
	• Oat (bran) (0.46–0.49 mg/100 g)	[53]
	• Oat (seed, bran) (15.2–115.3 mg/100 g)	[42]
	• Oat (seeds) (32.7 mg/100 g)	[56]
	• Oat (hull) (809.5 mg/100 g)	
	• Oat (bran) (33.0 mg/100 g)	[55]
	• Oat (hull, bran, endosperm, germ) (0.91–1.03 mg/100 g)	[48]
	• Oat (bran) (9 mg/100 g)	[55]
Sinapic acid	• Oat (Germ, endosperm) (2.4 mg/100 g)	[47]
	• Oat (husk, hull) (0.14 mg/100 g)	
	• Oat (Germ, endosperm) (2.81 mg/100 g)	
	• Oat (hull, husk) (0.27 mg/100 g)	

(Continued)

TABLE 4.1 (Continued) Phenolic Compounds in Oat

COMPOUND	PART	REFERENCE
Caffeic acid	• Oat (hull) (0.56 mg/100 g)	[49]
	• Oat (bran) (0.47–0.53 mg/100 g)	[53]
	• Oat (seed, bran) (1.89–8.03 mg/100 g)	[42]
	• Oat (germ, endosperm) (0.52–1.57 mg/100 g)	[48]
	• Oat (hull, bran, endosperm, germ) (1.68 mg/100 g)	[49]
	• Oat (hull, bran, endosperm, germ) (0.09–0.70 mg/100 g)	[51]
	• Oat (bran) (0.86–2.28 mg/100 g)	[53]
	• Oat (grains) (0.2–23.9 nmol/g)	[59]
	• Oat (seed, bran) (1.04–7.27 mg/100 g)	[42]
	• Oat (seed) (0.86 mg/100 g)	[56]
	• Oat (hull) (0.42 mg/100 g)	
	• Oat (bran) (0.5 mg/100 g)	[55]
Syringaldehyde	• Oat (hull, bran, endosperm, germ) (0.32–2.12 mg/100 g)	[48]
	• Oat (hull) (566 mg/100 g)	[60]
	• Oat (hull, bran, endosperm, germ) (0.11–0.17 mg/100 g)	[52]
Syringic acid	• Oat (bran) (2.8 mg/100 g)	[55]
	• Oat (hull, bran, endosperm, germ) (0.46–0.79 mg/100 g)	[48]
	• Oat (endosperm, germ) (0.34 mg/100 g)	[47]
	• Oat (hull) (0.68 mg/100 g)	
	• Oat (Germ, endosperm) (0.55 mg/100 g)	
	• Oat (Hull or husks) (0.43 mg/100 g)	
	• Oat (hull, bran, endosperm, germ) (0.39–0.89 mg/100 g)	[52]
	• Oat (bran, seed) (0.45–2.11 mg/100 g)	[42]
	• Oat (seed) (0.49 mg/100 g)	[56]
	• Oat (hull) (3.88 mg/100 g)	
Vanillic acid	• Oat (hull, bran, endosperm, germ) (0.39–9.38 mg/100 g)	[48]
	• Oat (endosperm, germ) (0.26 mg/100 g)	[47]
	• Oat (bran) (0.4 mg/100 g)	[55]
	• Oat (husk, hull) (1.12 mg/100 g)	[47]
	• Oat (germ, endosperm) (0.34 mg/100 g)	
	• Oat (husk, hull) (0.89 mg/100 g)	
	• Oat (hull, bran, endosperm, germ) (0.34 mg/100 g)	[49]
	• Oat (hull) (5.42 mg/100 g)	
	• Oat (hull, bran, endosperm, germ) 0.7–1.4 µg/seed	[50]

(Continued)

TABLE 4.1 (Continued) Phenolic Compounds in Oat

COMPOUND	PART	REFERENCE
	• Oat (hull, bran, endosperm, germ) (0.37–4.75 mg/100 g)	[51]
	• Oat (hull) (593 mg/100 g)	[60]
	• Oat (hull, bran, endosperm, germ) (0.46–0.71 mg/100 g)	[52]
	• Oat (bran) (1.01–1.25 mg/100 g)	[53]
	• Oat (seed, bran) (0.49–1.29 mg/100 g)	[42]
	• Oat (seed) (0.81 mg/100 g)	[56]
	• Oat (hull) (20.6 mg/100 g)	
	• Oat (naked) (0.51 mg/100 g)	[61]
Vanillin	• Oat (groats) (3.4 mg/kg) • Oat (hulls) (54.2 mg/kg)	[49]
Chlorogenic acid	• Oat (naked) (0.20 mg/100 g)	[61]
Gallic acid	• Oat (hull, bran, endosperm, germ) (1.43–7.05 mg/100 g)	[51]
Catechol	• Oat (groats) (0.1 mg/kg)	[49]
Coniferyl alcohol	• Oat (groats) (0.8 mg/kg)	[62]
p-Hydroxybenzoic acid	• Oat (groats) (3.5 mg/kg) • Oat (hulls) (50 mg/kg)	[49]
p-Hydroxybenzaldehyde	• Oat (groats) (0.3 mg/kg) • Oat (hulls) (7.7 mg/kg)	[63]
p-Hydroxyphenylacetic acid	• Oat (groats) (0.6 mg/kg) • Oat (hulls) (4.6 mg/kg)	[49]
Protocatechuic acid	• Oat (groats) (0.7 mg/kg) • Oat (hulls) (2.1 mg/kg)	[63]
Salicylic acid	• Oat (hulls) (3.1 mg/kg)	[49]
Rutin	• Oat (naked) (0.22–0.47 mg/100 g)	[61]

RE, Rutin equivalents; GAE, gallic acid equivalents.

effects of oat phenolic extracts are closely linked to their structure-activity relationships. Hydroxybenzoic and hydroxycinnamic acids possess free radical-scavenging abilities due to their polarity and the presence of hydroxyl groups. An example is ferulic acid, one of the most abundant phenolic acids in oats, which can react with free radicals due to a hydrogen atom in its hydroxyl group, exhibiting antioxidant properties.

Polyphenols of oats exert various physiological effects, such as antioxidative, anti-ageing, anticancer, and cardiovascular and cerebrovascular protective effects. During oat germination, the levels of polyphenols and GABA (Gamma-aminobutyric acid) significantly increase [39]. These compounds are primarily bound to cell wall cellulose or hemicellulose via ester bonds and are not readily hydrolysed by human digestive enzymes, resulting in low bioavailability. However, germination leads to the degradation of cellulose by cellulase, releasing phenols and GABA. Furthermore, germination reduces polyphenol oxidase activity while increasing anthrene amide synthase activity, promoting polyphenol synthesis and resulting in elevated levels of total polyphenols and free phenolic acids.

Ferulic acid in oats forms ester bonds with the arabinoxylans comprising the grain cell wall. Ferulic acid can exist in various forms in whole grains, including free, soluble, conjugated, and bound [40]. Notably, in oats, bound ferulic acid constitutes a significant majority (> 93% of the total), surpassing the levels of soluble conjugated ferulic acid. Ferulic acid is recognized for its potential health benefits, largely attributed to its antioxidant properties.

Coumaric acids, another class of phenolic compounds in oats, are hydroxyl derivatives of cinnamic acid. There are three distinct forms of coumaric acids: *p*-coumaric acid, *o*-coumaric acid, and *m*-coumaric acid, distinguished by the position of hydroxyl substitution on the phenolic group [30]. As *p*-coumaric acid is essentially a hydroxyl derivative of cinnamic acid, it is synonymous with *p*-hydroxycinnamic acid. *p*-Coumaric acid content is typically lower in the central part of the oat grain kernel and increases towards the outer layers. These compounds are primarily esterified with organic acids, sugars, and lipids. Coumaric acids are believed to possess antioxidant effects, with research indicating their ability to scavenge free radicals. Additionally, *p*-coumaric acid has shown promise in potentially inhibiting the growth of human malignant tumours, inducing cytostasis, and restraining the malignant properties of tumour cells in vitro. Concentrations ranging from 1 to 4.5 mmol/L resulted in a notable 50% reduction in cell proliferation. Furthermore, *p*-coumaric acids may have a protective effect against heart diseases, as they can reduce the resistance of low-density lipoproteins (LDL), prevent cholesterol oxidation and lipid peroxidation, and act on apo-protein B100.

Phenolic acids in oats are present in cereals in both free and bound forms. The majority of phenolic acids in oats are bound to cell walls, forming covalent bonds and becoming integral components of the cell wall structures. To extract these bound phenolic acids, one needs to use acid or alkaline conditions to break the covalent bonds. In contrast, free phenolic acids are primarily located in the outer layer of the pericarp and can be extracted using organic solvents. Free phenolic acids are concentrated in the outer layer of the pericarp, while bound phenolic acids are ester-linked to cell walls, necessitating acid, base, or enzymatic hydrolysis to release them from the cell matrix. Studies have reported low levels of free ferulic, vanillic, sinapic, and *p*-hydroxybenzoic acids in solid-liquid extracts using 70% ethanol in oat grains. However, the bulk of ferulic, sinapic, *p*-coumaric, and hydroxybenzoic acids are derived from soluble or insoluble bound forms, released through alkaline hydrolysis or the action of β-glucosidase. These findings suggest that these phenolic acids primarily exist as soluble esters and insoluble esters bound to polysaccharides, proteins, or cell walls. Also, the quantification of ferulic acid in oat grain revealed a content of 300 mg/kg, with the majority of it being in the bound form, firmly integrated into the oat's cell wall structure.

The biosynthesis of phenolic acids in oats primarily occurs through the shikimate/phenylpropanoid pathway, utilizing two aromatic amino acids: l-phenylalanine and/

or l-tyrosine. This pathway begins with the shikimate pathway, where plant phenolic compounds originate from a common intermediate, either phenylalanine or its close precursor, shikimic acid. The key enzyme in this process is PAL (Phenylalanine ammonialyase), which catalyses the conversion of the aromatic amino acid phenylalanine into phenolics, including hydroxycinnamic acids and coumarins. The biosynthesis of phenolic acids involves three essential processes: deamination, hydroxylation, and methylation [41] (Figure 4.3).

To briefly summarize, the deamination of amino acids phenylalanine and tyrosine results in the production of cinnamic acid (not considered a phenolic acid) and *p*-coumaric acid, respectively. The removal of the ethyl side chain from cinnamic acid leads to benzoic acid. Structurally, all phenolic acids are hydroxylated derivatives of either cinnamic acid or benzoic acid. Another pathway for phenolic acid biosynthesis is the polyketide (acetate) pathway, which can generate simple phenols and quinones.

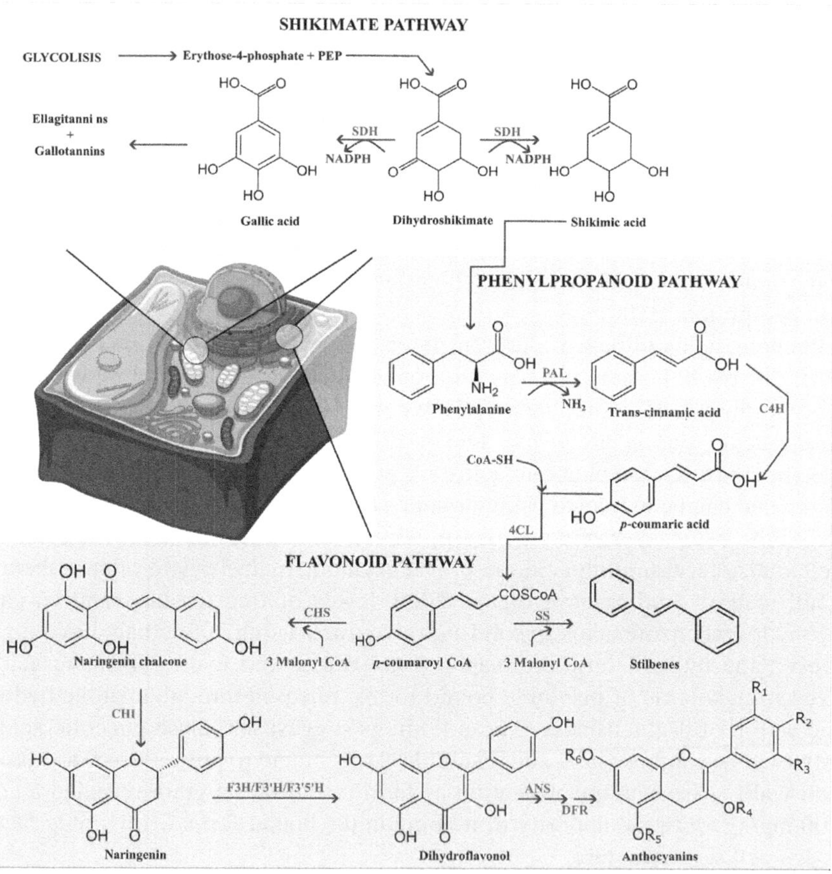

FIGURE 4.3   Biosynthesis of phenolic compounds.

Flavonoids, the largest group of phenolics, are typically derived from a combination of these two pathways, where one ring often originates from a molecule of resorcinol, and another ring is derived from the shikimate pathway. Phenolic acids are widely distributed in plants and can occur in various forms, including insoluble forms as structural components of the cell wall (associated with xylans, pectin, and lignin), in conjugate forms with sugars, as depsides, or as simple glycosides.

In a study conducted by Soycan et al. [42], they analysed 22 different commercial oat products and found that oat bran concentrate had the highest total phenolic acid content, followed by oat bran, flaked oats, rolled oats, and oatcakes. The majority of these phenolic compounds were detected in a bound form, with ferulic, sinapic, and caffeic acids being the most abundant among them [42]. The phenolic compounds in oat grains are as follows: 4-hydroxybenzoic acid, vanillic acid (4-hydroxy-3-methoxybenzoic acid), avenalumic acid and its 3′-hydroxy and 3′-methoxy derivatives, caffeic acid, 4-hydorxybenzaldeyhde, *p*-hydroxybenzoic acid, *p*-hydroxyphenylacetic acid, syringic acid, protocatechuic acid, *p*-hydroxybenzoic acid, salicylic acid, syringaldehyde, 2-hydroxycinnamic acid, catechol, coniferyl alcohol, *p*-coumaric acid, *o*-coumaric acid, sinapic acid, 3,5-dichloro-4-hydroxybenzoic acid, ferulic acid, AVAs, gallic acid, 2,4-dihydrobenzoic acid (protocatechuic acid), 4-hydroxyphenyl acetic acid, homovanillic acid, chlorogenic acid, rutin, luteolin, and apigenin [43]–[46] (Figure 4.2).

4.2.1 Mechanism of Antioxidant Activity

The effectiveness of polyphenolic compounds in combating oxidative stress is linked to their ability to neutralize reactive radical species. This neutralization occurs when antioxidants transfer either electrons or hydrogen atoms to these radicals. Phenolic compounds can scavenge free radicals through four different chemical pathways: adduct formation (AF), sequential proton loss electron transfer (SPLET), electron transfer-proton transfer (ET-PT), and proton coupled-electron transfer (PC-ET/HAT). The specific mechanism dominating the reaction depends on the surrounding conditions.

In the PC-ET/HAT mechanism, hydrogen atoms are rapidly donated to the radical species $R^\bullet$, leading to the following reaction:

- $ArOH + R^\bullet \rightarrow ArO^\bullet + RH$

The SPLET mechanism unfolds in two distinct steps. Firstly, the antioxidant undergoes dissociation, leading to the formation of the aroxyl anion (ArO^-). In the subsequent stage, an electron from the antioxidant anion can be transferred to the scavenged radical, leading to the creation of the radical anion (R^-). Finally, in the last phase of the reaction, the radical anion is protonated.

- $ArOH \rightarrow ArO^- + H^+$
- $ArO^- + R^\bullet \rightarrow ArO^\bullet + R^-$
- $R^- + H^+ \rightarrow RH$

Within the ET-PT mechanism, an electron is transferred from the antioxidant to the scavenged radical. This process results in the formation of the antioxidant cation radical ($ArOH^{\bullet+}$). Subsequently, this cation radical undergoes deprotonation, with the hydrogen cation being transferred to the radical anion (R^-).

- $ArOH + R^{\bullet} \rightarrow ArOH^{\bullet+} + R^-$
- $ArOH^{\bullet+} + R^- \rightarrow ArO^{\bullet} + RH$

The outcome of these mechanisms remains consistent, but they achieve it through different pathways. Several characteristics of antioxidants play a role in influencing these mechanisms: bond dissociation enthalpy, which is particularly crucial in the HAT/PC-ET mechanism; proton affinity coupled with the electron transfer energy of ArO^-, which is significant in the SPLET mechanism; and ionization potential of ArOH, along with proton dissociation enthalpy of $ArOH^{\bullet+}$ in the ET-PT mechanism. The balance between these mechanisms is contingent on the conditions of the reaction environment. The interaction between phenolic antioxidants and radicals primarily occurs through a combination of the PC-ET and SPLET mechanisms. The former is slower and prevails in non-polar solvents with low dielectric constants and low basicity. In contrast, the latter is faster and is characteristic of solvents with high dielectric constants and high basicity, which facilitate the ionization of antioxidants. The degree of ionization of phenolic antioxidants (ArOH) depends on both a bulk property of the solvent, namely its relative permittivity, and a molecular property related to its capacity to solvate and thus stabilize anions (ArO^-).

4.2.2 Flavonoids

Flavonoids constitute an extensive group of more than 5,000 polyphenolic compounds characterized by a common 15-carbon core structure. The term "flavonoids" serves as a collective descriptor for plant pigments, primarily derived from benzo-γ-pyrone, which is also referred to as chromone [64]. Typically, flavonoids are composed of two phenyl rings, denoted A and B, and a heterocyclic ring, known as C, that incorporates an embedded oxygen atom [65]. However, it's worth noting that chalcones deviate from this pattern, as they have a cleaved C-ring. The antioxidant capacity of flavonoids is influenced by the positioning of the catechol B-ring on the pyran C-ring and the number and location of hydroxy groups on the catechol portion of the B-ring [66]. Flavonoids exhibit various structural variations, and the primary skeletal structures include isoflavone, catechin, chalcone, flavandiol (flavanol), anthocyanidin, flavanonol, flavanone, flavonol, and flavone. Flavonoids can be encountered in oats in both *O*- and/or *C*-glycoside-bound forms and in free aglycone forms. Among these, flavones and flavonols are the most prevalent forms, widely found in diets across the globe.

Flavonoids, derived from the Latin word "flavus," meaning "yellow," play various roles in plants. These roles encompass antioxidative stress responses, defence against

UV-light-induced damage and phytopathogens, involvement in legume nodulation, pollination facilitation, support for male fertility, contribution to seed development, emission of visual signals, regulation of auxin transport, and allelopathy. In the case of oats, numerous genes involved in flavonoid biosynthesis are activated under stressful conditions. Consequently, the levels of flavonoids increase when plants are exposed to biotic and abiotic stressors such as injury, drought, metal toxicity, and nutrient deficiency. A common factor in these environmental stress scenarios is the generation and buildup of ROS, including superoxide anions ($O2^{-\bullet}$), hydrogen peroxide (H_2O_2), hydroxyl radicals ($OH^\bullet$), and singlet oxygen ($_1O^2$) [67]. The accumulation of ROS can result in oxidative stress, which has the potential to harm cellular components like DNA, lipids, proteins, and sugars. To mitigate the adverse effects of oxidative stress, plants employ a complex system of enzymatic and non-enzymatic antioxidants to maintain ROS homeostasis. Flavonoids are believed to function as antioxidants, shielding plants from the damaging effects of oxidative stress. The hydroxy groups within flavonoids can donate electrons through resonance, effectively stabilizing free radicals and offering antioxidant protection.

In the context of human health, flavonoids are sometimes referred to as "vitamin P," although this term is controversial because they do not strictly meet the criteria for being classified as vitamins. These compounds are linked to a wide array of health benefits attributable to their bioactive characteristics. These advantages encompass their anti-inflammatory, anticancer, anti-ageing, cardio-protective, neuroprotective, immunomodulatory, anti-diabetic, antibacterial, antiparasitic, urolithiasis-preventing, hypertension-regulating, venous insufficiency alleviating, and antiviral properties [68].

Oat flavonoids originate from two distinct biosynthetic pathways: the phenylpropanoid pathway, responsible for generating the phenylpropanoid skeleton (C6-C3), and the polyketide pathway, which produces building blocks for polymeric C2 units. The enzyme chalcone synthase plays a pivotal role by catalysing the formation of the 2'-hydroxychalcone scaffold, scientifically known as (*E*)-1-(2-hydroxyphenyl)-3-phenylprop-2-en-1-one, using *p*-coumaroyl CoA and malonyl CoA as substrates. Subsequent enzymatic reactions utilize this scaffold to produce various other flavonoid compounds [69].

Oat flavonoids typically share a common structural framework, featuring a C6–C3–C6 arrangement consisting of two benzene rings labelled as A and B, interconnected by a heterocyclic pyrene ring (C) that contains an oxygen atom. The classification of flavonoids can be based on the degree of saturation in the central heterocyclic ring. For instance, anthocyanidins, flavones, flavonols, and isoflavones exhibit a C2=C3 unsaturation, while flavanones, dihydroflavonols, and flavan-3-ols are examples of saturated flavonoids. Beyond this common classification, flavonoids can also be categorized based on their molecular size, particularly due to the presence of biflavonyls in gymnosperms. Additionally, the structure of flavonoids can vary in terms of substituents on the A and B rings, which may include hydroxy groups, alkyl groups, and methoxy groups [66].

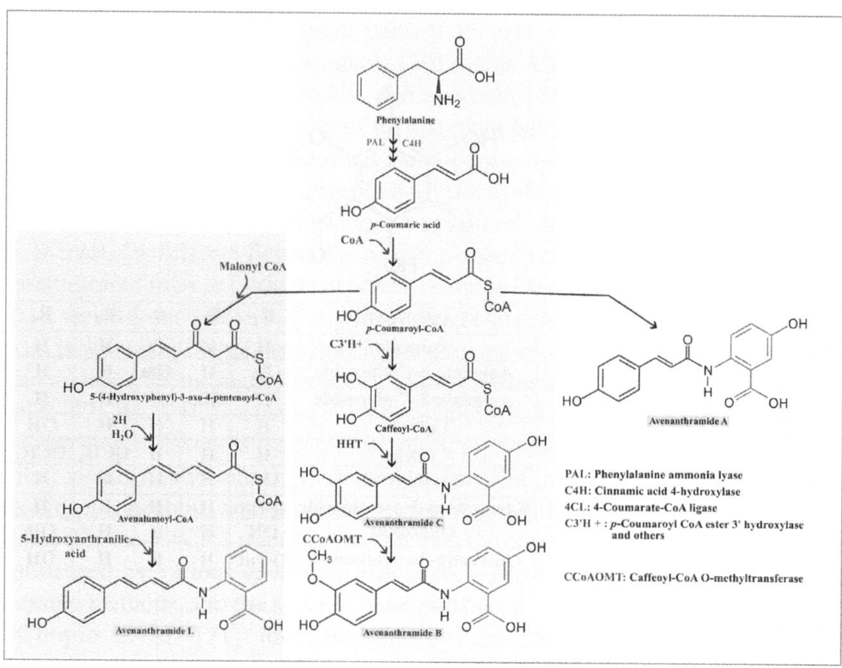

FIGURE 4.5   Biosynthesis pathway of avenanthramides.

TABLE 4.3   Avenanthramides in Oat

COMPOUND	PART	REFERENCE
Total avenanth-ramides (AVAs)	• Oat (hull, bran, endosperm, germ) (4.20–9.10 mg/100 g)	[48]
	• Oat (hull, bran, endosperm, germ) (0.50–21.43 mg/100 g)	[51]
	• Oat (hull, bran, endosperm, germ) (1.12–8.39 mg/100 g)	[52]
	• Oat (bran) (0.79–13.3 mg/100 g)	[74]
	• Oat (naked) (3.73–71.85mg/100 g)	[61]
AVA 2c	• Oat (hull, bran, endosperm, germ) (1.58–4.49 mg/100 g)	[48]
	• Oat (hull, bran, endosperm, germ) (74–115 nmol/g)	[75]
	• Oat (spikelet, leaves, hull, bran, endosperm, germ) (4.02–7.8 nmol/g)	[76]
	• Oat (hull, bran, endosperm, germ) (1.1–1.6 mg/100 g)	[77]
	• Oat (hull, bran, endosperm, germ) (0.7–2.1 mg/100 g)	
	• Oat (bran) (0.9–2.9 mg/100 g)	
	• Oat (bran) (0.41 mg/100 g)	[53]

(Continued)

TABLE 4.3   (Continued) Avenanthramides in Oat

COMPOUND	PART	REFERENCE
	• Oat (bran) (0.07–1.49 mg/100 g)	[74]
	• Oat (seeds) (0.66 mg/100 g)	[56]
	• Oat (hull) (6.37 mg/100 g)	
	• Oat (hulls, groats) (0.11 mg/100 g)	[78]
	• Oat (grains) (0.6–2.9 mg/100 g)	[58]
	• Oat (flakes, whole grain) (0.4–0.9 mg/100 g)	[55]
AVA 2p	• Oat (hull, bran, endosperm, germ) (1.3–3.0 mg/100 g)	[48]
	• Oat (hull, bran, endosperm, germ) (78–120 nmol/g)	[75]
	• Oat (spikelet, leaves, hull, bran, endosperm, germ) (3.93–74.26 nmol/g)	[76]
	• Oat (hull, bran, endosperm, germ) (0.6–1.5 mg/100 g) • Oat (bran) (0.7–1.6 mg/100 g)	[77]
	• Oat (hull, bran, endosperm, germ) (0.23–7.45 mg/100 g)	[51]
	• Oat (hull, bran, endosperm, germ) (0.60–3.96 mg/100 g)	[52]
	• Oat (bran) (0.06–3.32 mg/100 g)	[74]
	• Oat (seeds) (2.56 mg/100 g) • Oat (hull) (2.48 mg/100 g)	[56]
AVA 2f	• Oat (hulls, groats) (0.12 mg/100 g)	[78]
	• Oat (hull, bran, endosperm, germ) (62–65 nmol/g)	[75]
	• Oat (spikelet, leaves, hull, bran, endosperm, germ) (3.35–18.16 nmol/g)	[76]
	• Oat (hull, bran, endosperm, germ) (0.9–2.3 mg/100 g) • Oat (bran) (1.0–2.8 mg/100 g)	[77]
	• Oat (bran) (0.78–0.91 mg/100 g)	[53]
	• Oat (seeds) (2.18 mg/100 g) • Oat (hull) (3.03 mg/100 g)	[56]

Oat bran and flakes boast the highest concentration of AVAs, which are typically found in all milling fractions and are consequently present in various commercial oat products. When it comes to processing, steaming and flaking have a moderate impact on reducing the content of AVA-A in dehulled oat groats, while AVA-C and B remain largely unaffected by the steaming process. However, when oat grains undergo autoclaving or steamed rolled oats are subjected to drum drying, there is a significant decrease in the AVA content [79]. The synthesis of AVAs displays tissue-specific characteristics, with their presence being constitutive in grain parts such as the endosperm and scutellum, while inducible expression occurs in leaves.

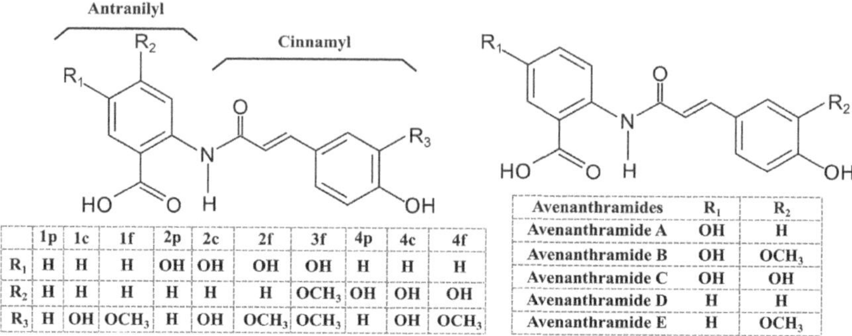

	1p	1c	1f	2p	2c	2f	3f	4p	4c	4f
R_1	H	H	H	OH	OH	OH	OH	H	H	H
R_2	H	H	H	H	H	H	OCH_3	OH	OH	OH
R_3	H	OH	OCH_3	H	OH	OCH_3	OCH_3	H	OH	OCH_3

Avenanthramides	R_1	R_2
Avenanthramide A	OH	H
Avenanthramide B	OH	OCH_3
Avenanthramide C	OH	OH
Avenanthramide D	H	H
Avenanthramide E	H	OCH_3

FIGURE 4.6   Avenanthramides in oat.

AVAs play a crucial role in protecting LDL cholesterol from the harmful effects of free radicals. When combined with vitamin C, an AVAs-enriched oat extract has been shown to effectively inhibit the oxidation of LDL cholesterol in laboratory settings. Both animal experiments and clinical trials involving humans have provided evidence that antioxidants found in oats have the potential to decrease cardiovascular risks. This is achieved by reducing serum cholesterol levels and preventing the oxidation and per-oxidation of LDL cholesterol. Research suggests that AVAs primarily work to prevent cancer by obstructing the action of reactive species [26]. Furthermore, they demonstrate promising therapeutic properties by influencing various pathways, including promoting apoptosis and senescence, impeding cell proliferation, and inhibiting processes such as epithelial-mesenchymal transition and metastasis. AVAs represent a hopeful class of chemopreventive and anticancer phytochemicals [80]. However, further clinical trials and toxicological studies are necessary to determine their effectiveness in preventing and mitigating cancer-related diseases.

4.2.3.1 Chemical Structure of AVAs

AVAs, or *N*-cinnamoyl anthranilic acids, possess a structural composition resulting from the fusion of two components: one originating from anthranilic acid (the left side) and the other from cinnamic acid (the right side). To streamline nomenclature, Dimberg introduced an alphanumeric system, assigning numbers to anthranilate derivatives and letters to accompanying cinnamate derivatives: "c" for caffeic acid, "f" for ferulic acid, and "p" for *p*-coumaric acid. This alphanumeric system is used in this chapter. The anthranilic acid segment includes variants such as anthranilic acid itself (1), 5-hydroxyanthranilic acid (2), 5-hydroxy-4-methoxyanthranilic acid (3), and 4-hydroxyanthranilic acid (4). Meanwhile, the cinnamic acid part comprises cinnamic acid (a), caffeic acid (c), ferulic acid (f), *p*-coumaric acid (p), and sinapic acid [73]. In oats, the most prevalent AVAs are 2c, 2f, and 2p. Nevertheless, oats can contain at least 25 distinct AVAs, albeit some exist in trace amounts and haven't been isolated from oats. AVA concentrations in oats typically range from 2 to 300 mg/kg, with higher levels observed in the bran and outer layers of oat kernels, gradually decreasing from the outer layer to the endosperm. Additionally, AVAs can be found in oat hulls and leaves, with concentrations varying significantly depending on oat cultivars and elicitors, spanning from 5 to 120 mg/kg. The concentration of AVAs in oat leaves can range from 5 to 120 mg/kg, with notable differences between cultivars and cultivation conditions, and particularly elevated concentrations in leaves subjected to elicitor treatments. Major AVAs in oats are N-(40-hydroxy-30-methoxycinnamoyl)-5-hydroxyanthranilic acid (2f), N-(40-hydroxycinnamoyl)-5-hydroxyanthranilic acid (2p), N-(30,40-dihydroxycinnamoyl)-5-hydroxyanthranilic acid (2c), (N-(40-hydroxycinnamoyl)-5-hydroxyanthranilic acid) (2p), (N-(30, 40-dihydroxycinnamoyl)-5-hydroxyanthranilic acid) (2c), and (N-(40-hydroxy-30-methoxycinnamoyl)-5-hydro-xyanthranilic acid) (2f) [81] (Figure 4.6).

4.3 TOCOLS

Tocols, which encompass tocopherols and tocotrienols, are natural antioxidants found in cereal grains and are well-known for their biological activity. Vitamin E is a broad term that represents a group of structurally similar compounds, consisting of two forms: tocopherol and tocotrienol [82]. There are eight variations of tocols, namely α-tocopherol (αTP), β-tocopherol (βTP), γ-tocopherol (γTP), δ-tocopherol (δTP), and α-tocotrienols (αTT), β-tocotrienol (βTT), γ-tocotrienol (γTT), and δ-tocotrienol (δTT). In general, tocols comprise a polar chromanol ring connected to an isoprenoid-derived hydrocarbon chain, with the only difference being the saturation level of the isoprenoid side chain. The typical structure of tocopherols consists of 2-methyl-2-(4, 8, 12-trimethyltridecyl) chroman-6-ol, whereas tocotrienols consist of 2-methyl-2-(4, 8, 12-trimethyltrideca-3, 7, 11-trienyl) chroman-6-ol [83] (Figure 4.7). The presence of the phenolic hydroxyl group in both tocopherols and tocotrienols is essential for their antioxidant activity within vitamin E. This is because they can donate a phenolic hydroxyl group from the chromanol ring to free radicals, thereby stabilizing them and interrupting the propagation phase of oxidative chain reactions.

Oat kernels contain varying concentrations of tocols, ranging from 13.6 to 36.1 mg/kg, and this distribution is not uniform throughout the kernel [48] (Table 4.4). This information is significant because oats are commonly consumed in their whole-grain form, such as oat flakes, rolled oats, or oatmeal. In oats, tocopherols are primarily found in the germ, while tocotrienols are mostly concentrated in the endosperm. When oats are in their unprocessed groat form, tocols remain stable for more than seven months when stored at room temperature. However, in all processed oat products, including dried groats, they degrade significantly within one to two months. Unlike barley, oats contain only α and β vitamers, with αTT being the predominant form, contributing to 57% to 69% of the total tocols. Similarly, according to a study by Fardet et al. [84], αTT is the major vitamer in oats, accounting for approximately 90% of the tocols.

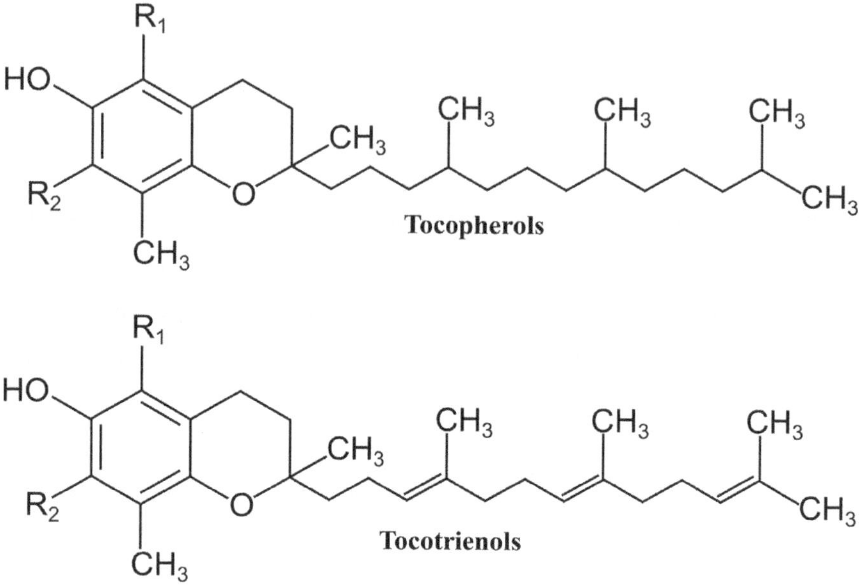

TOCOPHEROLS	R_1	R_2
α-Tocopherol	CH_3	CH_3
β-Tocopherol	CH_3	H
γ-Tocopherol	H	CH_3
δ-Tocopherol	H	H

FIGURE 4.7   Tocopherols and tocotrienols in oats.

Another study by White et al. [85] reported that αTT makes up around 66% of the total tocols in oat grains. Oat oil contains α-tocotrienol and α-tocopherol, along with small amounts of other tocols, and there is a positive correlation between tocotrienols and oil concentrations in various oat varieties. Studies indicate that oat grains typically contain (expressed as mg/kg): 6.6–14.9 αTP, 0.5–3.0 βTP, 0.4 γTP, 0.01 δTP, and 13.3–56.4 αTT [86], [87].

In addition to their antioxidant properties, oat tocols offer potential health benefits for humans by influencing degenerative diseases like cancer and cardiovascular diseases (CVD), as well as by reducing blood cholesterol levels. It has been observed in various reports that the vitamin E activity of these tocols depends on their chemical structure and physiological factors. For instance, different tocol isomers demonstrate varying levels of vitamin E activity, with the order being αTP > βTP > αTT > γTP > βTT > δTP, while γTT and δTT may not exhibit such activity [86]. Recent research has uncovered several novel benefits of tocotrienols, a subgroup of tocols. They may contribute to lowering LDL cholesterol by inhibiting cholesterol biosynthesis. Studies also indicate that

TABLE 4.4 Tocols in Oat

COMPOUND	PART	REFERENCE
Total tocols (TP)	• Oat (hull, bran, endosperm, germ) (1.61–3.61 mg/100 g)	[48]
	• Oat (germ, endospore, bran) (7.21 mg/100 g)	[86]
	• Oat (naked) (115 µg/g)	[92]
	• Oat (hulled) (122 µg/g)	
	• Total range (grains) (68.4 to 163 µg/g)	
	• Oat (germ, endospore, bran) (0.5 mg/100 g)	[93]
Trienols (TT)	• Oat (hull, bran, endosperm, germ) (1.09–2.57 mg/100 g)	[48]
	• Oat (germ, endosperm) (1.35 mg/100 g)	[93]
α-TT	• Oat (grains) (81.2 µg/g)	[92]
	• Oat (germ, endosperm, bran, hull) (0.94–2.30 mg/100 g)	[48]
	• Oat (germ, endospore, bran) (5.64 mg/100 g)	[86]
	• Oat (germ, endospore) (0.27 mg/100 g)	[93]
α-TP	• Oat (grains) (31.4 µg/g)	[92]
	• Oat (germ, endosperm, bran, hull) (0.45–0.98 mg/100 g)	[48]
	• Oat (germ, endosperm, bran) (0.72–0.94 mg/100 g)	[94]
	• Oat (germ, endospore, bran) (1.49 mg/100 g)	[86]
	• Oat (germ, endosperm, bran, hull) (0.56–4.14 mg/100 g)	[95]
β-TT	• Oat (grains) (5.47 µg/g)	[92]
	• Oat (germ, endosperm, bran, hull) (0.13–0.27 mg/100 g)	[48]
	• Oat (germ, endospore, bran) (0.54 mg/100 g)	[86]
	• Oat (germ, endospore) (0.11 mg/100 g)	[93]
β-TP	• Oat (germ, endosperm, bran, hull) (0.06–0.10 mg/100 g)	[48]
	• Oat (germ, endosperm, bran) (0.3 mg/100 g)	[86]
	• Oat (germ, endosperm, bran, hull) (0.08–0.84 mg/100 g)	[95]
	• Oat (grains) (1.88 µg/g)	[92]
γ-TP	• Oat (germ, endosperm, bran) (0.05–0.12 mg/100 g)	[94]
	• Oat (germ, endospore, bran) (0.04 mg/100 g)	[86]
	• Oat (germ, endosperm, bran, hull) (0.03–0.36 mg/100 g)	[95]

a high intake of α-tocopherols from oats can reduce lipid peroxidation, inhibit platelet aggregation, and serve as a potent anti-inflammatory agent. Besides their antioxidant properties, tocols present in oats have demonstrated anticancer and cancer-suppressing effects, immune system modulation, the moderation of cardiovascular disease (CVD) risk factors, and the promotion of apoptosis induction [88], [89]. One particularly notable finding about tocols is their potential to clear atherosclerotic blockages (stenosis) in the carotid artery, which could reduce the risk of stroke [90]. Tocols also protect against oxidative damage to polyunsaturated fatty acids in cell membranes, lipoproteins, DNA nucleotidic bases, and proteins [91]. Tocotrienols are generally considered to be stronger antioxidants compared to tocopherols.

4.4 PHYTOSTEROLS

Phytosterols, also known as plant sterols, play a crucial role as triterpenes in the structural makeup of plant membranes. Just as cholesterol does in animal cell membranes, free phytosterols help maintain the stability of phospholipid bilayers within plant cell membranes [96]. Most phytosterols typically consist of either 28 or 29 carbon atoms and may have one or two carbon-carbon double bonds. These double bonds are usually found in the sterol nucleus, and occasionally, there may be a second double bond in the alkyl side chain. Phytostanols, a subgroup of phytosterols, are fully saturated and contain no double bonds. They have a tetracyclic structure and a side chain at position C-17. The structure of phytosterols closely resembles that of cholesterol, which is the predominant sterol found in animal cells. Contrary to a common misconception, plant cells do contain some cholesterol, although their levels typically remain below 1% of the total sterol content. In contrast to animal cells, plant cells have been identified to contain numerous sterols, numbering in the hundreds. These sterols vary mainly in their substitutions at C-4 and C-24 on the side chain, the degree of unsaturation in the side chain and rings, and the presence of conjugation between the C-3 alcoholic hydroxyl group and not only fatty acids but also phenolic acids and carbohydrates [97] (Figure 4.8).

Apart from their free form, phytosterols exist in four distinct types of conjugates. In these conjugates, the 3β-OH group is linked through esterification to either a fatty acid or a hydroxycinnamic acid, or it can be glycosylated using a hexose, typically glucose, or a hexose that is acylated with a fatty acid (Table 4.5). Free phytosterols often possess a double bond in the B-ring, specifically between C-5 and C-6 or between C-7 and C-8. These are referred to as Δ^5-sterols and Δ7-sterols, respectively. The placement of this double bond in the ring is a distinguishing feature among different plant species. While Δ^5-sterols are prevalent in most plants, certain plant families, such as Cucurbitaceae and Amaranthaceae, predominantly contain Δ^7-sterols. Phytosterols that have a saturated ring structure are termed stanols, which are considered a subset of phytosterols and are typically included when calculating the total phytosterol content. Furthermore, phytosterols can be categorized based on the number of methyl substituents at C-4, dividing them into desmethyl-, 4-monomethyl-, or 4,4-dimethyl sterols [98] (Figure 4.8).

The structural diversity of phytosterols in higher plants is further enhanced by the alkylation of C-24, a characteristic that is largely unique to plant sterols, with some exceptions in fungi (primarily ergosterol), slime moulds, and a few other taxa. This alkylation at C-24 can involve the attachment of a methyl, methylene, ethyl, or ethylidene group. Among these C-24 substitutions, ethylation typically occurs as 24α-epimers and is more common, accounting for over 70% of sterols, whereas methyl substitution is less frequent, making up less than 30% of sterols and occurring as both 24α- and 24β-epimers. Moreover, phytosterols can feature double bonds in their side chains, most commonly between C-22 and C-23, leading to an increase in the sterol's polarity. The primary phytosterols found in plants include β-sitosterol (24α-ethylcholesterol), campesterol (24α-methylcholesterol), and stigmasterol (Δ^{22}, 24α-ethylcholesterol)

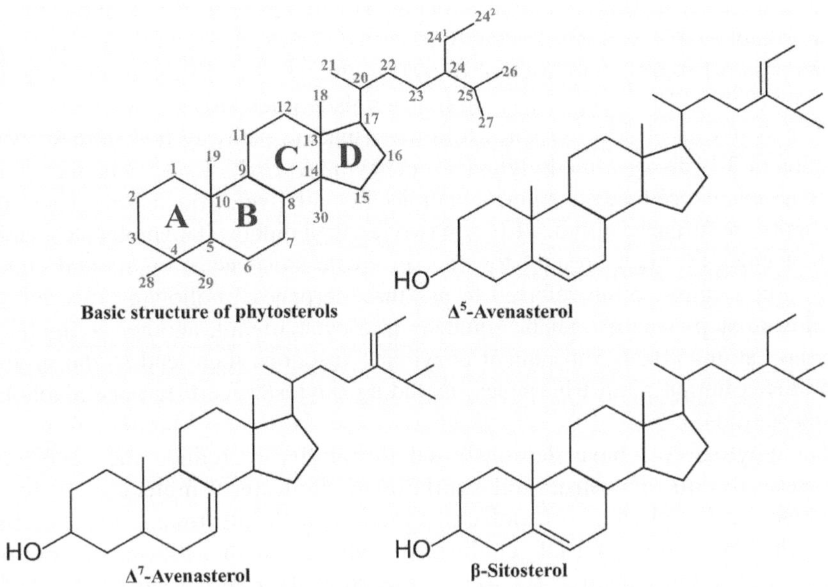

FIGURE 4.8 Phytosterols in oat.

TABLE 4.5 Phytosterols in Oat

COMPOUND	PART	REFERENCE
Total sterols	• Oat (karnel) (350–491 µg/g)	[100]
Stanols, %	• Oat (germ, endosperm, bran, hull) (1.3–1.6 mg/100 g)	[48]
Sitosterol	• Oat (germ, endosperm, bran, hull) (36.5–44.2 mg/100 g) • Oat (germ, endosperm, bran, hull) (30.6–42.9%) • Oat (karnel) (67–88 mg/g)	[48] [104]
ß-Sitosterol	• Oat (karnel) (237–321 mg/g)	[100]
Campesterol	• Oat (germ, endosperm, bran, hull) (5.0–6.2 mg/100 g) • Oat (karnel) (32–46 mg/g)	[48] [100]
Stigmasterol	• Oat (germ, endosperm, bran, hull) (3.9–4.6%) • Oat (karnel) (11–21 mg/g)	[104] [100]
Δ⁷-Stigmasterol	• Oat (1–2%)	[104]
Δ⁵-Avenasterol	• Oat (karnel) (29–45 mg/g)	[100]
Δ⁷-Avenasterol	• Oat (karnel) (7–14 mg/g)	[100]

[99]. The total phytosterol content in oats can range from 35 mg/100 g to 68.2 mg/100 g. Research indicates that in oat kernels, the most abundant phytosterol is typically β-sitosterol (237–321 µg/g), followed by campesterol (32–46 µg/g), Δ⁵-avenasterol (15–47 µg/g), and stigmasterol (11–21 µg/g) [100]. In oat bran, the primary phytosterols

include campesterol (0.22), campestanol (0.04), stigmasterol (0.13), sitosterol (1.56), and sitostanol (0.07), expressed as mg free sterols/g lipids. In oat hull, these phytosterols are campesterol (0.68), campestanol (0.09), stigmasterol (0.53), sitosterol (4.09), and sitostanol (0.49), also expressed as mg free sterols/g lipids [101].

The synthesis of all triterpenes follows a specific pathway that initiates with the reduction of 3-hydroxy-3-methylglutaryl coenzyme A (HMG-CoA), which contains six carbon atoms, to produce mevalonate, a molecule with five carbon atoms. These mevalonate units are further combined to form two farnesyl diphosphate molecules, and these two molecules are then brought together to create squalene, a compound composed of 30 carbon atoms, often referred to as "three terpenes." Following this, enzymatic ring closure steps occur to shape squalene into cycloartenol, another compound with 30 carbon atoms [102]. Subsequent enzymatic reactions then lead to the production of various common plant triterpenes, including phytosterols, triterpene alcohols, and brassinosteroids.

Oat phytosterols have demonstrated the ability to reduce the absorption of cholesterol due to their structural similarity to cholesterol molecules. It has been hypothesized that phytosterol molecules interact with intestinal cells, thereby hindering the absorption of LDL cholesterol, which can then be mostly eliminated through faeces. Only a small fraction of phytosterols, ranging from 0.1% to 5%, is absorbed in the intestines, and the majority of these molecules are excreted. Epidemiological studies conducted on representative groups of volunteers have revealed that consuming 1–3 g of plant sterols daily can lead to an average reduction of LDL cholesterol levels in blood serum by about 10%. Importantly, these changes in cholesterol levels did not significantly impact the levels of "good" high-density lipoprotein-cholesterol and triacylglycerols [103].

4.5 FATTY ACIDS

Oat fat is notably abundant in unsaturated fatty acids. Specifically, in naked oats, the linoleic acid content ranges from 38.1% to 52% of the total fat content, while oleic acid makes up around 30% to 40% of the total unsaturated fatty acid content. In terms of calorie content, oats have one of the highest among other food crops. They possess the highest fat content of any cereal, characterized by low levels of saturated fatty acids and a substantial presence of essential unsaturated fatty acids, which can contribute to reducing the risk of cardiovascular diseases. Oats are particularly high in linoleic acid and low in saturated fat, making them beneficial for heart and vascular health. Monounsaturated fatty acids (MUFA, C18:1) and polyunsaturated fatty acids (PUFA, C18:2) are the most prevalent fatty acids found in oats, followed by saturated fatty acids like palmitic acid (16:0) and lower levels of stearic acid (18:0) and linoleic acid (18:3) [105]. Triglycerides make up the primary component of lipids, with phospholipids also present, and notable amounts of glycolipids and sterols are found in oats. The high lipid content of oats makes them a valuable functional food ingredient in a wide range of industries. In terms of the fatty acid content per 100 g of oat flour sample, it ranges from 193.5–292.9 (C16:0), 11.5–33.3 (C18:0), 385.0–718.0 (C18:1), 532.3–748.9 (C18:2), and 12.3–16.1 (C18:3) [27] (Table 4.6).

Bioactive fatty acids (BFAs) present in oats, including polyunsaturated fatty acids (PUFAs), conjugated fatty acids, and medium-chain triglycerides (MCTs), have been extensively researched due to their potential health-promoting properties. These properties span a wide range of health concerns, including inflammation, cancer, oxidative stress, allergies, diabetes, thrombosis, obesity, hypertension, lipidemia, and various degenerative diseases [106]. Oats contain BFAs such as linoleic acid and its

TABLE 4.6 Bioactive Fatty Acids in Oat

COMPOUND	PART	REFERENCE
Myristic (C14:0)	• Oat (germ, endosperm, bran) (0.5–0.7%) • Oat (germ, endosperm, bran, hull) (0.2%) • Oat (germ, endosperm, bran) (0.2–0.3%)	[110] [111] [112]
Palmitic (C16:0)	• Oat (germ, endosperm, bran, hull) (21.4–22.8%) • Oat (flour) (31.8–262.3 mg/100 g) • Oat (germ, endosperm, bran, hull) (16.1–17.1%) • Oat (germ, endosperm, bran, hull) (12–20.9%) • Oat (germ, endosperm, bran, hull) (15.7–18.8%)	[110] [113] [111] [114] [95]
Palmitoleic (C16:1 *cis*-9)	• Oat (germ, endosperm, bran) (0.2–0.3%)	[110]
Stearic (C18:0)	• Oat (germ, endosperm, bran) (1.5–3-1%) • Oat (germ, endosperm, bran, hull) (1.7–2.5%)	[110] [111]
Oleic (C18:1)	• Oat (germ, endosperm, bran, hull) (36.2–37.8%)	[111]
Elaidic (C18:1 *trans*-9)	• Oat (germ, endosperm, bran) (0.1–0.5%)	[110]
Oleic (C18:1 *cis*-9)	• Oat (germ, endosperm, bran) (30.7–32.2%)	[110]
Cis-13-Octadecenoic (C18:1 *cis*-13)	• Oat (germ, endosperm, bran, hull) (1.5–1.8%)	[110]
Linoleic (C18:2)	• Oat (germ, endosperm, bran, hull) (1–1.2%) • Oat (flour) (1.2–17.1 mg/100 g)	[111] [113]
C18:2 (n-6)	• Oat (germ, endosperm, bran, hull) (39.4–41.6%)	[111]
Linoelaidic trans (C18:2 *trans, trans*-9,12)	• Oat (germ, endosperm) (<0.1–0.4%)	[110]
Linoelaidic *cis* (C18:2 *cis,cis*-9,12)	• Oat (germ, endosperm) (34.6–38.2%)	[110]
Linolenic (C18:3)	• Oat (germ, endosperm, bran) (1.1–1.9%)	[112]
Linolenic (C18:3 (n-3))	• Oat (germ, endosperm, bran, hull) (0.9–1.3%)	[111]
Alpha-Linolenic (C18:3 all *cis* 9,12,15)	• Oat (germ, endosperm, bran) (1.2–1.6%)	[110]
Linolenic (C18:3) isomers	• Oat (germ, endosperm, bran) (0.1–0.4%)	[110]
Arachidic (C20:0)	• Oat (germ, endosperm, bran) (0.2–0.4%)	[110]
Eicosapentanoic (C20:5)	• Oat (germ, endosperm, bran) (0.2–0.4%)	[111]

conjugated form (CLA), alphalinolenic acid (ALA, 18:3, n-3), eicosapentaenoic acid (EPA, 20:5, n-3), and docosahexaenoic acid (DHA, 22:6, n-3), which have been extensively studied.

Fatty acids like ARA, EPA, and DHA are transformed into eicosanoids, which play crucial roles in regulating various homeostatic and inflammatory processes associated with diseases like cancer and obesity. They also contribute to maintaining normal heart function and managing hypertriglyceridemia. Eicosanoids derived from omega-3 or 6 long-chain PUFAs (LC-PUFAs) exhibit anti-inflammatory and pro-inflammatory activities, respectively. Omega-3 FAs, for example, reduce the production of inflammatory cytokines such as TNF-α by immune cells and moderate the expression of inflammatory genes by inhibiting nuclear factor-kappa B (NF-κB), a transcription factor upstream of TNF-α. However, meeting the challenges posed by changing consumer preferences, niche market expansion, and reformulation strategies may require diversification and the identification of lipids with unique bioactivities for inclusion in functional foods. Oat oil serves as a source of natural antioxidants, including tocopherols, alk(en)iloresorcinols, phenolic acids and their derivatives, and AVAs. Notably, AVAs are unique to oats and are not found in other cereal grains.

Fatty acid esters of hydroxy fatty acids (FAHFAs) found in oats represent a relatively recent and intriguing class of bioactive lipids that are gaining substantial attention within the research community. These FAHFAs are drawing interest due to their promising health benefits and potential therapeutic applications in addressing diabetes, inflammation associated with obesity, lipid oxidation, and oxidative stress. In wholegrain oats, the levels of FAHFAs are approximately 0.32 µg/g fresh weight basis (FWB), while they are present at a lower concentration of 0.02 µg/g FWB in fine oat flakes [107]. Oat oil, on the other hand, contains a significantly higher concentration of FAHFAs, approximately 300 µg/g FWB [108]. These FAHFAs include POHPO: Palmitoleic acid hydroxy palmitoleic acid; PAHSA: Palmitic acid ester of hydroxy stearic acids; POHPA: Palmitoleic acid hydroxy palmitic acid; SAHSA: Stearic acid hydroxy stearic acid; PAHPA: Palmitic acid hydroxy palmitic acid [109]. Oat FAHFAs and their potential health benefits represent a promising avenue in the field of nutrition and health research.

4.6 BIOACTIVE POLYPEPTIDES

Dietary protein plays a crucial role as a macronutrient in our food, and it offers more than just nutritional value. It also provides additional health benefits by releasing active peptides that are originally concealed within the native protein structure [10], [11], [13], [14], [115]–[118]. Typically, these bioactive peptides, often referred to as "cryptides," are short chains of amino acids consisting of 2 to 20 units (~3 kDa molecular weight). These amino acids possess specific but dormant properties within the parent protein and need to be liberated to unleash their potential biological activities [10], [11], [13], [14], [18], [115], [118]. This liberation can occur through various processes, including in vitro hydrolysis of peptide bonds, which involves the use of proteolytic enzymes, as well as treatments with acid or alkali. Additionally, in vivo, gastrointestinal digestion and microbial fermentation are other means by which these bioactive peptides can be released [119]. It's worth noting that these hydrolysis methods result in the release of cryptides into a mixture containing several other peptides and free amino acids, collectively known as protein hydrolysates. Due to their high protein content, sustainability, and favourable nutritional profile, oats are regarded as a promising cereal for the extraction of plant-based proteins and the isolation of bioactive peptides. These peptides either naturally exist or are generated from precursor proteins through processes like gestational simulation, microbial fermentation, or enzymatic hydrolysis. Research has shown that bioactive peptides tend to have simpler structures, greater stability, and more notable physiological activities and functions when compared to their parent proteins [10], [13], [16], [115].

Depending on factors such as their amino acid sequence, composition, length, and charge, oat protein-based bioactive peptides can exhibit a diverse range of beneficial biological properties. These properties include antioxidant, antimicrobial, immuno-modulatory, anticancer, antihypertensive, anti-inflammatory, mineral binding, opiate, and anti-lipidemic activities [120]. These activities have the potential to impact various systems within the human body, including the cardiovascular, gastrointestinal, immune, and endocrine systems [119]. Furthermore, these peptides have the advantage of not accumulating in body tissues, thus posing minimal risk of serious side effects. Consequently, they offer promising alternatives to traditional drugs for preventing and treating lifestyle-related diseases. However, their practical application in the food industry is hindered by challenges such as relatively low chemical stability, bitter taste, interactions with food matrices, and susceptibility to gastrointestinal digestion. Nevertheless, these obstacles can be overcome by adopting well-designed delivery systems that enhance encapsulation and targeted release [121]. Given the wide range of beneficial biological functions they possess, it becomes imperative to harness the potential of food protein hydrolysates and peptides as valuable functional components for promoting human health.

Oat proteins have gained recognition as a valuable source of antioxidant capacity, holding the potential to enhance the management of conditions linked to oxidative stress, prolong the preservation of food items by inhibiting oxidation, and ultimately contribute to an improved quality of life [122]. When evaluated through various assays, including 2,2 azino-bis-ethylbenzoline-6-sulfonic acid (ABTS), hydroxyl radicals ($HO^{\bullet}$ and $O^{\bullet}_2$), and Fe^{2+} chelating, oat protein isolates and hydrolysates have demonstrated outstanding antioxidant properties [123]. Among the bioactive peptides derived from the globulin fraction of oats, specific sequences such as Asn–Ser–Lys–Asn–Phe–Pro–Thr–Leu, Leu–Ile–Gly–Arg–Pro–Ile–Ile–Tyr, Phe–Asn–Asp–Ile–Leu–Arg–Arg–Gly–Gln–Leu–Leu, Phe–Leu–Lys–Pro–Met–Thr, and Ile–Arg–Ile–Pro–Ile–Leu exhibited the most potent scavenging activity against 2,2-diphenyl-1-picryl-hydrazyl-hydrate (DPPH) radicals (with an IC_{50} value of 4.11 mg/mL) and hydroxyl radicals (with an IC_{50} value of 1.83 mg/mL) [124]. In another study, oat peptides including Gly–Gln–Thr–Val, Tyr–His–Asn–Ala–Pro, Gly–Leu–Val–Tyr–Ile–Leu and displayed notable cytoprotective effects and demonstrated the ability to scavenge peroxyl radicals, as evidenced by their significant oxygen radical absorbance capacity (ORAC) values of 0.67, 0.61, and 0.52 Trolox equivalent (TE)/µM, respectively. Interestingly, the cytoprotective activity of these peptides was found to be associated with their overall hydrophobicity rather than their ORAC values [125].

Oat hydrolysates have demonstrated a remarkable cytoprotective effect by shielding HepG2 cells from AAPH-induced oxidative stress. This protection was achieved by significantly enhancing the activities of key antioxidant enzymes such as GPx (glutathione peroxidase), CAT (catalase), and SOD (superoxide dismutase), while simultaneously reducing the levels of ROS [126]. Moreover, these hydrolysates exhibited a notable capacity to inhibit lipid oxidation and peroxidation of linolenic acid, with peptides Ser–Pro–Phe–Trp–Asn–Ile–Asn–Ala–His, Tyr–Phe–Asp–Glu–Gln–Asn–Glu–Gln–Phe–Arg, and Asn–Ile–Asn–Ala–His–Ser–Val–Val–Tyr and showing inhibition rates of up to 16%, 35%, and 52% respectively [127]. The presence of amino acids like tyrosine and histidine, whether at the *N*-terminal or *C*-terminal positions within the peptide sequences, contributed to their enhanced antioxidant activity. This effect is attributed to the electron or proton-donating ability of these amino acids. Additionally, the hydrophobic nature of the peptides played a crucial role in their interaction with lipids [127]. A recent development in addressing anaemia and oxidative stress involved the use of oat antioxidant peptides as carriers to create a novel oat peptide-ferrous (OP-Fe^{+2}) chelate. OP-Fe^{+2} has shown promise in alleviating anaemia, while also improving the activities of antioxidant enzymes, such as GSH (glutathione) and SOD, and reducing the malondialdehyde (MDA) content in the livers of iron-deficient anaemic rat models [128]. Furthermore, oat peptides demonstrated their effectiveness in mitigating H_2O_2-induced apoptosis and oxidative stress in human dermal fibroblasts by regulating cellular antioxidant enzymes [129]. Taken together, these findings underscore the potential of oat-derived peptides in reducing oxidative stress and associated disorders, making them valuable candidates for the development of nutraceuticals or functional foods with enhanced health benefits.

Oat GABA, or γ-aminobutyric acid, is a non-protein amino acid known for its reported health benefits, including the reduction of blood pressure, stress relief, and the inhibition of cancer cell proliferation. In crops, the production of GABA typically occurs through the decarboxylation of l-glutamic acid by residual enzymes. The GABA content in crops can be increased in response to various stress signals, such as cold shock, hypoxia, and specific germination processes.

4.7 PHYTIC ACID

Myo-inositol-1,2,3,4,5,6-hexakisphosphate, commonly known as phytic acid, is a member of the myo-inositol (Ins) phosphorylated derivatives family (Figure 4.9). It is characterized as a cyclic alcohol that serves as the carbon backbone for phytic acid biosynthesis. Phytic acid has a molar mass of 660.04 g/mol, and its molecular formula is $C_6H_{18}O_{24}P_6$. X-ray crystallographic analysis reveals that the phosphate groups are attached axially to carbons 1, 3, 4, 5, and 6, while they are attached equatorially to carbon 2 [130]. Phytic acid is an inert and highly stable molecule, allowing it to be stored in neutral or alkaline aqueous solutions as a solid for extended periods, often

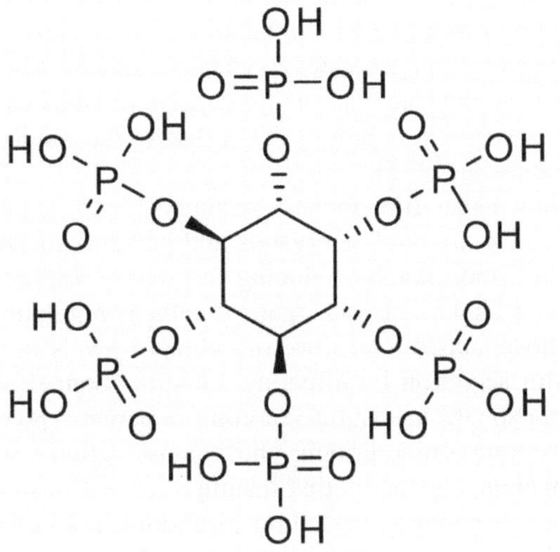

Phytic acid

FIGURE 4.9 Phytic acid structure.

months or years, before producing any decomposition products. When in the salt form, IP6 (inositol hexaphosphate) is also referred to as phytate. Inositol molecules with fewer phosphate groups, namely IP1 to IP5, are collectively known as phytates. IP6 and its lower phosphorylated forms (IP1–5) are found in nearly all mammalian cells. Phytic acid constitutes over 70% of the total phosphorus content in whole grains and makes up about 1–7% of the dry weight of the entire grain. It is primarily located in the bran fraction of whole-grain cereals, particularly within the aleurone layer [131]. In whole oat grains, phytic acid is present at concentrations ranging from 5.6 to 8.7 mg/g [132].

Phytic acid possesses a potent chelating ability, attributed to its structure which exhibits a strong affinity for polyvalent cations. This affinity follows a descending stability order: $Cu^{2+} > Zn^{2+} > Ni^{2+} > Co^{2+} > Mn^{2+} > Fe^{3+} > Ca^{2+}$. When phytic acid chelates with these cations, it forms water-insoluble phytate salts. The most commonly encountered mono- and divalent cations in this context are K^+, Mg^{2+}, and Ca^{2+}. Phytic acid also binds directly or indirectly with starch and protein. For many years, phytic acid was viewed as an antinutrient. However, numerous studies conducted on both human and animal models have demonstrated the preventive effects of phytic acid against various pathologies. It's worth noting that phytic acid is widespread in eukaryotic species, and lower levels of *myo*-inositol with fewer phosphate groups (IP1–5) play a significant role in regulating essential cellular functions, including cell division, cellular differentiation, exocytosis, and endocytosis [133].

Phytic acid in oats demonstrates strong antioxidant properties in vitro. It effectively inhibits iron (Fe)-catalysed oxidative reactions by chelating free iron ions, thus preventing the Fenton reaction, and it may function as a potent antioxidant in vivo by reducing lipid peroxidation [134]. Phytic acid also plays a role in reducing the incidence of colonic cancer by protecting the gut epithelium from oxidative damage, particularly in the colon, where bacteria can generate oxygenated radicals. Additionally, phytic acid inhibits xanthine oxidase-induced superoxide-dependent DNA damage. Xanthine oxidases, which produce superoxide anions (O_2^-) during the oxidation of xanthine, are abundant within the intestine [135].

Studies have shown that IP6 (inositol hexaphosphate) significantly inhibits the formation of urinary calcium oxalate crystals and prevents the crystallization of calcium oxalate salts in urine, thereby reducing the risk of kidney stone development. Phytic acid also plays a vital role in pancreatic β-cells by regulating stimulus-secretion coupling, protein phosphatases, and lowering glucose levels in vivo [136], [137]. It may modulate insulin secretion by affecting calcium channel activity, and it is the dominant inositol phosphate in insulin-secreting pancreatic β-cells. Studies suggest that IP6 inhibits serine-threonine protein phosphatase activity, which, in turn, opens intracellular calcium channels, facilitating insulin release. Consumption of phytic acid can have various health benefits, including promoting colon health and protecting against cardiovascular diseases, diabetes, and several cancers mediated by oxidative processes [137].

4.8 SAPONINS

The term "saponin" originates from the Latin word "sapo," meaning "soap." This is due to the fact that saponin molecules generate frothy, soap-like bubbles when agitated with water. They are a varied group of compounds with diverse structures, falling under the chemical categories of triterpene and steroid glycosides. These molecules consist of hydrophobic aglycones combined with one or more sugar units. The presence of both hydrophilic and hydrophobic components in their structures explains their ability to exhibit soap-like properties in aqueous solutions. Saponins are glycosides featuring a steroid or triterpenoid aglycone [138]. They constitute a structurally diverse class of substances found in numerous plant species, distinguished by a core structure derived from the 30-carbon precursor oxidosqualene, to which sugar residues are attached. Traditionally, saponins are categorized into triterpenoid and steroid glycosides, or further subdivided into triterpenoid, spirostanol, and furostanol saponins [139] (Table 4.7).

Saponins display a wide array of characteristics, encompassing qualities such as sweetness and bitterness, the ability to create foam and act as emulsifiers, pharmacological and medicinal attributes, and hemolytic properties, as well as antimicrobial, insecticidal, and molluscicidal activities. These compounds serve as protective mechanisms for plants and find pharmaceutical applications in humans due to their anti-thrombotic, anti-inflammatory, anticancer, anti-diabetic, and antihypertensive properties, as well as their efficacy in addressing reproductive disorders [140].

Saponins are present in various plant species, but oats are unique as they are the only cereal that accumulates saponins. Apart from contributing to the bitter taste of oats and

TABLE 4.7   Saponins in Oat

COMPOUND	PART	REFERENCE
Avenacoside A	• Oat (0.15–2.6 mg/100 g)	[144]
	• Oat (0.008–0.03% DW)	[145]
Avenacoside B	• Oat (0.06–2.51 mg/100 g)	[144]
	• Oat (0.003–0.01% DW)	[145]
26-Desglucoav-enacoside A	• Oat (grains) (0.07–0.7 mg/100 g)	[144]
Total avenacins	• Oat (roots) (1,280 mg/100 g)	[143]
Total saponins	• Oat (porridge) (130 mg/100 g)	[146]
	• Oat (porridge) (100 mg/100 g)	[147]

DW, dry weight.

serving as a defence mechanism against fungal attacks, saponins are believed to have potential health benefits for humans, such as lowering cholesterol levels and influencing the immune system [141], [142]. Oats produce two groups of saponins: steroidal avenacosides and triterpenoid avenacins. The saponin content in oat endosperm ranges from 0.02% to 0.13% (dry weight) [143]. Avenacins, found in their active form, are primarily located in oat roots, whereas avenacosides, which are inactive forms, are present in leaves and grains. Avenacosides A (1) and B (2) can be converted into their active counterparts: 26-desglucoavenacoside A (3) and 26-desglucoavenacoside B (4). Avenacoside A constitutes 41.9%–60.6% of the total saponin content in oat grain and 37.1%–57.7% in husks. Avenacoside B accounts for 35.8%–55.2% in oat grain and 13.8%–49.0% in husks of the total saponin content [144]. The content of 26-desglucoavenacoside A reaches 6.4% in grain and 48.3% in husks. However, the levels of avenacosides can vary due to differences in oat cultivars, growth conditions, and variations in the sensitivity and precision of quantification methods used in various studies.

4.9 CONCLUSION

Oats are recognized as significant sources of valuable nutrients, particularly protein and fat, enriched with healthy mono- and polyunsaturated fatty acids and a balanced amino acid composition. They also offer essential minerals, making them a vital part of a nutritious diet. Moreover, oat grains provide natural antioxidants that contribute to reducing the risk of various diseases, establishing their place in functional food formulations globally and promoting a healthier lifestyle. Oats contain numerous bioactive components, including protein, peptides, amino acids, β-glucan, resistant starch, polyunsaturated fatty acids, polyphenols, alkaloids, oat saponins, and β-sitosterol. These compounds offer a range of biological functions, such as antioxidative, anti-diabetic, antimicrobial, anticancer, anti-obesity, immunomodulatory, and cardiovascular protective effects. Given the increasing concern about obesity and its associated complications, dietary prevention through oat consumption is viewed as a preferable strategy. However, research gaps exist, including the limited study of oat alkaloids' separation and purification methods and the need to investigate their solubility, bioavailability, and mechanisms of action. Mechanistic studies on the lipid-lowering effects of oat proteins and the potential impact of oat-resistant starch on weight loss and lipid reduction are also areas for further exploration.

Beyond fibre, oats offer bioactive compounds with robust antioxidant and anti-inflammatory properties that may help prevent chronic diseases like cancer and cardiovascular disease. Nevertheless, research on the health benefits of these compounds, particularly AVAs and avenacosides A and B, is still in its early stages, leaving room for more discoveries. Increased consumption of whole-grain oats has shown associations with reduced risks of diet-related disorders such as type 2 diabetes, cancer, and cardiovascular diseases. However, inconsistencies in epidemiological studies result from difficulties in accurately assessing dietary intake and internal dosage. Factors like plant cultivar, processing methods, and storage affect bioactive component levels. Additionally, genetic variations and gut microbiota differences among individuals complicate the relationship between food intake and chronic diseases. Biomarkers for whole-grain oat exposure and effects are essential for a deeper understanding of their health benefits.

Future research directions in oat antioxidants include characterizing germplasm for antioxidant compound concentrations, determining the effects of growing environments, investigating bioavailability and physiological effects, and developing methods for fractionating oats to incorporate their components into food systems. Nutritional genomics offers opportunities to modify oat enzymes and pathways to enhance desired constituent production. In conclusion, oats stand as a promising plant food for the future, credited for their nutritional, medicinal, and therapeutic properties. Continued research and exploration of their bioactive compounds hold the potential to unlock even more health benefits, contributing to a healthier world.

REFERENCES

[1]   A. Patra, S. Abdullah and R. C. Pradhan, "Review on the extraction of bioactive compounds and characterization of fruit industry by-products," *Bioresour. Bioprocess.*, vol. 9, p. 14, 2022, doi: 10.1186/s40643-022-00498-3.

[2]   D. Liu et al., "Elderberry (Sambucus nigra L.): Bioactive compounds, health functions, and applications," *J. Agric. Food Chem.*, vol. 70, pp. 4202–4220, 2022, doi: 10.1021/acs.jafc.2c00010.

[3]   J. M. Macharia et al., "Medicinal plants with anti-colorectal cancer bioactive compounds: Potential game-changers in colorectal cancer management," *Biomed. Pharmacother.*, vol. 153, p. 113383, 2022, doi: 10.1016/j.biopha.2022.113383.

[4]   V. Ninkuu, L. Zhang, J. Yan, Z. Fu, T. Yang and H. Zeng, "Biochemistry of terpenes and recent advances in plant protection," *Int J Mol Sci.*, vol. 22, p. 5710, 2021, doi: 10.3390/ijms22115710.

[5]   A. Masyita et al., "Terpenes and terpenoids as main bioactive compounds of essential oils, their roles in human health and potential application as natural food preservatives," *Food Chem. X.*, vol. 13, p. 100217, 2022, doi: 10.1016/j.fochx.2022.100217.

[6] F. Rodríguez-Félix et al., "Trends in sustainable green synthesis of silver nanoparticles using agri-food waste extracts and their applications in health," *J Nanomater.*, vol. 2022, p. e8874003, 2022, doi: 10.1155/2022/8874003.

[7] L. P. Y. Lam et al., "Flavonoids in major cereal grasses: Distribution, functions, biosynthesis, and applications," *Phytochem. Rev.*, 2023, doi: 10.1007/s11101-023-09873-0.

[8] R. Gupta, M. Meghwal and P. K. Prabhakar, "Bioactive compounds of pigmented wheat (Triticum aestivum): Potential benefits in human health," *Trends Food Sci. Technol.*, vol. 110, pp. 240–252, 2021, doi: 10.1016/j.tifs.2021.02.003.

[9] X. Zhang et al., "Identification and quantitative analysis of phenolic glycosides with antioxidant activity in methanolic extract of Dendrobium catenatum flowers and selection of quality control herb-markers," *Food Res. Int.*, vol. 123, pp. 732–745, 2019, doi: 10.1016/j.foodres.2019.05.040.

[10] M. Tomar et al., "Interactome of millet-based food matrices: A review," *Food Chem.*, vol. 385, p. 132636, 2022, doi: 10.1016/j.foodchem.2022.132636.

[11] M. Tomar et al., "Nutritional composition patterns and application of multivariate analysis to evaluate indigenous Pearl millet ((*Pennisetum glaucum* (L.) R. Br.) germplasm," *J. Food Compos. Anal.*, vol. 103, p. 104086, 2021, doi: 10.1016/j.jfca.2021.104086.

[12] R. N. Tiozon Jr, K. J. D. Sartagoda, L. M. N. Serrano, A. R. Fernie and N. Sreenivasulu, "Metabolomics based inferences to unravel phenolic compound diversity in cereals and its implications for human gut health," *Trends Food Sci. Technol.*, vol. 127, pp. 14–25, 2022, doi: 10.1016/j.tifs.2022.06.011.

[13] M. Kumar et al., "Cottonseed feedstock as a source of plant-based protein and bioactive peptides: Evidence based on biofunctionalities and industrial applications," *Food Hydrocoll.*, vol. 131, p. 107776, 2022, doi: 10.1016/j.foodhyd.2022.107776.

[14] M. Kumar et al., "Cottonseed: A sustainable contributor to global protein requirements," *Trends Food Sci. Technol.*, vol. 111, pp. 100–113, 2021, doi: 10.1016/j.tifs.2021.02.058.

[15] M. Kumar et al., "Delineating the inherent functional descriptors and biofunctionalities of pectic polysaccharides," *Carbohydr. Polym.*, vol. 269, p. 118319, 2021, doi: 10.1016/j.carbpol.2021.118319.

[16] M. Tomar et al., "Development of NIR spectroscopy based prediction models for nutritional profiling of pearl millet (*Pennisetum glaucum* (L.)) R.Br: A chemometrics approach," *LWT.*, vol. 149, p. 111813, 2021, doi: 10.1016/j.lwt.2021.111813.

[17] M. Kumar, M. Tomar, S. Punia, R. Amarowicz and C. Kaur, "Evaluation of cellulolytic enzyme-assisted microwave extraction of punica granatum peel phenolics and antioxidant activity," *Plant Foods Hum Nutr.*, vol. 75, pp. 614–620, 2020, doi: 10.1007/s11130-020-00859-3.

[18] M. Kumar et al., "Functional characterization of plant-based protein to determine its quality for food applications," *Food Hydrocoll.*, p. 106986, 2021, doi: 10.1016/j.foodhyd.2021.106986.

[19] M. Kumar et al., "Phenolics as plant protective companion against abiotic stress," in Plant *Phenolics in Sustainable Agriculture : Volume 1*, R. Lone, R. Shuab and A. N. Kamili, Eds. Singapore, Singapore: Springer, 2020, pp. 277–308, doi: 10.1007/978-981-15-4890-1_12.

[20] M. A. Hassan et al., "Health benefits and phenolic compounds of Moringa oleifera leaves: A comprehensive review," *Phytomedicine.*, vol. 93, p. 153771, 2021, doi: 10.1016/j.phymed.2021.153771.

[21] R. M. Tomar, M. Kumar and D. Seva Nayak, "Role of phenolic metabolites in salinity stress management in plants," in *Plant Phenolics in Abiotic Stress Management*, R. Lone, S. Khan and A. Mohammed Al-Sadi, Eds. Singapore, Singapore: Springer Nature, 2023, pp. 353–368, doi: 10.1007/978-981-19-6426-8_16.

[22] J. Nishad et al., "Ultrasound-assisted development of stable grapefruit peel polyphenolic nano-emulsion: Optimization and application in improving oxidative stability of mustard oil," *Food Chem.*, vol. 334, p. 127561, 2021, doi: 10.1016/j.foodchem.2020.127561.

[23] S. W. C. Chung, "A critical review of analytical methods for ergot alkaloids in cereals and feed and in particular suitability of method performance for regulatory monitoring and epimer-specific quantification," *Food Addit. Contam. Part A.*, vol. 38, pp. 997–1012, 2021, doi: 10.1080/19440049.2021.1898679.

[24] H. Guo, H. Wu, A. Sajid and Z. Li, "Whole grain cereals: The potential roles of functional components in human health," *Crit. Rev. Food Sci. Nutr.*, vol. 62, pp. 8388–8402, 2022, doi: 10.1080/10408398.2021.1928596.

[25] I. Usman et al., "Traditional and innovative approaches for the extraction of bioactive compounds," *Int. J. Food Prop.*, vol. 25, pp. 1215–1233, 2022, doi: 10.1080/10942912.2022.2074030.

[26] Y. Tang et al., "Bioactive components and health functions of oat," *Food Rev. Int.*, vol. 39, pp. 4545–4564, 2023, doi: 10.1080/87559129.2022.2029477.

[27] G. F. Alemayehu, S. F. Forsido, Y. B. Tola and E. Amare, "Nutritional and phytochemical composition and associated health benefits of oat (*Avena sativa*) grains and oat-based fermented food products," *Sci. World J.*, vol. 2023, p. e2730175, 2023, doi: 10.1155/2023/2730175.

[28] L. Yang et al., "Recent advances in biosynthesis of bioactive compounds in traditional Chinese medicinal plants," *Sci. Bull.*, vol. 61, pp. 3–17, 2016, doi: 10.1007/s11434-015-0929-2.

[29] P. Choyal et al., "Chemical manipulation of source and sink dynamics improves significantly the root biomass and the with anolides yield in Withania somnifera, *Ind. Crops Prod.*, vol. 188, p. 115577, 2022, doi: 10.1016/j.indcrop.2022.115577.

[30] G. Rocchetti et al., "Functional implications of bound phenolic compounds and phenolics–food interaction: A review," *Compr. Rev. Food Sci. Food Saf.*, vol. 21, pp. 811–842, 2022, doi: 10.1111/1541-4337.12921.

[31] A. Wojdyło, J. Oszmiański and R. Czemerys, "Antioxidant activity and phenolic compounds in 32 selected herbs," *Food Chem.*, vol. 105, pp. 940–949, 2007, doi: 10.1016/j.foodchem.2007.04.038.

[32] A. P. G. da Silva, W. G. Sganzerla, O. D. John and R. Marchiosi, "A comprehensive review of the classification, sources, biosynthesis, and biological properties of hydroxybenzoic and hydroxycinnamic acids," *Phytochem. Rev.*, 2023, doi: 10.1007/s11101-023-09891-y.

[33] H. Punia, J. Tokas, A. Malik, Satpal and S. Sangwan, "Characterization of phenolic compounds and antioxidant activity in sorghum [Sorghum bicolor (L.) Moench] grains," *Cereal Res. Commun.*, vol. 49, pp. 343–353, 2021, doi: 10.1007/s42976-020-00118-w.

[34] M. Morzel, F. Canon and S. Guyot, "Interactions between salivary proteins and dietary polyphenols: Potential consequences on gastrointestinal digestive events," *J. Agric. Food Chem.*, vol. 70, pp. 6317–6327, 2022, doi: 10.1021/acs.jafc.2c01183.

[35] A. Rana, M. Samtiya, T. Dhewa, V. Mishra and R. E. Aluko, "Health benefits of polyphenols: A concise review," *J. Food Biochem.*, vol. 46, p. e14264, 2022, doi: 10.1111/jfbc.14264.

[36] B. Zhang, Y. Zhang, X. Xing and S. Wang, "Health benefits of dietary polyphenols: Insight into interindividual variability in absorption and metabolism," *Curr. Opin. Food Sci.*, vol. 48, p. 100941, 2022, doi: 10.1016/j.cofs.2022.100941.

[37] H. N. Rajha et al., "Recent advances in research on polyphenols: Effects on microbiota, metabolism, and health," *Mol. Nutr. Food Res.*, vol. 66, p. 2100670, 2022, doi: 10.1002/mnfr.202100670.

[38] M. Olszowy, "What is responsible for antioxidant properties of polyphenolic compounds from plants?" *Plant Physiol. Biochem.*, vol. 144, pp. 135–143, 2019, doi: 10.1016/j.plaphy.2019.09.039.

[39] X. Y. Lee, J. S. Tan and L. H. Cheng, "Gamma aminobutyric acid (GABA) enrichment in plant-based food – A mini review," *Food Rev. Int.*, vol. 39, pp. 5864–5885, 2023, doi: 10.1080/87559129.2022.2097257.

[40] A. Shehzad, R. Rabail, S. Munir, H. Jan, D. Fernández-Lázaro and R. M. Aadil, "Impact of oats on appetite hormones and body weight management: A review," *Curr. Nutr. Rep.*, vol. 12, pp. 66–82, 2023, doi: 10.1007/s13668-023-00454-3.

[41] R. Marchiosi et al., "Biosynthesis and metabolic actions of simple phenolic acids in plants," *Phytochem. Rev.*, vol. 19, pp. 865–906, 2020, doi: 10.1007/s11101-020-09689-2.

[42] G. Soycan et al., "Composition and content of phenolic acids and avenanthramides in commercial oat products: Are oats an important polyphenol source for consumers?" *Food Chem. X.*, vol. 3, p. 100047, 2019, doi: 10.1016/j.fochx.2019.100047.

[43] H. Boz, "Phenolic amides (avenanthramides) in oats – A review," *Czech J. Food Sci.*, vol. 33, pp. 399–404, 2015, doi: 10.17221/696/2014-CJFS.

[44] D. M. Peterson, "Oat antioxidants," *J. Cereal Sci.*, vol. 33, pp. 115–129, 2001, doi: 10.1006/jcrs.2000.0349.

[45] C. J. Pretorius and I. A. Dubery, "Avenanthramides, distinctive hydroxycinnamoyl conjugates of oat, Avena sativa L.: An update on the biosynthesis, chemistry, and bioactivities," *Plants.*, vol. 12, p. 1388, 2023, doi: 10.3390/plants12061388.

[46] P. F. Raguindin et al., "A systematic review of phytochemicals in oat and buckwheat," *Food Chem.*, vol. 338, p. 127982, 2021, doi: 10.1016/j.foodchem.2020.127982.

[47] I. Kerienė, A. Mankevičienė, S. Bliznikas, D. Jablonskytė-Raščė, S. Maikštėnienė and R. Česnulevičienė, "Biologically active phenolic compounds in buckwheat, oats and winter spelt wheat.," *Žemdirbystè (Agriculture).*, vol. 102, pp. 289–296, 2015, doi: 10.13080/z-a.2015.102.037.

[48] P. R. Shewry et al., "Phytochemical and fiber components in oat varieties in the health-grain diversity screen," *J. Agric. Food Chem.*, vol. 56, pp. 9777–9784, 2008, doi: 10.1021/jf801880d.

[49] Y. Xing and P. J. White, "Identification and function of antioxidants from oat groats and hulls," *J. Am. Oil Chem. Soc.*, vol. 74, pp. 303–307, 1997, doi: 10.1007/s11746-997-0141-x.

[50] R. S. Gallagher, R. Ananth, K. Granger, B. Bradley, J. V. Anderson and E. P. Fuerst, "Phenolic and short-chained aliphatic organic acid constituents of wild oat (Avena fatua L.) seeds," *J. Agric. Food Chem.*, vol. 58, pp. 218–225, 2010, doi: 10.1021/jf9038106.

[51] C. Chen et al., "Phenolic contents, cellular antioxidant activity and antiproliferative capacity of different varieties of oats," *Food Chem.*, vol. 239, pp. 260–267, 2018, doi: 10.1016/j.foodchem.2017.06.104.

[52] S. Multari, J.-M. Pihlava, P. Ollennu-Chuasam, V. Hietaniemi, B. Yang and J.-P. Suomela, "Identification and quantification of avenanthramides and free and bound phenolic acids in eight cultivars of husked oat (Avena sativa L) from Finland," *J. Agric. Food Chem.*, vol. 66, pp. 2900–2908, 2018, doi: 10.1021/acs.jafc.7b05726.

[53] L. F. Călinoiu and D. C. Vodnar, "Thermal processing for the release of phenolic compounds from wheat and oat bran," *Biomolecules.*, vol. 10, p. 21, 2020, doi: 10.3390/biom10010021.

[54] M. Holasova, V. Fiedlerova, H. Smrcinova, M. Orsak, J. Lachman and S. Vavreinova, "Buckwheat – The source of antioxidant activity in functional foods," *Food Res. Int.*, vol. 35, pp. 207–211, 2002, doi: 10.1016/S0963-9969(01)00185-5.

[55] P. Mattila, J. Pihlava and J. Hellström, "Contents of phenolic acids, alkyl- and alkenyl-resorcinols, and avenanthramides in commercial grain products," *J. Agric. Food Chem.*, vol. 53, pp. 8290–8295, 2005, doi: 10.1021/jf051437z.

[56] M. Varga, R. Jójárt, P. Fónad, R. Mihály and A. Palágyi, "Phenolic composition and antioxidant activity of colored oats," *Food Chem.*, vol. 268, pp. 153–161, 2018, doi: 10.1016/j.foodchem.2018.06.035.

[57] M. Kováčová and E. Malinová, "Ferulic and coumaric acids, total phenolic compounds and their correlation in selected oat genotypes," *Czech J. Food Sci.*, vol. 25, pp. 325–332, 2007. Accessed: Oct. 3, 2023. [Online]. Available: https://ideas.repec.org//a/caa/jnlcjf/v25y2007i6id746-cjfs.html

[58]   T. Dokuyucu, D. M. Peterson and A. Akkaya, "Contents of antioxidant compounds in turkish oats: Simple phenolics and avenanthramide concentrations," *Cereal Chem.*, vol. 80, pp. 542–543, 2003, doi: 10.1094/CCHEM.2003.80.5.542.

[59]   M. Skoglund, D. M. Peterson, R. Andersson, J. Nilsson and L. H. Dimberg, "Avenanthramide content and related enzyme activities in oats as affected by steeping and germination," *J. Cereal Sci.*, vol. 48, pp. 294–303, 2008, doi: 10.1016/j.jcs.2007.09.010.

[60]   K. A. Garleb, L. D. Bourquin, J. T. Hsu, G. W. Wagner, S. J. Schmidt and G. C. Fahey Jr., "Isolation and chemical analyses of nonfermented fiber fractions of oat hulls and cottonseed hulls," *J. Anim. Sci.*, vol. 69, pp. 1255–1271, 1991, doi: 10.2527/1991.6931255x.

[61]   L. Tong, L. Liu, K. Zhong, Y. Wang, L. Guo and S. Zhou, "Effects of cultivar on phenolic content and antioxidant activity of naked oat in China," *J. Integr. Agric.*, vol. 13, pp. 1809–1816, 2014, doi: 10.1016/S2095-3119(13)60626-7.

[62]   L. H. Dimberg, E. L. Molteberg, R. Solheim and W. Frølich, "Variation in oat groats due to variety, storage and heat treatment. I: Phenolic compounds," *J. Cereal Sci.*, vol. 24, pp. 263–272, 1996, doi: 10.1006/jcrs.1996.0058.

[63]   C. L. Emmons and D. M. Peterson, "Antioxidant activity and phenolic contents of oat groats and hulls," *Cereal Chem.*, vol. 76, pp. 902–906, 1999, doi: 10.1094/CCHEM.1999.76.6.902.

[64]   S. Kumar and A. K. Pandey, "Chemistry and biological activities of flavonoids: An overview," *Sci. World J.*, vol. 2013, p. e162750, 2013, doi: 10.1155/2013/162750.

[65]   A. N. Panche, A. D. Diwan and S. R. Chandra, "Flavonoids: An overview," *J. Nutr. Sci.*, vol. 5, p. e47, 2016, doi: 10.1017/jns.2016.41.

[66]   N. Shen, T. Wang, Q. Gan, S. Liu, L. Wang and B. Jin, "Plant flavonoids: Classification, distribution, biosynthesis, and antioxidant activity," *Food Chem.*, vol. 383, p. 132531, 2022, doi: 10.1016/j.foodchem.2022.132531.

[67]   I. Hernández, L. Alegre, F. V. Breusegem and S. Munné-Bosch, "How relevant are flavonoids as antioxidants in plants?" *Trends Plant Sci.*, vol. 14, pp. 125–132, 2009, doi: 10.1016/j.tplants.2008.12.003.

[68]   H. Tao et al., "Comparative metabolomics of flavonoids in twenty vegetables reveal their nutritional diversity and potential health benefits," *Food Res. Int.*, vol. 164, p. 112384, 2023, doi: 10.1016/j.foodres.2022.112384.

[69]   J. Naik, P. Misra, P. K. Trivedi and A. Pandey, "Molecular components associated with the regulation of flavonoid biosynthesis," *Plant Sci.*, vol. 317, p. 111196, 2022, doi: 10.1016/j.plantsci.2022.111196.

[70]   K. K. Adom and R. H. Liu, "Antioxidant activity of grains," *J. Agric. Food Chem.*, vol. 50, pp. 6182–6187, 2002, doi: 10.1021/jf0205099.

[71]   J. Chopin, G. Dellamonica, M. L. Bouillant, A. Besset, G. Popovici and G. Weissenböck, "C-Glycosylflavones from Avena sativa," *Phytochemistry.*, vol. 16, pp. 2041–2043, 1977, doi: 10.1016/0031-9422(77)80131-3.

[72]   Q. Bei, Y. Liu, L. Wang, G. Chen and Z. Wu, "Improving free, conjugated, and bound phenolic fractions in fermented oats (Avena sativa L.) with Monascus anka and their antioxidant activity," *J. Funct. Foods.*, vol. 32, pp. 185–194, 2017, doi: 10.1016/j.jff.2017.02.028.

[73]   Y. Yu et al., "The progress of nomenclature, structure, metabolism, and bioactivities of oat novel phytochemical: Avenanthramides," *J. Agric. Food Chem.*, vol. 70, pp. 446–457, 2022, doi: 10.1021/acs.jafc.1c05704.

[74]   C. Hu, Y. Tang, Y. Zhao and S. Sang, "Quantitative analysis and anti-inflammatory activity evaluation of the A-type avenanthramides in commercial sprouted oat products," *J. Agric. Food Chem.*, vol. 68, pp. 13068–13075, 2020, doi: 10.1021/acs.jafc.9b06812.

[75]   L. H. Dimberg, C. Gissén and J. Nilsson, "Phenolic compounds in oat grains (Avena sativa L.) grown in conventional and organic systems," *Ambio.*, vol. 34, pp. 331–337, 2005. Accessed: Oct. 5, 2023. [Online]. Available: www.jstor.org/stable/4315611

[76] D. M. Peterson and L. H. Dimberg, "Avenanthramide concentrations and hydroxy-cinnamoyl-CoA:hydroxyanthranilate N-hydroxycinnamoyltransferase activities in developing oats," *J. Cereal Sci.*, vol. 47, pp. 101–108, 2008, doi: 10.1016/j.jcs.2007.02.007.

[77] A. A. Pridal, W. Böttger and A. B. Ross, "Analysis of avenanthramides in oat products and estimation of avenanthramide intake in humans," *Food Chem.*, vol. 253, pp. 93–100, 2018, doi: 10.1016/j.foodchem.2018.01.138.

[78] F. Ortiz-Robledo, I. Villanueva Fierro, B. D. Oomah, I. Lares Asseff, J. B. Proal Nájera and J. D. J. Návar Cháidez, "Avenanthramides and nutritional components of four Mexican oat (Avena sativa L.) varieties," *Agrociencia.*, vol. 47, pp. 225–232, 2013. Accessed: Oct. 5, 2023. [Online]. https://dialnet.unirioja.es/servlet/articulo?codigo=5385551

[79] K. Liu and M. L. Wise, "Distributions of nutrients and avenanthramides within oat grain and effects on pearled kernel composition," *Food Chem.*, vol. 336, p. 127668, 2021, doi: 10.1016/j.foodchem.2020.127668.

[80] W. Wang, H. D. Snooks and S. Sang, "The chemistry and health benefits of dietary phenolamides," *J. Agric. Food Chem.*, vol. 68, pp. 6248–6267, 2020, doi: 10.1021/acs.jafc.0c02605.

[81] D. Ryan, M. Kendall and K. Robards, "Bioactivity of oats as it relates to cardiovascular disease," *Nutr. Res. Rev.*, vol. 20, pp. 147–162, 2007, doi: 10.1017/S0954422407782884.

[82] U. Tiwari and E. Cummins, "Nutritional importance and effect of processing on tocols in cereals," *Trends Food Sci. Technol.*, vol. 20, pp. 511–520, 2009, doi: 10.1016/j.tifs.2009.06.001.

[83] N. Rodrigues et al., "Olive oil characteristics of eleven cultivars produced in a high-density grove in Valladolid province (Spain)," *Eur. Food Res. Technol.*, vol. 247, pp. 3113–3122, 2021, doi: 10.1007/s00217-021-03858-z.

[84] A. Fardet, E. Rock and C. Rémésy, "Is the in vitro antioxidant potential of whole-grain cereals and cereal products well reflected in vivo?" *J. Cereal Sci.*, vol. 48, pp. 258–276, 2008, doi: 10.1016/j.jcs.2008.01.002.

[85] D. A. White, I. D. Fisk and D. A. Gray, "Characterisation of oat (Avena sativa L.) oil bodies and intrinsically associated E-vitamers," *J. Cereal Sci.*, vol. 43, pp. 244–249, 2006, doi: 10.1016/j.jcs.2005.10.002.

[86] G. Panfili, A. Fratianni and M. Irano, "Normal phase high-performance liquid chromatography method for the determination of tocopherols and tocotrienols in cereals," *J. Agric. Food Chem.*, vol. 51, pp. 3940–3944, 2003, doi: 10.1021/jf030009v.

[87] H. Zielinski, H. Kozlowska and B. Lewczuk, "Bioactive compounds in the cereal grains before and after hydrothermal processing," *Innov. Food Sci. Emerg. Technol.*, vol. 2, pp. 159–169, 2001, doi: 10.1016/S1466-8564(01)00040-6.

[88] S. Kumari et al., "Ethnobotany and phytopharmacology of Avena sativa: A qualitative review," *Sciphy.*, vol. 2, pp. 56–74, 2023, doi: 10.58920/sciphy02010056.

[89] D. Paudel, B. Dhungana, M. Caffe and P. Krishnan, "A review of health-beneficial properties of oats," *Foods.*, vol. 10, p. 2591, 2021, doi: 10.3390/foods10112591.

[90] E. Llanaj et al., "Effect of oat supplementation interventions on cardiovascular disease risk markers: A systematic review and meta-analysis of randomized controlled trials," *Eur. J. Nutr.*, vol. 61, pp. 1749–1778, 2022, doi: 10.1007/s00394-021-02763-1.

[91] A. Durazzo et al., "Occurrence of tocols in foods: An updated shot of current databases," *J. Food Qual.*, vol. 2021, p. e8857571, 2021, doi: 10.1155/2021/8857571.

[92] Z. Kotíková et al., "Tocol content in oat varieties grown under different environmental conditions and farming systems," *J. Cereal Sci.*, vol. 113, p. 103733, 2023, doi: 10.1016/j.jcs.2023.103733.

[93] H. Zielinski, E. Ciska and H. Kozlowska, "The cereal grains: Focus on vitamin E," *Czech J. Food Sci.*, vol. 19, pp. 182–188, 2001. Available: https://EconPapers.repec.org/RePEc:caa:jnlcjf:v:19:y:2001:i:5:id:6605-cjfs.

[94] D. M. Peterson and A. A. Qureshi, "Genotype and environment effects on tocols of barley and oats," *Cereal Chem.*, vol. 70, pp. 157–162, 1993.

[95] M. Musa Özcan, G. Özkan and A. Topal, "Characteristics of grains and oils of four different oats (Avena sativa L.) cultivars growing in Turkey," *Int. J. Food Sci. Nutr.*, vol. 57, pp. 345–352, 2006, doi: 10.1080/09637480600802363.

[96] B. Salehi et al., "Phytosterols: From preclinical evidence to potential clinical applications," *Front. Pharmacol.*, vol. 11, 2021. Accessed: Oct. 6, 2023. [Online]. Available: www.frontiersin.org/articles/10.3389/fphar.2020.599959

[97] R. Zhang, Y. Han, D. J. McClements, D. Xu and S. Chen, "Production, characterization, delivery, and cholesterol-lowering mechanism of phytosterols: A review," *J. Agric. Food Chem.*, vol. 70, pp. 2483–2494, 2022, doi: 10.1021/acs.jafc.1c07390.

[98] R. A. Moreau et al., "Phytosterols and their derivatives: Structural diversity, distribution, metabolism, analysis, and health-promoting uses," *Prog. Lipid Res.*, vol. 70, pp. 35–61, 2018, doi: 10.1016/j.plipres.2018.04.001.

[99] D. Kritchevsky and S. C. Chen, "Phytosterols – Health benefits and potential concerns: A review," *Nutr. Res.*, vol. 25, pp. 413–428, 2005, doi: 10.1016/j.nutres.2005.02.003.

[100] K. Määttä, A.-M. Lampi, J. Petterson, B. M. Fogelfors, V. Piironen and A. Kamal-Eldin, "Phytosterol content in seven oat cultivars grown at three locations in Sweden," *J. Sci. Food Agric.*, vol. 79, pp. 1021–1027, 1999, doi: 10.1002/(SICI)1097-0010(19990515)79:7<1021::AID-JSFA316>3.0.CO;2-E.

[101] Y. Jiang and T. Wang, "Phytosterols in cereal by-products," *J. Am. Oil Chem. Soc.*, vol. 82, pp. 439–444, 2005, doi: 10.1007/s11746-005-1090-5.

[102] X. Zhang, K. Lin and Y. Li, "Highlights to phytosterols accumulation and equilibrium in plants: Biosynthetic pathway and feedback regulation," *Plant Physiol. Biochem.*, vol. 155, pp. 637–649, 2020, doi: 10.1016/j.plaphy.2020.08.021.

[103] E. Nattagh-Eshtivani et al., "Biological and pharmacological effects and nutritional impact of phytosterols: A comprehensive review," *Phytother. Res.*, vol. 36, pp. 299–322, 2022, doi: 10.1002/ptr.7312.

[104] W. Eichenberger and B. Urban, "Sterols in seeds and leaves of oats (Avena sativa L.)," *Plant Cell Rep.*, vol. 3, pp. 226–229, 1984, doi: 10.1007/BF00269298.

[105] K. Banaś and J. Harasym, "Current knowledge of content and composition of oat oil – Future perspectives of oat as oil source," *Food Bioprocess Technol.*, vol. 14, pp. 232–247, 2021, doi: 10.1007/s11947-020-02535-5.

[106] B. M. Akonjuen, J. O. Onuh and A. N. A. Aryee, "Bioactive fatty acids from non-conventional lipid sources and their potential application in functional food development," *Food Sci. Nutr.*, pp. 1–12, 2023, doi: 10.1002/fsn3.3521.

[107] A.-M. Liberati-Čizmek et al., "Analysis of fatty acid esters of hydroxyl fatty acid in selected plant food," *Plant Foods Hum. Nutr.*, vol. 74, pp. 235–240, 2019, doi: 10.1007/s11130-019-00728-8.

[108] M. J. Kolar et al., "Faster protocol for endogenous fatty acid esters of hydroxy fatty acid (FAHFA) measurements," *Anal. Chem.*, vol. 90, pp. 5358–5365, 2018, doi: 10.1021/acs.analchem.8b00503.

[109] T. M. Olajide and W. Cao, "Exploring foods as natural sources of FAHFAs – A review of occurrence, extraction, analytical techniques and emerging bioactive potential," *Trends Food Sci. Technol.*, vol. 129, pp. 591–607, 2022, doi: 10.1016/j.tifs.2022.11.005.

[110] L. Kouřimská, M. Sabolová, P. Horčička, S. Rys and M. Božik, "Lipid content, fatty acid profile, and nutritional value of new oat cultivars," *J. Cereal Sci.*, vol. 84, pp. 44–48, 2018, doi: 10.1016/j.jcs.2018.09.012.

[111] V. Sterna, S. Zute, L. Brunava and Z. Vicupe, "Lipid composition of oat grain grown in Latvia," 9th Baltic Conference on Food Science and Technology "Food for Consumer Well-Being" FOODBALT 2014, Jelgava, Latvia, 8–9 May 2014, pp. 77–80. Accessed: October 6, 2023. [Online]. Available: www.cabdirect.org/cabdirect/abstract/20143210623

[112] L. Brindzová, M. Čertík, P. Rapta, M. Zalibera, A. Mikulajová and M. Takácsová, "Antioxidant activity, β-glucan and lipid contents of oat varieties," *Czech J. Food Sci.*, vol. 26, pp. 163–173, 2008. Accessed: Oct. 6, 2023. [Online]. Available: https://ideas.repec.org//a/caa/jnlcjf/v26y2008i3id2564-cjfs.html

[113] H. C. Van den Broeck, D. M. Londono, R. Timmer, M. J. M. Smulders, L. J. W. J. Gilissen and I. M. Van der Meer, "Profiling of nutritional and health-related compounds in oat varieties," *Foods.*, vol. 5, p. 2, 2016, doi: 10.3390/foods5010002.

[114] A. Banaś et al., "Lipids in grain tissues of oat (Avena sativa): Differences in content, time of deposition, and fatty acid composition," *J. Exp. Bot.*, vol. 58, pp. 2463–2470, 2007, doi: 10.1093/jxb/erm125.

[115] M. Kumar et al., "Advances in the plant protein extraction: Mechanism and recommendations," *Food Hydrocoll.*, vol. 115, p. 106595, 2021, doi: 10.1016/j.foodhyd.2021.106595.

[116] S. Kumar, V. Kumar, T. Singh, A. Maity and V. K. Yadav, "Diurnal and temporal activity of pronubial insects on berseem flowers in a subtropical environment," *J. Apic. Res.*, pp. 1–6, 2021, doi: 10.1080/00218839.2021.1963123.

[117] M. Kumar et al., "Recent trends in extraction of plant bioactives using green technologies: A review," *Food Chem.*, vol. 353, p. 129431, 2021, doi: 10.1016/j.foodchem.2021.129431.

[118] M. Kumar et al., "Plant-based proteins and their multifaceted industrial applications," *LWT.*, vol. 154, p. 112620, 2022, doi: 10.1016/j.lwt.2021.112620.

[119] M. Chalamaiah, S. Keskin Ulug, H. Hong and J. Wu, "Regulatory requirements of bioactive peptides (protein hydrolysates) from food proteins," *J. Funct. Foods.*, vol. 58, pp. 123–129, 2019, doi: 10.1016/j.jff.2019.04.050.

[120] H. Rafique et al., "Dietary-nutraceutical properties of oat protein and peptides," *Front. Nutr.*, vol. 9, 2022. Accessed: Sept. 23, 2023. www.frontiersin.org/articles/10.3389/fnut.2022.950400.

[121] Y. Wang and C. Selomulya, "Spray drying strategy for encapsulation of bioactive peptide powders for food applications," *Adv. Powd. Technol.*, vol. 31, pp. 409–415, 2020, doi: 10.1016/j.apt.2019.10.034.

[122] J. Chen, Y. Hu, J. Wang, H. Hu and H. Cui, "Combined effect of ozone treatment and modified atmosphere packaging on antioxidant defense system of fresh-cut green peppers," *J. Food Process. Preserv.*, vol. 40, pp. 1145–1150, 2016, doi: 10.1111/jfpp.12695.

[123] R. Esfandi, W. G. Willmore and A. Tsopmo, "Peptidomic analysis of hydrolyzed oat bran proteins, and their in vitro antioxidant and metal chelating properties," *Food Chem.*, vol. 279, pp. 49–57, 2019, doi: 10.1016/j.foodchem.2018.11.110.

[124] S. Ma, M. Zhang, X. Bao and Y. Fu, "Preparation of antioxidant peptides from oat globulin," *CyTA J. Food.*, vol. 18, pp. 108–115, 2020, doi: 10.1080/19476337.2020.1716076.

[125] Y. Du, R. Esfandi, W. G. Willmore and A. Tsopmo, "Antioxidant activity of oat proteins derived peptides in stressed hepatic HepG2 cells," *Antioxidants.*, vol. 5, p. 39, 2016, doi: 10.3390/antiox5040039.

[126] R. Esfandi, W. G. Willmore and A. Tsopmo, "Antioxidant and anti-apoptotic properties of oat bran protein hydrolysates in stressed hepatic cells," *Foods.*, vol. 8, p. 160, 2019, doi: 10.3390/foods8050160.

[127] R. Esfandi, I. Seidu, W. Willmore and A. Tsopmo, "Antioxidant, pancreatic lipase, and α-amylase inhibitory properties of oat bran hydrolyzed proteins and peptides," *J. Food Biochem.*, vol. 46, p. e13762, 2022, doi: 10.1111/jfbc.13762.

[128] H. Yuanqing et al., "The preparation, antioxidant activity evaluation, and iron-deficient anemic improvement of oat (Avena sativa L.) peptides–ferrous chelate," *Front. Nutr.*, vol. 8, 2021. Accessed: Oct. 6, 2023. [Online]. Available: www.frontiersin.org/articles/10.3389/fnut.2021.687133.

[129] B. Feng, L. Ma, J. Yao, Y. Fang, Y. Mei and S. Wei, "Protective effect of oat bran extracts on human dermal fibroblast injury induced by hydrogen peroxide," *J. Zhejiang Univ. Sci. B.*, vol. 14, pp. 97–105, 2013, doi: 10.1631/jzus.B1200159.

[130] A. P. M. Bloot, D. L. Kalschne, J. A. S. Amaral, I. J. Baraldi and C. Canan, "A review of phytic acid sources, obtention, and applications," *Food Rev. Int.*, vol. 39, pp. 73–92, 2023, doi: 10.1080/87559129.2021.1906697.

[131] A. Kumar et al., "Phytic acid: Blessing in disguise, a prime compound required for both plant and human nutrition," *Food Res. Int.*, vol. 142, p. 110193, 2021, doi: 10.1016/j.foodres.2021.110193.

[132] C. Martínez-Villaluenga and E. Peñas, "Health benefits of oat: Current evidence and molecular mechanisms," *Curr. Opin. Food Sci.*, vol. 14, pp. 26–31, 2017, doi: 10.1016/j.cofs.2017.01.004.

[133] A. K. M. Shamsuddin and I. Vucenik, "IP6 & inositol in cancer prevention and therapy," *Curr. Cancer Ther. Rev.*, vol. 1, pp. 259–269, 2005, doi: 10.2174/157339405774574216.

[134] A. Zajdel, A. Wilczok, L. Węglarz and Z. Dzierżewicz, "Phytic acid inhibits lipid peroxidation *In Vitro*," *BioMed Res. Int.*, vol. 2013, p. e147307, 2013, doi: 10.1155/2013/147307.

[135] S. Muraoka and T. Miura, "Inhibition of xanthine oxidase by phytic acid and its antioxidative action," *Life Sci.*, vol. 74, pp. 1691–1700, 2004, doi: 10.1016/j.lfs.2003.09.040.

[136] C. H. Fox and M. Eberl, "Phytic acid (IP6), novel broad spectrum anti-neoplastic agent: A systematic review," *Complement Ther Med.*, vol. 10, pp. 229–234, 2002, doi: 10.1016/s0965-2299(02)00092-4.

[137] A. Gani, S. M. Wani, F. A. Masoodi and G. Hameed, "Whole-grain cereal bioactive compounds and their health benefits: A review," *J. Food Process. Technol.*, vol. 3, 2012, doi: 10.4172/2157-7110.1000146.

[138] K. Sharma et al., "Saponins: A concise review on food related aspects, applications and health implications," *Food Chem. Adv.*, vol. 2, p. 100191, 2023, doi: 10.1016/j.focha.2023.100191.

[139] J.-P. Vincken, L. Heng, A. de Groot and H. Gruppen, "Saponins, classification and occurrence in the plant kingdom," *Phytochemistry.*, vol. 68, pp. 275–297, 2007, doi: 10.1016/j.phytochem.2006.10.008.

[140] M. Garutti et al., "The impact of cereal grain composition on the health and disease outcomes," *Front. Nutr.*, vol. 9, 2022. Accessed Oct. 7, 2023. [Online]. Available: www.frontiersin.org/articles/10.3389/fnut.2022.888974

[141] A. E. Osbourn, B. R. Clarke, P. Lunness, P. R. Scott and M. J. Daniels, "An oat species lacking avenacin is susceptible to infection by Gaeumannomyces graminis var. tritici," *Physiol Mol Plant Pathol.*, vol. 45, pp. 457–467, 1994, doi: 10.1016/S0885-5765(05)80042-6.

[142] J. Shi, K. Arunasalam, D. Yeung, Y. Kakuda, G. Mittal and Y. Jiang, "Saponins from edible legumes: Chemistry, processing, and health benefits," *J. Med. Food.*, vol. 7, pp. 67–78, 2004, doi: 10.1089/109662004322984734.

[143] W. Mary, L. Crombie and L. Crombie, "Distribution of avenacins A-1, A-2, B-1 and B-2 in oat roots: Their fungicidal activity towards 'take-all' fungus," *Phytochemistry.*, vol. 25, pp. 2069–2073, 1986, doi: 10.1016/0031-9422(86)80068-1.

[144] Ł. Pecio, A. Wawrzyniak-Szołkowska, W. Oleszek and A. Stochmal, "Rapid analysis of avenacosides in grain and husks of oats by UPLC–TQ–MS," *Food Chem.*, vol. 141, pp. 2300–2304, 2013, doi: 10.1016/j.foodchem.2013.04.094.

[145] G. Önning and N.-G. Asp, "Analysis of saponins in oat kernels," *Food Chem.*, vol. 48, pp. 301–305, 1993, doi: 10.1016/0308-8146(93)90145-6.

[146] R. Tschesche and G. Wulff, "Chemie und Biologie der Saponine," in *Fortschritte Der Chemie Organischer Naturstoffe: Progress in the Chemistry of Organic Natural Products*, M. J. Cormier et al., Eds. Vienna, Austria: Springer, 1973, pp. 461–606, doi: 10.1007/978-3-7091-7102-8_7.

[147] D. E. Fenwick and D. Oakenfull, "Saponin content of food plants and some prepared foods," *J. Sci. Food Agric.*, vol. 34, pp. 186–191, 1983, doi: 10.1002/jsfa.2740340212.

Milling, Processing, and Storage of Oats

Strategies and Effect on Nutritional Properties

Racheal John, Rakesh Bhardwaj,
Archana T. Janamatti, and Prabha Singh

5.1 INTRODUCTION

Mankind has engaged in the practice of grain milling since the dawn of civilization. The initial milling methods employed were notably rudimentary [1]. These early human endeavours in grain milling ultimately led to the evolution of mortar and pestle. In this ancient technique, grain was crushed between two stones; one possessed a flat, somewhat concave surface, while the other, a pounding stone, was oval with a rounded base and a top that comfortably fit into the hand [2]. A significant advancement came with the advent of the burr mill. This innovative milling apparatus involved grinding the grain between a stationary, flat, circular stone and a complementary rotating stone positioned directly above it [3]. The spacing between these stones determined the coarseness of the resulting flour. It wasn't until the latter part of the nineteenth century that milling technology made notable strides. As technology progressed, iron or porcelain rolls gradually replaced the traditional stone mills. These advancements, combined with changes in power sources, led to the development of more efficient mills, which yielded more refined and superior-quality flours and meals.

Among the diverse grains, oats presented a distinct challenge for millers. The conventional oat kernel, as it is harvested, is encased in a hull comprising two layers known botanically as the lemma and the palea, respectively [4]. These hulls must be removed before processing the grain into finished products. Fortunately, the hull and kernel are not fused, unlike barley and rice, and can be separated with minimal disruption to the kernel tissue. The first significant enhancement in oat milling came in the form of a dehuller patented by a U.S. miller in 1840. The next milestone occurred in 1875 when Ferdinand Schumacher of the United States patented a cutting machine. This invention facilitated the division of oats into three or four pieces with minimal production of fines. The resulting steel-cut oats swiftly supplanted the coarse meal produced by burr mills, becoming the preferred choice for oat porridge. Despite their longer cooking time, steel-cut oats possessed a considerably extended shelf life. During that era, processed oats were stored in open barrels and were susceptible to rancidity. The crushed meal, due to its larger surface area, was more prone to oxidative rancidity [5]. The capability to cut oats, in combination with the advent of roller mills, laid the groundwork for the production of rolled oats as we know them today. Subsequently, steam was introduced to the process to act as a binder and reduce the production of fines during rolling. The steaming process partially precooked the flakes and marked the initial step in the development of "instantized" products. The first "instantized" ready-to-cook product, bearing the symbol "3 minutes," was introduced in 1877 [6].

Processing, including preparation, contributes to the improvement of food in terms of health, safety, taste, and shelf stability. A fundamental question remains regarding the influence of whole oat grain processing on the content of nutrients and phytochemicals [7]. While processing is often seen as detrimental to nutrition, and some forms of processing do indeed diminish nutritional value, several factors emphasize the significance of grain processing in enhancing oat grain consumption [8]. Firstly, whole grains as they are harvested are generally not directly consumable by humans and necessitate some form of processing before consumption. While refining, which involves removing the bran and germ, diminishes the nutrient content of grains, milling of grains concentrates desirable grain components and eliminates poorly digestible compounds and contaminants [9]. The concentrations of nutritional constituents in oats undergo alterations through various processing methods, including milling, fermentation, germination (sprouting), extrusion, and thermal processing. Vitamins, notably ascorbic acid, thiamin, and folic acid, are highly susceptible to the same processing techniques [10]. The duration and temperature of processing, the composition of the product, and storage conditions are all significant factors that affect the vitamin content of our foods. Cooking grains generally increases the digestibility of nutrients and phytochemicals. Studies, in both animal models and humans, support the notion that processed grains often offer superior nutrition compared to unprocessed grains, likely due to enhanced nutrient bioavailability in processed grains [11]. Grain processing also yields shelf-stable products that are convenient and pleasing to consumers.

While agricultural productivity has experienced significant growth in recent years, this alone is insufficient to ensure global food security. There exists a pressing need to enhance food availability, and reducing postharvest losses at farm, retail, and consumer levels represents a crucial step in this direction. The majority of cereal crops are seasonal, and following harvest, surplus grains are stored for varying durations as food reserves. The primary goal of storage should be to preserve the initial quality of the produce to the greatest extent possible. During storage, respiratory and metabolic processes persist, utilizing the stored grain's nutrients to generate energy and sustain metabolism [12]. The quality of cereal grains during storage is influenced by physical factors like temperature and humidity, biological factors such as microflora, arthropods, and vertebrates, as well as technical factors like storage conditions, methods, and duration. These factors collectively lead to physicochemical and organoleptic changes, which result in significant qualitative and quantitative losses [13].

This chapter offers a comprehensive exploration of modern oat storage, handling, and processing, in addition to a thorough examination of specifications for milling-quality oats. Most oat mill products are whole grain items containing the entire kernel and all its components. Typical products include rolled oats, steel-cut groats, various flakes produced from cut groats, oat flour, and oat bran are also discussed in detail. This chapter also introduces and compares various strategies aimed at enhancing the production of stable oat products. These strategies encompass both thermal methods, such as kilning, hot-air dry roasting, extrusion, superheat steam treatment, and microwave treatment, and non-thermal approaches, including ultrasound, cold plasma, high-pressure processing, and irradiation. By exploring and evaluating these strategies, the objective is to advance the development of high-quality oat-based food products. Additionally, the study offers insights and recommendations for future applications of oats in the production of food items, further contributing to the enhancement of oat-based products.

5.2 MILLING OF OATS

Oats present distinct attributes that differentiate their milling process from that of other cereal grains. Notably, their hull is not firmly attached to the endosperm, they possess a higher fat content in comparison to most cereal grains, and they are rich in soluble dietary fibres [14]. The oat hull primarily consists of cellulose, hemicelluloses, and lignin. Nestled within the hull is the groat, which constitutes a substantial 68–72% of the entire kernel. Oats are typically processed as whole grains, primarily due to the groat's softer nature compared to other grains like wheat, making it challenging to separate into distinct germ, endosperm, and bran fractions. The outer layer of the groat holds significant quantities of protein, neutral lipids, β-glucan, phenolics, and niacin. Occasionally, this outer layer is isolated from the groat to create oat bran. The inner endosperm is composed of proteins, starch, and β-glucan, while the germ primarily contains lipids and proteins. These distinctive components of oats, combined with their unique physiological structure, necessitate an altered processing method in contrast to other grains. Furthermore, they bestow upon oats certain exceptional nutritional qualities, rendering them a valuable, albeit sometimes underappreciated, food product, occasionally employed as an ingredient in various other food products.

Oat milling is a comprehensive process comprising multiple sequential steps aimed at the elimination of extraneous matter (field contaminants), hull removal, stabilization of the groat, flavour development, and the transformation of the grain into finished products. While the fundamental stages have remained constant through time, technological advancements have brought changes in their sequencing. The quality of milled oats is contingent upon various factors including plant genetics (varieties), agricultural practices, chemical composition, and storage and handling conditions [15]. Oat genetics play a significant role in milling efficiency, with factors like kernel size and groat percentage directly impacting yield. Furthermore, the growing environment and climatic variables like rainfall and frost can exert their influence [16]. Chemical composition is a pivotal determinant of both nutritional content and quality; for instance, elevated levels of non-esterified fatty acids (NEFA) often indicate improper storage and handling, leading to kernel damage and subsequent lipase-mediated triacylglycerol (TAG) hydrolysis. NEFA's presence diminishes quality by imparting off-flavours and heightening susceptibility to oxidative rancidity. Proper storage and handling are paramount to curbing nutrient loss and averting the formation of off-flavours arising from lipid oxidation.

When oats are stored in bulk, the moisture content of each individual kernel adapts to reach equilibrium with its immediate environment, making storage conditions a critical food preservation factor. Inadequate moisture control can foster microbial growth and spoilage, introducing food safety risks such as the development of aflatoxins from mould proliferation. Elevated temperatures can also compromise quality by accelerating enzyme reactions, nutrient degradation, and microbial growth. Therefore, it is advisable to store oats at a water activity of approximately 0.65 (equivalent to roughly 13% moisture content in the kernels) within a temperature range of 5–20°C. Overall, the milling process is meticulously structured to eliminate foreign matter, isolate and stabilize the groat, and render it suitable for cooking. The sequential steps include cleaning, grading, dehulling, hull removal, groat separation, kilning, cutting and/or flaking, flour production, and oat bran production.

Processing methodologies are employed within the food industry to enhance the nutritional profile, texture, and sensory attributes, all of which serve to appeal to consumers. In the context of oats, the processing regimen encompasses the following key steps: (a) cleaning and heat treatment, (b) dehulling and cutting, and (c) flaking or milling. It's worth noting that there might be some variations in this process contingent on factors like the oat sample (e.g., covered or naked oats) or the intended final oat product. Consequently, oat cereals are available in a diverse array of forms, including whole groats, steel-cut oats, rolled oats, quick oats, oat flour, and oat bran, each designed to cater to different consumer preferences and culinary applications (Figure 5.1 and Table 5.1).

5.2.1 Cleaning

In the case of oats, as is common with various agricultural products, the harvesting process introduces an amalgamation of oats with extraneous components encountered in the field and during transportation. The presence of these foreign materials necessitates their elimination to render oats suitable for human consumption [17]. Common

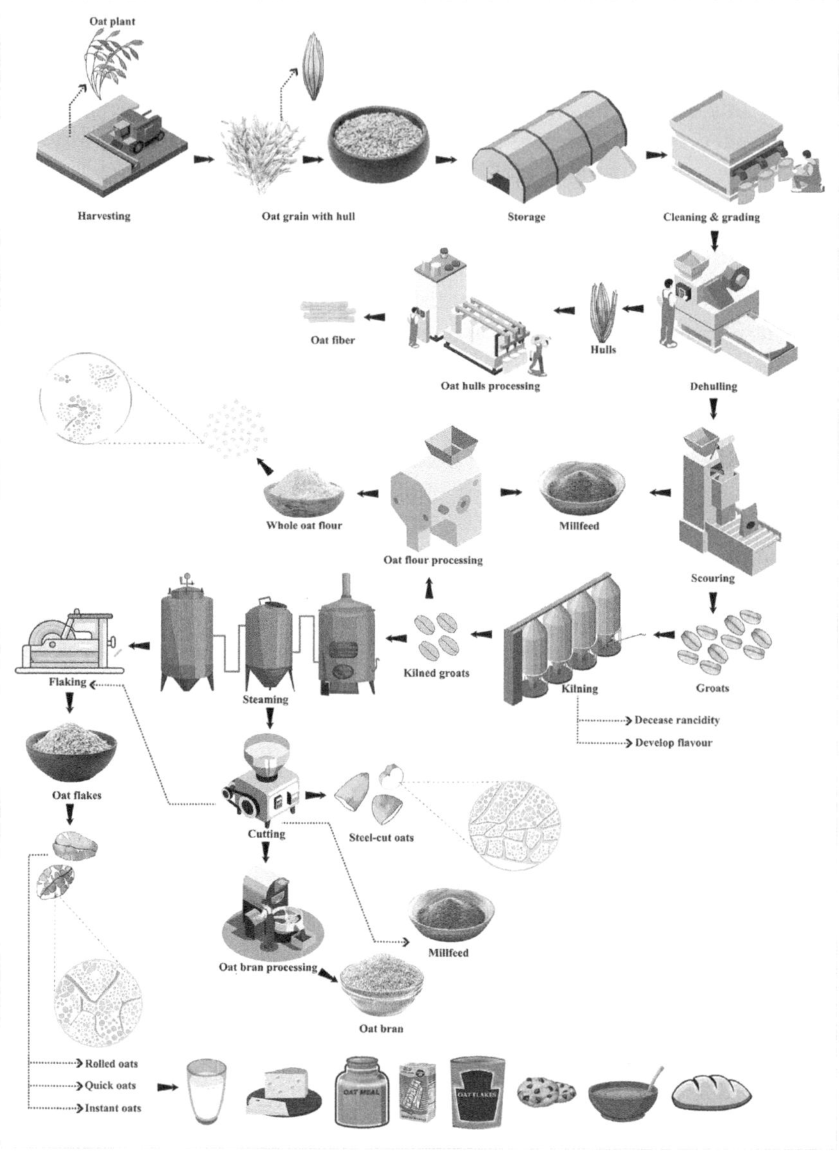

FIGURE 5.1 Various methods for oat milling and processing.

contaminants in the cleaning process encompass both biological and non-biological materials. These include weed seeds, straw, and other grains, as well as additional foreign elements such as sticks, stones, metal fragments, dirt or sand, and residual dust that persists after the initial cleaning stages [18]. Furthermore, during the cleaning process, fractions of oats with poor milling quality are segregated from the high-quality milling oats. (a) Pin oats: they are characterized by their diminutive size and thinness. They often possess a small or even no groat inside; (b) double (bosom) oats: they arise when

TABLE 5.1   Sequential Stages in Oat Processing

STEP	DESCRIPTION
Cleaning and sorting	Oats are subjected to a rigorous purification process to eliminate extraneous impurities, including stones, foreign matter, and fractured grains. Subsequently, they are meticulously categorized based on their size and quality.
Hulling	In this stage, the outer husk or hull is meticulously separated from the oat groat, resulting in the pristine oat kernel.
Kilning or steaming	Oat kernels are exposed to controlled heating to stabilize the innate enzymes within oats. This thermal treatment not only enhances the shelf life but also contributes to flavour maturation. Both kilning and steaming methods can be employed to achieve this goal.
Rolling or flaking	The oat kernels undergo specialized rolling processes to attain a flattened, flake-like structure. The thickness of these flakes can be finely adjusted to produce a variety of oat products, including old-fashioned oats or quick oats.
Cutting and sifting	Rolled oats may undergo further refinement through precision cutting into smaller fragments, followed by meticulous sifting. This process yields oatmeal with distinctive textures, such as steel-cut oats or instant oats.
Toasting (optional)	Certain oat products may undergo an optional toasting procedure to elevate their flavour profile. Toasting can be applied either before or following the cutting and sifting phases.
Packaging	The final oat products are systematically weighed, expertly packaged, and prepared for distribution to consumers.

the hull of the primary kernel envelops a secondary grain. In such cases, both kernels are usually underdeveloped, resulting in a notably high hull percentage; (c) light oats: they are generally of a similar size to regular oats but feature a significantly smaller groat [10]. Consequently, they can be easily separated through aspiration. Additional undesirable oat fractions may encompass oats that are discoloured, green, or damaged with hulls, and twins, which may or may not be removed in the cleaning process based on their size. Twins refer to two kernels that have grown closely together, appearing as a single unit. Their removal during cleaning depends on their size, as smaller twins may escape the cleaning process.

Cleaning is primarily executed through a process known as screening. In its simplest form, the cleaning of oats involves two fundamental procedures: aspiration and size separation. (a) Aspiration: in the aspiration phase, the air is employed to lift lighter particles such as dust and chaff from the heavier grain stream. This effectively separates impurities from the oats; (b) size separation: in the size separation step, scalping screens are utilized to eliminate oversized and undesired materials [19]. This includes contaminants like other grains (e.g., corn, soybeans), stones, sticks, or straw. These screens ensure that only oats of the desired size proceed further in the process. Upon entering the mill, the oats undergo additional refinement steps to ensure their purity:

(a) magnetic separator: as a standard practice in many food-processing operations, oats pass under a magnetic separator, which removes foreign metal objects; (b) rotating or oscillating screens: these screens serve a dual purpose. They retain large objects such as straw, sticks, and stones while allowing smaller objects like underdeveloped oats, dirt, weed seeds, and dust to pass through; (c) aspiration: retained oat stream is subjected to another round of aspiration to further eliminate lightweight materials; (d) dry stoner: a dry stoner is employed to remove high-density, similarly sized particles, such as rocks and other grains (e.g., maize) [20].

In certain instances, oats undergo a clipping process before cleaning. Clipping involves removing the tips of the oats to enhance subsequent dehulling efficiency. This is done prior to cleaning so that the clipped-off portions can be effectively removed before further milling. Clipping is executed using a meshed screen through which the narrow end of the oat can penetrate [21]. A rotating bar displaces the oat from the mesh, causing the tip to break off. The clipped-off tips are subsequently removed by aspiration. To enhance milling efficiency, a rotary separator may be used to sort the oats into various size classes. An indented rotary drum is employed for this purpose. The indents on the inner face of the rotating cylinder correspond to the size of the seeds that need to be removed. For example, an indent separator designed to eliminate weed seeds has smaller indents than the oats [22]. Weed seeds fit snugly into these indents and are carried up the side of the rotating cylinder. Ultimately, the pull of gravity deposits the weed seeds into a central trough. A screw conveyor then removes the seeds from the trough, while the larger oats, which are not lifted high enough up the side walls, continue moving out of the bottom of the cylinder [23]. The size of the particles removed by the screw conveyor can be adjusted by altering the height of the catch trough. Lowering the trough results in the removal of larger particles since even particles that don't fit tightly in the indents will ascend the cylinder's sides due to friction [19]. This process can also remove small oats such as light oats, double oats, and pin oats, which are subsequently used as animal feed. Many oat mills perform a third round of size separation to eliminate thin or pin oats [24]. These are either processed separately or directed to a by-product stream for conversion into animal feed. Additionally, a final aspiration step may be executed to remove oats without groats, known as "empties," and oats with very small groats, referred to as "light oats." These have limited or no milling value for subsequent food production.

5.2.2 Grading

The principal objective of the grading operation is to categorize clean oats into two to four fractions based on their density and weight. Typical oat samples exhibit a range of sizes, which is a natural and expected variation but must be effectively managed to maximize the efficiency of an oat mill [25]. Hence, millers must exercise meticulous control over the grading process to optimize hulling efficiency and minimize groat breakage. The grading process is typically guided by either grain width or length. In modern mills employing impact dehullers, oats are sorted into size classes based on width, as this approach generates streams with similar kernel weights [26]. Historically, mills using stone dehullers would classify fractions based on kernel length. The grading process, following a mill flow that utilizes an impact dehuller, entails weighing the clean oats and directing them to the width graders, which consist of a series of slowly rotating horizontal slotted cylinders. Slot sizes are chosen in accordance with the initial oat quality [27]. The first cylinder usually features an intermediate slot size. The over-tail includes the largest kernel size, while the throughs from this cylinder encompass the small and medium oat size categories. These throughs are conveyed to the subsequent cylinder, which employs slightly smaller slot sizes to once again separate the oat stream into two distinct size categories. Medium-sized oats are directed over, while smaller oats pass through the slots. In high-capacity mills, further size separations might occur. The output streams from the width graders are subsequently directed to the dehullers. It's worth noting that millers typically incorporate some form of magnetic separators at the entry and exit points of the cleaning and grading system to eliminate ferrous metal particles that may have chipped or detached from combines or other handling equipment during the harvesting and transportation of the oats.

5.2.3 Dehulling

Dehulling is a pivotal process in oat milling, aimed at extracting the groat or oat kernel by removing the indigestible hull. This process hinges on a combination of impact and abrasion forces, as oat hulls are not firmly bound to the kernel and can be effectively dislodged by mechanical means that crack or shatter the hull. Typically, oat hulls constitute around one-third of the oat seed's weight. Before dehulling, oats may undergo sorting into two to four fractions, either by width or length, to enhance uniformity in size and bolster dehulling efficiency. Plumper oats, characterized by their ease of dehulling, necessitate less aggressive operating conditions than thinner oats. Longer oats are generally plumper than shorter ones and, therefore, dehull more effortlessly than shorter varieties often referred to as "stub oats." Presently, impact dehulling is the predominant method employed. In modern mills, the initial dehulling step involves a rotating disc with numerous fins extending from the centre to the periphery. Oats descend into the centre of this disc and are propelled into a series of impact rings on the dehuller's wall, resulting in the separation of the groat from the hull. The oat stream is introduced to the dehuller's centre and falls onto a spinning rotor comprised of two horizontal flat plates with vanes that direct the oats lengthwise and outwards into the impact ring at high velocity. The force of impact leads to the fragmentation of the hulls, releasing the groats. Subsequently, the mixture of oats, groats, and hulls undergoes aspiration to remove a significant portion of the hulls. The groats then proceed to a scouring operation where trichomes, hair-like fibres, are polished off. This process can be carried out by machines like scourers, clippers, debearders, pearlers, or similar abrasion-based machines. Some millers may opt to retain a portion of the hulls with the groats to enhance polishing. A second aspiration step is employed to eliminate the remaining hulls and loosened trichomes. The residual mixture of oats and groats is further divided into their respective fractions. This is typically achieved through length grading using indent cylinders, which can lift the shorter groats out of the generally longer oat stream.

Alternatively, density separation machines like gravity tables isolate the lighter oat fraction from the heavier groat fraction. A paddy table sorter, which separates heavy and light components, also removes any barley contamination, which is crucial for oat flaking operations. Dehulling is typically a recursive operation; oats that aren't dehulled in the initial pass may be reprocessed in the second, third, or fourth dehulling cycles. For multi-pass dehulling, the dehuller's speed is progressively increased with each pass as the remaining oat stream becomes more resistant to dehulling. The collective output of the dehulling process is termed "raw groats," and the process is typically terminated when approximately 85% of the oats are dehulled, as excessive dehulling can lead to groat breakage, reducing overall yield.

The efficiency of dehulling is contingent upon factors such as oat weight and moisture content, as well as the throughput of the dehulling machine. Hence, oats are graded to ensure similar weights before dehulling. The rotation speed of the disc can be adjusted to enhance dehulling efficiency without causing groat breakage. For example, larger oats require a slower rotation speed to separate the hull compared to the speed needed for smaller oats. Moisture significantly affects dehulling efficiency; high moisture levels decrease dehulling, while low moisture increases groat breakage rates, making a moisture content of 12–13% ideal. Subsequently, the oat stream is subjected to aspiration to eliminate hulls and fines – small particles resulting from breakage. The mostly dehulled oats are then passed through a cylinder with a rough interior to scour off any adhering hulls, followed by a second aspiration. The oat stream proceeds to a table or paddy separator, which differentiates groats from unhulled oats based on differences in density and particle smoothness. Groats, characterized by a smoother texture and higher density than unhulled oats, pass through the separator at a quicker pace. The oat stream enters an inclined table with a series of bumpers, similar to a pinball machine, rocking back and forth, causing the oat stream to rebound off the bumpers. Smoother and denser groats gravitate towards the bottom, while unhulled oats rise to the top. The unhulled oats are then returned to the dehuller. In cases where high levels of dehulled oat removal are required, such as in cut oats, several table separators are used in succession. Ultimately, a perforated drum separator is employed to eliminate larger contaminating grains like wheat and barley, which are larger than the groats.

5.2.4 Kiln Drying

Oats possess a unique quality by containing a relatively high fat content, ranging from 6% to 8%, in contrast to the more typical fat content of 2% to 3% found in most other grains. Additionally, they are distinguished by their significant concentration of polyunsaturated fatty acids (PUFA), notably linoleic acid, constituting approximately 35% of their fatty acid composition [28]. Furthermore, oats exhibit elevated levels of lipid-digesting enzymes. The primary lipid forms in oats comprise phospholipids and TAG, which are notably susceptible to hydrolysis by lipases, resulting in the formation of NEFA [29]. Oats are recognized for their heightened lipase activity in comparison to other grain varieties. It is worth noting that NEFA generated by lipase not only impart an undesirable soapy taste but can also engage with lipoxygenases, which catalyse the conversion of unsaturated fatty acids, predominantly linoleic acid, into fatty acid hydroperoxides [30]. These hydroperoxides can subsequently decompose into a series of volatile fatty acid decomposition products, including hexanal, contributing to the development of rancid odours [31]. In the natural state of the grain kernel, lipase and lipoxygenase are compartmentalized, ensuring that they do not interact with TAG and phospholipids. Nevertheless, during the milling process, this compartmentalization is disrupted, facilitating the interaction between the enzymes and lipids [10]. Consequently, to preempt the onset of off-flavours prior to decompartmentalization, it is imperative to inactivate lipase and lipoxygenase through heat denaturation. This is achieved through a two-step procedure: initial live steam application, referred to as steaming, followed by prolonged heating, known as kilning [32].

Kilning confers an additional advantage by enhancing the Maillard reaction, an interaction between proteins and carbohydrates that yields favourable flavours, browning, and the generation of antioxidant compounds that further bolster lipid stability [33]. Kilning is conventionally executed by placing groats in lengthy vertical cylinders, subsequently introducing steam and air into these columns. Live steam is introduced at the upper end of the column, expeditiously elevating the temperature of the groats [34]. The steam augments the moisture content of the groats, a beneficial attribute as enzyme inactivation efficiency augments with increased moisture levels. Nonetheless, augmented moisture content within the groats may compromise the quality and storage longevity of the final products. Consequently, lower down the column, groats undergo radiant heating (dry heat) to eliminate excess moisture [35]. Radiant heating also accelerates the Maillard reaction, giving rise to appealing nutty flavours and caramel hues. Towards the conclusion of this process, the air is introduced to lower the temperature and reduce the moisture content to a final value of 10%. The effectiveness of enzyme inactivation is monitored by evaluating peroxidase activity, which, being more heat-resistant than lipase and lipoxygenase, assures their comprehensive inactivation [36].

Furthermore, kilning offers an advantageous facet in terms of oat quality by inactivating potentially detrimental bacteria, yeasts, and moulds, which could otherwise diminish shelf-life and pose food safety risks. However, akin to other thermal processing treatments, kilning does lead to the destruction of certain heat-sensitive vitamins, such as B vitamins [37]. Nevertheless, the benefits of kilning, particularly its capacity to extend shelf-life, greatly outweigh these undesirable consequences. Kilning is an operation primarily focused on enzyme deactivation to enhance the stability of groats against oxidative degradation. Among the various enzymes present and active in raw oats, peroxidase stands out as the marker of heat treatment efficacy due to its high heat resistance and ease of measurement. It is essential to note that shelf-stable oat ingredients can be manufactured without kilning, although some form of heat treatment is indispensable in downstream processes to deactivate oxidative enzymes. The term "roasting," as it appears in older literature, has essentially evolved into kilning. Initially, roasting was used to describe the dry pan method, reliant solely on dry heat. However, dry pans have now been largely supplanted by kilns, also known as conditioners.

A contemporary oat kiln constitutes a vertical tower wherein raw groats are introduced at the top, descending into a steaming zone where live steam is introduced to raise both temperature and moisture levels. Detailed time-temperature-moisture profiles essential for accomplishing enzyme inactivation have been documented in the literature [24]. Subsequently, the groats progress into one or more lower zones, where dry heat is administered via internal radiators, impacting drying, roasting, and flavour development. Finally, the groats advance into a cooling zone, where ambient air passes through the grain bed, further facilitating drying. Ideally, the exit moisture content approximates the inlet moisture content, typically within the 12% to 14% range, thus minimizing yield losses. Rate and total residence time are meticulously regulated through screw conveyors or other feeder mechanisms at the kiln's bottom discharge point. Kilned groats, commercially known as kiln-dried husked oat groats (KDHOs) or "cooked groats," may be placed in in-process storage or directly forwarded for subsequent processing [38]. The storage interval permits temperature and moisture equilibrium within the groats themselves, mitigating certain operational issues downstream.

5.3 TRANSFORMING GROATS INTO CULINARY INGREDIENTS AND FOOD PRODUCTS

Following the milling process, the resultant products encompass a range of distinct forms. These forms comprise whole groats, characterized by their assorted sizes, fragmented groats, and finely powdered fines. These diverse product outputs serve as valuable raw materials for the production of a variety of oat-based products, including oat flakes, steel-cut oats, oat flour, and oat bran. Furthermore, in specific instances, these milled components can also be harnessed for the development of oat-derived ingredients, such as dietary fibre.

5.3.1 Cutting

Steel-cut oats, an integral product in the cereal industry, are generated by the straightforward process of fragmenting whole oat groats into smaller segments. This process is facilitated by a rotary granulator, comprising a perforated drum outfitted with steel blades on its periphery [39]. The drum's rotation, in conjunction with the knives, acts to sever the sections of the groat that extend through the perforations. Ordinarily, each groat undergoes two to four cutting operations. Several variables exert influence over the dimensions of the resulting cut groats, encompassing the speed of drum rotation, the placement of the knives, the dimensions of the perforations, and the initial size of the groat [14]. It is noteworthy that this procedure generates a minor proportion of fines, typically amounting to less than 2%, which are subsequently eliminated via a sifting process. Furthermore, the segregation of cut oats into distinct sizes is carried out employing an indented cylinder, a device akin to the one described in the cleaning process.

The aforesaid cutting operation is instrumental in the production of steel-cut oats. The raw material for this operation includes the undersized and fragmented groats stemming from the grading phase, in conjunction with an adequate quantity of larger groats to meet the requisites for steel-cut groats [15]. Notably, the preceding grading phase may be omitted when groats are not required for the production of whole oat flakes.

The machinery responsible for creating steel-cut oats, known as a rotary granulator, is characterized by a revolving perforated drum and an array of stationary knives positioned externally on the lower section of the drum [40]. The perforations are circular and countersunk, allowing the groats to align themselves upright and extend through the drum's surface. The drum rotates at a rate of approximately 36 to 40 revolutions per minute. As the groats descend through the perforations, their tips are excised upon encountering the initial knife. The groat, as the drum rotates, may traverse through the perforation for a second or even a third time, culminating in groats being typically divided into two to four pieces. The size of the individual pieces is subject to various factors, including the drum's rotational speed, the adjustable knife blade spacing, the sharpness of the blades, the diameter of the drum perforations, and the initial size of the groats. Notably, a reduction in the drum's rotational speed results in fewer cuts and an augmented average piece size. The sharpness and positioning of the knives hold pivotal importance in regulating process efficiency, as improperly positioned or dulled knives are liable to generate an excess of fines exceeding 2%. Consequently, a well-maintained rotary granulator typically yields a minor fraction of fines, approximating 1% to 1.5%.

Moreover, it is imperative to underscore that the moisture content of the groats plays a role in determining fines production [41]. Processors may opt for either steam or water conditioning to enhance the durability of the groats, thereby diminishing fine levels. The amalgam of steel-cut groats encompasses segments of varied dimensions, a few uncut groats, and fines (including middlings and flour). These fines are systematically sieved out by passing the stream of steel-cut oats through a sifter. Subsequently, an additional process involving a length-sizing mechanism, such as an indented cylinder or a disc separator, is executed to segregate the uncut groats and reincorporate them into the cutting process. If necessary, the processor may implement a size-based separation of the cut stock to yield different fractions of cut groats distinguished by their sizes. The ultimate step in the steel-cut groat production process involves aspiration, a procedure designed to eliminate any remaining hull fragments or residual fines.

5.3.2 Flaking

Historically, oat flakes and oat flour represent the culminating outcomes of the oat milling process. Oat flakes, a staple in the realm of cereal production, are fashioned by flattening either whole or steel-cut groats through the action of two revolving rollers. Upon exiting the kilning process, the groats typically possess a moisture content ranging from 9% to 12%. At these moisture levels, the groats exhibit heightened fragility. To address this issue, steam nozzles are strategically situated at the entry point of the live steam chamber, effectively instating a uniform moisture infusion into the incoming stream of groats. However, a notable challenge arises with groats emerging from the kiln drying process; their minimal moisture content renders them exceedingly susceptible to disintegration into a fine powder. To circumvent this issue, a pre-rolling step is introduced, wherein the groats are subjected to steam infusion during agitation [42].

Furthermore, an agitator within the chamber meticulously blends the groats, ensuring an even distribution of moisture. The prevailing goal is to introduce 3–5% moisture at the uppermost section of the steamer. The balance of the steamer then functions as a tempering chamber, facilitating the equilibration of moisture throughout the groats or steel-cut groats. Temperature-monitoring probes, strategically positioned throughout the steamer, play a pivotal role in precise process control. The groats spend approximately

20–30 minutes within the steamer, during which their temperature escalates from ambient conditions to a range of 203–220°F (95–102°C). In the ideal scenario, moisture equilibrium is achieved with the least possible increase in temperature over the shortest possible duration, thereby mitigating the degradation of essential nutrients.

The thickness of the resultant flakes can be meticulously regulated by adjusting the gap between the rolling rollers. In essence, the thinner the flakes, the quicker their cooking time [43]. In practice, quick-cooking flakes are intentionally rolled to thinner dimensions, typically measuring between 0.36 and 0.46 mm, in contrast to whole oat flakes, which range from 0.51 to 0.76 mm. Furthermore, for specific products like muesli, even thicker flakes are engineered. Notably, flake thickness may fluctuate from 0.7 to 1.2 mm for particular applications, to as thin as 0.4 mm for quick-cooking oats. Subsequent to the rolling process, the flakes traverse an air stream, serving the dual purpose of reducing both their temperature and moisture content, ultimately restoring the flakes to a water content of 10–12%. To finalize the production, the flakes undergo a thorough separation procedure using a shaking shifter. This phase not only serves to disintegrate clumps of flakes but also efficiently sieves out fines and smaller flakes.

It is pertinent to recognize that the combination of steam conditioning and subsequent drying can lead to a partial pre-gelatinization of the starch within the oat flakes. Pre-gelatinized starch exhibits the distinct advantage of a heightened water absorption rate in comparison to unprocessed starch, thus considerably reducing the cooking time. Managing this process is akin to a delicate balancing act, wherein the retention time must be judiciously calibrated to allow uniform moisture equilibration and reach the desired final temperature. This minimizes the generation of fines during the flaking process and subsequent handling. It is essential to note that flake strength, or toughness, progressively intensifies with tempering time, reaching an optimal level after approximately 20–30 minutes in the steamer. Simultaneously, it is imperative to minimize vitamin loss.

The flaking operation follows the tempering process. The stream of groats passes through a feed gate that uniformly disperses a curtain of groats or steel-cut groats across the entire nip length of a pair of flaking rolls. Industrial flaking rolls vary in size, with diameters ranging from approximately 300 mm (12 inches) by 760 mm (30 inches) to 710 mm (28 inches) by 1320 mm (53 inches). While sizes are tailored to specific mill production requirements, typical diameters typically fall within the 400–500 mm range (16–20 inches). The gap between the rolls, crucial in determining flake thickness, is controlled by hydraulic pressure. In the United States, flake dimensions range from 0.356 to 0.457 mm (0.014–0.018 inches) for quick-cooking flakes, extending to 0.508–0.762 mm (0.020–0.030 inches) for whole oat flakes. In Europe, slightly larger flakes are produced, especially for use in muesli and oatmeal. Various flake designations and sizes include jumbo flakes (0.7–1.2 mm or 0.028–0.047 inches), small flakes (0.4–0.5 mm or 0.016–0.020 inches), and quick-cooking flakes (0.3–0.4 mm or 0.012–0.016 inches).

5.3.3 Flour

The transformation of groats or oat flakes into oat flour can be achieved through the process of milling, employing either a pin mill or a hammer mill. The grinding operation poses a unique challenge as oat flour, rich in fat content, has a tendency to clump [44].

To mitigate this, air is introduced to facilitate the movement of the flour through the mill, thereby preventing the accumulation of excessive heat. Upon exiting the mill, the flour is subsequently subjected to a vibrating sifter, an essential step aimed at eliminating any remaining larger particles. These larger particles are commonly recycled into a secondary milling process. Oat flour, as a product, finds its principal utility in the realm of baby food and ready-to-eat cereals.

Generally, flour originating from groats is characterized by a coarser texture compared to flour milled from flakes. However, the specific texture achieved is also influenced by the type of grinding equipment used. A pin mill or a hammer mill is conventionally employed for this purpose. To cater to the distinctive attributes of oats, a robust exhaust system is imperative to draw a significant volume of air through the mill housing. This serves the dual purpose of averting clogging of the grinder's screen and preventing clumping of the product, in addition to curbing excessive heat generation. The product emerging from the mill undergoes further processing within a sifting system, typically involving a vibroduster or a gyratory sifter equipped with a screen of appropriate size. Any product that does not successfully pass through the screen is channelled back either to the primary grinder or, in the case of larger mills, to a secondary grinder. In certain specialized scenarios, millers may employ a series of three or four corrugated break rolls to progressively reduce particle size, with fines sifted out between each rolling stage. The unique fat content of oats necessitates a gradual reduction to prevent the oat particles from obstructing the grooves. Often, a smooth roll is utilized as the final step in achieving the desired size reduction. The primary applications for oat flour are in the manufacture of baby food and ready-to-eat cereals, with the granulation of baby food flours typically falling under 0.5 mm.

Oat flour may be procured directly from KDHOs or alternatively, by grinding rolled oats. Notably, the fines resulting from groat cutting and flaking processes typically become part of the oat flour stream. The grinding operation is typically accomplished using hammermills, although pin mills and other forms of size reduction equipment may be employed individually or in sequence. It is worth highlighting that corrugated rolls, commonly employed in wheat milling, are ill-suited for oat milling due to the inherent risk of groove plugging caused by the high fat content of oat groats. Whole oat flour is typically sourced from clean, 100% groats or from products derived from whole groats, ensuring minimal material loss through stabilization and size reduction processes. Oat flour may be considered either a by-product of oat bran production or a composite of the sifting losses described earlier. In instances where the market demand for oat flour as a standalone ingredient is insufficient, it is often blended with millfeed to enhance its overall value.

5.3.4 Oat Bran

Oat flour can be further partitioned into two distinct fractions: the coarse fraction, recognized as bran, and the fine fraction, referred to as flour. Bran is predominantly sourced from the outer aleurone and sub-aleurone layers of the groat, and it boasts elevated levels of fibre, protein, vitamins, minerals, and slightly higher fat content. To derive bran from groats, oat flakes, or steel-cut groats, as previously delineated, the process involves grinding in an impact mill or passage through a roller mill. The resultant oat flour undergoes sieving to segregate it into coarse (bran) and fine (flour) fractions. In the case of impact mills, the granulation of the ground material is influenced by the mill speed and the screen size employed [10].

Oat bran is the product obtained by grinding clean oat groats or rolled oats, followed by the separation of the resulting oat flour through sieving, bolting, or other appropriate techniques. This separation process ensures that the oat bran fraction does not exceed 50% of the original starting material. It also stipulates specific nutritional criteria, necessitating that oat bran must contain a total-glucan content of at least 5.5% (on a dry weight basis) and a total dietary fibre content of at least 16.0% (on a dry weight basis). Significantly, a minimum of one-third of the total dietary fibre should be in the form of soluble fibre [14].

Oat bran, as derived from flaked or bumped groats, is notably enriched in dietary fibre, protein, vitamins, minerals, and phenolic compounds typically associated with the aleurone-sub-aleurone regions. It is pertinent to highlight that its fat content exhibits a slight increase relative to the starting groat content. On the other hand, the fine flour fraction is characterized by lower levels of these components but a higher starch content [45]. The yield and characteristics of bran are intrinsically linked to the speed of the hammer mill and the screen size employed. Subsequent to the grinding process, the flour stream is directed towards a sifter that effectively separates it into fine and coarse fractions. The most commonly used screen sizes are either 25 mesh (0.710 mm) or 36 mesh (0.538 mm), with variations in screen size giving rise to changes in the yield and quality attributes of the oat bran fraction [46]. As bran fraction yields increase, there is a concomitant reduction in the levels of total dietary fibre and β-glucan content.

The fine fraction is notably high in starch content. The coarser bran fraction is separated through a sifting process. According to standards set forth by the American Association of Cereal Chemists and the U.S. Food and Drug Administration, oat bran must encompass a minimum of 16% total dietary fibre, with one-third of the fibre constituting soluble fibre, and it must contain at least 5.5% β-glucan.

5.3.5 Concentrated ß-Glucan

Various techniques can be employed to process oat grain into fractions with elevated β-glucan content. One approach involves dry milling methods designed to separate the starch from oat bran. This is achieved by initially drying the oat bran and subsequently subjecting it to additional grinding or rolling processes to facilitate the release of starch from the β-glucan. The fibre and starch fractions are then segregated through sieving and aspiration, resulting in β-glucan concentrations ranging from 12% to 22%. Alternatively, β-glucan concentrations can be increased through the solubilization of β-glucan with the use of water, heat, and shearing, thereby reducing viscosity. This resultant slurry can be passed through a sieve or subjected to centrifugation to isolate non-solubilized components, such as starch. Another method involves the use of enzymes to degrade starch, protein, and lipids. This can be achieved by adding water to the oats and allowing the endogenous enzymes to break down the non-fibre components. Exogenous enzymes like α-amylase and trypsin can also be incorporated to aid in the hydrolysis of starch. These techniques not only serve to increase β-glucan concentrations in high-fibre foods but also have the potential to replace fats in certain food products due to their ability to increase viscosity. It is important to note, however, that these methods are multi-step processes, and as a result, the enrichment of β-glucan leads to a net increase in the price per kilogram when compared to the original oat product.

5.4 BY-PRODUCTS OF OAT MILLING

Oat processing and milling yield two primary by-products: oat hulls and oat millfeed. In certain instances, light oats are also isolated from the screening process as a distinct by-product. These by-products find their way into various commodity markets and serve a range of secondary applications. Oat screenings, essentially a conglomerate of materials rejected during the cleaning process, encompass scalpings, siftings, and potentially, light oats. These screenings can be ground into animal feed or subjected to further cleaning to extract higher-value constituents such as corn, soybeans, and canola. This multi-pronged utility serves both economic and sustainability objectives, optimizing the utilization of these materials. Light oats, when generated, can be integrated into commodity oats to enhance the overall product mix for marketing purposes. Alternatively, they can be employed as bedding material for livestock or poultry, serving as a viable alternative to conventional straw. This dual-purpose approach ensures that all by-products from the oat processing and milling cycle are efficiently repurposed, reducing waste and contributing to economic viability.

5.4.1 Oat Hulls

Oat hulls, also referred to as husks, represent the most voluminous by-product stemming from oat milling operations. While high-quality milling oats may exhibit as low as 25% hull content, variations ranging from 20% to 36% have been reported. The elemental composition of oat hulls comprises approximately 30–35% crude fibre, 30–35% pentosans, 10–15% lignin, around 4% protein, and 5% ash (including 3–4% silicic acid). When finely ground, oat hulls have diverse applications, ranging from high-fibre animal feed to human food ingredient incorporation [10]. Due to their substantial volume, the disposal of oat hulls can pose a significant challenge for oat millers. In the past, oat hulls were primarily utilized for furfural production [47]. However, the preference has shifted towards alternative pentosan sources such as corncobs and sugarcane bagasse for furfural production. Moreover, an increasingly prevalent utilization involves oat hulls as a biomass fuel for power plants. A case in point is the partnership between General Mills, where oat hulls from a food-processing plant are utilized in a nearby biomass power plant, generating electricity sufficient to power over 17,000 homes. A similar initiative is pursued by the University of Iowa in collaboration with Quaker Oats, where oat hulls are employed as a substitute for coal, supplying more than 10% of the university's energy requirements. Another avenue for oat hull utilization entails their conversion into a source of cellulosic fibre through alkaline treatments.

Numerous alternative applications for oat hulls have been explored. The two most prevalent are their utilization as finely ground high-fibre animal feed and as processed high dietary fibre food ingredients [48]. In certain regions of northern Europe, oat mills have implemented a hull combustion process to harness energy. Notably, the University of Iowa conducted a study examining the utilization of oat hulls as a biomass fuel replacement for coal, resulting in a significant reduction in CO_2 and SO_2 emissions. As a consequence, the university now employs oat hulls for steam generation on its main campus, thereby producing approximately 10 million kWh of "green" power. Oat hulls contribute to 20% of the fuel utilized (comprising coal, natural gas, and biomass) in the University of Iowa's primary power plant.

Oat hulls are undeniably among the most versatile by-products. A substantial portion is used as clean-burning biomass for electricity and steam generation. They can also be subjected to chemical processing to yield furfural, a renewable, non-petroleum-based feedstock for adhesives, plastics, and nylon. Alternatively, oat hulls can be treated with alkali to extract food-grade oat fibre. Lastly, a smaller quantity finds application as a fibre supplement in animal feeds.

5.4.2 Oat Millfeed

Oat millfeed, a comprehensive term encompassing all materials rejected during the oat milling process, is primarily directed towards animal feed applications. This conglomerate comprises a mixture of processing dust, minimal trichomes, oat hulls that have not been entirely eliminated during the dehulling phase, and, on occasion, oat flour. This composite consists of fine fragments derived from flakes, chips, and flour, obtained in the course of steel-cutting and flaking operations. In a well-managed milling facility, the millfeed yield should ideally remain within the range of 3–5% of the original starting material. The compositional attributes of this fraction are akin to those of the initial raw material. Depending on its hull content, it can be channelled into the oat flour process or is marketed as a premium-quality animal feed.

5.5 ENHANCING OAT-BASED FOOD QUALITY AND NUTRITION: EFFECTIVE STRATEGIES

5.5.1 Thermal Processing

The use of various thermal treatments in oat processing is important not only for extending storage stability but also for enhancing sensory qualities. These treatments can impart a pleasant roasted flavour to oats. Different methods, such as microwave, hot-air roasting, infrared roasting, and normal- or high-pressure steaming, are utilized to achieve these effects [49]. Interestingly, it has been observed that all dry heat treatments can improve the sensory quality of oats. Some of the thermal processes mentioned in this context include kilning, hot-air dry roasting, extrusion, superheat steam treatment, and microwave treatment. Each of these methods has its own impact on the sensory and nutritional quality of oat-based products (Table 5.2).

TABLE 5.2   Effect of Thermal Processing Techniques on the Influence of Oat Cereals

PROCESSING METHOD	OAT PRODUCT	EFFECTS AND OUTCOMES
Kilning	Oat flour	• Inactivates peroxygenase, reducing lipid oxidation – controls lipid degradation through enzyme inactivation
	Oat groat	• Enhances flavour, browning, and antioxidant capacity – extends shelf-life but may degrade heat-sensitive vitamins
	Dehulled oat after kilning	• Marked increase in volatile compounds after kilning
Hot-air dry roasting	Oat groats and oat flour	• High temperatures retain lipase activity, leading to free fatty acids – epoxy fatty acids accumulate
	Naked oat flour	• Inactivates lipase, improving storage properties
	Naked oat kernel	• No significant impact on oat β-glucan and lipids – enhances starch gelatinization
	Oat grain	• Reduces ochratoxin A levels with temperature and time – enhanced reduction with added sugars
Extrusion	Oat bran	• Increases oat bran oil extraction efficiency – moderate influence on fatty acids and lipid oxidation
	Oat flour	• Creates a homogeneous matrix and enhances water solubility – moderately affects oat proteins – inactivates lipase
	Whole meal oat flour from dehulled oat grains	• Prevents enzymatic degradation – stabilizes lipids even at low extrusion temperature
Superheated steam treatment	Oat flour and oat noodles	• Reduces lipase activity and damaged starch – improves water properties and product texture and taste
	Naked oat	• Dramatically reduces microbes – maintains shelf stability
	Oat groats	• Minimal changes in properties during storage – inhibits hexanal formation – shelf-stable
Microwave	Oat grains	• Enhances flour properties and disrupts starch crystals – suitable for quality oat noodles
	Oat hull	• Increases calorific values but reduces mass yield – higher power saves energy
	Naked oat kernels	• Inactivates lipase, maintaining triglyceride stability – improves storage properties

5.5.1.1 Microwave

Microwaves are non-ionizing electromagnetic waves with a frequency range spanning from 300 MHz to 300 GHz. They induce thermal effects in materials through the response of the material to the electric and magnetic fields of microwaves. The utility of microwave-assisted techniques has evolved significantly, transitioning from alternative roles to a wide array of applications, with particular effectiveness in food processing [50]. This can be attributed to their user-friendly operation, ability for selective heating, high efficiency, and relatively high energy-saving capacity.

In the context of oat hull processing, an increase in microwave power levels, ranging from 400 W to 650 W, results in reduced energy consumption due to the abbreviated processing time [51]. Also, the investigation revealed that subjecting biomass to high temperatures for a residence time of 3 minutes or undergoing an intense torrefaction process, led to a remarkable enhancement in calorific values of oat hulls, elevating them by as much as 35% relative to their initial values. However, this boost in energy content was coupled with a substantial reduction in mass yield, which plummeted to 60.77%. Furthermore, the application of severe torrefaction exerted a notable influence on several key parameters. It notably diminished moisture absorption and moisture content, resulting in the mitigation of grinding energy consumption. Conversely, this process adversely impacted energy yield and bulk density. Interestingly, the residence time, when examined independently, did not impart any significant alterations to the physico-chemical properties of the biomass. Nevertheless, it is imperative to underscore that prolonged residence times may impose substantial financial burdens, as they are inclined to substantially augment production costs.

Similar to other thermal treatments, microwave treatment is utilized to produce stable oat products, with a primary focus on inactivating enzyme activity and safeguarding lipids from degradation. A study was conducted to unravel the principal factors influencing the efficacy of microwave heating pretreatments in deactivating lipase within naked oat kernels [52]. The investigation meticulously scrutinized the impact of various parameters. These included temperature, heating duration, moisture content of the oat kernels, tempering time, and packaging conditions on the lipase activity inactivation. Remarkably, the application of microwave heat treatment for a mere 45 seconds yielded impressive results, leading to the deactivation of approximately 98–99% of the lipase content within oat kernels containing 20 g of material enclosed in a polyethylene package and possessing an 11.1% moisture content. This outcome effectively conferred stability to the oat kernels, effectively guarding against triglyceride lipolysis. The quantity of steam generated emerged as a pivotal determinant in lipase inactivation. A discernible trend surfaced: as the quantity of evaporated steam escalated, the residual lipase activities within the entire kernels diminished proportionally. Moreover, several advantageous pretreatment strategies were identified. These included the application of vacuum packaging, elevating the moisture content of the oat kernels from 11.1% to a range of 17.0–25.0%, and promptly initiating heat treatments once the kernel moisture content was adjusted. These measures facilitated the expedited evaporation of steam, thereby augmenting the effectiveness of microwave heating in deactivating lipase.

Additionally, research has demonstrated a significant reduction in lipase activity following microwave treatment for both oat flour and kernels, even at a relatively low temperature of 105°C. This process, in turn, enhances the storage properties and sensory quality of oat [53]. Furthermore, aside from steaming and hot-air drying treatments, microwave treatment has the capacity to enhance the storage stability of oat bran by mitigating lipid deterioration [54]. The results exhibited notable enhancements in sensory scores as well as L^*, a^*, and b^* values. Concurrently, the decrease in lipase activity within the oat bran resulted in a gradual increase in their fatty acid values. It's worth noting that the malondialdehyde content demonstrated a mild, gradual rise, consistently remaining lower than the corresponding values observed in unprocessed oat bran.

Numerous studies have delved into the influence of microwave treatment on the physicochemical properties, nutritional quality, and functionality of oat fractions. Microwave treatment can fortify the nutritional quality of native cereals by releasing nutritional compounds such as β-glucan and glucose into the water phase of the oat food matrix [55]. This can be attributed to the enhanced solubility of these compounds. Some of these released compounds, like phenolics, may possess antioxidant activity, thereby augmenting the overall antioxidant capacity of oats. Moreover, microwave treatment finds potential application in oat by-products. For instance, microwave treatment affects the structural and functional properties of oat dietary fibres derived from oat bran [54]. Additionally, microwave-assisted alkali treatment of oat bran enhances glucose yield, offering potential benefits for bioethanol production [56]. The results demonstrated a significant increase in pellet density and tensile strength for samples treated with microwave-assisted alkali pretreatment in comparison to untreated or microwave-only treated samples.

This treatment also improves the hydration and gelatinization properties of oats for the preparation of noodles made from oat flour, indicating its considerable potential in oat processing [57]. This study established a model to determine the optimal microwave pregelatinization conditions for varying degrees of gelatinization (DG) in oat and subsequently examined the characteristics of oat flour at different DG levels [57]. The results unveiled several significant improvements in the oat flour's properties. Hydration, as indicated by water solubility index and water absorption index, increased to 5.43 g/100 g and 4.33 g/g, respectively. Additionally, the thermodynamic properties of the oat flour exhibited enhancements. Notably, scanning electron microscopy (SEM) and X-ray diffraction results highlighted the transformative effects of high-frequency electromagnetic fields and thermal factors generated by microwaves. These effects disrupted the crystal structure of starch, resulting in the formation of aggregates with lower gelatinization temperature and enthalpy. Remarkably, oat flour with a DG of 88.5 g/100 g, which would typically be unsuitable for extrusion into strips, was successfully transformed into high-quality noodle strips. This outcome serves as compelling evidence for the significant potential of microwave technology in advancing the development of oat-based products.

Despite the high lipid content of oats and the challenges posed by large-scale industrial production, microwave treatment in oat processing remains relatively underexplored. Therefore, there is a clear need for further research in this area, as microwave treatment holds promise as an effective method for enhancing various aspects of oat processing.

5.5.1.2 Hot-Air Dry Roasting

Dry roasting with hot-air stands as a readily accessible and straightforward thermal treatment, holding considerable promise for enhancing the storage quality of cereals and augmenting the attributes of cereal-based food products, oat being no exception. Preceding the dry roasting process, oat kernels traditionally undergo a tempering step spanning 2 to 3 hours, aimed at achieving an even distribution of water and moisture adjustment. Following this, the oats are subjected to high-temperature roasting in a hot-air oven or roaster [53]. Notably, the roasting conditions, encompassing temperature and duration, exhibit variation depending on the morphology and moisture content of the oat kernels. These variables, in turn, exert a significant influence on the ultimate quality and storage stability of oat-derived products [58].

In parallel with kilning treatments, dry roasting offers the advantageous capability to efficiently mitigate undesirable off-flavours in cereals, oat included [59]. In a comprehensive study, the presence of oxygenated fatty acids within oat grains was meticulously characterized utilizing gas chromatography-mass spectrometry [58]. The concentration of these fatty acids was quantified subsequent to subjecting oat groats or oat flour to hydrothermal treatments and extended storage under conditions of 37°C and 65% relative humidity for a duration of 22 weeks. It is noteworthy that steam treatments demonstrated a pronounced ability to deactivate lipases, whereas roasting at 106°C did not yield the same effect. Consequently, a rapid accumulation of free fatty acids (FFAs) was observed in untreated or roasted flour, while this phenomenon was conspicuously absent in the case of steamed flour or groats. The analysis identified a total of six distinct hydroxy and epoxy fatty acids. Intriguingly, these oxidized fatty acids were detected in both esterified lipids and FFAs, a discovery of particular significance, as it indicates that the process of lipid oxidation does not mandate the involvement of lipase activity. Furthermore, the abundance of oxidation products was markedly higher in flour compared to groats, with a discernible reduction in their presence following steamed treatments. It is plausible that the enzyme, lipoxygenase, played a pivotal role in the formation of these oxidation products, although it is essential to acknowledge the potential contribution of non-enzymatic mechanisms as well. Of paramount importance is the fact that the hydroxy fatty acids that were identified were intimately linked with the development of intensely bitter flavours and are considered undesirable in oat-based products. This set of findings underscores the critical significance of inactivating enzymes before embarking on the storage of processed oat products. In stark contrast, a low level of lipase activity perseveres over an eight-week storage period following hot-air roasting at 155°C for 20 minutes, resulting in an improved storage profile for oats [53].

Similar findings ascertained that the activities of lipase and peroxidase were notably inhibited in naked oats following hot-air roasting at 155°C for 30 minutes. Importantly, this process did not adversely affect the levels of β-glucan and lipids, while concurrently enhancing starch gelatinization properties. In a comparative study, two distinct heat treatment methods, namely stirring roasting (at 240°C for 15 minutes; referred to as OFG) and kiln roasting (at 140°C for 45 minutes; referred to as OMG), were employed to investigate their respective impacts on the structure and digestibility properties of oat globulins. The outcomes of this investigation revealed that when compared with the control oat globulin, both of these heat treatments resulted in a reduction in the amino acid content within the oat globulins. Of particular note, it was observed that elevating the roasting temperature, from 140°C to 240°C, induced significant alterations in the secondary structure of oat globulins. This manifested as a decrease in the β-sheet and β-turn components, concomitant with an increase in α-helix and random coil proportions. Furthermore, a close examination under SEM unveiled that the structure of oat flour subjected to stirring roasting (OFG) exhibited fragmentation into smaller clumps. Comparative analysis between kiln roasting at 140°C and stirring roasting at 240°C demonstrated that the latter led to a reduction in average molecular weight, peak viscosity, and denaturation enthalpy. Concurrently, it gave rise to an increase in viscosity and the in vitro digestibility of oat globulin. Notably, stirring roasting not only enhanced the in vitro digestibility of oat globulin compared to kiln roasting, thus contributing to the taste profile, but it also entailed a greater loss of nutritional value [60].

Furthermore, it is noteworthy that dry roasting has been harnessed as a means to mitigate potential human carcinogens present in oat-based food products [61]. Ochratoxin A (OTA), a potential human carcinogen, is notably prevalent in oats and their processed derivatives. Due to its remarkable heat stability, OTA has been detected in thermally processed food products, including breakfast cereals and cereal grains. In a dedicated study, the reduction of OTA during the roasting of oats was explored under conditions mimicking industrial applications, which also involved the addition of sugars. The experiment involved conditioning oat grains to attain a uniform moisture content (16% wet weight basis, wb), with an initial OTA concentration of 100 µg/kg wb. Subsequently, the grains were subjected to roasting at temperatures of 120°C and 180°C for durations of 30 and 60 minutes, respectively. Notably, the concentration of OTA observed in the roasted oat-based cereals exhibited a decrease ranging from 2% to 18%, with an increase in both roasting temperature and time. The reduction of OTA was notably more pronounced when oat grains were roasted in the presence of reducing sugars, specifically glucose (11%) and fructose (15%), in comparison to oat-based cereal samples with no added sugar (10%). Furthermore, it is pertinent to highlight that the formation of previously identified degradation products of OTA, such as OTA isomer, OTα, and OTα amide, did not occur during the roasting process. These findings underscore the feasibility of achieving a heightened reduction of OTA in oats through roasting in the presence of sugars, a methodology that can be readily implemented in the commercial production of oat-based snack foods.

5.5.1.3 Extrusion

Extrusion, a multifaceted thermal process, exerts various effects on food products. It possesses the capacity to mitigate antinutritional compounds, hinder starch gelatinization, enhance soluble dietary fibre content, and retard lipid oxidation [62]. Notably, this technique leads to improved oil extraction efficiency in oat bran, making it a promising method for oat bran oil production. Significantly, extrusion does not adversely affect the fatty acid composition, acid, peroxide, or iodine values of oats when compared to other methods [63]. Cereal brans are inherently complex matrices, leading to diverse chemical reactions that can influence the flavour and chemical stability of products.

Extrusion markedly reduces hydrolytic degradation and the release of FFAs in oat flour. It also effectively prevents the formation of volatile lipid oxidation products during storage [64].

The utility of extrusion in the oat processing industry should not be underestimated. However, it's worth noting that the effectiveness of extrusion is contingent on various factors, including moisture content, extrusion temperature, and the composition of food materials. For instance, an investigation was to assess the potential of extrusion to ameliorate the storage stability of dried oat noodles through the inhibition of lipid-degrading enzyme activity and lipid degradation [65]. To this end, noodles were fabricated from oat subjected to extrusion treatment under two distinct conditions, and subsequently subjected to a 12-week storage period. Remarkably, the process of extrusion achieved complete inactivation of lipase and peroxidase in oat flour, with lipoxygenase activity remaining at a notably low level. The preparation of dried oat noodles also exerted a significant impact on enzyme activity. Most notably, lipase activity experienced a substantial reduction, dropping to approximately 11 U/min/g in the freshly produced noodles originating from oat flour that had not undergone heat treatment. It is noteworthy that the extrusion-treated noodles effectively controlled lipid hydrolysis, as evidenced by the absence of an increase in fatty acid values during storage. Additionally, the total lipids exhibited a more pronounced reduction in the extrusion-treated groups in comparison to the control sample. This phenomenon might signify that extrusion promotes non-enzymatic reactions, especially as the initial levels of volatile compounds were notably higher in the extrusion-treated samples. Significantly, the occurrence of non-enzymatic lipid oxidation during storage is expected to be mild, as evidenced by the moderate reduction in tocols and the accumulation of volatile compounds observed in the extrusion-treated oat noodles. The findings indicated that extrusion is a valuable method for improving the storage stability of dried oat noodles by deactivating lipase activity without triggering severe non-enzymatic lipid oxidation.

Moreover, extrusion preserves the structure of oat proteins, which remain partially denatured even at high extrusion temperatures of up to 130°C. The research focused on exploring the impact of extrusion temperature, screw speed, and specific mechanical energy (SME) on the reorganization of oat components, encompassing starch, proteins, and lipids, during the extrusion process of whole oat flour [66]. Notably, the application of high SME resulted in the transformation of whole oat flour into a more uniform and consistent matrix. However, the utilization of confocal laser scanning microscopy revealed that high SME caused the separation of lipids from the oat matrix, especially at high screw speeds, while this effect was not as pronounced at lower extrusion temperatures. Furthermore, the cellular structures within the oat material underwent fragmentation and degradation, leading to an increase in the water solubility of oat components. The study also identified specific extrusion conditions necessary for the complete melting and solubilization of oat starch, with a minimum extrusion temperature of 110°C and a screw speed of 200 rpm required for this transformation. In contrast, cell wall polysaccharides exhibited solubility at lower extrusion temperatures, a consequence of the elevated friction generated during the process. Oat proteins, particularly globulins, displayed remarkable resilience to denaturation, even under extreme conditions, such as temperatures as high as 130°C. However, their solubility in water substantially decreased under milder extrusion conditions. Moreover, the extrusion process proved effective in the inactivation of endogenous lipases, even at relatively low extrusion temperatures (around 70°C). Additionally, the native amylose-lipid complexes were found to be partially disrupted during the extrusion process. The study shed light on how varying extrusion parameters impact the reorganization of oat components, highlighting the importance of SME, extrusion temperature, and screw speed in achieving desired transformations in oat flour. Additionally, extrusion offers an avenue to fortify the nutritional value of oats. It has been established that extrusion can enhance the nutritional quality by ameliorating the functional properties of oat bran, leading to slower gut transit and prolonged satiety [10].

Wet extrusion represents a widely employed technology for generating meat-like structures. This process involves the introduction of protein-water mixtures into an extruder, which creates a microenvironment characterized by elevated pressure, robust shear forces, and high temperatures. These conditions promote the unfolding and aggregation of proteins, resulting in their texturization into fibres that resemble meat-like structures. For instance, a study delved into the functionality of oat fibre concentrate and faba bean protein concentrate in crafting plant-based substitutes for minced meat (SMs) [67]. The ultimate objective was to develop a product that emulates the mechanical and physicochemical attributes of beef minced meat (BM), suitable for various applications, such as frying and burger patty production. Remarkably, the mechanical properties, including attributes like chewiness and Young's modulus, exhibited by the original and fried SMs were on par with or even exceeded those of their BM counterparts. However, it's worth noting that the structural integrity of SM patties (comprising 45% SMs) was comparatively weaker when juxtaposed with beef burger patties constituted entirely of BM. Intriguingly, rheological analysis unveiled that the inclusion of oat fibre concentrate in the blend bolstered the gel-like properties of the mixture, a characteristic that was positively correlated with the overall strength of the original SMs, particularly reflected in Young's modulus. Consequently, these findings suggest that SMs could effectively serve as substitutes for BM in the formulation of vegetarian meat-like products, underscoring their potential in the realm of plant-based culinary endeavours. Nevertheless, it's imperative to acknowledge that the properties of meat analogues can be influenced by a multitude of factors, including the oat-to-pea protein ratios, moisture content, extrusion temperature, and screw speed [68]. Hence, optimization of extrusion processing conditions is essential. In summation, extrusion emerges as an effective and versatile technique extensively employed in food processing to enhance the desirable characteristic cereal flavour and the stability of food products, including meat analogues.

5.5.1.4 Superheated Steam Treatment

Superheated steam treatment (SST) is an innovative method that involves the application of dry steam generated by adding sensible thermal energy to wet saturated steam within food materials [69]. The introduction of thermal energy allows for elevating the steam temperature beyond the boiling or saturation point at a specific pressure. Consequently, SST offers several advantages compared to conventional processing techniques. Notably, it can be employed effectively for processing dry food materials, as long as the temperature remains above the saturation point, allowing for moisture absorption.

Moreover, SST boasts high energy transfer capacity, facilitating rapid and efficient heat transfer within food materials.

In recent times, SST has gained prominence in the production of plant-based foods. For instance, Head et al. [70] assessed the storage stability of oat groats processed through two distinct methods: commercially (involving conditioning with saturated steam followed by kiln drying) and with SST. The evaluation was conducted at both room temperature (21°C) for 26 weeks and elevated temperature (38°C) for 13 weeks. Various parameters, including hexanal and FFA levels, moisture content, colour, cold paste viscosity, and sensory evaluation, were monitored throughout the storage period. Both the SST-processed and commercially processed groats demonstrated remarkable shelf stability over the duration of the study. Notable observations included minimal changes in colour, cold paste viscosity, and FFA content in groats that had undergone different heat treatments as time elapsed. The fluctuations in moisture content in the stored groats corresponded to seasonal variations in humidity. One interesting finding was that, at both storage temperatures, the release of hexanal from groats processed either with SST or commercially increased as storage time extended. However, groats processed with SS released lower amounts of hexanal compared to their commercially processed counterparts. Additionally, as the storage period progressed, both SS-processed and commercially processed groats exhibited a diminishing flavour profile, becoming progressively less distinguishable to sensory panellists. In summary, the study highlighted the enduring shelf stability of groats processed using both SST and commercial methods. Despite variations in hexanal release and sensory attributes over time, the groats remained viable for extended storage periods, with both processing methods yielding comparably stable results.

Furthermore, SST has demonstrated its ability to enhance the quality characteristics (texture, tensile force, chewiness, hardness) of oat and whole grain wheat flour products [71], improve lipid stability (deactivation of peroxidase, lipoxygenase, and lipase) in black soybean and dried whole wheat noodles during storage [72], and control surface microbes (bacteria and mould) and enzyme activity in naked oat [73]. Nevertheless, the precise impact of high-energy capacity SST on oat-based foods remains somewhat unclear. Therefore, additional research is warranted to investigate the effects of SST processing on the flavour, physicochemical attributes, and nutritional properties of oats, further elucidating its potential in food processing and preservation.

5.5.1.5 Kilning

Kilning has long been acknowledged as a traditional yet highly effective method for large-scale oat product production, which confers augmented lipid stability during storage [10]. In the kilning process, oat groats are arranged vertically within cylindrical vessels, followed by the infusion of steam and air throughout the material. The swift introduction of hot steam from the cylinder's apex rapidly elevates moisture levels and effectively deactivates enzymatic activity. The development of desirable flavours and appealing colours is achieved through chemical transformations, notably the Maillard reaction and lipid degradation, occurring during kilning. The primary function of kilning lies in the prevention of the accumulation of lipid-derived off-flavours during oat product manufacturing and subsequent storage, achieved by enzymatic inactivation. Notably, volatile lipid oxidation compounds, including hexanal and 2-pentylfuran, as well as non-volatile lipid oxidation by-products such as epoxy and hydroxy fatty acids, are substantially suppressed in kilning-treated oat grain flours [74]. Additionally, the release of FFAs is curtailed due to the inactivation of lipase activity following kilning treatment. Consequently, the combination of heat treatment and elevated moisture levels effectively mitigates rancidity and off-flavour development [75].

Nevertheless, it is worth noting that one study observed higher levels of lipid volatile oxidation products in heating-dried oat fractions during prolonged storage, despite low lipase activity [76]. A discernible trend emerged, indicating that as the residual lipase activity within whole oat kernels or kernel fractions decreased, there was a concomitant increase in lipid oxidation and the generation of volatile oxidation products during extended storage of these dry fractions. Specifically, when bran underwent a heat treatment to completely eliminate lipase activity, the quantity of headspace hexanal detected after 12 months of storage exceeded that found in untreated bran by a factor of 5 to 7. This heightened production of hexanal was attributed to the oxidation of polar lipids. Significantly, when heat treatment was entirely omitted, the oxidation of unsaturated fatty acids within polar lipids remained absent, even during prolonged storage. This occurrence hints at heat-induced breakdown of membrane structures and the deactivation of thermally sensitive antioxidants. The findings of this investigation underscore the critical role of heat treatments as pivotal control points in the quest for oat products characterized by enhanced self-stability.

Similarly, another investigation found to evaluate the impact of different heat treatment procedures on the flavour and volatile compounds of oats, an analysis was conducted on various oat forms, including raw oats, kilned and dried oats, dehulled oats, and oat flakes. A sensory profiling method was employed to monitor changes in flavour, transitioning from a hay-like profile in raw oats to a nutty, bread-like character in oat flakes. For the isolation of aroma compounds, two techniques were utilized: headspace solid-phase microextraction and solvent-assisted flavour evaporation. Among the compounds detected in the headspace, hexanal was the most abundant, exhibiting concentration fluctuations ranging from 176 to 1671 mg/kg, contingent on the specific processing stage. Identification of the primary aroma compounds in oat flakes was achieved through gas chromatography-olfactometry and aroma extract dilution analysis, highlighting the presence of 2-methyl-3-furanthiol with a roast/cooked oatmeal aroma, alongside methional, dimethyl trisulphide, 1-octen-3-ol, and 2-methyl-3,5-diethylpyrazine. The hydrothermal process resulted in an elevation of volatile compound concentration, increasing from 1409.9 mg/kg in raw oats to 2457.9 mg/kg in kilned and dried oats. Intriguingly, the dehulling process led to a reduction in the total volatile content, dropping to 430.8 mg/kg. This decline may be attributed to the removal of bran, a component where volatiles are also found. Furthermore, it's essential to note that the composition of volatile compounds is highly sensitive to the parameters of heat treatment, especially when Maillard reactions occur. These reactions can introduce pyrazines, pyrroles, and furans, which have the potential to impact the overall flavour profile [77]. It is imperative to emphasize that, despite some drawbacks such as the potential loss of heat-sensitive components like vitamins, the advantages brought to the oat industry by kilning vastly outweigh these limitations.

5.5.2 Non-Thermal Processing

Numerous thermal treatments employed in food processing harbour inherent drawbacks, primarily stemming from their propensity to trigger the formation of undesirable chemical compounds, induce alterations in the physical attributes, and culminate in the loss of organoleptic qualities within food products [78]. As a result, recent research endeavours have been directed towards the exploration of innovative approaches aimed at developing eco-friendly, non-thermal processing techniques that circumvent these challenges, without exacerbating preexisting issues. To exemplify, both thermal and non-thermal methodologies have demonstrated proficiency in managing microbial contamination, restraining enzyme activity, and extending the shelf-life of millet-based products. However, it is crucial to acknowledge that thermal treatments, albeit effective in these aspects, can inadvertently impair the physical and functional attributes of millet-derived goods.

The contemporary landscape of non-thermal food processing encompasses several prominently utilized techniques, notably ultrasound, cold plasma, high-pressure processing, and irradiation. A wealth of research studies has undertaken a comprehensive investigation into the repercussions of these treatments on the characteristics of oat cereals. Consequently, the adoption of non-thermal methods signifies a burgeoning trend that holds significant potential in ameliorating the deficiencies wrought by conventional thermal treatments within the oat industry.

5.5.2.1 γ-Ray Irradiation

Irradiation, an exceptionally versatile technology, has found applications across a broad spectrum of food processing procedures. Among the various irradiation techniques, γ-ray irradiation, typically emanating from a Co^{60} source, is a prevailing choice [79]. It simultaneously emits two types of γ-rays, possessing energies of approximately 1.17 MeV and 1.33 MeV, along with a low-energy electron exhibiting a maximum energy of 0.3 MeV. γ-Irradiation has garnered significant attention due to its merits, which encompass unparalleled penetrability, energy efficiency, and minimal impact on the physical attributes of food products [80]. Importantly, an overarching consensus has emerged that an irradiation dose of 10 kGy, as stipulated by the Codex General Standard for Irradiated Foods No. 106–1983, does not introduce noteworthy nutritional or microbiological concerns in food items.

Studies have probed the effects of γ-irradiation on a diverse array of cereals, including oat and rice [81], [82]. The impact of γ-ray irradiation extends to the physico-chemical, structural, and thermal properties of oat starch. Evidently, a comprehensive investigation was conducted on three distinct varieties of oat grains, namely Sabzaar, SKO-20, and SKO-90 [83]. These oat samples, each maintaining a moisture level of 12%, were subjected to γ-irradiation at four distinct dosage levels, namely 5, 10, 15, and 20 kGy. Subsequently, starch extraction was performed, and a multifaceted analysis was undertaken to scrutinize the alterations in physicochemical, structural, thermal, and antioxidant properties. Among the array of physicochemical characteristics assessed, parameters such as syneresis, solubility index, swelling index, and light transmittance values exhibited notable deviations from their unirradiated counterparts. Notably, irradiation also exerted a discernible impact on the rapid visco analyser profiles, manifesting as a reduction in peak, trough, final, and setback viscosities, while the pasting temperatures underwent a marked and statistically significant ($P \leq 0.05$) decrease. To gain further insights into the structural changes induced by irradiation, an analysis via Attenuated Total Reflection Fourier Transform Infrared Spectroscopy (ATR FT-IR) was performed, confirming the exposure of hydroxyl groups within the starch chain. Furthermore, a striking observation emerged from SEM analysis, which disclosed the formation of distinctive ridges on the starch surface as a direct consequence of γ-irradiation. Intriguingly, the application of γ-irradiation engendered a significant enhancement in the antioxidant activity of the extracted starches. This multifaceted study underscores the profound impact of irradiation on the physicochemical, structural, thermal, and antioxidant attributes of oat starch, illuminating its potential as a transformative technology in the realm of oat-based products.

Similarly, another study was undertaken to elucidate the impact of gamma irradiation (0 to 20 kGy) on the physicochemical, rheological, and thermal characteristics of both buckwheat and oat starch [84]. The findings of this study unveiled compelling insights into the transformative effects of irradiation on these starches. An interesting revelation was that as the irradiation dose increased, the transition temperature and gelatinization enthalpy of the starches exhibited a noteworthy reduction. This decrease signifies a consequential alteration in the thermal properties of the starches due to gamma irradiation. Furthermore, the pasting properties, including peak, trough, setback, pasting temperature, and final viscosity, experienced a consistent decline in response to gamma irradiation. This phenomenon suggests that irradiation significantly influenced the rheological properties of the starches, leading to alterations in their viscoelastic behaviour. Gamma irradiation also induced a reduction in the percentage of crystallinity of both starch types. Notably, the apparent amylose content and swelling index showed a decrease with increasing irradiation dose, highlighting a structural transformation within the starch granules. On the other hand, the solubility index increased with gamma irradiation, indicating a greater solubility of the starches following exposure to irradiation. Intriguingly, despite these profound changes, no discernible surface fissures were observed in the irradiated starches, indicating the preservation of their structural integrity. Additionally, the Fourier transform infrared (FTIR) spectra patterns remained unaltered following gamma irradiation, suggesting that the fundamental chemical structure of the starches remained largely unaffected. These findings underscore the potential of gamma irradiation as a transformative technology in the context of starch modification and offer valuable insights for further applications in food and industrial processes.

Remarkably, γ-ray irradiation may bolster the antioxidant activity of starch and β-glucan in oat [81], [83]. This enhancement could potentially be attributed to radiolysis-induced depolymerization of larger molecules, exposing hydroxyl groups and reducing intramolecular hydrogen bonding, thus facilitating the accessibility of smaller molecules like β-glucan. Nevertheless, the full-scale implementation of irradiation techniques in the cereal industry confronts formidable challenges, partly stemming from public apprehension and regulatory restrictions surrounding irradiation. Consequently, the potential of this technology has been somewhat underestimated. More extensive research efforts are warranted to focus on irradiation as a novel approach to understanding the physicochemical and functional alterations in cereals such as oats. A more comprehensive understanding of irradiation could pave the way for its expanded industrial application, thereby contributing to the development of safe and stable oat-based food products.

5.5.2.2 Cold Plasma

Plasma represents a complex amalgamation of excited atomic, ionic, molecular, and radical species intermingled with various reactive components, including ions, electrons, gas atoms, and ground or excited molecules [85]. Cold plasma, also referred to as non-thermal or non-equilibrium plasma, has emerged as an innovative, cost-effective, and eco-friendly non-thermal technology. Its suitability for processing sensitive biomaterials has rendered it particularly advantageous in the food industry. Cold plasma is renowned for its remarkable efficiency in the inactivation of enzymes, microbial decontamination, and extension of the shelf-life of food products.

However, the high lipid content found in oats introduces certain limitations to the application of cold plasma. Notably, cold plasma has been known to induce lipid oxidation, particularly in lipid-rich food matrices, including cereals such as oat, wheat, and rice [86]. It has been established that both atmospheric pressure and exposure time exert an influence on oxidative stability, as exemplified in both white and brown cooked rice. Extended processing times (e.g., 20 minutes) and higher treatment powers (e.g., 250 W) have been observed to accelerate lipid oxidation, thereby negatively impacting the quality of the final rice-based food products. Cold plasma has also found applications in various other cereal and cereal-derived products, including fresh-wet noodles [87]. It holds promise as a novel technology for the modification of wheat flour functionality.

When applied at lower levels (e.g., air, power levels of 15 and 20 V, treatment times of 60 and 120 s), cold plasma treatment has shown minimal influence on total aerobic bacteria and mould counts, as well as non-starch lipids, non-polar, and glycolipids. However, it was associated with a decrease in the levels of total FFAs and an increase in lipid oxidation compounds. Achieving stable food products through cold plasma processing necessitates meticulous consideration of appropriate processing parameters. Enzyme inactivation through cold plasma is intricately dependent on variables such as discharge power, the degree of exposure to reactive species, mass transfer in plasma-liquid phases, and the specific properties of the enzyme [88]. The mechanism of enzyme inactivation primarily involves alterations in the secondary structure of proteins, resulting from the breakdown of specific bonds or chemical reactions. Consequently, it is imperative to investigate the impact of the cold plasma technique on oat and to optimize the relevant parameters to ensure the production of high-quality oat-based products.

A recent study assessed the effects of novel pin-to-plate atmospheric cold plasma treatment, considering two different input voltages (170 and 230 V) and exposure times (15 and 30 minutes), on oat protein [89]. An array of analytical techniques was employed to explore the structural, morphological, chemical, and foaming properties of the oat protein. The plasma treatment induced a reduction in the pH of the dispersions while simultaneously elevating the oxidation-reduction potential. These shifts in the ionic environment had discernible repercussions on the ζ potential and particle size distribution. The outcome was the formation of larger aggregates in cases such as the

170 V treatment for 15 minutes and the 230 V treatment for 15 minutes, as well as the distortion of smaller aggregates, notably following the 170 V treatment for 30 minutes and the 230 V treatment for 30 minutes. These structural alterations were corroborated by SEM analysis. The FTIR spectra exhibited a reduction in intensity within specific amide bands (1600–1700 cm^{-1}) and an increase in carbonyl stretching (1743 cm^{-1}). This heightened carbonyl content signified oxidative carbonylation, reflecting an increase in carbonyl groups. Consequently, the partial exposure of hydrophobic amino acids led to an augmentation of surface hydrophobicity. Furthermore, changes in the secondary and tertiary structures of the oat protein were observed. Circular dichroism analysis revealed an increase in α-helix content, while β-sheet and turns showed a decrement. The UV absorbance and fluorescence characteristics of proteins also displayed noticeable changes, indicative of transformations in their tertiary structures. The plasma treatment significantly influenced the content of free sulfhydryl groups and disulphide bonds within the oat protein. These changes were attributed to protein unfolding and the formation of aggregates. Additionally, the treatment led to increased solubility and reduced surface tension, contributing to improved foaming characteristics. In summary, the study demonstrated that plasma processing has a substantial impact on the structure of oat proteins, subsequently affecting their overall characteristics and functionalities.

5.5.2.3 *High Hydrostatic Pressure*

High hydrostatic pressure (HHP) treatment, a non-thermal technique, has emerged as an innovative approach to food processing. This method involves the application of pressures, typically ranging from 100 MPa to 600 MPa, often using water as the transmitting medium, within a controlled chamber at a moderate temperature. HHP has proven to be highly effective in inactivating microorganisms and enzymes, modifying the structures and properties of starch and proteins, while simultaneously mitigating the quality loss of food [90].

For instance, a study indicated that when oat and rice grains were treated with HHP across a range of pressures (300–600 MPa) and durations, changes in microorganism counts, enzyme inactivation, and specific physicochemical properties were investigated [91]. The results provided valuable insights into the effects of HHP treatment on these grains. HHP treatment at an elevated pressure of 600 MPa for a brief duration of 5 minutes yielded a significant reduction in the total bacterial count, indicating its effectiveness in microbial inactivation. At pressure levels ranging from 300 MPa to 500 MPa and exposure times from 0 to 15 minutes, lipase activity (LA) was noticeably inhibited, and the response to HHP treatment adhered to a first-order kinetics model. Furthermore, the application of HHP treatment at 600 MPa for 5 minutes led to the remarkable inactivation of 97.5% of LA and 92.0% of catalase activity in oats, highlighting its potential in enzyme inactivation. In terms of physicochemical properties, the pasting rate of both rice and oats exhibited substantial increases when subjected to HHP treatment at 600 MPa for 5 minutes, with rice showing a 75% increase, and oats displaying a 68% rise. In contrast, the time required to reach a pasting degree of 85% was reduced by 46%, and the heat absorption capacities of rice and oats decreased by 36% and 43%, respectively. These findings emphasize the impact of HHP treatment on microorganism counts, enzyme activity, and selected physicochemical properties in oat and rice grains, underscoring the potential of HHP as a valuable tool for enhancing food safety and modifying grain properties.

The impact of HHP treatment on proteins is primarily mediated through non-covalent bonds, encompassing hydrophobic, hydrogen, and ionic bonds [92]. The results are pressure-dependent; for instance, in the range of 200 MPa to 300 MPa, HHP induces conformational changes in proteins, while pressures exceeding 500 MPa lead to protein unfolding [93]. Furthermore, HHP significantly influences protein extraction, as evidenced by the fact that pressures above 350 MPa result in a substantial reduction in protein extraction, and no proteins are extracted at 500 MPa. This phenomenon is associated with the potential build-up of urea-insoluble complexes, disulphide bonds, and protein aggregates under high-pressure conditions. In breadmaking, an extreme treatment pressure of 500 MPa yields an exceptionally stiff, low-cohesive, and inextensible dough, rendering it unsuitable for bread production [94]. Conversely, a pressure of 200 MPa reduces the staling rate of bread, which is thought to have a positive impact on oat bread quality by weakening the protein structure, redistributing moisture, and altering interactions between proteins and starch [95].

HHP treatment also induces significant modifications in the physicochemical properties and structure of starch, with the extent of modification contingent on treatment conditions, starch types, and concentrations. HHP facilitates the penetration and diffusion of water molecules into the amorphous regions of starch, disrupting its crystal structure and leading to changes in starch properties. Furthermore, the level of pressure has a substantial influence on the crystal structure of oat starch. Treatment conditions within the range of 300 to 400 MPa increase the short-range ordered structure, double helix structure, and crystallinity of starch. However, when the pressure level rises to 500–600 MPa, these structural properties decline, and the crystal structure shifts to a V-type [96]. Differential scanning calorimetry analysis reveals that starch gelatinization begins at 300 MPa and is nearly complete at 500 MPa. In summary, when employing HHP treatment in oat and other cereal processing, it is imperative to consider its influence on food products, particularly with regard to macromolecular components such as proteins and starch.

5.5.2.4 Ultrasound

Ultrasound treatment, commonly referred to as ultrasonication, represents a promising methodology for the application of mechanical waves across a range of frequencies exceeding the human auditory threshold (>16 kHz). These ultrasound waves encompass both expansion and compression phases, wherein molecules are subjected to positive pressure during compression, while negative pressure generates cavities during expansion [97]. In recent years, ultrasound treatment has garnered substantial attention within the domain of food processing, primarily attributed to its utilization of high-frequency and high-power attributes. It offers a multitude of advantages, including heightened product yield, accelerated reaction rates, diminished temperature and processing duration, energy efficiency, and superior throughput [98]. Consequently, ultrasound treatment has emerged as a common practice in the modification of macromolecular compounds, such as proteins and starch, with a particular emphasis on the enhancement of oat-based cereal products and the optimization of oat by-products, notably oat bran [99].

Ultrasound treatment significantly impacts the composition, structure, and properties of starch derived from diverse cereal sources, bringing about alterations in physicochemical characteristics contingent upon specific treatment conditions. A corresponding observation was made concerning oat starch, wherein amylose content, solubility, swelling capacity, water absorption, and lipid-holding capability increased, while gel hardness exhibited a decrease post-sonication treatment. In a study, oat starch granules underwent ultrasound treatment utilizing either a 20 kHz horn sonicator at intensities of 39, 48, and 63 W/cm^2 or an ultrasound bath operating at an intensity of 5 W/cm^2 for durations of 10 and 20 minutes [100]. This comprehensive investigation encompassed an assessment of the morphological, structural, and functional properties of both the native and sonicated samples. SEM analysis unveiled the emergence of discernible fissures and pores on the surface of starch granules subjected to treatment with the horn sonicator. Notably, the highest sonication intensity induced a noticeable reduction in granule size. The ultrasound treatment engendered an increase in amylose content, swelling power, solubility, transmittance, water absorption capacity, and lipid retention ability, while simultaneously resulting in a reduction in gel hardness following sonication. Investigations into syneresis revealed that, during a 5-day storage period, sonicated starch gels expelled greater quantities of water in comparison to their native counterparts. Furthermore, the ultrasound treatment led to an elevation in the onset, peak, and conclusion temperatures of gelatinization. Simultaneously, the range of gelatinization temperature exhibited a decrease as a consequence of sonication. An examination of the crystalline properties exposed a reduction in the degree of crystallinity, as well as a decrease in the enthalpy of gelatinization, indicating that the crystalline structures within oat starch granules had been partially disrupted due to the ultrasound treatment. Notably, the A-type crystalline pattern remained unaltered throughout this process.

Within a starch-water system, ultrasonication generates localized strong shear forces, elevated temperatures, and free radicals, all of which collectively instigate profound alterations in the structure and properties of starch. The extent of these modifications is contingent upon several factors, including the frequency and intensity of the ultrasound, the duration and specific parameters of the ultrasonication process, the temperature and moisture content of the system, and the type of starch involved. This comprehensive review serves to consolidate existing knowledge regarding the impact of ultrasonication on the composition, structure, physicochemical attributes, and overall modifications observed in starch [101]. On the other hand, the utilization of power ultrasound as an emerging processing technology has garnered considerable attention for its potential to stimulate seed germination and enhance the accumulation of health-promoting metabolites, notably γ-aminobutyric acid (GABA) and phenolic compounds [102]. This research endeavours to assess the impact of power ultrasound at a frequency of 25 kHz on the nutritional characteristics of germinated oats and the microstructural changes within oat groats subsequent to treatment. To delve into the alterations in both the external and internal microstructures of ultrasound-treated oat kernels, we employed environmental scanning electron microscopy and 3D X-ray micro-computed tomography. The physicochemical attributes of oats exhibited notable improvements during germination. This encompassed enhancements in GABA, free sugars, avenanthramides, total phenolic content, and antioxidant capacities. Furthermore, the application of power ultrasound for a duration of 5 minutes following soaking significantly elevated the levels of GABA (within the 48–96 hour timeframe), alanine (from 24 to 96 hours), succinic acid (within 48–72 hours), total phenolic content (at 24 hours), and total avenanthramides (at 24 hours) in the germinated oats.

In the realm of oats, ultrasound-assisted extraction techniques have demonstrated remarkable efficiency in recovering compounds from oat bran, encompassing phenolics and β-glucan; nevertheless, the intensity of treatment necessitates careful consideration [103].

Moreover, a study was aimed to comprehensively characterize the solubility, structural, thermal, and aggregation properties of oat protein when subjected to high-intensity ultrasound (HIU) treatment. Suspensions of oat protein isolate (OPI) across a pH range of 2.0–8.0 were subjected to HIU for a 5-minute duration at 70% amplitude [104]. Various parameters, including solubility, particle size, surface characteristics, UV–Vis absorption, intrinsic fluorescence, polypeptide profiles, calorimetric properties, and thermal aggregation, were meticulously analysed. The results of this study revealed several significant outcomes. Notably, HIU treatment led to a considerable reduction in particle size, with a maximum reduction of up to 37%. Simultaneously, the surface charge of OPI increased, resulting in significant solubility enhancements of up to 48% at pH levels of 2.0–3.0 and 5.5–8.0 ($P < 0.05$). It is imperative to note that HIU treatment did not induce alterations in the protein profile or disrupt the disulphide linkages between the α and β subunits. Moreover, a decrease in the enthalpy of denaturation was observed in HIU-treated samples, with no discernible shift in the thermal transition temperature. This observation held true unless disulphide bonds were cleaved prior to treatment. It is noteworthy that while control OPI exhibited variable changes in particle size when subjected to heating within the temperature range of 20–95°C, the HIU-treated sample maintained a relatively uniform and smaller particle size. Collectively, these findings signify that HIU treatment, through the disruption of protein particles and the weakening of intermolecular forces, contributed to the improvement of the physicochemical and thermal properties of OPI. These advancements hold particular relevance for the development of oat protein-based beverages and other food products.

Furthermore, ultrasound was used as an emerging technology, exhibiting the capability to effectively disrupt the structure of biofilms and, to some extent, inactivate microorganisms within these biofilms. It's important to note that low-frequency and low-intensity ultrasound treatment may paradoxically stimulate microbial growth after application [105]. When ultrasound is combined with chemical disinfectants, particularly in the case of low-frequency and HIU, a synergistic effect is observed, resulting in a relatively high proportion of inactivated microbes within the biofilms compared to using either strategy in isolation.

In a study, two innovative food packaging films were developed: one composed of oat protein and pullulan (Op/Pul), and the other was Nisin-loaded oat protein and pullulan (Nis@Op/Pul) films [106]. To enhance the mechanical, structural, and physicochemical properties of these films, ultrasound was incorporated as a processing technique. The Op/Pul film exhibited several advantageous characteristics when compared to films made from pure oat protein and pullulan. It displayed lower light transmittance, reduced water vapour permeability, and lower oxygen permeability (OP). Additionally, Op/Pul films showed improved uniformity in comparison to their counterparts. The introduction of Nisin, however, led to a significant reduction in the transparency of the composite films, along with decreased moisture content and total soluble matter (TSM). The application of ultrasound treatment played a pivotal role in enhancing the properties of the Nis@Op/Pul film. It notably increased the film's elongation at the break by 18.37% and its transparency by 8.03%. Moreover, ultrasound treatment resulted in an 8.33% reduction in TSM and a 2.78% reduction in OP when compared to the conventional preparation method. An analysis of the film structure unveiled that ultrasound treatment strengthened intermolecular hydrogen bonding, reduced crystallinity, and created a more regular and uniform surface. Remarkably, the Nis@Op/Pul film prepared using ultrasound treatment proved effective in delaying the decay and deterioration of fresh strawberries, thereby extending their shelf life. In summation, ultrasound treatment stands as an emerging technology offering efficacious avenues for the extraction of oat components for food-related applications, while simultaneously showcasing promising prospects in diverse fields, notably in the realm of biofilms.

5.6 CONCLUSION

This chapter offers an in-depth exploration of the rich history and evolution of grain milling, with a specific focus on the milling and processing of oats. It takes us on a journey from the rudimentary methods of grain crushing using a mortar and pestle to the revolutionary invention of the burr mill, and the subsequent transition to more efficient iron and porcelain mills. The unique challenges posed by oats, particularly their hulls, are discussed, and we learn how innovative dehulling techniques and cutting machines paved the way for the production of steel-cut oats and the rolled oats we are familiar with today. This chapter also underscores the crucial role of processing in enhancing the nutritional content, safety, taste, and shelf stability of oat-based products. It emphasizes that while processing may sometimes be viewed as detrimental to nutrition, it is often indispensable for making grains suitable for consumption and can even improve the bioavailability of nutrients. Furthermore, the convenience and shelf stability provided by processed grain products are essential in today's fast-paced food industry. Food security is an escalating concern, and the chapter highlights the significance of mitigating postharvest losses to ensure a steady food supply. It explores the various factors affecting the quality of cereal grains during storage and offers insights into strategies for preserving the quality of oat products. Additionally, the chapter offers a comprehensive examination of modern oat storage, handling, and processing. It provides insights into milling-quality oat specifications and various oat mill products. Beyond traditional processing methods, the chapter introduces both thermal and non-thermal approaches to enhance the production of stable oat-based products. The objective is to promote the development of high-quality oat-based food items and lay the groundwork for future innovations in the field. In summary, this chapter makes a valuable contribution to our understanding of oat milling, processing, and the potential for creating high-quality oat-based food products, ultimately advancing the broader goal of improving the oat-based food industry.

REFERENCES

[1]   A. Bhargava and S. Srivastava, "Human civilization and agriculture," in *Participatory Plant Breeding: Concept and Applications*, A. Bhargava and S. Srivastava, Eds. Singapore, Singapore: Springer, 2019, pp. 1–27, doi: 10.1007/978-981-13-7119-6_1.

[2]   A. Fišteš, "The evolution of milling process," in *Cereal-Based Foodstuffs: The Backbone of Mediterranean Cuisine*, F. Boukid, Ed. Cham, Switzerland: Springer International Publishing, 2021, pp. 19–45, doi: 10.1007/978-3-030-69228-5_2.

[3]   O. A. Adetola, B. J. Akindinola and A. M. Sedara, "Development and optimization of double compartments grinding machine for agricultural processes," *Adeleke Univ. J. Eng. Technol.*, vol. 5, pp. 61–71, 2022.

[4]   P. R. Shewry, U. H. Mantila and S. O. Serna-Saldivar, "Structure and development of cereal grains," in *ICC Handbook of 21st Century Cereal Science and Technology*, Elsevier, 2023, pp. 17–30, doi: 10.1016/B978-0-323-95295-8.00001-0.

[5]   P. E. T. Prabhasankar Pichan, "Nutritional potential of cereals," in *Cereal Processing Technologies (First Edition)*, Boca Raton, Florida: CRC Press, 2023.

[6]   D. Burnette, M. Lenz, P. F. Sisson, S. Sutherland and S. H. Weaver, "Marketing, processing, and uses of oat for food," in *Oat Science and Technology*, John Wiley & Sons, Ltd, 1992, pp. 247–263, doi: 10.2134/agronmonogr33.c9.

[7]   D. Knorr and H. Watzke, "Food processing at a crossroad," *Front. Nutr.*, vol. 6, pp. 1–8, 2019, doi: 10.3389/fnut.2019.00085.

[8]   W. Biel, K. Kazimierska and U. Bashutska, "Nutritional value of wheat, triticale, barley and oat grains," *Acta Sci. Pol. Zootech.*, vol. 19, pp. 19–28, 2020.

[9]   C. J. Seal, C. M. Courtin, K. Venema and J. de Vries, "Health benefits of whole grain: Effects on dietary carbohydrate quality, the gut microbiome, and consequences of processing," *Compr. Rev. Food Sci. Food Saf.*, vol. 20, pp. 2742–2768, 2021, doi: 10.1111/1541-4337.12728.

[10] E. A. Decker, D. J. Rose and D. Stewart, "Processing of oats and the impact of processing operations on nutrition and health benefits," *Br. J. Nutr.*, vol. 112, pp. S58–S64, 2014, doi: 10.1017/S000711451400227X.

[11] A. S. Saleh, Q. Zhang, J. Chen and Q. Shen, "Millet grains: Nutritional quality, processing, and potential health benefits," *Compr. Rev. Food Sci. Food Saf.*, vol. 12, pp. 281–295, 2013.

[12] S. A. O. Adeyeye, "The role of food processing and appropriate storage technologies in ensuring food security and food availability in Africa," *Nutr. Food Sci.*, vol. 47, pp. 122–139, 2017, doi: 10.1108/NFS-03-2016-0037.

[13] M. Taddese et al., "Assessment of quantitative and qualitative losses of stored grains due to insect infestation in Ethiopia," *J. Stored Prod. Res.*, vol. 89, p. 101689, 2020, doi: 10.1016/j.jspr.2020.101689.

[14] N. Girardet and F. H. Webster, "Oat milling: Specifications, storage, and processing," *Oats Chem. Technol.*, pp. 301–319, 2011. Accessed: May 18, 2022. [Online]. Available: www.cabdirect.org/cabdirect/abstract/20113242313

[15] T. P. Shukla and G. H. Wells, "Chemistry of oats: Protein foods and other industrial products," *Crit. Rev. Food Sci. Nutr.*, vol. 6, pp. 383–431, 1975, doi: 10.1080/10408397509527196.

[16] W. Yan, S. J. Molnar, J. Fregeau-Reid, A. McElroy and N. A. Tinker, "Associations among oat traits and their responses to the environment," *J. Crop Improv.*, vol. 20, pp. 1–29, 2007, doi: 10.1300/J411v20n01_01.

[17] K. Vander Mijnsbrugge, A. Bischoff and B. Smith, "A question of origin: Where and how to collect seed for ecological restoration," *Basic Appl. Ecol.*, vol. 11, pp. 300–311, 2010, doi: 10.1016/j.baae.2009.09.002.

[18] S. Frischie, A. L. Miller, S. Pedrini and O. A. Kildisheva, "Ensuring seed quality in ecological restoration: Native seed cleaning and testing," *Restor. Ecol.*, vol. 28, pp. S239–S248, 2020, doi: 10.1111/rec.13217.

[19] F. G. Sayyad, H. K. Sharma and N. Kumar, "Cleaning and separation," in *Agro-Processing and Food Engineering: Operational and Application Aspects*, H. K. Sharma and N. Kumar, Eds. Singapore, Singapore: Springer, 2022, pp. 307–352, doi: 10.1007/978-981-16-7289-7_8.

[20] M. Papageorgiou and A. Skendi, "Introduction to cereal processing and by-products," in *Sustainable Recovery and Reutilization of Cereal Processing By-Products*, C. M. Galanakis, Ed. Woodhead Publishing, 2018, pp. 1–25, doi: 10.1016/B978-0-08-102162-0.00001-0.

[21] G. Brodal, H. U. Aamot, M. Almvik and I. S. Hofgaard, "Removal of small Kernels reduces the content of Fusarium mycotoxins in oat grain," *Toxins.*, vol. 12, p. 346, 2020, doi: 10.3390/toxins12050346.

[22] X. Hao et al., "Study on radial segregation of whole and broken rice in an indented cylinder separator," *Powder Technol.*, vol. 422, p. 118499, 2023, doi: 10.1016/j.powtec.2023.118499.

[23] M. Dadlani and D. K. Yadava, *Seed Science and Technology: Biology, Production, Quality*, Singapore: Springer Nature, 2023.

[24] R. Menon, T. Gonzalez, M. Ferruzzi, E. Jackson, D. Winderl and J. Watson, "Oats – From farm to fork, in *Advances in Food and Nutrition Research*, J. Henry, Ed. Academic Press, 2016, pp. 1–55, doi: 10.1016/bs.afnr.2015.12.001.

[25] D. C. Doehlert and D. P. Wiessenborn, "Influence of physical grain characteristics on optimal rotor speed during impact dehulling of oats," *Cereal Chem.*, vol. 84, pp. 294–300, 2007, doi: 10.1094/CCHEM-84-3-0294.

[26] D. C. Doehlert, "Quality improvement in oat," *J. Crop Prod.*, vol. 5, pp. 165–189, 2008, doi: 10.1300/J144v05n01_07.

[27] N. Ames, C. Rhymer and J. Storsley, "Food oat quality throughout the value chain," in: *Oats Nutrition and Technology*, John Wiley & Sons, Ltd, 2013, pp. 33–70, doi: 10.1002/9781118354100.ch3.

[28] L. Kouřimská, M. Sabolová, P. Horčička, S. Rys and M. Božik, "Lipid content, fatty acid profile, and nutritional value of new oat cultivars," *J. Cereal Sci.*, vol. 84, pp. 44–48, 2018, doi: 10.1016/j.jcs.2018.09.012.

[29] M. Vahvaselkä, P. Lehtinen, S. Sippola and S. Laakso, "Enrichment of conjugated linoleic acid in oats (Avena sativa L.) by microbial isomerization," *J. Agric. Food Chem.*, vol. 52, pp. 1749–1752, 2004, doi: 10.1021/jf034996j.

[30] H. Jung and S. Moon, "Purification, distribution, and characterization activity of lipase from oat seeds (Avena sativa L.)," *J. Korean Soc. Appl. Biol. Chem.*, vol. 56, pp. 639–645, 2013, doi: 10.1007/s13765-013-3119-4.

[31] C. Cognat, T. Shepherd, S. R. Verrall and D. Stewart, "Relationship between volatile profile and sensory development of an oat-based biscuit," *Food Chem.*, vol. 160, pp. 72–81, 2014, doi: 10.1016/j.foodchem.2014.02.170.

[32] D. S. Head, S. Cenkowski, S. Arntfield and K. Henderson, "Superheated steam processing of oat groats," *LWT Food Sci. Technol.*, vol. 43, pp. 690–694, 2010, doi: 10.1016/j.lwt.2009.12.002.

[33] M. van Boekel et al., "A review on the beneficial aspects of food processing," *Mol. Nutr. Food Res.*, vol. 54, pp. 1215–1247, 2010, doi: 10.1002/mnfr.200900608.

[34] A. Alfy, B. V. Kiran, G. C. Jeevitha and H. U. Hebbar, "Recent developments in superheated steam processing of foods – A review," *Crit. Rev. Food Sci. Nutr.*, vol. 56, pp. 2191–2208, 2016, doi: 10.1080/10408398.2012.740641.

[35] D. M. Londono, M. J. M. Smulders, R. G. F. Visser, L. J. W. J. Gilissen and R. J. Hamer, "Effect of kilning and milling on the dough-making properties of oat flour," *LWT.*, vol. 63, pp. 960–965, 2015, doi: 10.1016/j.lwt.2015.04.033.

[36]   X. Li, I. Oey and B. Kebede, "Effect of industrial processing on the volatiles, enzymes and lipids of wholegrain and rolled oats," *Food Res. Int.*, vol. 157, p. 111243, 2022, doi: 10.1016/j.foodres.2022.111243.

[37]   P. Rasane, A. Jha, L. Sabikhi, A. Kumar and V. S. Unnikrishnan, "Nutritional advantages of oats and opportunities for its processing as value added foods – A review," *J. Food Sci. Technol.*, vol. 52, pp. 662–675, 2015, doi: 10.1007/s13197-013-1072-1.

[38]   A. Sides, K. Robards, S. Helliwell and M. An, "Changes in the volatile profile of oats induced by processing," *J. Agric. Food Chem.*, vol. 49, pp. 2125–2130, 2001, doi: 10.1021/jf0010127.

[39]   F. M. Al Hasawi et al., "In vitro measurements of luminal viscosity and glucose/maltose bioaccessibility for oat bran, instant oats, and steel cut oats," *Food Hydrocoll.*, vol. 70, pp. 293–303, 2017, doi: 10.1016/j.foodhyd.2017.04.015.

[40]   W. Ganßmann and K. Vorwerck, "Oat milling, processing and storage," in *The Oat Crop: Production and Utilization*, R. W. Welch, Ed. Dordrecht, The Netherlands: Springer Netherlands, 1995, pp. 369–408, doi: 10.1007/978-94-011-0015-1_12.

[41]   A. Lapveteläinen et al., "Relationships of selected physical, chemical, and sensory parameters in oat grain, rolled oats, and cooked oatmeal – A three-year study with eight cultivars," *Cereal Chem.*, vol. 78, pp. 322–329, 2001, doi: 10.1094/CCHEM.2001.78.3.322.

[42]   I. Jokinen, P. Silventoinen-Veijalainen, M. Lille, E. Nordlund and U. Holopainen-Mantila, "Variability of carbohydrate composition and pasting properties of oat flakes and oat flours produced by industrial oat milling process – Comparison to non-heat-treated oat flours," *Food Chem.*, vol. 405, p. 134902, 2023, doi: 10.1016/j.foodchem.2022.134902.

[43]   Z. Yang, C. Xie, Y. Bao, F. Liu, H. Wang and Y. Wang, "Oat: Current state and challenges in plant-based food applications," *Trends Food Sci. Technol.*, vol. 134, pp. 56–71, 2023, doi: 10.1016/j.tifs.2023.02.017.

[44]   K. Zhang, R. Dong, X. Hu, C. Ren and Y. Li, "Oat-based foods: Chemical constituents, glycemic index, and the effect of processing," *Foods.*, vol. 10, p. 1304, 2021, doi: 10.3390/foods10061304.

[45]   D. C. Doehlert and W. R. Moore, "Composition of oat bran and flour prepared by three different mechanisms of dry milling," *Cereal Chem.*, vol. 74, pp. 403–406, 1997, doi: 10.1094/CCHEM.1997.74.4.403.

[46]   R. Wang, A. A. Koutinas and G. M. Campbell, "Dry processing of oats – Application of dry milling," *J. Food Eng.*, vol. 82, pp. 559–567, 2007, doi: 10.1016/j.jfoodeng.2007.03.011.

[47]   K. J. Yong et al., "Furfural production from biomass residues: Current technologies, challenges and future prospects," *Biomass. Bioenerg.*, vol. 161, p. 106458, 2022, doi: 10.1016/j.biombioe.2022.106458.

[48]   S. K. Sharma, S. Bansal, M. Mangal, A. K. Dixit, R. K. Gupta and A. K. Mangal, "Utilization of food processing by-products as dietary, functional, and novel fiber: A review," *Crit. Rev. Food Sci. Nutr.*, vol. 56, pp. 1647–1661, 2016, doi: 10.1080/10408398.2013.794327.

[49]   N. U. Sruthi, Y. Premjit, R. Pandiselvam, A. Kothakota and S. V. Ramesh, "An overview of conventional and emerging techniques of roasting: Effect on food bioactive signatures," *Food Chem.*, vol. 348, p. 129088, 2021, doi: 10.1016/j.foodchem.2021.129088.

[50]   P. Viji, B. Madhusudana Rao, J. Debbarma and C. N. Ravishankar, "Research developments in the applications of microwave energy in fish processing: A review," *Trends Food Sci. Technol.*, vol. 123, pp. 222–232, 2022, doi: 10.1016/j.tifs.2022.03.010.

[51]   E. Valdez, L. G. Tabil, E. Mupondwa, D. Cree and H. Moazed, "Microwave torrefaction of oat hull: Effect of temperature and residence time," *Energies.*, vol. 14, p. 4298, 2021, doi: 10.3390/en14144298.

[52] Q. Keying, R. Changzhong and L. Zaigui, "An investigation on pretreatments for inactivation of lipase in naked oat kernels using microwave heating," *J. Food Eng.*, vol. 95, pp. 280–284, 2009, doi: 10.1016/j.jfoodeng.2009.05.002.

[53] C. Ruge, R. Changzhong and L. Zaigui, "The effects of different inactivation treatments on the storage properties and sensory quality of naked oat," *Food Bioprocess Technol.*, vol. 5, pp. 1853–1859, 2012, doi: 10.1007/s11947-011-0551-5.

[54] X. Bai et al., "Effects of steaming, microwaving, and hot-air drying on the physicochemical properties and storage stability of oat bran," *J. Food Qual.*, vol. 2021, p. e4058645, 2021, doi: 10.1155/2021/4058645.

[55] J. Harasym and R. Olędzki, "The mutual correlation of glucose, starch, and beta-glucan release during microwave heating and antioxidant activity of oat water extracts," *Food Bioprocess Technol.*, vol. 11, pp. 874–884, 2018, doi: 10.1007/s11947-018-2065-x.

[56] O. S. Agu, L. G. Tabil and T. Dumonceaux, "Microwave-assisted alkali pre-treatment, densification and enzymatic saccharification of canola straw and oat hull," *Bioengineering.*, vol. 4, p. 25, 2017, doi: 10.3390/bioengineering4020025.

[57] M. Zhang et al., "Effects of microwave on microscopic, hydration, and gelatinization properties of oat and its application on noodle processing," *J. Food Process. Preserv.*, vol. 46, p. e16470, 2022, doi: 10.1111/jfpp.16470.

[58] D. C. Doehlert, S. Angelikousis and B. Vick, "Accumulation of oxygenated fatty acids in oat lipids during storage," *Cereal Chem.*, vol. 87, pp. 532–537, 2010, doi: 10.1094/CCHEM-05-10-0074.

[59] N. U. Sruthi and P. S. Rao, "Effect of processing on storage stability of millet flour: A review," *Trends Food Sci. Technol.*, vol. 112, pp. 58–74, 2021, doi: 10.1016/j.tifs.2021.03.043.

[60] T. He, J. Wang and X. Hu, "Effect of heat treatment on the structure and digestion properties of oat globulin," *Cereal Chem.*, vol. 98, pp. 740–748, 2021, doi: 10.1002/cche.10417.

[61] H. J. Lee, "Stability of ochratoxin A in oats during roasting with reducing sugars," *Food Control.*, vol. 118, p. 107382, 2020, doi: 10.1016/j.foodcont.2020.107382.

[62] D. Zhang et al., "Effect of extrusion on the structural and flavor properties of oat flours," *J. Cereal Sci.*, vol. 113, p. 103742, 2023, doi: 10.1016/j.jcs.2023.103742.

[63] J. Liu et al., "Effect of extrusion pretreatment on extraction, quality and antioxidant capacity of oat (Avena Sativa L.) bran oil," *J. Cereal Sci.*, vol. 95, p. 102972, 2020, doi: 10.1016/j.jcs.2020.102972.

[64] A.-M. Lampi et al., "Changes in lipids and volatile compounds of oat flours and extrudates during processing and storage," *J. Cereal Sci.*, vol. 62, pp. 102–109, 2015, doi: 10.1016/j.jcs.2014.12.011.

[65] Z. Yang, Y. Zhou, J.-J. Xing, X.-N. Guo and K.-X. Zhu, "Influence of extrusion on storage quality of dried oat noodles: Lipid degradation and off-flavours," *J. Cereal Sci.*, vol. 101, p. 103316, 2021, doi: 10.1016/j.jcs.2021.103316.

[66] T. Moisio, P. Forssell, R. Partanen, A. Damerau and S. E. Hill, "Reorganisation of starch, proteins and lipids in extrusion of oats," *J. Cereal Sci.*, vol. 64, pp. 48–55, 2015, doi: 10.1016/j.jcs.2015.04.001.

[67] J. M. Ramos-Diaz, K. Kantanen, J. M. Edelmann, K. Jouppila, T. Sontag-Strohm and V. Piironen, "Functionality of oat fiber concentrate and faba bean protein concentrate in plant-based substitutes for minced meat," *Curr. Res. Food Sci.*, vol. 5, pp. 858–867, 2022, doi: 10.1016/j.crfs.2022.04.010.

[68] A. Kaleda, K. Talvistu, H. Vaikma, M.-L. Tammik, S. Rosenvald and R. Vilu, "Physico-chemical, textural, and sensorial properties of fibrous meat analogs from oat-pea protein blends extruded at different moistures, temperatures, and screw speeds," *Future Foods.*, vol. 4, p. 100092, 2021, doi: 10.1016/j.fufo.2021.100092.

[69] Y. Liu, M. Li, D. Jiang, E. Guan, K. Bian and Y. Zhang, "Superheated steam processing of cereals and cereal products: A review," *Compr. Rev. Food Sci. Food Saf.*, vol. 22, pp. 1360–1386, 2023, doi: 10.1111/1541-4337.13114.

[70] D. Head, S. Cenkowski, S. Arntfield and K. Henderson, "Storage stability of oat groats processed commercially and with superheated steam," *LWT.*, vol. 44, pp. 261–268, 2011, doi: 10.1016/j.lwt.2010.05.022.

[71] X.-N. Guo, F. Gao and K.-X. Zhu, "Effect of fresh egg white addition on the quality characteristics and protein aggregation of oat noodles," *Food Chem.*, vol. 330, p. 127319, 2020, doi: 10.1016/j.foodchem.2020.127319.

[72] W.-T. Jia, Z. Yang, X.-N. Guo and K.-X. Zhu, "Effect of superheated steam treatment on the lipid stability of dried whole wheat noodles during storage," *Foods.*, vol. 10, p. 1348, 2021, doi: 10.3390/foods10061348.

[73] Y. Chang et al., "Effect of processing in superheated steam on surface microbes and enzyme activity of naked oats," *J. Food Process. Preserv.*, vol. 39, pp. 2753–2761, 2015, doi: 10.1111/jfpp.12526.

[74] Z. Yang, V. Piironen and A.-M. Lampi, "Epoxy and hydroxy fatty acids as non-volatile lipid oxidation products in oat," *Food Chem.*, vol. 295, pp. 82–93, 2019, doi: 10.1016/j.foodchem.2019.05.052.

[75] R. J. McGorrin, "Key aroma compounds in oats and oat cereals," *J. Agric. Food Chem.*, vol. 67, pp. 13778–13789, 2019, doi: 10.1021/acs.jafc.9b00994.

[76] P. Lehtinen, K. Kiiliäinen, I. Lehtomäki and S. Laakso, "Effect of heat treatment on lipid stability in processed oats," *J. Cereal Sci.*, vol. 37, pp. 215–221, 2003, doi: 10.1006/jcrs.2002.0496.

[77] D. Klensporf and H. H. Jeleń, "Effect of heat treatment on the flavor of oat flakes," *J. Cereal Sci.*, vol. 48, pp. 656–661, 2008, doi: 10.1016/j.jcs.2008.02.005.

[78] N. N. Misra, S. K. Pankaj, A. Segat and K. Ishikawa, "Cold plasma interactions with enzymes in foods and model systems," *Trends Food Sci. Technol.*, vol. 55, pp. 39–47, 2016, doi: 10.1016/j.tifs.2016.07.001.

[79] R. N. Pereira and A. A. Vicente, "Environmental impact of novel thermal and non-thermal technologies in food processing," *Food Res. Int.*, vol. 43, pp. 1936–1943, 2010, doi: 10.1016/j.foodres.2009.09.013.

[80] X. Pi et al., "Food irradiation: A promising technology to produce hypoallergenic food with high quality," *Crit. Rev. Food Sci. Nutr.*, vol. 62, pp. 6698–6713, 2021, doi: 10.1080/10408398.2021.1904822.

[81] A. Shah, F. A. Masoodi, A. Gani and B. A. Ashwar, "Effect of γ-irradiation on antioxidant and antiproliferative properties of oat β-glucan," *Radiat. Phys. Chem.*, vol. 117, pp. 120–127, 2015, doi: 10.1016/j.radphyschem.2015.06.022.

[82] Y. Zhai, L. Pan, X. Luo, Y. Zhang, R. Wang and Z. Chen, "Effect of electron beam irradiation on storage, moisture and eating properties of high-moisture rice during storage," *J. Cereal Sci.*, vol. 103, p. 103407, 2022, doi: 10.1016/j.jcs.2021.103407.

[83] R. Mukhtar et al., "γ-Irradiation of oat grain – Effect on physico-chemical, structural, thermal, and antioxidant properties of extracted starch," *Int. J. Biol. Macromol.*, vol. 104, pp. 1313–1320, 2017, doi: 10.1016/j.ijbiomac.2017.05.092.

[84] M. Z. Dar et al., "Modification of structure and physicochemical properties of buckwheat and oat starch by γ-irradiation," *Int. J. Biol. Macromol.*, vol. 108, pp. 1348–1356, 2018, doi: 10.1016/j.ijbiomac.2017.11.067.

[85] S. Punia Bangar et al., "Recent developments in cold plasma-based enzyme activity (browning, cell wall degradation, and antioxidant) in fruits and vegetables," *Compr. Rev. Food Sci. Food Saf.*, vol. 21, pp. 1958–1978, 2022, doi: 10.1111/1541-4337.12895.

[86] M. Gavahian, Y.-H. Chu, A. Mousavi Khaneghah, F. J. Barba and N. N. Misra, "A critical analysis of the cold plasma induced lipid oxidation in foods," *Trends Food Sci. Technol.*, vol. 77, pp. 32–41, 2018, doi: 10.1016/j.tifs.2018.04.009.

[87] Y. Chen, G. Chen, R. Wei, Y. Zhang, S. Li and Y. Chen, "Quality characteristics of fresh wet noodles treated with nonthermal plasma sterilization," *Food Chem.*, vol. 297, p. 124900, 2019, doi: 10.1016/j.foodchem.2019.05.174.

[88] N. N. Misra et al., "Landmarks in the historical development of twenty first century food processing technologies," *Food Res. Int.*, vol. 97, pp. 318–339, 2017, doi: 10.1016/j.foodres.2017.05.001.

[89] G. Eazhumalai, R. G. T. Kalaivendan and U. S. Annapure, "Effect of atmospheric pin-to-plate cold plasma on oat protein: Structural, chemical, and foaming characteristics," *Int. J. Biol. Macromol.*, vol. 242, p. 125103, 2023, doi: 10.1016/j.ijbiomac.2023.125103.

[90] H.-W. Huang, C.-P. Hsu and C.-Y. Wang, "Healthy expectations of high hydrostatic pressure treatment in food processing industry," *J. Food Drug Anal.*, vol. 28, pp. 1–13, 2020, doi: 10.1016/j.jfda.2019.10.002.

[91] J. Gao, H. Yang, A. Rong, X. Bao and M. Zhang, "Effects of HHP on microorganisms, enzyme inactivation and physicochemical properties of instant oats and rice," *J. Food Process Eng.*, vol. 37, pp. 191–198, 2014, doi: 10.1111/jfpe.12062.

[92] K. Aganovic et al., "Aspects of high hydrostatic pressure food processing: Perspectives on technology and food safety," *Compr. Rev. Food Sci. Food Saf.*, vol. 20, pp. 3225–3266, 2021, doi: 10.1111/1541-4337.12763.

[93] E. K. Hüttner, F. Dal Bello, K. Poutanen and E. K. Arendt, "Fundamental evaluation of the impact of high hydrostatic pressure on oat batters," *J. Cereal Sci.*, vol. 49, pp. 363–370, 2009, doi: 10.1016/j.jcs.2008.12.005.

[94] A. Angioloni and C. Collar, "Promoting dough viscoelastic structure in composite cereal matrices by high hydrostatic pressure," *J. Food Eng.*, vol. 111, pp. 598–605, 2012, doi: 10.1016/j.jfoodeng.2012.03.010.

[95] E. K. Hüttner, F. Dal Bello and E. K. Arendt, "Fundamental study on the effect of hydrostatic pressure treatment on the bread-making performance of oat flour," *Eur. Food Res. Technol.*, vol. 230, pp. 827–835, 2010, doi: 10.1007/s00217-010-1228-4.

[96] J. Zhang, M. Zhang, Y. Zhang, X. Bai and C. Wang, "Effects of high hydrostatic pressure on the structure and retrogradation inhibition of oat starch," *Int. J. Food Sci. Technol.*, vol. 57, pp. 2113–2125, 2022, doi: 10.1111/ijfs.15642.

[97] N. Bhargava, R. S. Mor, K. Kumar and V. S. Sharanagat, "Advances in application of ultrasound in food processing: A review," *Ultrason. Sonochem.*, vol. 70, p. 105293, 2021, doi: 10.1016/j.ultsonch.2020.105293.

[98] M. Singla and N. Sit, "Application of ultrasound in combination with other technologies in food processing: A review," *Ultrason Sonochem.*, vol. 73, p. 105506, 2021, doi: 10.1016/j.ultsonch.2021.105506.

[99] H. Kaur and B. S. Gill, "Effect of high-intensity ultrasound treatment on nutritional, rheological and structural properties of starches obtained from different cereals," *Int. J. Biol. Macromol.*, vol. 126, pp. 367–375, 2019, doi: 10.1016/j.ijbiomac.2018.12.149.

[100] S. R. Falsafi, Y. Maghsoudlou, H. Rostamabadi, M. M. Rostamabadi, H. Hamedi and S. M. H. Hosseini, "Preparation of physically modified oat starch with different sonication treatments," *Food Hydrocoll.*, vol. 89, pp. 311–320, 2019, doi: 10.1016/j.foodhyd.2018.10.046.

[101] F. Zhu, "Impact of ultrasound on structure, physicochemical properties, modifications, and applications of starch," *Trends Food Sci. Technol.*, vol. 43, pp. 1–17, 2015, doi: 10.1016/j.tifs.2014.12.008.

[102] J. Ding, J. Johnson, Y. F. Chu and H. Feng, 'Enhancement of γ-aminobutyric acid, avenanthramides, and other health-promoting metabolites in germinating oats (Avena sativa L.) treated with and without power ultrasound," *Food Chem.*, vol. 283, pp. 239–247, 2019, doi: 10.1016/j.foodchem.2018.12.136.

[103] N. Milićević et al., "Kinetic modelling of ultrasound-assisted extraction of phenolics from cereal brans," *Ultrason. Sonochem.*, vol. 79, p. 105761, 2021, doi: 10.1016/j. ultsonch.2021.105761.

[104] R. Li and Y. L. Xiong, "Ultrasound-induced structural modification and thermal properties of oat protein," *LWT.*, vol. 149, p. 111861, 2021, doi: 10.1016/j.lwt.2021.111861.

[105] H. Yu et al., "Ultrasound-involved emerging strategies for controlling foodborne microbial biofilms," *Trends Food Sci. Technol.*, vol. 96, pp. 91–101, 2020, doi: 10.1016/j.tifs.2019.12.010.

[106] L. Kang et al., "Insights into ultrasonic treatment on the properties of pullulan/oat protein/nisin composite film: Mechanical, structural and physicochemical properties," *Food Chem.*, vol. 402, pp. 134237, 2023, doi: 10.1016/j.foodchem.2022.134237.

Health Benefits and Medicinal Properties of Oats

Molecular Mechanisms and Disease Management

Muzaffar Hasan, Chirag Maheshwari,
Nand Lal Meena, Nitin Kumar Garg,
Kailashpati Tripathi, and Dilshad Ahmad

6.1 INTRODUCTION

Oats, scientifically known as *Avena sativa* L., hold a prominent position as a functional cereal grain with a global appeal and an increasingly recognized array of health advantages. These grains are cultivated worldwide and serve as a dietary cornerstone in numerous regions. Within the realm of oats, a wide spectrum of varieties exists [1]. Oats exhibit a remarkable richness in protein content, featuring a host of vital minerals, lipids, and the pivotal β-glucan, a mixed-linkage polysaccharide constituting a substantial component of oat dietary fibre [2]. Furthermore, oats encompass a plethora of additional phytoconstituents, such as avenanthramides, the indole alkaloid gramine, flavonoids, flavonolignans, triterpenoid saponins, sterols, and tocols. The bounty of bioactive compounds found in oats, most notably β-glucan, makes them an ideal candidate for the development of functional foods and health products aimed at diabetes prevention and management [3]. These bioactive constituents grant oats an extensive array of properties, including antioxidant, anti-diabetic, antimicrobial, anticancer, antihypertensive, immunomodulatory, anti-hyperlipidemic, anti-obesity, and cardioprotective attributes [4].

Oats are a veritable treasure trove of essential nutrients, offering an abundance of protein, fibre, calcium, vitamins (B, C, E, and K), amino acids, and antioxidants (such as β-carotene, polyphenols, chlorophyll, and flavonoids) [5]. Notably, β-glucan and avenanthramides fortify the immune system, facilitate detoxification, reduce blood cholesterol levels, and support weight loss by optimizing lipid profiles and fat metabolism. β-Glucan also regulates insulin secretion, which plays a pivotal role in diabetes prevention [6]. Progladins, another constituent, contribute to cholesterol reduction, triglyceride control, inflammation suppression, and enhanced skin health [7]. Saponin-based avanacosidase and flavone glycosides bolster immune function, curb inflammation, and enhance skin health. Lignin and phytoestrogens offer protection against hormone-related cancers and enhance the quality of life for postmenopausal women. Furthermore, sprouted oats are a rich source of saponarin, aiding in liver detoxification [8].

Avenanthramides (AVAs), exclusive to oats, serve as phenolic alkaloids and exhibit antioxidant, anti-inflammatory, antiproliferative, and anti-itching properties. The most prevalent AVAs in oats include 2c, 2f, and 2p, although oats harbour a total of 25 distinct AVAs [9]. Oats also boast steroidal saponins, primarily avenacins and avenacosides, which not only function as plant defence mechanisms but also offer potential in cholesterol reduction, immunoregulation, and anticancer activities [10]. Saponins have demonstrated efficacy against colon cancer cell growth [11]. While the saponin content in rolled oats and oat porridge is reported as 0.9 g/kg and 0.1 g/kg (as consumed), respectively, in-depth research on saponin content, chemical composition, and their associated health benefits in oats remains an open avenue for exploration.

Cancer ranks as one of the leading causes of global mortality, with common types including lung, breast, colorectal, and stomach cancers. Lifestyle and dietary factors significantly influence cancer incidence and progression, contributing to 30% of cancer-related deaths [12]. High body mass index, physical inactivity, tobacco use, alcohol consumption, and insufficient fruit and vegetable intake are the five primary behavioural and dietary risk factors. Recently, dietary polyphenols have emerged as promising contributors to health, with their potent antioxidant properties and associations with the prevention of oxidative stress-related diseases, such as cardiovascular and neurodegenerative conditions and cancer [13]. As the field of cancer treatment advances, challenges like undesirable side effects and drug resistance persist. Natural products, including polyphenols, offer a promising avenue for novel anticancer strategies. Polyphenols, recognized for their antioxidant properties, exert anticancer effects by modulating multiple pathways and mechanisms [14]. They have the potential to activate apoptosis and senescence, inhibit cell proliferation, hinder epithelial mesenchymal transition, metastatization, and influence various enzymes and cell receptors. This multifaceted nature positions polyphenols as not only antioxidants but also valuable allies in the prevention and treatment of diseases such as cancer [9]. AVAs are emerging as promising chemopreventive and anticancer phytochemicals, with further clinical trials and toxicological studies needed to establish their efficacy in reducing the cancer burden [3].

Oats find applications beyond nutrition, extending to the realm of dermatology. AVAs, unique oat metabolites, endow oats with anti-inflammatory, antipruritic, antioxidant, and antifungal properties, rendering them effective in addressing conditions like atopic dermatitis, contact dermatitis, pruritic dermatoses, sunburn, drug eruptions, and various skin afflictions [15]. Colloidal oatmeal, in particular, offers relief for minor skin irritations and itching associated with eczema, functioning as a cleanser, moisturizer, and skin protectant. Oat flavonoids safeguard against ultraviolet A radiation, while tocopherol protects against inflammation and photodamage. Histopathological evidence supports improved wound healing with topical oat extract application [16].

Coeliac disease (CD), a widespread ailment affecting about 1% of the global population, stems from chronic inflammation of the proximal small intestine and occurs in genetically susceptible individuals exposed to gluten [17]. Symptoms vary but often encompass headaches, diarrhoea, abdominal discomfort, unexplained weight loss, and iron-deficiency or unspecified anaemia. Dermatitis herpetiformis may also manifest. Diagnosis involves blood tests and small intestine biopsy. Treatment necessitates a lifelong gluten-free diet [18]. Oats, boasting low levels of prolamins responsible for gluten-related toxicity, are considered a valuable fibre source for those adhering to a gluten-free regimen [17]. Numerous CD organizations and clinical studies endorse the consumption of oats by individuals with the condition, without adverse effects.

Phytic acid (PA), known scientifically as myo-inositol hexakisphosphate, is the primary phosphorus storage compound in seeds, constituting 65% to 85% of the total phosphorus content. PA's negatively charged nature enables it to chelate metal cations, forming insoluble phytate salts that render divalent cations like Fe^{2+}, Zn^{2+}, Mg^{2+}, and Ca^{2+} unavailable for absorption by monogastric animals [19]. This may lead to micronutrient deficiencies in humans, given their lack of the phytase enzyme needed to hydrolyse phytate and release bound micronutrients. PA's presence in the diet poses two primary concerns: its impact on mineral bioavailability and its inhibition of proteases essential for protein digestion. However, PA's positive attributes have been underestimated, as it serves as a potent natural plant antioxidant, offering protection against oxidative stress in seeds and playing a preventive role in various human diseases. Recent reports suggest beneficial roles of PA as an anti-diabetic and antibacterial agent [20]. Fine-tuning seed content allows the development of grains with low PA, potentially modified distribution patterns, and enhanced properties. Despite potential drawbacks, the consumption of PA also offers notable benefits. PA exhibits antioxidant activity by curbing free radicals and lipid peroxidation associated with iron. Its association with zinc reduces non-specific DNA synthesis and influences starch digestibility by inhibiting α-amylase, benefitting diabetics through blood glucose level control and colon health promotion [21]. The PA-zinc interaction also reduces serum cholesterol levels, lowering the zinc-to-copper ratio and preventing cancer and coronary heart disease. Moreover, PA reduces renal stone formation by inhibiting calcification.

Diabetes stands as a global health concern with an escalating incidence, and nutritional therapy emerges as a pivotal factor in its prevention and treatment. Epidemiological and short-term interventional studies underscore the connection between higher fibre intake and improvements in lipid profiles, fasting and postprandial glycaemic control, obesity management, dyslipidemia, hypertension, and various cancers [22]. Soluble fibres, like β-glucans, have garnered heightened interest for their multifunctional and bioactive attributes and can be readily sourced from oats and barley grains. The fermentability and high-viscosity solutions created by β-glucans in the human intestine underpin their health benefits [23]. β-Glucans contribute to reduced postprandial glucose and insulin responses through various mechanisms. The degree of their effect on glycaemic control hinges on factors such as dosage, consumption duration, physicochemical attributes, processing methods, and food forms. An emphasis on the consumption of β-glucans and products containing them has the potential to play a vital role in diabetes management, lowering the risk of diabetes-related complications [24].

The gut microbiota, comprising a consortium of microorganisms residing in the intestinal tract, plays a pivotal role in digestion and disease prevention when dominated by beneficial species. Imbalances in the gut microbiota can contribute to various diseases [25]. Diet plays a critical role in determining the composition of the gut microbiota, with a fibre-rich diet offering positive modulation. Oats, being a source of both soluble and insoluble fibre, hold functional ingredient status with prebiotic potential [26]. Additionally, they contain plant proteins, unsaturated fats, and antioxidants. The impact of oat consumption on the gut microbiota is an emerging area of study, with observed associations between oat consumption and the abundance of beneficial microorganisms like *Akkermansia muciniphila*, *Roseburia*, *Lactobacillus*, *Bifidobacterium*, and *Faecalibacterium prausnitzii* [27].

In the ensuing chapter, we embark on a comprehensive exploration of oat bioactive compounds, delving into their mechanistic foundations and diverse biological functions. This exhaustive examination covers a wide array of bioactive components, encompassing proteins, peptides, amino acids, β-glucans, resistant starch, dietary fibres, polyunsaturated fatty acids, vitamins, minerals, polyphenols, AVAs, oat saponins, and β-sitosterol. Their multifaceted roles are unveiled, from providing antioxidative and anti-diabetic properties to their potential in combatting microbial threats, cancer, hypertension, obesity, and heart health. This in-depth exploration offers a comprehensive understanding of oats' multifaceted contributions to human health and nutrition.

6.2 UNLOCKING THE HEALING POTENTIAL OF OAT BIOACTIVES FOR OPTIMAL HEALTH MANAGEMENT

6.2.1 Exploring Oats as a Potential Option for Managing Coeliac Disease

6.2.1.1 Coeliac Disease

CD constitutes a persistent immune-mediated enteropathy, ignited by the consumption of wheat, rye, and barley. It is demarcated by a distinctive clinical trait: the atrophy of the intestinal mucosa and the dearth of conventional villi, culminating in a pervasive deficiency in nutrient absorption [28] (Figure 6.1). The prevalence of CD within

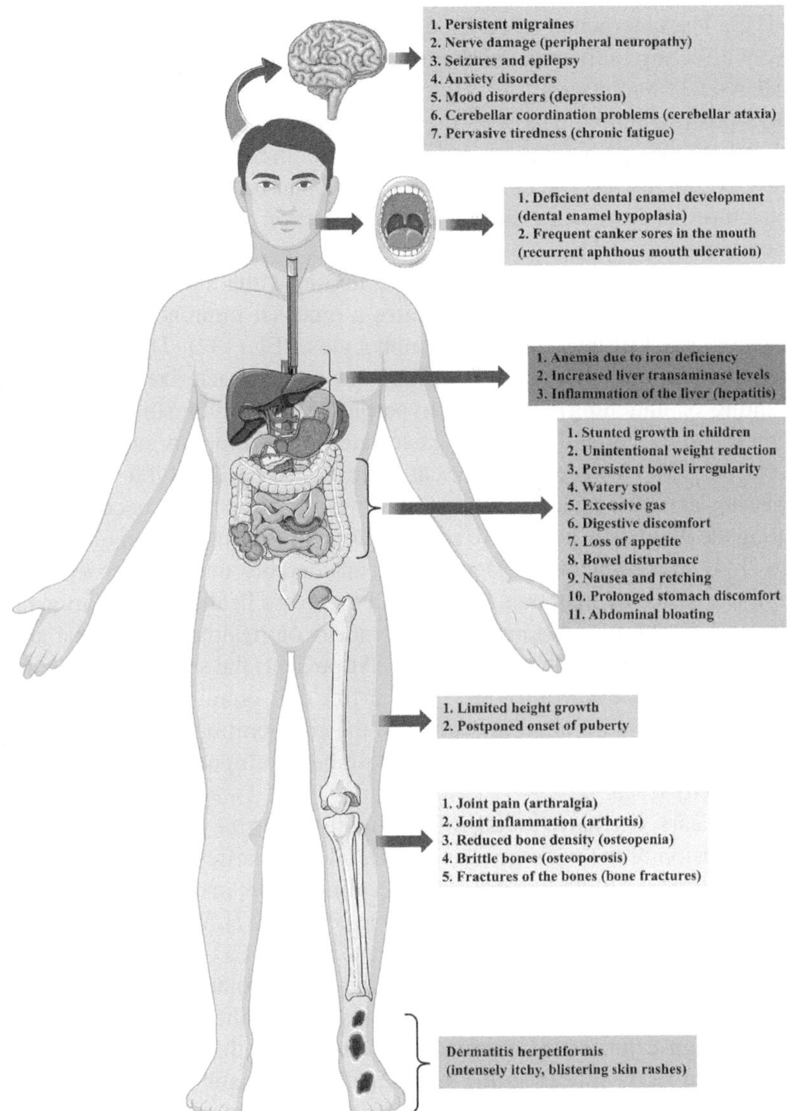

FIGURE 6.1 Diverse Manifestations of CD. CD, conventionally recognized for gastrointestinal symptoms, exhibits a spectrum of clinical presentations illustrated in this figure. Beyond digestive issues, manifestations encompass neurological complications such as migraines and peripheral neuropathy, mental health challenges including anxiety and depression, oral and dental abnormalities, hepatic conditions, diverse paediatric symptoms, musculoskeletal issues, and dermatological manifestations like dermatitis herpetiformis. This visual emphasizes the broad clinical spectrum of CD, underlining the necessity for a comprehensive understanding to facilitate accurate diagnosis and appropriate therapeutic strategies.

the Caucasian population is estimated to reside between 1 in 100 and 1 in 300 individuals [17]. The emergence of celiac disease hinges on genetic susceptibility, almost exclusively affecting individuals harbouring the human leukocyte antigen (HLA)-DQ2 and/or HLA-DQ8 haplotypes [29]. Remarkably, a mere fraction of HLA-DQ2 and/or HLA-DQ8-positive individuals who ingest gluten succumb to the ailment, suggesting the implication of supplementary genetic and environmental constituents in its inception [30]. The CD demonstrates an escalated prevalence among females, is liable to manifest at any juncture subsequent to dietary gluten induction, and is not constrained to any specific ethnic cohort [31].

The predominant target of CD is the mucosa of the small intestine. In susceptible individuals, gluten consumption incites a mucosal immune response typified by an augmented count of intraepithelial lymphocytes (IEL) [32]. This immune rejoinder eventuates in structural amendments in the intestine, characterized by villous atrophy (villi blunting or flattening) and crypt hyperplasia (crypt elongation). Celiac disease-linked enteropathy frequently exhibits gastrointestinal symptoms and manifestations of malabsorption [33]. However, the clinical indications of CD exhibit a broad spectrum, encompassing extraintestinal symptoms and even asymptomatic occurrences, thereby convoluting the diagnostic procedure and potentially resulting in postponed or neglected diagnoses [34]. Consequently, CD remains considerably underdiagnosed on a global scale. In the absence of treatment, it can lead to severe health complications, elevated morbidity and mortality, substantial encumbrances on healthcare systems, and a deterioration in the patient's quality of life [35]. At present, the sole efficacious remedy is unwavering compliance with a rigorous gluten-free diet, culminating in the recuperation of mucosal integrity in the small intestine and the amelioration of symptoms [36]. Early initiation of a gluten-free diet may also forestall the development of complications connected to celiac disease.

In recent years, extensive biochemical investigations have considerably augmented our comprehension of the pathogenesis of CD. Gluten, particularly the storage proteins known as gliadins and glutenins in wheat, secalins in rye, and hordeins in barley, have been identified as the instigating agents in toxic cereals [37]. While there remains ongoing contention concerning the toxicity of oat avenins, all CD toxic proteins share structural attributes, primarily domains rich in glutamine (Gln) and proline (Pro) sequences [38]. The high Pro content endows these proteins with resilience against full proteolytic degradation by gastrointestinal enzymes, culminating in the accumulation of substantial Pro- and Gln-rich peptides in the subepithelial lymphatic tissue of the small intestine. Depending on their amino acid sequences, these peptides can incite two distinct immune responses.

The swift innate response is distinguished by the secretion of interleukin-15 and a substantial augmentation in IELs. The slower adaptive response entails the binding of gluten peptides (either in their native state or partially deamidated by tissue transglutaminase) to HLA-DQ2 or HLA-DQ8 on APCs [39]. This interaction prompts T cells, resulting in the release of pro-inflammatory cytokines such as interferon-γ and the activation of matrix metalloproteinases. Both immune responses culminate in mucosal impairment and epithelial apoptosis. Moreover, activated T cells induce B cells to generate serum IgA and IgG antibodies targeting gluten proteins (the antigen) and tissue transglutaminase (the autoantigen). These antibodies can be harnessed in noninvasive screening assays for the diagnosis of CD.

The prevailing pillar of CD treatment revolves around unwavering adherence to a lifelong gluten-free diet. Dietetic gluten-free products for CD patients align with the Codex Alimentarius Standard for Gluten-Free Foods, prescribing a maximum gluten content of 20 mg/kg for naturally gluten-free products (e.g., those predicated on rice or corn flour) and 200 mg/kg for gluten-reduced products (e.g., wheat starch) [40]. A plethora of analytical techniques for gluten detection have been conceived, mainly grounded in immunochemical assays, mass spectrometry, or polymerase chain reaction. Solely two enzyme-linked immunosorbent assay (ELISA) have undergone rigorous cross-validation and are commercially accessible [41]. Recent years have witnessed the proposition of several methodologies for the prevention and management of CD. These approaches encompass the elimination of toxic epitopes through enzymatic degradation or genetic engineering, along with the modulation of the immune system [42]. Nonetheless, any alternative therapeutic modality must demonstrate a safety profile that competes with that of a gluten-free diet.

6.2.1.2 The Significance of Dietary Gluten as the Provocative Antigen

Gluten, a nomenclature closely affiliated with the chief storage proteins, denominated prolamins, which inhabit wheat, rye, and barley, stands as a pivotal concern for those afflicted with CD. Gluten assumes a pivotal role, not solely in the compositional integrity of these cereals, but also in the formation of dough, courtesy of its distinctive viscoelastic attributes [43]. Wheat gluten, to elucidate, represents a multifaceted amalgamation of alcohol-soluble gliadins (categorized into α-gliadins, γ-gliadins, and ω-gliadins) and alcohol-insoluble glutenins (comprising high-molecular-mass and low-molecular-mass glutenins) [44]. Gliadins and glutenins gain eminence owing to their abundance of proline and glutamine amino acids, rendering them recalcitrant to complete enzymatic cleavage by gastric, pancreatic, and small intestinal brush-border membrane enzymes [45]. Consequently, they instigate the generation of protracted gliadin peptides within the confines of the gastrointestinal tract, endowed with the potential to incite immune responses characteristic of CD. Within this milieu of peptides, the extensively scrutinized "33mer" holds prominence, characterized by six partially overlapping, putatively detrimental epitopes, frequently acclaimed as the preeminent coeliac immunogenic sequence within gluten [46].

In addition to kindling immune responses in CD, these indigested peptides operate as a reservoir of nourishment for the intestinal bacterial metabolism of gluten, thereby influencing the intestinal microbiota. Oats, notwithstanding their botanical proximity to *Triticeae* cereals (wheat, rye, and barley), bear conspicuously diminished prolamins, denominated avenin [17]. Furthermore, avenins exhibit a paucity of proline and glutamine residues when juxtaposed with prolamins, thereby conferring a diminished proclivity for adverse effects on individuals with CD, thereby explicating their benign nature for the majority of patients.

The development of CD requisites the dual presence of gluten consumption and genetic predisposition. Genetic susceptibility is underscored by an augmented average prevalence of CD among first-degree kin of patients, approximating 8%. Among the array of identified genetic elements, the HLA-DQ haplotypes, specifically HLA-DQ2 and HLA-DQ8, underpin the most substantial risk, contributing an estimated 25–40%

of the genetic liability [18]. Nevertheless, it is imperative to underscore that roughly 40% of the North American and European populations harbour these haplotypes, yet the majority remains unaffected by CD. Hence, while HLA-DQ2 or HLA-DQ8 serves as a prerequisite, it remains insufficient, independently, to instigate the manifestation of CD [30].

Gluten peptides originating from incomplete digestion within the gut lumen possess the capability to traverse the epithelial barricade, infiltrating the lamina propria, either through the transcellular or paracellular route. In individuals afflicted with CD, these peptides function as stimulants for both adaptive and innate immune responses.

6.2.1.3 The Origination of Gluten-Specific T Cell Responses

The adaptive immune rejoinder in CD is emblematic of distinct CD4+ T cell retorts to gluten, manifesting within the mucosa of the small intestine, in tandem with antibodies targeting wheat gliadin and transglutaminase 2 (TG2), a product encoded by *TGM2* [47]. In 1997, TG2 was ascertained as a pivotal autoantigen, culminating in improved comprehension of the ailment's pathogenesis and the formulation of diagnostic assays [48]. TG2 demonstrates the capacity to deamidate gluten peptides, substituting glutamine with glutamic acid, thus heightening their affinity for binding to HLA-DQ2 or HLA-DQ8 molecules on antigen-presenting cells (APCs). These HLA-bound gliadin peptides are subsequently presented to gluten-specific CD4+ T cells [49]. While dendritic cells were once postulated to be the primary APCs in CD, it is now posited that gliadin-specific and TG2-specific B cells might undertake analogous roles. Intriguingly, individuals with coeliac disease harbour distinctive gluten-specific T cells featuring distinctive gliadin epitope recognition modalities, potentially attributable to the stochastic genesis of T cell receptors (TCRs) [50]. This stochasticity implies that only a fraction of HLA-DQ2-positive or HLA-DQ8-positive individuals may generate high-affinity TCRs specific to gliadin, conceivably elucidating the discerning development of coeliac disease [51]. Once galvanized, gluten-specific CD4+ T cells emit cytokines such as IFNγ and IL-21, thereby engendering an inflammatory milieu in the small intestine, thereby contributing to mucosal damage.

6.2.1.4 Autoantibodies Generation

Gluten-specific CD4+ cells in CD not only contribute to the pro-inflammatory cytokine network within the small intestine but also incite characteristic antibody reactions. Following activation upon encountering HLA-bound gliadin on APCs, CD4+ cells deliver assistance signals to both gluten-specific and TG2-specific B cells, inciting their activation and differentiation into plasma cells [17]. These plasma cells generate antibodies against deamidated gliadin peptides (DGPs) and TG2, observable in the systemic circulation of CD patients. TG2 antibodies (TG2-Abs) also appear in the mucosa of the small intestine, accumulating around the subepithelial basement membrane and the mucosal vasculature.

While traditionally, it was surmised that both circulating and intestinally deposited TG2-Abs were locally produced within the small intestine by plasma cells, contemporary data posit that serum TG2-Abs emanate from plasma cells affiliated with intestinal

TG2-specific plasma cells but located extraintestinally [52]. Irrespective of their origin, both gliadin antibodies and TG2-Abs are conjectured to exert an impact on the pathogenesis of CD, as they are believed to augment the permeability of the epithelial barrier, thereby enabling gliadin peptides to access the lamina propria and exerting influence on epithelial cell biology [53]. Notably, autoimmune responses targeting other members of the transglutaminase family have been linked to distinct manifestations of CD. Antibodies targeting TG3 and TG6, identified in dermatitis herpetiformis and gluten ataxia, respectively, are deemed potential contributors to the pathogenesis of these extraintestinal expressions.

6.2.1.5 The Function of Cytokines in Modulating Intestinal Mucosal Immunity

In CD, particular cytokines produced by gluten-specific CD4+ T cells, such as IFNγ and IL-21, operate as intermediaries between the adaptive and innate immune reactions. The innate immunological facet of the malady is denoted by amplified mucosal expression of IL-15, IL-18, and type I interferons, posited to be engendered by distressed intestinal epithelial cells and/or dendritic cells [54]. Among these cytokines, IL-15 assumes a pivotal role in the ailment's development. IL-15 obstructs the regulatory functions of regulatory CD4+ T (Treg) cells, leading to a diminishment in oral tolerance and immune regulation. IL-15 also empowers IELs to assail and eliminate intestinal epithelial cells [55].

6.2.1.6 The Role of Oats in the Management of Celiac Disease

Individuals afflicted with CD manifest adverse reactions upon the ingestion of gluten, a protein ensconced in select cereal grains. The foremost gluten protein factions that bear paramount relevance to those enduring CD are the prolamins and glutenins. Predominantly, the alcohol-soluble prolamins derived from wheat (gliadins), rye (secalins), and barley (hordeins) pose the most noteworthy risk. It is noteworthy that oats also encompass a prolamin fraction denoted avenin, which structurally aligns with gliadins, secalins, and hordeins [56]. Nevertheless, oat avenins exhibit distinctive characteristics when juxtaposed with the prolamin factions found in wheat, rye, and barley. Primarily, oat avenins represent a minor proportion of the total oat protein composition, constituting a mere 10–15%, a divergence from the prolamin content in wheat, which may ascend to 40–50% [57]. Secondly, oat avenins present a diminished proportion of proline and glutamine when contrasted with prolamins originating from other cereal grains. While maize, sorghum, and rice prolamins customarily comprise 25–30% proline and glutamine, the prolamins in the Triticeae tribe (wheat, barley, and rye) may exceed 70% of these amino acids [58]. In contradistinction, proline and glutamine constitute 35–50% of the amino acids in oat prolamins. In addition, oat avenins harbour two abbreviated domains that are rich in proline and glutamine, distinct from the singular, extensive repetitive domain discerned in Triticeae prolamins. Moreover, the disulphide linkage pattern in oat prolamins diverges from that found in wheat γ-gliadins and low-molecular-weight (LMW) glutenins. Oat prolamins partake in disulphide bonding between contiguous cysteines at positions 145–146, in contradistinction to wheat proteins, wherein these proximate cysteines form connections with more distant cysteines within the prolamin structure.

However, despite these recorded disparities, avenins have remained underinvestigated, with existing genetic databases offering descriptions of merely a few genotypes, thus not affording a comprehensive representation of the variability inherent in oat avenin genes. At present, the singular therapeutic recourse for CD remains a lifelong gluten-free diet (GFD) [59]. Individuals grappling with CD must meticulously scrutinize food product labels to discern gluten-containing constituents, thereby averting undesirable health repercussions. Accurate food labelling assumes a critical role in ensuring the absence of concealed sources of gluten within packaged foodstuffs designated as "gluten-free." Nevertheless, adhering to a GFD is arduous and can potentially engender nutritional deficiencies in essential vitamins, calcium, iron, and dietary fibre [60]. Oats, replete with valuable nutrients and fibre, proffer a viable nutritional option and can be seamlessly integrated into the dietary regimen. However, the inclusion of oats within the GFD of individuals affected by CD, encompassing both adults and children, has remained a topic of dispute, principally in light of historical concerns regarding potential cross-contamination during oat cultivation and processing, involving gluten sources such as barley and wheat.

In a study new gluten isolation technique yielding celiac-safe avenin from wheat-free oats was used [61]. The novel gluten isolation method enabled the extraction of 2 kg of avenin from 400 kg of wheat-free oats under strict gluten-free and food-grade conditions. The resulting avenin extract contained 85% protein, with 96% of it being avenin. Starch, β-glucan, and free sugars were present at low levels. Comprehensive analyses confirmed the absence of gluten-containing cereals. This high-quality avenin preparation is suitable for definitive studies on oat consumption safety for individuals with celiac disease. In another study, the isolation and sequencing of genes that could potentially pose issues, specifically avenins, globulins, and α-amylase/trypsin inhibitors, within six distinct oat cultivars were assessed [62]. The study harnessed PacBio sequencing technology to assess genetic diversity and subsequently contrasted these results with the preexisting gene sequences accessible in genetic repositories. In totality, the research successfully pinpointed and mapped 21 avenin genes, 75 globulin genes, and 25 α-amylase/trypsin inhibitor genes on the chromosomes of hexaploid oats. Within each gene family, slight variations in the gene sequences were discerned among oat varieties. It is noteworthy that avenin epitopes were discerned across all four categories of avenin genes within all the scrutinized oat varieties. Nonetheless, it is worth highlighting that the number of avenin genes was substantially lower when juxtaposed with globulin genes, comprising a mere 10% of the cumulative storage proteins at the protein level.

A concurrent investigation was undertaken to delve into the variance observed in the composition of oat proteins, with specific regard to their influence on health-related and techno-functional attributes [63]. This comprehensive study encompassed a diverse assemblage of oat samples, comprising 162 cultivated varieties hailing from 20 distinct nations. The central objective of this inquiry resided in characterizing the protein compositions within these diverse samples. To evaluate the size distribution of total protein extracts, we employed size exclusion-high-performance liquid chromatography (SE-HPLC), while the proteins extracted with 70% ethanol underwent rigorous analysis via reversed-phase high-performance liquid chromatography (RP-HPLC). The SE-HPLC column adeptly segregated protein extracts into three predominant categories: polymeric proteins, avenins (each categorized into three subgroups based on their size), and soluble proteins, collectively constituting 68.79% to 86.60%, 8.86% to 27.72%, and 2.89% to 11.85% of the total protein content, respectively. The ratio of polymeric to monomeric proteins exhibited a range of variability from 1.37 to 3.73. Significantly, a total of 76 distinct peaks were discerned through RP-HPLC analysis, effectively discriminating the ethanol-extractable proteins within the entire sample population. These peaks demonstrated divergent distributions across the spectrum of oat cultivars, with the number of peaks per cultivar ranging from 6 to 23. Furthermore, the frequency of appearance of these peaks exhibited notable disparities, with one peak identified in 107 samples and 15 peaks appearing in fewer than five cultivars. To estimate the avenin-epitope content of the samples, we devised a method that harnessed mass spectrometric data obtained from the RP-HPLC peaks, in conjunction with advanced bioinformatics techniques. Additionally, through the implementation of ELISA methodology employing the R5 antibody, a significant proportion of the analysed samples revealed the presence of trace levels of wheat, barley, or rye contamination.

Both long-term cohort studies and short-term intervention studies have consistently demonstrated that individuals with CD can safely include uncontaminated oats or specially produced oat products in their diets, provided that these products adhere to the internationally recognized gluten contamination threshold of 20 ppm. This is because oats lack the epitopes found in wheat, barley, and rye, rendering them non-reactive for the majority of celiac patients. Although a small subset of patients may exhibit immune responses to specific avenin

6.2.2 Oats and Hypertension

Hypertension, characterized by high blood pressure, is now widespread in all Western societies and ranks among the top causes of cardiovascular-related deaths in both men and women. It is important to note that hypertension is a risk factor for diabetes, and conversely, diabetes can also exacerbate hypertension. These conditions often coexist and can mutually influence each other, making their management and control vital for overall cardiovascular health [64].

The inclusion of oats in one's diet can contribute to a reduction in hypertension, primarily because of the presence of soluble fibres, specifically $(1\rightarrow3)$ $(1\rightarrow4)$-β-D-glucans, which play a role in promoting a sense of satiety. Clinical trials involving foods containing oat β-glucan have demonstrated a decrease in blood pressure, particularly in individuals with high blood pressure or stage-1 hypertension. Research conducted by Keenan et al. [65] found that incorporating oats into the regular diet of individuals with hypertension led to significant reductions in both systolic and diastolic blood pressure. The study suggested that oat cereals rich in soluble fibre could impact blood pressure by modulating changes in insulin metabolism. This mechanism is believed to involve the slow absorption of macronutrients from the gastrointestinal tract, resulting in a flattening of the post-meal glycaemic curve.

In a study conducted by Pins et al. [66], the consumption of whole-grain oat cereals containing β-glucan was found to have a positive impact on blood pressure. When whole oats were added to the daily diet, there was a significant reduction in the need for antihypertensive medication, and blood pressure control notably improved over the course of the twelve-week intervention. Furthermore, the inclusion of whole oats in the diet led to improvements in blood lipid profiles and fasting glucose levels. Additionally, it resulted in a reduction in the incidence of side effects related to the study. These findings suggest that increasing the consumption of whole oats in the diet can have a substantial positive effect in reducing the risk of cardiovascular disease among individuals with hypertension.

A study involving patients with high blood pressure who followed a diet containing oat β-glucan for a three-month period revealed that only individuals with high body mass indices (BMI) experienced a reduction in their blood pressure as a result of this dietary intervention. The authors of the study concluded that oat β-glucan may be effective in treating hypertensive individuals who are also obese, given that it had a positive impact on this specific subgroup [67]. Another study conducted by Saltzman et al. [68] investigated the effects of a six-month trial involving a hypocaloric diet with and without oat supplementation in healthy subjects. Their findings showed that the diet supplemented with oats led to greater improvements in blood pressure control and lipid profiles when compared to the non-oat diet. This suggests that incorporating oats into the diet can have favourable effects on blood pressure and overall cardiovascular health, especially when included as part of a balanced diet plan.

In a review conducted by Evans et al. [69], the effects of consuming fibre isolate or fibre-rich diets on the blood pressure of healthy individuals were examined. This meta-analysis encompassed studies with randomized, controlled trials lasting at least 6 weeks. Upon analysing specific fibre types, the authors found that the consumption of fibre with high concentrations of β-glucan, such as those found in barley and oats, had the potential to reduce both systolic and diastolic blood pressure. In contrast, other types of fibre did not demonstrate significant positive effects on the blood pressure of the individuals studied, even when consumed in substantial quantities. The review suggested that a diet rich in β-glucan, especially from sources like barley and oats, is recommended, particularly for individuals with a high risk of cardiovascular conditions. Such a dietary approach may be beneficial in managing and improving blood pressure levels in these individuals.

6.2.3 Immunomodulation

The immunomodulatory activity of oat β-glucans is triggered by intracellular pathways initiated after β-glucan binds to specific receptors on the surface of immune cells [70]. These receptors include pattern recognition receptors (PRRs) such as toll-like receptors (TLRs), C-lectin receptor (CLR) 1, and dectin-1 found on various types of immune cells. The specificity of recognition and the subsequent signalling pathways activated depend on the specific carbohydrate structures and morphology exposed by the microorganism. For example, β-glucan that is initially exposed can become masked by mannan during the formation of hyphae. Interestingly, dectin-1 signalling is activated only by particulate β-glucan, despite its ability to bind both soluble and particulate β-glucan polymers. This means that insoluble whole glucan particles, as opposed to soluble glucans, are effective in eliciting dectin-1 signalling. The recognition of β-glucan also varies depending on the specific type of immune cell and the microenvironment, which can be influenced by external factors such as the fungal species encountered, the pathogens present, and the host's response. Dectin-1, unlike other PRRs, plays a crucial role in the innate immune response by distinguishing between direct binding to microbes and binding to substances released by microorganisms [71]. Notably, the literature suggests that the molecular weight (MW) of β-glucan is related to its immunomodulatory activity. Specifically, purified β-1.3 glucan backbones with a high degree of β-1.6 branching and higher MW are more likely to exert immunomodulatory properties.

In addition to their recognition, orally administered β-glucans are engulfed and processed by macrophages and dendritic cells. These immune cells then migrate to various immune organs and release fragmented soluble β-glucan particles, as indicated in a study by Marco Castro et al. [70]. This process primes leukocytes, primarily through the action of receptors like Dectin-1 and other cooperating receptors. This priming enhances immunosurveillance and equips the host's immune system to better combat pathogen attacks. The enhanced activation of the complement system and the improved functions of innate immune cells result in heightened antimicrobial and inflammatory responses. Many studies have investigated the potential of β-glucans as modifiers of the immune response, aiming to bolster host resistance to pathogens. This approach offers a non-specific form of protection and has the potential to be used for preventing and treating infections. It is particularly valuable in enhancing immune resistance in immunocompromised populations, including both the very young and the elderly.

AVAs represent a group of phenolic alkaloid compounds synthesized within oat plants, characterized by their origin as derivatives or conjugates of hydroxyanthranilic acid (hydroxylated 2-amino-benzoic acids) and hydroxycinnamic acids. Oat bran and flakes contain the highest concentration of AVAs, and they are typically found in all milling fractions, rendering them a ubiquitous component of commercial oat products [72]. Notably, AVAs exhibit a remarkable approximate 30-fold higher antioxidant activity in comparison to other phenolic compounds. AVAs in oats are categorized into different types primarily based on their association with N-cinnamoyl anthranilic acid: Avn A combined with p-coumaric acid, Avn B combined with ferulic acid, and Avn C combined with caffeic acid. The structural similarity between Avn and tranilast, a commercially available anti-allergic drug, has spurred extensive research into the anti-inflammatory and anti-atherogenic properties of Avn. Importantly, Avn is known to impede the release of inflammatory substances by macrophages, diminish the adhesion of monocytes to vascular endothelial cells, and exhibit anticancer effects through antiproliferative and pro-apoptotic activities.

In the context of skeletal muscle C2C12 cells, AVAs play a pivotal role in mediating anti-inflammatory activities. These unique polyphenolic molecules primarily exert their anti-inflammatory effects by deactivating nuclear factor-kappaB (NF-κB) within C2C12 cells. AVAs have been found to reduce the expression of IκB kinase beta (IKKβ), an inhibitor of the NF-κB kinase subunit beta, in response to tert-butyl hydroperoxide (tBHP)-induced oxidative stress. Furthermore, they decrease the transcriptional expression of inflammatory cytokines such as tumour necrosis factor-alpha (TNFα) and interleukin 1β (IL-1β) under similar conditions. Additionally, AVAs lead to a reduction in the levels of cyclooxygenase-2 (COX-2) protein and subsequently prostaglandin E2 (PGE2). The inhibition of the COX2/PGE2 pathway results in the suppression of various cellular processes, encompassing cell proliferation, migration, apoptosis, angiogenesis, and carcinogenesis across diverse cell lines. In summary, AVAs exhibit significant potential as inhibitors of the NF-κB-mediated inflammatory response through the down-regulation of IKKβ activity in C2C12 cells [73], [74].

Research by Arena et al. [75] observed that when oats and barley β-glucans were used to incubate human lipopolysaccharide (LPS)-stimulated THP-1 macrophages, the expression of pro-inflammatory cytokines like IL-6, IL-8, and IL-1b was reduced. This suggests that β-glucans from cereals possess immunomodulatory properties that can mitigate the pro-inflammatory response. Similarly, Chaiyasut et al. [76] conducted an in vivo study comparing the immunomodulatory activity of β-glucans from three different sources: yeast, mushrooms, and oats. They found that yeast β-glucans were more effective at stimulating the expression of IL-6, IL-17, IFN-γ, IL-10, and TGF-β compared to oat and mushroom β-glucans. This study indicated that yeast β-glucan is a potent immune activator and enhances the host's antioxidant capacity to a greater extent than oat and mushroom β-glucans. Importantly, the type of immune modulation observed varied depending on the specific strain and source of β-glucan.

Collectively, the findings suggest a connection between the structure and immunomodulatory activity of β-glucans from various sources. This aspect should be taken into account when formulating products containing β-glucans. To gain a deeper understanding of the mechanisms behind β-glucans' "immunomodulation," it is imperative to conduct well-designed human intervention trials. These trials should assess immunity endpoints that provide insights into the processes through which β-glucans exert their effects on immune function. Such research can contribute to the development of more targeted and effective immune-boosting products.

6.2.4 Gut Microbiota Regulation

The physicochemical properties of β-glucan can have an impact on the composition of the gut microbiota, as suggested by Dong et al. [77]. Additionally, research demonstrated that oat β-glucan can serve as a substrate for fermentation by the human gut microbiota, leading to the production of beneficial metabolites, including short-chain fatty acids (SCFA), and the modulation of beneficial microbes in the intestines. Furthermore, β (1→3)/β(1→4)-glucan can undergo degradation by the resident microbiota in the human gut, which can result in changes to the composition of the gut microbiota, as highlighted by Tamura et al. [78]. They elucidated the complex molecular mechanism of β-glucan metabolization by *Bacteroides ovatus* and found that a significant portion of the human population analysed possessed *Bacteroidetes* capable of utilizing β-glucan. This suggests that β-glucan can influence the gut microbiota composition through microbial metabolism in the digestive system.

A recent research investigation compared the impacts of two different processing methods, namely steaming and microwave processing, on the physical and chemical characteristics of oat β-glucan and its prebiotic effects. The findings revealed that microwave-processed oat β-glucan, which had a lower average MW, had a more pronounced influence in promoting the growth of *Lactobacillus* and *Bifidobacterium* when compared to steaming-processed oat β-glucan with a higher MW. The researchers suggest that microwave processing contributed to the breakdown and fermentation of oat β-glucan, leading to the increased production of SCFA, such as butyrate. Additionally, higher levels of Blautia and Dialister, known as butyrate producers, were observed [79]. Consequently, this study has shed light on the prebiotic role of β-glucans. Furthermore, as a component of dietary fibre, β-glucans serve as a vital energy source that stimulates the growth, activity, and survival of beneficial bacterial strains like *Lactobacillus* and *Bifidobacterium*, while inhibiting the proliferation of harmful bacteria like *E. coli* and *Clostridium celatum* [80]. Despite the need for the expression of glucanase enzymes for the fermentation of β-glucan by gut microbiota bacterial strains, cell-surface glycan-binding proteins play a pivotal role in recognizing β-glucan and facilitating its transport to the gut microbiota. This evidence helps elucidate the prebiotic activity of β-glucans [81]. Indeed, further research will be required to fully understand the prebiotic activity of β-glucans. Studies designed to unravel the molecular pathways through which microbiota microorganisms utilize β-glucan are indispensable for developing novel therapeutic interventions and targeted prebiotic-based therapies.

6.2.5 Antitumor/Anticancer Effect

The immunogenic properties of β-glucans have been linked to their structural characteristics, water solubility, elevated viscosity, composition, and substantial MW. For a considerable time now, β-glucans have been a subject of interest as a potential tool in the fight against tumours. Their antitumor activity operates through a unique mechanism that involves neutrophils, a predominant type of white blood cell in humans crucial for the innate immune system's function [82]. What sets this approach apart is the priming of these neutrophils with a substance called betafectin, a process not typically associated with defending against cancer. Recent research has introduced the concept that when orally administered, β-glucan can augment the immune response, especially when used in conjunction with externally administered antitumor antibodies that activate specific components. This combined approach has shown promise in combatting a broad spectrum of cancers, particularly when paired with monoclonal antibodies designed to either activate certain responses or promote complement binding to the tumour. The complement system facilitates the attachment of these primed neutrophils to the tumour, ultimately leading to its destruction. Ordinarily, neutrophils do not actively engage in attacking cancerous tissue because they recognize cancer as "self" rather than foreign or "nonself." Current cancer immunotherapies primarily involve monoclonal antibodies and vaccines, which stimulate the adaptive immune response but do not alter the innate immune system's perception of cancer as "self." Consequently, monoclonal antibodies alone do not fully harness the innate immune system's potential to eliminate cancer cells, as this system is primarily designed to defend against bacterial and fungal infections. International research has effectively demonstrated that orally administered yeast β-1,3-d glucan provides similar protective effects as its injectable counterpart, offering protection against both infectious diseases and cancer. Furthermore, recent findings indicate that orally delivered β-glucan significantly enhances the proliferation and activation of monocytes in the peripheral blood of patients with advanced breast cancer.

AVAs are distinguished for their potent antiproliferative and pro-apoptotic activities. Upon administration of AVAs, they instigate the activation of crucial regulatory proteins, including p53, p27kip1, and p21cip1. These activated proteins collaboratively function to repress the expression of components related to the cell cycle, such as cyclin E and cyclin-dependent kinase 2 (CDK2), as well as cyclin A and CDK2. This concerted action leads to a halt in the cell cycle progression, specifically at the G1 to S phase transition. Additionally, AVAs downregulate the expression of cyclin D1 and its associated CDK4 and CDK6 while promoting the phosphorylation of the Rb protein (pRb), a tumour suppressor. Consequently, AVAs bring about cell cycle arrest at the M phase [74], [83]. These findings underscore the pivotal role of AVAs in positively regulating the cell cycle while inhibiting tumour progression.

In terms of their pro-apoptotic activity, AVAs have been demonstrated to upregulate the expression of caspase 3 (CASP3) and caspase 8 (CASP8), pivotal components in the apoptotic pathway. Concurrently, they downregulate the expression of insulin-like growth factor 2 mRNA-binding protein 3 (IGF2BP3), hypoxia-inducible factor 1-alpha (HIF1α), vascular endothelial growth factor (VEGF), cyclooxygenase 2 (COX2), and prostaglandin E2 (PGE2) in tumour cell lines. This multifaceted impact strengthens their anticancer effects by bolstering antioxidative capacity, restraining cell proliferation, promoting programmed cell death (apoptosis), instigating cellular senescence, and hindering extracellular matrix degradation, metastasis, and the epithelial mesenchymal transition [8]. The collective action of AVAs presents promising avenues for both cancer therapy and prevention.

In a comparative study assessing the antioxidant effects and the inhibition of cancer cell proliferation in oat extract using various extraction solvents, the antioxidant activity of the extract was evaluated by quantifying its capacity to neutralize 2,2′-azinobis 3-ethylbenzothiazoline-6-sulphonic acid (ABTS) and 1,1-diphenyl-1-picrylhydrazyl (DPPH) radicals, as well as its reducing power [84]. Additionally, the study investigated its impact on the proliferation of cancer cells, focusing on colorectal, lung, and breast cancer cell lines. The outcomes revealed that methanol extracts exhibited the highest values for total polyphenol content, along with superior scavenging abilities against ABTS and DPPH radicals, as well as robust reducing power. Furthermore, methanol extracts demonstrated the most substantial inhibitory effects on the proliferation of colorectal cancer (HCT116), lung cancer (NCI-H460), and breast cancer (MCF7) cells. While variations were observed in the antioxidant effects and the inhibition of cancer cell proliferation depending on the choice of extraction solvent, the findings strongly underscore the antioxidant and anticancer properties of oats. Significantly, it is noteworthy that, as of the present, no studies have reported any adverse effects associated with AVA supplementation, further emphasizing its safety and potential health benefits.

The study was conducted to investigate the antitumor properties of newly developed high and low-molecular-weight oat β-glucans [85]. These were tested using two human epithelial lung cancer (HELC) lines (A549 and H69AR) as well as normal keratinocytes (HaCaT). The impact of these high and low MW β-glucans from oats was assessed through various parameters, including cellular viability assessment, evaluation of lipid peroxidation, measurement of manganese superoxide dismutase activity, visualization of cytoskeletal structures, and examination of red blood cell haemolysis. The findings suggested that oat β-glucans developed β-glucans from oats possess potent antitumor properties, while simultaneously demonstrating no toxicity towards normal cells.

Yeast-derived β-glucan has demonstrated tumour-inhibiting effects without harming normal mouse cells [86]. (1→3,1→6)-β-d-Glucans, produced by *Diaporthe* sp. endophytes, exhibit antiproliferative properties against human breast carcinoma (MCF-7) and hepatocellular carcinoma (HepG2-C3A) cells [87]. Lentinan, a representative β-(1→3,1→6)-glucan found in *Lentinus edodes*, can induce apoptosis in S180 cells through mitochondrial pathways. A novel low-molecular-weight β-glucan from oats demonstrates strong anti-tumour attributes, possibly due to its ability to significantly increase caspase-12 expression in Me45 and A431 cancer cell lines [88]. Pro-apoptotic characteristics have been reported for (1→3) (1→4)-β-d-glucan from oats against human melanoma HTB-140 cells in vitro. Oat β-d-glucan induces apoptosis in a concentration-dependent manner, leading to increased caspase-3/7 activation and the externalization of phosphatidylserine on cellular membranes, where it binds to annexin V-FITC, indicating apoptosis induction. Intracellular ATP levels decrease alongside diminishing mitochondrial potential, suggesting a mitochondrial pathway for apoptosis. Cell cycle analysis reveals an increase in apoptotic cells and cells in the G1 phase, as well as a decrease in cells in the G2/M phase. The antiproliferative effect of β-glucan is believed to involve the repression of genes associated with the G1 phase of the cell cycle and potential interactions with the CCR5 receptor.

Similarly, the growth-inhibitory effect of polysaccharide Oat β-glucan was observed on human skin melanoma HTB-140 cells in vitro. The Oat β-glucan exhibited a cytotoxic effect on HTB-140 cells. After 24 hours of incubation, we determined the LD50 (the concentration at which 50% of the cells were found to be deceased) to be 194.6 ± 9.8 µg/mL. Oat β-glucan induced apoptosis in a concentration-dependent manner, as evidenced by an increase in caspase-3/-7 activation and the presence of phosphatidylserine on the external surface of cellular membranes, where it bound to annexin V-FITC. These findings suggested that oat β-glucan triggers apoptosis. Furthermore, there was a decrease in intracellular ATP levels and mitochondrial potential, indicating the involvement of a mitochondrial pathway in apoptosis. Cell cycle analysis revealed an increase in apoptotic cells, a rise in the number of cells in the G1 phase, and a decrease in the number of cells in the G2/M phase. These results collectively suggested that oat β-glucan (OBG) exerts its anti-tumour effect through the induction of apoptosis in HTB-140 cells.

The potential for (1→3) (1→6)-β-d-glucan from *Saccharomyces cerevisiae* to combat tumours likely stems from its capacity to boost the immune system and trigger apoptosis, or programmed cell death. β-Glucan has been observed to hinder the activity of legumain, a process involving the internalization of legumain into macrophages through the dectin-1 receptor. When tested in RAW 264.7 macrophages, particulate β-glucans proved more effective at inducing TNF-α compared to partially water-soluble and water-soluble variants. Furthermore, β-Glucan derived from Baker's yeast (BBG) engaged with CR3 and TLR2 receptors on the surface of macrophage-like RAW264.7 cells, leading to their activation and significant production of TNF-α and monocyte chemoattractant protein 1 (MCP-1). Notably, BBG also spurred the activation of nuclear factor kappa B p65 (NF-κB p65), c-Jun N-terminal kinase, and extracellular signal-regulated kinase in RAW264.7 cells, confirming its stimulating impact on these cells. Imprime Poly-(1,6)-beta-Glucopyranosyl-(1,3)-beta-Glucopyranose (PGG), a soluble yeast β-(1→3) (1→6)-glucan, has been effectively administered intravenously. It possesses a unique β-glucan PAMP (pathogen-associated molecular pattern) that binds to and activates innate immune effector cells, triggering a series of immune activation events that coordinate an immune response against cancer. In preclinical studies, Imprime PGG enhances the effectiveness of treatments targeting tumours, angiogenesis inhibition, and immune checkpoint inhibitors.

Though the precise mechanisms behind the antiproliferative effects of β-glucans are not fully elucidated, it appears that having a (1→3)-β-glucopyranose main chain, with substitutions at O-6 positions by β-glucopyranose, is vital for their inhibitory activity. This branched structure may facilitate more effective interactions with cell receptors in tumour cells, ultimately playing a significant role in triggering cell death.

6.2.6 Regulation of Postprandial Blood Glucose and Insulin Levels for Diabetes

Diabetes is a persistent medical condition marked by elevated blood glucose levels, posing a significant risk to one's overall health. It serves as a key contributing factor to several cardiovascular diseases, including atherosclerosis, hypertension, peripheral vascular disease, coronary artery disease, and cardiomyopathy. Globally, the occurrence of diabetes among adults stands at approximately 8.5% [89]. Regardless of the type of diabetes mellitus (be it type 1, type 2, or even the pre-diabetic condition that precedes type 2, which is glucose intolerance), several interventions can be employed for patient treatment. These interventions encompass maintaining a suitable diet, implementing an appropriate regimen of physical exercise, and, when deemed necessary, administering relevant medications like metformin. Effective management of diabetes is crucial to reduce or prevent the onset of other health conditions, notably those associated with cardiovascular diseases.

The primary focus in managing diabetes centres on the regulation of hyperglycaemia, a condition associated with the insufficient secretion of insulin by the pancreatic β cells within the endocrine system, and/or the presence of insulin resistance. When peripheral tissues like the liver, adipose tissue, and muscle exhibit incomplete responsiveness to insulin signals, this can lead to a heightened risk of cardiovascular complications, contributing to increased morbidity rates among individuals with diabetes. Hyperglycemia also leads to the generation of reactive oxygen species and reactive nitrogen species, which can significantly determine both the diabetic condition itself and the development of cardiovascular-related diseases [90].

Natural products, including cereals and mushrooms, and their extracted polysaccharides like β-glucans, have anti-glycaemic properties. They offer a drug-free option for managing diabetes and reducing the risk of developing it, without the common side effects of pharmaceutical drugs. These natural products can effectively lower blood glucose levels through dietary adjustments, providing valuable support for individuals with diabetes and reducing the risk of coronary heart disease. Dyslipidemia, characterized by lipid metabolism disturbances, is common in diabetics and can increase the risk of heart disease. Lowering cholesterol levels can positively impact cardiovascular health and prevent atherosclerosis. Additionally, impaired fatty acid oxidation contributes to insulin resistance and the development of type 2 diabetes.

Cereal β-glucans have garnered significant attention due to their ability to regulate postprandial blood glucose and insulin levels, which is beneficial for preventing diabetes. Research has demonstrated that even low levels of oat β-glucan can substantially reduce both blood sugar and insulin levels, the treatment effects of β-glucan on diabetes can vary depending on the dose and physicochemical characteristics of the β-glucan used [91]. As the MW of β-glucan increases, it tends to have a more pronounced effect in reducing oxidative stress and hyperlipidemia in diabetic mice. β-Glucan with higher viscosity also can suppress the expression of intestinal glucose transporters, specifically glucose transporter 2 and transport protein 1 in epithelial cells (IEC-6), thereby regulating the activity of these key transporters [92], [93]. A meta-analysis of randomized controlled trials has also shown that β-glucan from barley has a positive impact on postprandial blood sugar levels in the healthy human population [94]. While one study has suggested a connection between the reduction in plasma glucose and the dose of cereal β-glucans, substantial evidence indicates that the viscosity of β-glucans is the primary factor responsible for lowering postprandial blood sugar, insulin, and LDL-cholesterol levels [95]. Another potential mechanism for cereal β-glucans in regulating postprandial blood glucose and insulin levels is their interaction with intestinal mucus [96]. However, data on blood glucose response suggests that the primary role of these mechanisms in reducing postprandial blood sugar response by β-glucan is related to coil overlap [97].

One of the mechanisms underlying the beneficial effects of β-glucans is their capacity to create a viscous solution, which slows down the rate of gastric emptying and extends the time it takes for food to move through the intestines. This, in turn, reduces the digestion and absorption of glucose. When the viscosity of the solution is high, the uptake of glucose into the bloodstream is diminished. This effect is supported by research by [98]. The presence of high digesta viscosity hinders the diffusion of enzymes and promotes the formation of an unstirred water layer, which, in turn, reduces the transport of glucose to enterocytes. Consequently, there is a net decrease in the rate of glucose absorption into the bloodstream, leading to lower post-meal insulin concentrations, as reported by [99]. Clinical studies have also revealed a delay in gastric emptying following the consumption of β-glucans. For example, in overweight individuals who consumed 5 g of oat β-glucan, the amount of exogenous glucose detected in the bloodstream over 120 minutes was found to be 18% lower compared to a control group, as indicated by [100].

Another descriptive mechanism explaining the protective effects of dietary fibre on glucose and insulin regulation involves the production of SCFA as a result of anaerobic fermentation of soluble fibres, such as β-glucan, in the colon. These SCFAs may play a role in mediating the effects on post-meal glucose levels in subsequent meals. Specifically, SCFA-like butyric acid, propionic acid, and acetic acid have been shown to increase the expression of insulin-sensitive glucose transporter type 4 (GLUT-4) by activating peroxisome proliferator receptor-γ (PPAR-γ). GLUT-4 is responsible for facilitating the transport of glucose into adipose tissue, consequently lowering plasma blood glucose levels. Additionally, research has indicated that oat β-glucan can increase the concentrations of sodium-glucose transporter-1 (SGLT-1) and glucose transporter-2 (GLUT-2). GLUT-2 plays a significant role in regulating blood glucose levels. It transports glucose absorbed after a meal into the portal circulation, facilitating its transport to the pancreas and liver. On the other hand, SGLT-1 is primarily found in the small intestine and the distal part of the proximal tubule in the kidneys. Its main function is the reabsorption of glucose, further influencing blood glucose levels. Another potential mechanism by which β-glucans can reduce blood glucose levels is by activating the PI3K/Akt signalling pathway. Decreased PI3K/Akt activity has been linked to the pathogenesis of diabetes. Studies have shown that the administration of β-glucans can increase PI3K/Akt activity, which tends to decrease in diabetes, through several receptors. These receptors stimulated by β-glucans include dectin-1, CR3 (complement receptor 3), lactocylceramide, scavenger receptors, and toll-like receptors. These receptors are particularly crucial for recognizing β-glucan polymers that have branching $(1{\rightarrow}6)$ on a $(1{\rightarrow}3)$ chain. The activation of the PI3K/Akt pathway through these receptors can contribute to improved glucose metabolism and regulation, potentially assisting in the management of diabetes [101].

Battilana et al. [102] conducted a study to investigate the mechanism of action of β-glucans. The oat β-glucans used displayed high viscosity (96 mPa s or 96 cP) and high MW (2.275×10^6 Da). The study involved ten healthy adult men who were placed on a diet, with or without the addition of β-glucans (8.9 g/day), for three days. On the third day, the diet was administered as fractionated meals consumed every hour over 9 hours. This approach allowed the researchers to examine the effects on metabolism that were unrelated to delayed carbohydrate absorption, such as potential fermentation effects. The findings of the study indicated that glucose metabolism, including glucose and insulin concentrations, remained similar for both the diet with and without added β-glucans. The primary effect of the β-glucans appeared to be in delaying the intestinal absorption of carbohydrates.

The consumption of oat β-glucan during breakfast for four weeks among adult males with type 2 diabetes had a notable impact. It not only led to a reduction in cholesterol levels but also resulted in lower spikes in post-meal glucose levels. However, this treatment did not have any significant influence on fasting plasma glucose, insulin levels, or HbA1c (glycated haemoglobin, a measure of average plasma glucose levels over three months) [103]. The four-week intervention period was too brief to observe changes in glucose metabolism during fasting. In contrast, a longer 12-week pilot study involving bread containing oat bran concentrate showed improvements in post-meal glucose metabolism in individuals with type 2 diabetes. In a study conducted by Würsch et al. [104], it was found that incorporating 10% β-glucan into a cereal-based food resulted in a substantial 50% reduction in post-meal glucose spikes.

Gut hormones play a crucial role in controlling appetite and satiety, and they are closely linked to the improvement of insulin levels by β-glucan. Clinical trials have shown that β-glucan supplementation for 12 weeks can effectively increase the levels of peptide YY (PYY) while decreasing glucagon-like peptide-1 (GLP-1) in individuals with type 2 diabetes (T2D) [105]. Another mechanism through which β-glucan improves insulin homeostasis is by promoting the production of SCFAs through the fermentation of β-glucan. Studies have demonstrated that β-glucan treatment can elevate the level of butyrate in faeces, increase the expression of PPAR-γ in the ileum, and activate PPAR-γ signalling. PPAR-γ, in turn, enhances insulin sensitivity by regulating specific insulin signalling molecules [106]. The composition of gut microbiota is closely linked to diabetes, and β-glucan administration has been observed to influence this composition. It can increase the abundance of beneficial bacteria like *Lachnobacterium*, *Bacteroides*, and *Akkermansia* which can improve intestinal barrier integrity and produce SCFAs that protect against metabolic syndrome. Additionally, β-glucan has been found to increase the relative abundance of *Akkermansia*, leading to improvements in the microenvironment of visceral adipose tissues (VATs) by reducing fibrosis and angiogenesis. These findings suggest that polysaccharide treatments, like β-glucan, can alleviate type-2 diabetes by regulating the gut microbiota [107].

Studies conducted by Wood et al. [108] and Wood et al. [109] proposed that the decrease in glucose and insulin responses after a meal could be primarily attributed to the viscous nature of oats. They examined mixtures of oat β-glucans with varying viscosities and found a strong and significant linear relationship between viscosity and the responses of glucose and insulin. Their explanation suggested that the high viscosity of β-glucans caused a delay in the absorption of carbohydrates, contributing to these effects. The findings of Liu et al. [110] supported the observations of Wood and colleagues, confirming that the hypoglycaemic effects of oat β-glucans were indeed linked to their high viscosity. They reported that oat β-glucan increased insulin secretion, reduced insulin resistance, and improved hepatic glycometabolism. Interestingly, oat β-glucans with a higher MW (5.687×10^6 Da) exhibited more pronounced antidiabetic effects compared to those with medium (4.61×10^5 Da) and low (6.82×10^4 Da) MWs. Another mechanism proposed by Abbasi et al. [92] involved an in vitro assay using intestinal epithelial IEC-6 cells. They demonstrated that treatment with oat β-glucans reduced post-meal glucose levels by altering the activity of intestinal glucose transporters. The physical properties of β-glucan were suggested to contribute to the decreased expression of glucose transporters, specifically SGLT-1 and glucose transporter 2 (GLUT-2), thereby inhibiting the uptake of glucose. Additionally, oat β-glucans were suggested to delay gastric emptying, offering another potential mechanism for reducing glucose levels and improving the insulin response.

Oat β-glucan was also found to have a beneficial impact on the internal environment of the intestinal tract by effectively inhibiting the activities of mucosal intestinal α-disaccharidases, specifically lactase, maltase, and sucrase, in streptozotocin-induced diabetic mice [111]. In a six-week trial, mice with induced diabetes were administered three different levels of oat β-glucan. Following the treatment, improvements in glucose metabolism were observed across all three levels, with the highest inhibition of intestinal disaccharidases observed in the group receiving the highest dose of oat β-glucan. Furthermore, oat β-glucan exhibited inhibitory effects on all three enzyme activities when tested in vitro. This in vitro testing involved adding a solution of β-glucan to each of the three disaccharidases in test tubes, confirming the ability of oat β-glucan to effectively inhibit these enzyme activities.

Research also indicates that oat β-glucan particles, as part of the cell wall, form a network-like native structure that may encapsulate proteins and starch, creating a complex matrix within the cell wall. This matrix could limit enzyme access, leading to reduced starch digestion and a lower postprandial blood sugar response [112]. The high viscosity of oat β-glucan (OBG) may act as a physical barrier to glucose uptake in normal gut epithelial cells (IEC-6) by influencing the expression of SGLT-1 and 2 (GLUT-2) [92]. Furthermore, β-glucans have been shown to increase insulin secretion and reduce insulin resistance, primarily due to the high viscosity of the solution, which significantly enhances the integrity of pancreatic islet β-cells and tissue structures. Additionally, the reduction in glucose or insulin levels by β-glucans is influenced by gut peptides like YY and ghrelin, which can affect gut hormones and play a crucial role in glucose homeostasis [110], [113].

Studies examining the effects of β-glucan consumption in individuals with type 1 diabetes are quite limited, as noted in the research by Frid et al. [114]. The scarcity of such studies could be attributed to the predominant use of this type of fibre for obesity and type 2 diabetes in general. Additionally, evaluating the impact of β-glucan on blood glucose levels in individuals with type 1 diabetes can be challenging because they receive exogenous insulin injections. However, despite these challenges, promising outcomes have been observed in studies involving animals with type 1 diabetes. These studies have shown that β-glucan can enhance glycaemic control and improve the antioxidant profile, which is vital in reducing oxidative stress associated with diabetes. This improvement is characterized by the upregulation of enzymes like superoxide dismutase and catalase in the liver and kidneys. Furthermore, β-glucans have been found to increase Akt kinase levels and reduce the activation of pro-caspase-3. It has also been reported that β-glucans activate survival pathways and contribute to overall recovery by enhancing the body's resistance to the onset of diabetic complications, as demonstrated in research by Mirjana et al. [115].

6.2.7 Amyloid Formation

AVA-C exhibits notable potential in the prevention of amyloid formation. Amyloid fibrils, characterized by their extensive β-sheet-rich secondary structure, are implicated in a wide range of human diseases, encompassing neurodegenerative conditions like Parkinson's, Alzheimer's, and Huntington's disease, amyotrophic lateral sclerosis, type 2 diabetes, and disorders linked to the accumulation of insoluble serum amyloid A protein in organs such as the liver, spleen, and kidney. Despite relentless efforts to comprehend the underlying mechanisms of these diseases and develop effective therapeutic strategies, there remains a dearth of definitive evidence for the treatment and prevention of amyloid-related disorders. Polyphenols, including AVAs, have garnered considerable attention as potential inhibitors of amyloid aggregation. Their bioactive properties are intricately linked to the quantity and positioning of hydroxyl groups within the flavone backbone. Avn C, in particular, emerges as a promising biomolecule with the capability to hinder protein aggregation by curtailing the formation of the β-sheet structure within protein aggregates [116]. This presents a promising avenue for the potential prevention and treatment of amyloid-related diseases. Various studies related to disease management through oats are described in Table 6.1.

TABLE 6.1 Disease Management Using Oat-Based Foods

DISEASE TYPE	MODEL USED	NOTEWORTHY OBSERVATIONS	
Celiac disease	Human subjects	• Isolated oat prolamin proteins (avenins) with gluten-free purity. • New technique produced 2 kg of avenin from 400 kg of wheat-free oats. • Avenin had 85% protein content and 96% avenin purity. • Low levels of starch (1.8%), β-glucan (0.2%), and free sugars (1.8%). • Used liquid chromatography tandem mass spectrometry (LC-MS/MS) to verify uncontaminated oat proteins. • Proteomic analysis revealed five primary avenin protein groups, some with immune-stimulatory peptides. • High-quality avenin with the DQ2.5-ave-1a epitope for studies on oat safety for individuals with celiac disease.	[61]
Celiac disease	Not applicable	• Studied 162 oat varieties from 20 countries for protein content. • Used size exclusion-high-performance liquid chromatography (SE-HPLC) for protein analysis. • Identified three main protein groups: polymeric proteins (68.79–86.60%), avenins (8.86–27.72%), and soluble proteins (2.89–11.85%). • The polymeric to monomeric protein ratio ranged from 1.37 to 3.73. • Reversed-phase HPLC differentiated 76 peaks in ethanol-extracted proteins. • Developed a method to estimate avenin-epitope content using mass spectrometry and bioinformatics. • Used ELISA with the R5 antibody to detect contamination with wheat, barley, or rye in some samples. • Emphasized the importance of assessing oat varieties for protein and epitope composition to ensure gluten-free safety for individuals with celiac disease.	[63]
Celiac disease	Not applicable	• Oats are nutritionally rich with protein, lipids, fibre, antioxidants, and AVAs that make them unique among grains. • A study used PacBio sequencing to extract and sequence potentially harmful genes for individuals with CD in six oat varieties, including avenins, globulins, and α-amylase/trypsin inhibitors. • Identified 21 avenin, 75 globulin, and 25 α-amylase/trypsin inhibitor genes, and mapped them on hexaploid oat chromosomes.	[62]

(Continued)

TABLE 6.1 (Continued) Disease Management Using Oat-Based Foods

DISEASE TYPE	MODEL USED	NOTEWORTHY OBSERVATIONS	
		• Minor sequence differences were found within genes of oat varieties, mainly within individual genes. • Avenin epitopes were detected in all types of avenin genes across oat varieties, though they represented only 10% of storage proteins. • The suitability of oat consumption for individuals with CD remains uncertain and depends on specific criteria.	
Celiac disease	Human subjects	• Study compared healthy adults ($n = 14$), adults with CD ($n = 19$), and adults with non-celiac gluten sensitivity (NCGS) (n = 10). • Examined the impact of a gluten-free diet on faecal microbiota. • NCGS subjects had more gut symptoms, higher fat intake, and lower carbohydrate intake compared to healthy and CD subjects. • Oat consumption met recommended fibre intake without disrupting microbiota in CD or NCGS subjects. • Gut symptoms in NCGS were not linked to microbiota. • Healthy subjects had a higher proportion of faecal acetate, possibly due to increased Bifidobacterium. • Production of propionate, butyrate, ammonia, and β-glucuronidase activity was similar across groups. • Pure oats could be a foundation for a gluten-free diet, but further research is needed for minor microbiota imbalances.	[117]
Celiac disease	Human subjects	• A study examined oat consumption's safety and long-term effects in 312 long-term treated dermatitis herpetiformis (DH) patients, a skin condition associated with celiac disease. • 82% of patients included oats in their gluten-free diet. • Oat consumers and non-consumers had similar rates of long-term illnesses, CD complications, and medication usage. • Oat consumers reported a better quality of life and experienced ongoing gastrointestinal symptoms less frequently (4% vs. 19%, p = 0.004) compared to non-consumers. • The study suggests that oats can be safely included in the gluten-free diet of DH patients, improving their quality of life and reducing gastrointestinal symptoms over the long term.	[118]

(Continued)

TABLE 6.1   (Continued) Disease Management Using Oat-Based Foods

DISEASE TYPE	MODEL USED	NOTEWORTHY OBSERVATIONS	
Celiac disease	Not applicable	• Study assessed the safety of 26 oat cultivars and landraces for CD patients. • Total protein content ranged from 15.3% to 23.1%, with avenins accounting for 6.8% to 10.9%. • Avenin immunological activity tested using monoclonal antibodies (mAb) R5 and G12. • No immunological activity was detected with mAb R5 in immunoblotting and ELISA. • mAb G12 showed no activity in immunoblotting but had ELISA responses ranging from 13 to 53 mg/kg for total avenin extract. • Avenin fractionation revealed one fraction with a higher G12 response. • Protein sequence analysis suggested no direct binding to avenin-specific T cell epitopes, but differences in repetitive avenin regions may explain variations in G12 ELISA results. • Concludes that the oat cultivars tested did not display immunological activity related to celiac disease, though differences in G12 responses may be linked to avenin repetitive regions.	[119]
Hypertension	Human subjects	• Study on essential hypertension (HTN) divided 50 participants into a dietary fibre (DF) group and a control group. • DF group received dietary guidance and a daily oat bran supplement (30 g) with 8.9 g of DF. • After three months, the DF group showed significant reductions in office systolic blood pressure (oSBP) and office diastolic blood pressure (oDBP) compared to the control group. • DF group had greater improvements in 24-hour maximum systolic blood pressure (SBP) and diastolic blood pressure (DBP), as well as average 24-hour SBP and DBP. • DF group also reduced their use of antihypertensive drugs. • Gut microbiota analysis revealed significant differences in beta diversity between the groups, and the DF group exhibited changes in Bifidobacterium and Spirillum in their gut microbiota. • Supplementing with dietary fibre (oat bran) improved blood pressure, reduced the need for antihypertensive drugs, and positively influenced gut microbiota composition in essential hypertension patients.	[120]

TABLE 6.1 (Continued) Disease Management Using Oat-Based Foods

DISEASE TYPE	*MODEL USED*	*NOTEWORTHY OBSERVATIONS*	
Hypertension	Rats (spontaneously hypertensive)	• Study in spontaneously hypertensive rats (SHR) examined the effects of oat AVA-C and β-glucan, individually and in combination, on blood pressure and cardioprotection. • β-glucan alone prevented an increase in systolic and diastolic blood pressure in SHR. • AVA-C alone or in combination did not have the same antihypertensive effect on blood pressure. • Rats treated with β-glucan (without AVA-C or the combination) showed a reduction in isovolumetric relaxation time compared to those treated with the vehicle, indicating potential cardioprotection. • Both β-glucan and AVA-C reduced levels of malondialdehyde, a marker of oxidative stress in SHR. • Suggests that β-glucan may have potential as an antihypertensive agent with cardiovascular benefits, while AVA-C did not exhibit the same antihypertensive effect in this context.	[121]
Hypertension	Human subjects	• Meta-analysis of 21 randomized controlled trials with 1,569 participants examined the impact of oat consumption on blood pressure (BP) in adults. • Oat consumption led to a significant reduction in SBP by an average of −2.82 mm Hg. • Subgroup analyses showed that oat consumption was particularly effective in reducing SBP in hypertensive participants and when compared to control group participants consuming refined grains. • Although the overall reduction in DBP after oat consumption was not statistically significant, sensitivity analyses suggested a significant reduction in DBP, implying that the initial result might not have been robust. • Subgroup analyses also demonstrated that oat consumption significantly reduced DBP in participants with baseline BP in the prehypertensive range. • Significant reductions in both SBP and DBP were observed when the dosage of oat consumption was ≥5 g/day of β-glucan or the duration of oat consumption was ≥8 weeks. • In conclusion, oat consumption has a positive impact on reducing SBP levels, especially in individuals with hypertension or when compared to those consuming refined grains at matched total energy intake.	[122]

(*Continued*)

TABLE 6.1   (Continued) Disease Management Using Oat-Based Foods

DISEASE TYPE	MODEL USED	NOTEWORTHY OBSERVATIONS	
Hypertension	Human subjects	• A study investigated the impact of DF supplementation with oat bran on heart rate (HR) in patients with essential hypertension (HTN). • Seventy patients were divided into a control group (n = 34) and an intervention group (n = 36) receiving regular Dietary Approaches to Stop Hypertension (DASH) dietary care. • The intervention group also received a daily oat bran supplement (30 g) with 8.9 g of dietary fibre. • After 3 months, the intervention group showed a significantly lower 24-hour maximum heart rate (24h maxHR) compared to the control group. • Within the intervention group, significant reductions were observed in various HR parameters, including 24h aveHR, 24h maxHR, average heart rate during the daytime (D-aveHR), minimum heart rate during the daytime (D-minHR), and maximum heart rate during the daytime (D-maxHR). • No similar differences were found in the control group. • Suggests that dietary fibre supplementation, especially with oat bran, has a beneficial effect on reducing heart rate in patients with essential hypertension.	[123]
Immune response	Human peripheral blood mononuclear cells (PBMCs) and monocytes	• A study investigated the cardiovascular benefits of oat β-glucan extract, alone and in combination with the antihypertensive medication hydrochlorothiazide, in male and female spontaneously hypertensive rats (SHRs). • Male and female SHRs, along with Wistar–Kyoto (WKY) rats, were treated with oat β-glucan and hydrochlorothiazide for 15 weeks. • At 20 weeks of age, male and female SHRs exhibited high BP, cardiac remodelling, cardiac dysfunction, increased levels of malondialdehyde (MDA), angiotensin II, and norepinephrine. • Treatment with β-glucan, either alone or in combination with hydrochlorothiazide, had different effects in preventing high BP, cardiac dysfunction, and alterations in MDA, angiotensin II, and norepinephrine in 20-week-old male and female SHRs. • The study suggests that oat β-glucan shows promise for managing hypertension and reducing related cardiac complications, with potential sex-specific roles in the cardiovascular benefits of this treatment.	[124]

(Continued)

TABLE 6.1 (Continued) Disease Management Using Oat-Based Foods

DISEASE TYPE	MODEL USED	NOTEWORTHY OBSERVATIONS	
Immune response	Human monocytes	• Study in female BALB/c mice investigated the immunomodulatory activity of oat-derived oligopeptides (OOPs). • Mice received OOPs at various doses (0.25, 0.5, 1.0, and 2.0 g/kg body weight) via intragastric administration. • The study assessed OOPs' effects on immune responses through seven assays, including immune organ ratios, cellular and humoral immune responses, macrophage phagocytosis, natural killer (NK) cell activity, spleen T lymphocyte subpopulations, and serum cytokine and immunoglobulin levels. • Results showed that OOPs significantly enhanced both innate and adaptive immune responses in mice. • Enhancement included boosting cell-mediated and humoral immunity, increasing macrophage phagocytosis capacity, and enhancing NK cell activity. • These effects were associated with increased percentages of T and Th cells and elevated secretion of various cytokines and immunoglobulins. • The study suggests that dietary OOPs have promising immunomodulatory effects at various doses, enhancing immune responses, cytokine secretion, and immunoglobulin production in mice.	[125]
Immune response	Mouse spleeno-cytes	• This study investigated trained immunity in innate immune cells and the impact of (1, 3)/(1, 4)-β-glucan, found in dietary fibre from oats, on trained immunity. • Trained immunity involves long-term epigenetic and metabolic reprogramming of innate immune cells after exposure to pathogens, leading to enhanced protection against secondary infections. • While (1, 3)/(1, 6)-β-glucan from fungi was known to induce trained immunity, the effect of (1, 3)/(1, 4)-β-glucan from oats had not been previously reported. • The study validated two cell culture systems for inducing trained immunity in monocytes/macrophages from mouse bone marrow and human THP-1 cells using positive inducers like β-glucan from Trametes versicolor and human-oxidized low-density lipoprotein.	[126]

(Continued)

TABLE 6.1 (Continued) Disease Management Using Oat-Based Foods

DISEASE TYPE	MODEL USED	NOTEWORTHY OBSERVATIONS	
		• Priming with oat β-glucan led to a significant increase in mRNA expression and production of pro-inflammatory cytokines (TNF-α and IL-6) when re-stimulated with TLR ligands (TLR-4/2).	
		• Oat β-glucan also upregulated the expression of key enzymes involved in glycolytic and tricarboxylic acid cycle pathways.	
		• Inhibiting these enzymes reduced the production of TNF-α and IL-6, indicating that metabolic reprogramming is involved in oat β-glucan-induced trained immunity.	
Immune response	Rats (TNBS-induced colitis)	• The study explored oat milk fermentation to enhance its nutritional value and its impact on the immune response in OVA-sensitized mice.	[127]
		• Fermented oat milk (FOM) was created using specific bacterial strains and glucose for improved fermentation.	
		• FOM remained stable at 4°C for up to seven days.	
		• Oral administration of FOM (0.4 and 2 g/kg body weight) didn't affect serum OVA-specific IgG levels or spleen index.	
		• FOM exhibited similar efficacy to commercial dairy yogurt in reducing stimulation index, IL-2, IFN-γ, and IL-4 production, while promoting TGF-β and IL-10 secretion by OVA-stimulated splenocytes.	
		• Suggests that FOM has immune-modulatory effects comparable to dairy yogurt, making it a potential nutritional option with immune benefits.	
Immune response	Mice (high-fat diet model)	• The study explored the potential use of non-digestible carbohydrates in infant formula to mimic the effects of human milk oligosaccharides, with a focus on β-glucans for supplementation.	[128]
		• In vitro fermentation of native and endo-1,3(4)-β-glucanase-treated oat β-glucan was investigated using faecal samples from 2- and 8-week-old infants.	
		• Results indicated that native oat β-glucan was not utilized, but enzyme-treated oat β-glucan oligomers with β(1→4)-linkages were specifically fermented.	
		• Fermentation was most effective in the microbiota of 2-week-old infants, leading to increased lactate production.	
		• Fermentation of media with oat β-glucans increased the relative abundance of Enterococcus and reduced the production of pro-inflammatory cytokines (IL-1β, IL-6, TNFα) in immature dendritic cells.	

(Continued)

TABLE 6.1 (Continued) Disease Management Using Oat-Based Foods

DISEASE TYPE	MODEL USED	NOTEWORTHY OBSERVATIONS	
		• This anti-inflammatory effect was more pronounced after enzyme treatment, possibly due to the enhanced ability of fermented oat β-glucan to stimulate Dectin-1 receptors. • Suggests that enzyme-treated oat β-glucans have promise for supplementation in infant formula, offering potential anti-inflammatory benefits.	
Immune response	Mice (HFD-fed)	• The study investigated the impact of oat β-glucans with varying molar masses on colon inflammation (colitis) in the early stages of 2,4,6-trinitrobenzene sulphonic acid (TNBS)-induced Crohn's disease (CrD) using an animal model. • Sprague–Dawley rats, both control and TNBS-induced CD models, were divided into three dietary groups and fed for 3 days (acute inflammation) or 7 days (remission). • Diets included 1% low molar mass oat β-glucan (βGl), high molar mass oat β-glucan (βGh), or a diet without β-glucan. • CD induction led to increased inflammatory markers, disruptions in cytokine signalling pathways, and histological colon tissue changes. • Consumption of oat β-glucans helped mitigate inflammatory markers, restore signalling pathways, and improve histological changes, with more pronounced effects for βGl after 7 days of colitis. • Suggests that dietary oat β-glucans have potential to reduce colitis at both molecular and organ levels and expedite CD remission, indicating their therapeutic potential.	[129]
Microbiota regulation	Mice (DSS-induced)	• The study focused on the impact of flavonoids from whole-grain oats (FO) on bile acid (BA) metabolism and gut microbiota in high-fat diet (HFD)-induced hyperlipidemic mice. • FO improved serum lipid profiles, reduced body weight, and decreased lipid deposition in HFD-fed mice. • RT-qPCR and Western blot assays showed that FO modulated the expression of genes and proteins related to lipid metabolism and bile acid regulation. • This modulation suppressed lipogenesis, promoted lipolysis, facilitated bile acid synthesis, and enhanced excretion via the farnesoid X receptor (FXR) pathway.	[130]

(Continued)

TABLE 6.1   (Continued) Disease Management Using Oat-Based Foods

DISEASE TYPE	MODEL USED	NOTEWORTHY OBSERVATIONS	
		• Spearman's correlation analysis indicated strong associations between these bacteria and hyperlipidemia-related parameters. • The study suggests that FO has an anti-hyperlipidemic effect by regulating the gut–liver axis, involving bile acid metabolism and gut microbiota.	
Microbiota regulation	Mice (HFD-fed)	• 16S rRNA sequencing revealed that FO significantly altered the gut microbiota composition, increasing beneficial bacteria (e.g., Akkermansia) and decreasing potentially harmful ones (e.g., Lachnoclostridium, Blautia, Colidextribacter, and Desulfovibrio). • The study aimed to investigate the positive impact of oat phenolic compounds (OPC) on alleviating metabolic syndrome by regulating metabolites and gut microbiota composition. • Oral administration of OPC effectively mitigated several metabolic syndrome symptoms in mice induced by a high-fat diet, including weight gain, glucose intolerance, elevated serum lipid levels, oxidative stress markers, and adipocyte hypertrophy. • OPC-treated mice exhibited reduced chronic inflammation and influenced the expression of genes related to glycolipid metabolism. • A high-fat diet disrupted the balance of gut microbiota, while OPC supplementation counteracted this negative effect. • OPC increased the abundance of Bacteroidetes and reduced the diversity of Firmicutes, indicating a positive shift in gut microbiota composition. • OPC treatment also led to higher levels of Eubacterium and decreased numbers of Alistipes and Lachnospiraceae NK4A136 groups in HFD-fed mice. • These findings suggest that polyphenols from whole grains, like OPC, have the potential to ameliorate glycolipid metabolism disorders through their effects on metabolic syndrome symptoms and gut microbiota composition.	[131]
Microbiota regulation	Human subjects	• The study explored the potential of oat β-glucan in mitigating ulcerative colitis (UC), an inflammatory bowel disease (IBD), and aimed to uncover the underlying mechanisms, with a focus on gut microbiota. • The dextran sulphate sodium model was used to induce colitis in mice.	

TABLE 6.1 (Continued) Disease Management Using Oat-Based Foods

DISEASE TYPE	MODEL USED	NOTEWORTHY OBSERVATIONS	
		• β-glucan treatment effectively alleviated colitis symptoms, including rectal bleeding, splenomegaly, colon shortening, and colonic inflammation.	[132]
		• Apoptosis levels in colon tissues were reduced following β-glucan treatment, and the expression of pro-inflammatory factors was significantly decreased.	
		• β-glucan treatment upregulated both protein and mRNA expression levels of tight junction proteins, enhancing gut barrier integrity.	
		• Analysis of gut microbiota demonstrated that β-glucan treatment influenced microbial composition and structure at the operational taxonomic unit (OTU) level in colitis mice.	
		• Further examination of gut microbial metabolism revealed increased concentrations of acetate, propionate, and butyrate SCFAs, which played a crucial role in affecting pro-inflammatory factor expression and tight junction protein levels.	
		• These findings suggest that β-glucan may have therapeutic potential in alleviating UC by influencing gut microbiota and their metabolic products.	
Microbiota regulation	Mice	• The study aimed to investigate the role of OPC and oat β-glucan (OBG) in regulating lipid metabolism and gut microbiota.	[133]
		• Both OPC and OBG reduced body weight, fasting blood glucose levels, and regulated serum and hepatic lipid levels in HFD-fed mice.	
		• There was no significant difference in the regulatory effects of OPC and OBG.	
		• The combination of OPC and OBG (OPC + OBG) had a synergistic effect, significantly reducing body weight, blood glucose, and lipid profile levels.	
		• Real-time quantitative PCR (RT-qPCR) studies showed that OPC + OBG significantly altered mRNA expression related to lipid metabolism.	
		• Histopathological analysis demonstrated that OPC + OBG improved liver lipid deposition and reduced liver oxidative stress.	
		• OPC + OBG had a positive impact on the gut microbiota community, increasing the abundance of probiotics and shifting the composition by increasing Bacteroidetes and reducing Firmicutes.	
		• This finding supports the benefits of whole grains in preventing hyperlipidemia by influencing both lipid metabolism and gut microbiota composition.	

(Continued)

TABLE 6.1   (Continued) Disease Management Using Oat-Based Foods

DISEASE TYPE	MODEL USED	NOTEWORTHY OBSERVATIONS	
Microbiota regulation	Human subjects	• In a study involving 210 mildly hypercholesterolemic subjects, the impact of daily consumption of oats (80 g) compared to rice over 45 days was assessed. • Both grains effectively reduced total and non-HDL cholesterol levels, with oats exhibiting a stronger effect. • Oat consumption led to favourable changes in the gut microbiota, including an increase in Akkermansia muciniphila and Roseburia and a decrease in unclassified f-Sutterellaceae. • Bifidobacterium was negatively correlated with LDL-C, and total cholesterol (TC) and LDL-C were negatively correlated with Faecalibacterium prausnitzii. • These gut microbiome changes were linked to alterations in plasma short-chain fatty acid concentrations. • The study highlights the potential of oats as prebiotics, contributing to their cholesterol-lowering effects.	[134]
Type 2 diabetes	Mice	• Oat β-d-glucan demonstrates potential in ameliorating diabetes by affecting multiple mechanisms. • Oat β-d-glucan enhances glycogen synthesis by increasing glycogen content, reducing glycogen synthase (GS) phosphorylation, and promoting hepatic GS kinase 3β (GSK3β) phosphorylation. • These effects are mediated through the PI3K/AKT/GSK3 pathway, leading to improved glycogen storage. • Oat β-d-glucan inhibits gluconeogenesis by suppressing the phosphoenolpyruvate carboxykinase (PEPCK) enzyme via the PI3K/AKT/Foxo1 pathway, contributing to glucose control. • The compound enhances glucose catabolism by elevating the protein levels of key complexes involved in oxidative phosphorylation. • The study highlights the role of the TLR4-mediated intracellular signalling pathway in maintaining hepatic glucose balance, as evidenced by the reduced impact of oat β-d-glucan when TLR4 is blocked with anti-TLR4 antibody. • Oat β-d-glucan's multifaceted actions offer potential therapeutic implications for diabetes management, addressing various aspects of glucose regulation.	[135]

(Continued)

TABLE 6.1   (Continued) Disease Management Using Oat-Based Foods

DISEASE TYPE	MODEL USED	NOTEWORTHY OBSERVATIONS	
Type 2 diabetes	Human subjects	• In 2012, global pre-diabetes prevalence was 280 million, with a projected increase to 400 million by 2030. • Oat-based foods, rich in β-glucans known to lower postprandial blood glucose, are promising for managing pre-diabetes. • A multicentre intervention study is being conducted with adults (40–70 years old) with a BMI of ≥27 kg/m2 and HbA1c levels between 35 and 50 mmol/mol in Norway, Sweden, and Germany. • Specially designed intervention breads are employed, and the goal is to recruit 250 participants. • The primary outcome measures the difference in HbA1c between the intervention and control groups. • The study protocol has received ethical approval from participating countries, and the findings will be shared through publication in international scientific journals and presentations at national and international conferences. • This study addresses a pressing global health concern with significant implications for diabetes prevention.	[136]
Type 2 diabetes	Human subjects	• The study explores the impact of oat β-glucan, a soluble dietary fibre, on glycaemic control, appetite-regulating hormones, and gut microbiota in type-2 diabetes (T2D). • Thirty-seven T2D subjects enriched their regular diets with daily oat β-glucan or microcrystalline cellulose (control) for 12 weeks (5 g/day). • Results revealed a decrease in HbA1c levels in the β-glucan group, indicating improved glycaemic control. • Insulin, C-peptide, HOMA, Lactobacillus spp, and butyrate-producing bacteria were reduced in the β-glucan group, while leptin, GLP-1, and PYY differed significantly between groups. • A 12-week intake of 5 g of oat β-glucan can enhance glycaemic control, enhance feelings of satiety, and induce favourable changes in gut microbiota composition among individuals with T2D. • The findings support the potential role of oat β-glucan-enriched diets as a functional food for T2D management.	[137]

(Continued)

TABLE 6.1   (Continued) Disease Management Using Oat-Based Foods

DISEASE TYPE	MODEL USED	NOTEWORTHY OBSERVATIONS	
Type 2 diabetes	Human subjects	• This meta-analysis aimed to reconcile conflicting findings in individual studies regarding the impact of oat β-glucan (OBG) on type 2 diabetes mellitus (T2DM). • Four articles meeting inclusion criteria were analysed, involving a total of 350 T2DM patients. • Results showed that T2DM patients who consumed OBG at a daily dose of 2.5 to 3.5 g for 3 to 8 weeks experienced a significant reduction in fasting plasma glucose (FPG) and glycosylated haemoglobin (HbA1c) compared to the control group. • OBG intake did not have a significant effect on fasting plasma insulin (FPI) concentration. • In summary, medium-term OBG consumption (3–8 weeks) improved glycaemic control in T2DM patients but did not enhance insulin sensitivity. • Data on the effects of long-term OBG intake on glycaemic control and insulin sensitivity are limited and warrant further investigation.	[138]

6.3 CONCLUSION

In conclusion, *A. sativa* L., commonly known as oats, emerges as a versatile and remarkable cereal grain celebrated for its manifold health benefits. Oats exhibit an impressive nutritional profile, serving as a rich source of essential nutrients, including proteins, fibres, vitamins, and an assortment of bioactive compounds such as β-glucan, AVAs, saponins, and polyphenols. These bioactive constituents endow oats with a wide spectrum of advantageous properties, encompassing antioxidant, anti-diabetic, antimicrobial, anticancer, antihypertensive, immunomodulatory, anti-hyperlipidemic, anti-obesity, and cardioprotective attributes. Furthermore, oats have discernible applications in dermatology, offering relief for various skin conditions. It is worth highlighting that oats are a valuable dietary option for individuals afflicted by CD due to their low gluten-related toxic prolamins content. Furthermore, the presence of AVAs and other bioactive compounds in oats positions them as potential contributors to the prevention and treatment of cancer. Their antioxidant and anti-inflammatory properties render them promising contenders in the battle against various types of cancer. Oats also play a pivotal role in the management of diabetes, primarily owing to their high content of soluble fibre, notably β-glucans. These compounds assist in the regulation of blood glucose levels and the overall enhancement of glycaemic control. Additionally, oats exert positive influences on the gut microbiota, displaying prebiotic potential and promoting the proliferation of beneficial microorganism populations. In the subsequent section, we delved into the diverse array of bioactive compounds within oats and their multifaceted roles in promoting human health and nutrition. Oats transcend their status as a mere staple cereal grain, emerging as a valuable source of potential health benefits, awaiting further exploration and utilization in the domains of food science, medicine, and nutrition.

REFERENCES

[1]   V. K. Sood et al., "Health benefits of oat (Avena sativa) and nutritional improvement through plant breeding interventions," *Crop Pasture Sci.*, 2022, doi: 10.1071/CP22268.

[2]   G. F. Alemayehu, S. F. Forsido, Y. B. Tola and E. Amare, "Nutritional and phytochemical composition and associated health benefits of oat (*Avena sativa*) grains and oat-based fermented food products," *Sci. World J.*, p. e2730175, 2023, doi: 10.1155/2023/2730175.

[3]   S. Kumari et al., "Ethnobotany and phytopharmacology of Avena sativa: A qualitative review," *Sciphy.*, vol. 2, pp. 56–74, 2023, doi: 10.58920/sciphy02010056.

[4]   X. Li, L. Zhou, Y. Yu, J. Zhang, J. Wang and B. Sun, "The potential functions and mechanisms of oat on cancer prevention: A review," *J. Agric. Food Chem.*, vol. 70, pp. 14588–14599, 2022, doi: 10.1021/acs.jafc.2c06518.

[5]   V. Sterna, S. Zute and L. Brunava, "Oat grain composition and its nutrition benefice," *Agric. Agric. Sci. Proc.*, vol. 8, pp. 252–256, 2016, doi: 10.1016/j.aaspro.2016.02.100.

[6]   R. B. Panhwar, A. Akbar, M. F. Ali, Q. Yang and B. Feng, "Phytochemical components of some minor cereals associated with diabetes prevention and management," *J. Biosci. Med.*, vol. 6, p. 9, 2018, doi: 10.4236/jbm.2018.62002.

[7]   P. Sousa, D. Tavares-Valente, M. Amorim, J. Azevedo-Silva, M. Pintado and J. Fernandes, "β-glucan extracts as high-value multifunctional ingredients for skin health: A review," *Carbohydr. Polym.*, vol. 322, p. 121329, 2023, doi: 10.1016/j.carbpol.2023.121329.

[8]   I.-S. Kim, C.-W. Hwang, W.-S. Yang and C.-H. Kim, "Multiple antioxidative and bioactive molecules of oats (Avena sativa L.) in human health," *Antioxidants.*, vol. 10, p. 1454, 2021, doi: 10.3390/antiox10091454.

[9]   E. Turrini, F. Maffei, A. Milelli, C. Calcabrini and C. Fimognari, "Overview of the anticancer profile of avenanthramides from oat," *Int. J. Mol. Sci.*, vol. 20, p. 4536, 2019, doi: 10.3390/ijms20184536.

[10]   D. Paudel, B. Dhungana, M. Caffe and P. Krishnan, "A review of health-beneficial properties of oats," *Foods.*, vol. 10, p. 2591, 2021, doi: 10.3390/foods10112591.

[11]   T. A. Quiñones-Muñoz, S. J. Villanueva-Rodríguez and J. G. Torruco-Uco, "Nutraceutical properties of Medicago sativa L., Agave spp., Zea mays L. and Avena sativa L.: A review of metabolites and mechanisms," *Metabolites.*, vol. 12, p. 806, 2022, doi: 10.3390/metabo12090806.

[12]   C. Mattiuzzi and G. Lippi, "Current cancer epidemiology," *J. Epidemiol. Glob. Health.*, vol. 9, pp. 217–222, 2019, doi: 10.2991/jegh.k.191008.001.

[13]   M. D. A. Fagundes, A. R. C. Silva, G. A. Fernandes and M. P. Curado, "Dietary polyphenol intake and gastric cancer: A systematic review and meta-analysis," *Cancers.*, vol. 14, p. 5878, 2022, doi: 10.3390/cancers14235878.

[14]   P. Maleki Dana, F. Sadoughi, Z. Asemi and B. Yousefi, "The role of polyphenols in overcoming cancer drug resistance: A comprehensive review," *Cell. Mol. Biol. Lett.*, vol. 27, p. 1, 2022, doi: 10.1186/s11658-021-00301-9.

[15]   J. Makdisi, A. Kutner and A. Friedman, "Oats and skin health," in *Oats Nutrition and Technology*, John Wiley & Sons, Ltd, 2013, pp. 311–331, doi: 10.1002/9781118354100.ch15.

[16] K. A. Reynertson et al., "Anti-inflammatory activities of colloidal oatmeal (Avena sativa) contribute to the effectiveness of oats in treatment of itch associated with dry, irritated skin," *J. Drugs Dermatol.*, vol. 14, pp. 43–48, 2015.

[17] K. Lindfors et al., "Coeliac disease," *Nat. Rev. Dis. Primers.*, vol. 5, pp. 1–18, 2019, doi: 10.1038/s41572-018-0054-z.

[18] G. M. Pes, S. Bibbò and M. P. Dore, "Coeliac disease: Beyond genetic susceptibility and gluten. A narrative review," *Ann. Med.*, vol. 51, pp. 1–16, 2019, doi: 10.1080/07853890.2019.1569254.

[19] A. Kumar et al., "Phytic acid: Blessing in disguise, a prime compound required for both plant and human nutrition," *Int. Food Res. J.*, vol. 142, p. 110193, 2021, doi: 10.1016/j.foodres.2021.110193.

[20] I. Abdulwaliyu, S. O. Arekemase, J. A. Adudu, M. L. Batari, M. N. Egbule and S. I. R. Okoduwa, "Investigation of the medicinal significance of phytic acid as an indispensable anti-nutrient in diseases," *Clin. Nutr. Exp.*, vol. 28, pp. 42–61, 2019, doi: 10.1016/j.yclnex.2019.10.002.

[21] E. Feizollahi, R. S. Mirmahdi, A. Zoghi, R. T. Zijlstra, M. S. Roopesh and T. Vasanthan, "Review of the beneficial and anti-nutritional qualities of phytic acid, and procedures for removing it from food products," *Food Res. J.*, vol. 143, p. 110284, 2021, doi: 10.1016/j.foodres.2021.110284.

[22] A. B. Evert et al., "Nutrition therapy recommendations for the management of adults with diabetes," *Diabetes Care.*, vol. 37, pp. S120–S143, 2013, doi: 10.2337/dc14-S120.

[23] D. El Khoury, C. Cuda, B. L. Luhovyy and G. H. Anderson, "Beta glucan: Health benefits in obesity and metabolic syndrome," *J. Nutr. Metab.*, vol. 2012, p. e851362, 2011, doi: 10.1155/2012/851362.

[24] M. S. Popoviciu et al., "Correlations between diabetes mellitus self-care activities and glycaemic control in the adult population: A cross-sectional study," *Healthcare.*, vol. 10, p. 174, 2022, doi: 10.3390/healthcare10010174.

[25] A. E. V. Quaglio, T. G. Grillo, E. C. S. De Oliveira, L. C. Di Stasi and L. Y. Sassaki, "Gut microbiota, inflammatory bowel disease and colorectal cancer," *World J. Gastroenterol.*, vol. 28, pp. 4053–4060, 2022, doi: 10.3748/wjg.v28.i30.4053.

[26] E. S. V. Rezende, G. C. Lima and M. M. V. Naves, "Dietary fibers as beneficial microbiota modulators: A proposed classification by prebiotic categories," *Nutrition.*, vol. 89, p. 111217, 2021, doi: 10.1016/j.nut.2021.111217.

[27] E. Valido et al., "Systematic review of the effects of oat intake on gastrointestinal health," *J. Nutr.*, vol. 151, pp. 3075–3090, 2021, doi: 10.1093/jn/nxab245.

[28] S. Varma and S. Krishnareddy, "Uncomplicated celiac disease," in *Refractory Celiac Disease*, G. Malamut and N. Cerf-Bensussan, Eds. Cham, Germany: Springer International Publishing, 2022, pp. 5–19, doi: 10.1007/978-3-030-90142-4_2.

[29] A. Lomash et al., "Utility of human leukocyte antigen DQ2 and DQ8 genotypes in Celiac disease: Two sides of the coin," *Med. Res. Arch.*, vol. 11, 2023, doi: 10.18103/mra.v11i1.2864.

[30] R. P. Anderson, "Review article: Diagnosis of coeliac disease: A perspective on current and future approaches," *Aliment Pharmacol Ther.*, vol. 56, pp. S18–S37, 2022, doi: 10.1111/apt.16840.

[31] L. Masucci et al., "Celiac disease predisposition and genital tract microbiota in women affected by recurrent pregnancy loss," *Nutrients.*, vol. 15, p. 221, 2023, doi: 10.3390/nu15010221.

[32] V. Vincenzo, S. Gloria, M. Melissa, C. Alessandro and D. S. Rachele, "Histopathological assessment of celiac disease," in *Advances in Celiac Disease: Improving Paediatric and Adult Care*, J. Amil-Dias and I. Polanco, Eds. Cham, Germany: Springer International Publishing, 2022, pp. 79–97, doi: 10.1007/978-3-030-82401-3_7.

[33] C. Catassi, E. F. Verdu, J. C. Bai and E. Lionetti, "Coeliac disease," *Lancet.*, vol. 399, pp. 2413–2426, 2022, doi: 10.1016/S0140-6736(22)00794-2.

[34] M. V. Lenti et al., "Diagnostic delay in adult coeliac disease: An Italian multicentre study," *Diges. Liver Dis.*, vol. 55, pp. 743–750, 2023, doi: 10.1016/j.dld.2022.11.021.

[35] L. M. Ailioaie, C. Ailioaie, G. Litscher and D. A. Chiran, "Celiac disease and targeting the molecular mechanisms of autoimmunity in COVID pandemic," *Int. J. Mol. Sci.*, vol. 23, p. 7719, 2022, doi: 10.3390/ijms23147719.

[36] G. Caio, R. Ciccocioppo, G. Zoli, R. De Giorgio, U. Volta, Therapeutic options for coeliac disease: What else beyond gluten-free diet?, Digestive and Liver Disease., vol. 52, pp. 130–137, 2020, doi: 10.1016/j.dld.2019.11.010.

[37] K. A. Scherf, P. Koehler, H. Wieser, Gluten and wheat sensitivities – An overview," *J. Cereal Sci.*, vol. 67, pp. 2–11, 2016, doi: 10.1016/j.jcs.2015.07.008.

[38] A. Abbasi et al., "A critical review on the gluten-induced enteropathy/celiac disease: Gluten-targeted dietary and non-dietary therapeutic approaches," *Food Rev. Int.*, 2023, pp. 1–41, doi: 10.1080/87559129.2023.2202405.

[39] X. Yu, J. Vargas, P. H. R. Green and G. Bhagat, "Innate lymphoid cells and celiac disease: Current perspective," *Cell. Mol. Gastroenterol. Hepatol.*, vol. 11, pp. 803–814, 2021, doi: 10.1016/j.jcmgh.2020.12.002.

[40] H. Wieser, Á. Ruiz-Carnicer, V. Segura, I. Comino and C. Sousa, "Challenges of monitoring the gluten-free diet adherence in the management and follow-up of patients with celiac disease," *Nutrients.*, vol. 13, p. 2274, 2021, doi: 10.3390/nu13072274.

[41] M. M. P. da Silva Neves, M. B. González-Garcia, H. P. A. Nouws, C. Delerue-Matos, A. Santos-Silva and A. Costa-García, "Celiac disease diagnosis and gluten-free food analytical control," *Anal Bioanal Chem.*, vol. 397, pp. 1743–1753, 2010, doi: 10.1007/s00216-010-3753-1.

[42] P. D'Avino, G. Serena, V. Kenyon and A. Fasano, "An updated overview on celiac disease: From immuno-pathogenesis and immuno-genetics to therapeutic implications," *Expert Rev. Clin. Immunol.*, vol. 17, pp. 269–284, 2021, doi: 10.1080/1744666X.2021.1880320.

[43] J. R. Biesiekierski, "What is gluten?" *J. Gastroenterol. Hepatol.*, vol. 32, pp. 78–81, 2017, doi: 10.1111/jgh.13703.

[44] N. Chaudhary, A. S. Virdi, P. Dangi, B. S. Khatkar, A. K. Mohanty and N. Singh, "Protein, thermal and functional properties of α-, γ- and ω-gliadins of wheat and their effect on bread making characteristics," *Food Hydrocoll.*, vol. 124, p. 107212, 2022, doi: 10.1016/j.foodhyd.2021.107212.

[45] K. Pourmohammadi and E. Abedi, "Hydrolytic enzymes and their directly and indirectly effects on gluten and dough properties: An extensive review," *Food Sci. Nutr.*, vol. 9, pp. 3988–4006, 2021, doi: 10.1002/fsn3.2344.

[46] K. Y. Woldemariam et al., "Celiac disease and immunogenic wheat gluten peptides and the association of gliadin peptides with HLA DQ2 and HLA DQ8," *Food Rev. Int.*, vol. 38, pp. 1553–1576, 2022, doi: 10.1080/87559129.2021.1907755.

[47] J. Voisine and V. Abadie, "Interplay between gluten, HLA, innate and adaptive immunity orchestrates the development of coeliac disease," *Front. Immunol.*, vol. 12, 2021. [Online]. Accessed: Nov. 1, 2023. Available: www.frontiersin.org/articles/10.3389/fimmu.2021.674313.

[48] W. Dieterich et al., "Identification of tissue transglutaminase as the autoantigen of celiac disease," *Nat. Med.*, vol. 3, pp. 797–801, 1997, doi: 10.1038/nm0797-797.

[49] C. B. Lindstad, A. E. Dewan, J. Stamnaes, L. M. Sollid and M. F. du Pré, "TG2-gluten complexes as antigens for gluten-specific and transglutaminase-2 specific B cells in celiac disease," *PLoS One.*, vol. 16, p. e0259082, 2021, doi: 10.1371/journal.pone.0259082.

[50] M. F. du Pré and L. M. Sollid, "T-cell and B-cell immunity in celiac disease," *Best Pract Res Clin Gastroenterol.*, vol. 29, pp. 413–423, 2015, doi: 10.1016/j.bpg.2015.04.001.

[51] F. Koning, R. Thomas, J. Rossjohn and R. E. Toes, "Coeliac disease and rheumatoid arthritis: Similar mechanisms, different antigens," *Nat. Rev. Rheumatol.*, vol. 11, pp. 450–461, 2015, doi: 10.1038/nrrheum.2015.59.

[52] S. Caja, M. Mäki, K. Kaukinen and K. Lindfors, "Antibodies in celiac disease: Implications beyond diagnostics," *Cell. Mol. Immunol.*, vol. 8, pp. 103–109, 2011, doi: 10.1038/cmi.2010.65.

[53] G. K. Makharia et al., "The global burden of coeliac disease: Opportunities and challenges," *Nat. Rev. Gastroenterol. Hepatol.*, vol. 19, pp. 313–327, 2022, doi: 10.1038/s41575-021-00552-z.

[54] B. Meresse, J. Verdier and N. Cerf-Bensussan, "The cytokine interleukin 21: A new player in coeliac disease?" *Gut.*, vol. 57, pp. 879–881, 2008, doi: 10.1136/gut.2007.141994.

[55] B. D. McDonald, B. Jabri and A. Bendelac, "Diverse developmental pathways of intestinal intraepithelial lymphocytes," *Nat. Rev. Immunol.*, vol. 18, pp. 514–525, 2018, doi: 10.1038/s41577-018-0013-7.

[56] H. Wieser and P. Koehler, "The biochemical basis of celiac disease," *Cereal Chem.*, vol. 85, pp. 1–13, 2008, doi: 10.1094/CCHEM-85-1-0001.

[57] L. Kumar, R. Sehrawat and Y. Kong, "Oat proteins: A perspective on functional properties," *LWT.*, vol. 152, 2021, p. 112307, doi: 10.1016/j.lwt.2021.112307.

[58] O.D. Anderson, "The spectrum of major seed storage genes and proteins in oats (Avena sativa)," *PLoS One.*, vol. 9, p. e83569, 2014, doi: 10.1371/journal.pone.0083569.

[59] A. Real et al., "Molecular and immunological characterization of gluten proteins isolated from oat cultivars that differ in toxicity for celiac disease," *PLoS One*, vol. 7, p. e48365, 2012, doi: 10.1371/journal.pone.0048365.

[60] G. Di Nardo et al., "Nutritional deficiencies in children with celiac disease resulting from a gluten-free diet: A systematic review," *Nutrients.*, vol. 11, p. 1588, 2019, doi: 10.3390/nu11071588.

[61] G. Tanner et al., "Preparation and characterization of avenin-enriched oat protein by chill precipitation for feeding trials in celiac disease," *Front. Nutr.*, vol. 6, 2019. Accessed: Nov. 1, 2023. [Online]. Available: www.frontiersin.org/articles/10.3389/fnut.2019.00162.

[62] L. Leišová-Svobodová, T. Sovová and V. Dvořáček, "Analysis of oat seed transcriptome with regards to proteins involved in celiac disease," *Sci Rep.*, vol. 12, p. 8660, 2022, doi: 10.1038/s41598-022-12711-6.

[63] G. Gell et al., "Investigation of protein and epitope characteristics of oats and its implications for celiac disease," *Front. Nutr.*, vol. 8, 2021. Accessed: Nov. 1, 2023. [Online]. Available: www.frontiersin.org/articles/10.3389/fnut.2021.702352.

[64] Z. Gai, S. Hu, G. Gong and J. Zhao, "Recent advances in understanding dietary polyphenols protecting against hypertension," *Trends Food Sci. Technol.*, vol. 138, pp. 685–696, 2023, doi: 10.1016/j.tifs.2023.07.008.

[65] J. M. Keenan, J. J. Pins, C. Frazel, A. Moran and L. Turnquist, "Oat ingestion reduces systolic and diastolic blood pressure in patients with mild or borderline hypertension: A pilot trial," *J. Fam. Pract.*, vol. 51, p. 369, 2002.

[66] J. J. Pins, D. Geleva, J. M. Keenan, C. Frazel, P. J. O'Connor and L. M. Cherney, "Do whole-grain oat cereals reduce the need for antihypertensive medications and improve blood pressure control," *J. Fam. Pract.*, vol. 51, pp. 353–359, 2002.

[67] K. C. Maki et al., "Effects of consuming foods containing oat β-glucan on blood pressure, carbohydrate metabolism and biomarkers of oxidative stress in men and women with elevated blood pressure," *Eur. J. Clin. Nutr.*, vol. 61, pp. 786–795, 2007, doi: 10.1038/sj.ejcn.1602562.

[68] E. Saltzman et al., "An oat-containing hypocaloric diet reduces systolic blood pressure and improves lipid profile beyond effects of weight loss in men and women," *J. Nutr.*, vol. 131, pp. 1465–1470, 2001, doi: 10.1093/jn/131.5.1465.

[69] C. E. L. Evans et al., "Effects of dietary fibre type on blood pressure: A systematic review and meta-analysis of randomized controlled trials of healthy individuals," *J. Hypertens.*, vol. 33, p. 897, 2015, doi: 10.1097/HJH.0000000000000515.

[70] E. De Marco Castro, P. C. Calder and H. M. Roche, "β-1,3/1,6-glucans and immunity: State of the art and future directions," *Mol. Nutr. Food Res.*, vol. 65, p. 1901071, 2021, doi: 10.1002/mnfr.201901071.

[71] K. Sivieri, S. M. de Oliveira, A. de S. Marquez, J. Pérez-Jiménez and S. N. Diniz, "Insights on β-glucan as a prebiotic coadjuvant in the treatment of diabetes mellitus: A review," *Food Hydrocoll. Heal.*, vol. 2, p. 100056, 2022, doi: 10.1016/j.fhfh.2022.100056.

[72] C. J. Pretorius and I. A. Dubery, "Avenanthramides, distinctive hydroxycinnamoyl conjugates of oat, Avena sativa L.: An update on the biosynthesis, chemistry, and bioactivities," *Plants.*, vol. 12, p. 1388, 2023, doi: 10.3390/plants12061388.

[73] C. Kang, W. S. Shin, D. Yeo, W. Lim, T. Zhang and L. L. Ji, "Anti-inflammatory effect of avenanthramides via NF-κB pathways in C2C12 skeletal muscle cells," *Free Radic. Biol. Med.*, vol. 117, pp. 30–36, 2018, doi: 10.1016/j.freeradbiomed.2018.01.020.

[74] V. Tripathi, A. Singh, M. Ashraf and M. Ashraf, "Avenanthramides of oats: Medicinal importance and future perspectives," *Phcog. Rev.*, vol. 12, pp. 66–71, 2018, doi: 10.4103/phrev.phrev_34_17.

[75] M. P. Arena et al., "Combinations of cereal β-glucans and probiotics can enhance the anti-inflammatory activity on host cells by a synergistic effect," *J. Funct. Foods.*, vol. 23, pp. 12–23, 2016, doi: 10.1016/j.jff.2016.02.015.

[76] C. Chaiyasut et al., "Extraction of β-glucan of Hericium erinaceus, Avena sativa L., and Saccharomyces cerevisiae and in vivo evaluation of their immunomodulatory effects," *Food Sci. Technol.*, vol. 38, pp. 138–146, 2018, doi: 10.1590/fst.18217.

[77] J. Dong, X. Yu, L. Dong and R. Shen, "In vitro fermentation of oat β-glucan and hydrolysates by fecal microbiota and selected probiotic strains," *J. Sci. Food Agric.*, vol. 97, pp. 4198–4203, 2017, doi: 10.1002/jsfa.8292.

[78] K. Tamura et al., "Molecular mechanism by which prominent human gut bacteroidetes utilize mixed-linkage beta-glucans, major health-promoting cereal polysaccharides," *Cell Rep.*, vol. 21, pp. 417–430, 2017, doi: 10.1016/j.celrep.2017.09.049.

[79] J. Dong, M. Yang, Y. Zhu, R. Shen and K. Zhang, "Comparative study of thermal processing on the physicochemical properties and prebiotic effects of the oat β-glucan by in vitro human fecal microbiota fermentation," *Food Res. J.*, vol. 138, p. 109818, 2020, doi: 10.1016/j.foodres.2020.109818.

[80] J. Zhao and P. C. K. Cheung, "Comparative proteome analysis of bifidobacterium longum subsp. Infant is grown on β-glucans from different sources and a model for their utilization," *J. Agric. Food Chem.*, vol. 61, pp. 4360–4370, 2013, doi: 10.1021/jf400792j.

[81] K. Tamura, G. Dejean, F. V. Petegem and H. Brumer, "Distinct protein architectures mediate species-specific beta-glucan binding and metabolism in the human gut microbiota," *J. Biol. Chem.*, vol. 296, 2021, doi: 10.1016/j.jbc.2021.100415.

[82] S. Trivedi, K. Patel, V. Belgamwar and K. Wadher, "Functional polysaccharide lentinan: Role in anti-cancer therapies and management of carcinomas," *Pharmacol. Res. Mod. Chin. Med.*, vol. 2, p. 100045, 2022, doi: 10.1016/j.prmcm.2022.100045.

[83] C. Giacinti and A. Giordano, "RB and cell cycle progression," *Oncogene.*, vol. 25, pp. 5220–5227, 2006, doi: 10.1038/sj.onc.1209615.

[84] E.S. Scarpa, M. Mari, E. Antonini, F. Palma and P. Ninfali, "Natural and synthetic avenanthramides activate caspases 2, 8, 3 and downregulate hTERT, MDR1 and COX-2 genes in CaCo-2 and Hep3B cancer cells," *Food Funct.*, vol. 9, pp. 2913–2921, 2018, doi: 10.1039/C7FO01804E.

[85] A. Choromanska, J. Kulbacka, J. Harasym, R. Oledzki, A. Szewczyk and J. Saczko, "High- and low-molecular weight oat beta-glucan reveals antitumor activity in human epithelial lung cancer," *Pathol. Oncol. Res.*, vol. 24, pp. 583–592, 2018, doi: 10.1007/s12253-017-0278-3.

[86] L. Mo et al., "Anti-tumor effects of (1→3)-β-d-glucan from Saccharomyces cerevisiae in S180 tumor-bearing mice," *Int. J. Biol. Macromol.*, vol. 95, pp. 385–392, 2017, doi: 10.1016/j.ijbiomac.2016.10.106.

[87] R.C. Orlandelli et al., "β-(1→3,1→6)-d-glucans produced by Diaporthe sp. Endophytes: Purification, chemical characterization and antiproliferative activity against MCF-7 and HepG2-C3A cells," *Int. J. Biol. Macromol.*, vol. 94, pp. 431–437, 2017, doi: 10.1016/j.ijbiomac.2016.10.048.

[88] A. Choromanska et al., "Anticancer properties of low molecular weight oat beta-glucan – An in vitro study," *Int. J. Biol. Macromol.*, vol. 80, pp. 23–28, 2015, doi: 10.1016/j.ijbiomac.2015.05.035.

[89] R. Pop-Busui et al., "Heart failure: An underappreciated complication of diabetes. A consensus report of the American Diabetes Association," *Diabetes Care.*, vol. 45, pp. 1670–1690, 2022, doi: 10.2337/dci22-0014.

[90] A. Abot, S. Fried, P. D. Cani and C. Knauf, "Reactive oxygen species/reactive nitrogen species as messengers in the gut: Impact on physiology and metabolic disorders," *Antioxid. Redox Signal.*, vol. 37, pp. 394–415, 2022, doi: 10.1089/ars.2021.0100.

[91] L. M. N. K. Ekström, E. A. E. Henningsson Bok, M. E. Sjöö and E. M. Östman, "Oat β-glucan containing bread increases the glycaemic profile," *J. Funct. Foods.*, vol. 32, pp. 106–111, 2017, doi: 10.1016/j.jff.2017.02.027.

[92] N. N. Abbasi, P. P. Purslow, S. M. Tosh and M. Bakovic, "Oat β-glucan depresses SGLT1- and GLUT2-mediated glucose transport in intestinal epithelial cells, IEC-6)," *Nutr. Res.*, vol. 36, pp. 541–552, 2016, doi: 10.1016/j.nutres.2016.02.004.

[93] Q. Zhao et al., "Physicochemical properties and regulatory effects on db/db diabetic mice of β-glucans extracted from oat, wheat and barley," *Food Hydrocoll.*, vol. 37, pp. 60–68, 2014, doi: 10.1016/j.foodhyd.2013.10.007.

[94] S. AbuMweis, S. J. Thandapilly, J. Storsley and N. Ames, "Effect of barley β-glucan on postprandial glycaemic response in the healthy human population: A meta-analysis of randomized controlled trials," *J. Funct. Foods.*, vol. 27, pp. 329–342, 2016, doi: 10.1016/j.jff.2016.08.057.

[95] T. H. Gamel, E.-S. M. Abdel-Aal, N. P. Ames, R. Duss and S. M. Tosh, "Enzymatic extraction of beta-glucan from oat bran cereals and oat crackers and optimization of viscosity measurement," *J. Cereal Sci.*, vol. 59, pp. 33–40, 2014, doi: 10.1016/j.jcs.2013.10.011.

[96] A. Mackie, N. Rigby, P. Harvey and B. Bajka, "Increasing dietary oat fibre decreases the permeability of intestinal mucus," *J. Funct. Foods.*, vol. 26, pp. 418–427, 2016, doi: 10.1016/j.jff.2016.08.018.

[97] A. Rieder, S. H. Knutsen and S. I, "In vitro digestion of beta-glucan rich cereal products results in extracts with physicochemical and rheological behavior like pure beta-glucan solutions – A basis for increased understanding of in vivo effects," *Food Hydrocoll.*, vol. 67, pp. 74–84, 2017, doi: 10.1016/j.foodhyd.2016.12.033.

[98] N. Ames and J. Storsley, "Effects of barley on post-prandial glycemic response," *Diabesity.*, vol. 1, pp. 21–23, 2015, doi: 10.15562/diabesity.2015.15.

[99] V. de O. Silva, N. O. de Moura, L. J. R. de Oliveira, A. P. Peconick and L. J. Pereira, "Promising effects of beta-glucans on metabolism and on the immune responses: Review article," *Am. J. Immunol.*, vol. 13, pp. 62–72, 2017, doi: 10.3844/ajisp.2017.62.72.

[100] J.-A. Nazare, S. Normand, A. Oste Triantafyllou, A. Brac de la Perrière, M. Desage and M. Laville, "Modulation of the postprandial phase by β-glucan in overweight subjects: Effects on glucose and insulin kinetics," *Mol. Nutr. Food Res.*, vol. 53, pp. 361–369, 2009, doi: 10.1002/mnfr.200800023.

[101] R. Bozbulut and N. Sanlier, "Promising effects of β-glucans on glyceamic control in diabetes," *Trends Food Sci. Technol.*, vol. 83, pp. 159–166, 2019, doi: 10.1016/j.tifs.2018.11.018.

[102] P. Battilana et al., "Mechanisms of action of β-glucan in postprandial glucose metabolism in healthy men," *Eur. J. Clin. Nutr.*, vol. 55, pp. 327–333, 2001, doi: 10.1038/sj.ejcn.1601160.

[103] M. Kabir et al., "Four-week low-glycemic index breakfast with a modest amount of soluble fibers in type 2 diabetic men," *Metabolism.*, vol. 51, pp. 819–826, 2002, doi: 10.1053/meta.2002.33345.

[104] P. Würsch and F. X. Pi-Sunyer, "The role of viscous soluble fiber in the metabolic control of diabetes: A review with special emphasis on cereals rich in β-glucan," *Diabetes Care.*, vol. 20, pp. 1774–1780, 1997, doi: 10.2337/diacare.20.11.1774.

[105] M. Biörklund, A. van Rees, R. P. Mensink and G. Önning, "Changes in serum lipids and postprandial glucose and insulin concentrations after consumption of beverages with β-glucans from oats or barley: a randomised dose-controlled trial," *Eur. J. Clin. Nutr.*, vol. 59, pp. 1272–1281, 2005, doi: 10.1038/sj.ejcn.1602240.

[106] C. Chen, X. Huang, H. Wang, F. Geng and S. Nie, "Effect of β-glucan on metabolic diseases: A review from the gut microbiota perspective," *Curr. Opin. Food Sci.*, vol. 47, p. 100907, 2022, doi: 10.1016/j.cofs.2022.100907.

[107] Y. Cao, Y. Sun, S. Zou, B. Duan, M. Sun and X. Xu, "Yeast β-glucan suppresses the chronic inflammation and improves the microenvironment in adipose tissues of ob/ob mice," *J. Agric. Food Chem.*, vol. 66, pp. 621–629, 2018, doi: 10.1021/acs.jafc.7b04921.

[108] P. Wood, J. T. Braaten, F. W. Scott, K. D. Riedel, M. S. Wolynetz and M. W. Collins, "Effect of dose and modification of viscous properties of oat gum on plasma glucose and insulin following an oral glucose load," *Br. J. Nutr.*, vol. 72, pp. 731–743, 1994, doi: 10.1079/BJN19940075.

[109] P. J. Wood, M. U. Beer and G. Butler, "Evaluation of role of concentration and molecular weight of oat β-glucan in determining effect of viscosity on plasma glucose and insulin following an oral glucose load," *Br. J. Nutr.*, vol. 84, pp. 19–23, 2000, doi: 10.1017/S0007114500001185.

[110] M. Liu et al., "The anti-diabetic activity of oat β-d-glucan in streptozotocin–nicotinamide induced diabetic mice," *Int. J. Biol. Macromol.*, vol. 91, pp. 1170–1176, 2016, doi: 10.1016/j.ijbiomac.2016.06.083.

[111] J. Dong, F. Cai, R. Shen and Y. Liu, "Hypoglycaemic effects and inhibitory effect on intestinal disaccharidases of oat beta-glucan in streptozotocin-induced diabetic mice," *Food Chem.*, vol. 129, pp. 1066–1071, 2011, doi: 10.1016/j.foodchem.2011.05.076.

[112] J. Zhang, K. Luo and G. Zhang, "Impact of native form oat β-glucan on starch digestion and postprandial glycemia," *J. Cereal Sci.*, vol. 73, pp. 84–90, 2017, doi: 10.1016/j.jcs.2016.11.013.

[113] S. Baldassano, G. Accardi and S. Vasto, "Beta-glucans and cancer: The influence of inflammation and gut peptide," *Eur. J. Med. Chem.*, vol. 142, pp. 486–492, 2017, doi: 10.1016/j.ejmech.2017.09.013.

[114] A. Frid, A. Tura, G. Pacini and M. Ridderstråle, "Effect of oral pre-meal administration of betaglucans on glycaemic control and variability in subjects with Type 1 diabetes," *Nutrients.*, vol. 9, p. 1004, 2017, doi: 10.3390/nu9091004.

[115] M. Mirjana et al., "β-glucan administration to diabetic rats reestablishes redox balance and stimulates cellular pro-survival mechanisms," *J. Funct. Foods.*, vol. 5, pp. 267–278, 2013, doi: 10.1016/j.jff.2012.10.016.

[116] M. G. Quiroz Vazquez, D. Montiel Condado, B. Gonzalez Hernandez and A. Gonzalez-Horta, "Avenanthramide-C prevents amyloid formation of bovine serum albumin," *Biophys. Chem.*, vol. 263, pp. 106391, 2020, doi: 10.1016/j.bpc.2020.106391.

[117] L. Nylund et al., "Diet, perceived intestinal well-being and compositions of fecal microbiota and short chain fatty acids in oat-using subjects with celiac disease or gluten sensitivity," *Nutrients.*, vol. 12, p. 2570, 2020, doi: 10.3390/nu12092570.

[118] A. Alakoski et al., "The long-term safety and quality of life effects of oats in dermatitis herpetiformis," *Nutrients.*, vol. 12, p. 1060, 2020, doi: 10.3390/nu12041060.

[119] H. G. Ahola, T. S. Sontag-Strohm, A. H. Schulman, P. Tanhuanpää, S. Viitala and X. Huang, "Immunochemical analysis of oat avenins in an oat cultivar and landrace collection," *J. Cereal Sci.*, vol. 95, p. 103053, 2020, doi: 10.1016/j.jcs.2020.103053.

[120] Y. Xue et al., "The effect of dietary fiber (oat bran) supplement on blood pressure in patients with essential hypertension: A randomized controlled trial," *Nutr. Metab. Cardiovasc. Dis.*, vol. 31, pp. 2458–2470, 2021, doi: 10.1016/j.numecd.2021.04.013.

[121] P. Raj, N. Ames, S. Joseph Thandapilly, L. Yu and T. Netticadan, "The effects of oat ingredients on blood pressure in spontaneously hypertensive rats," *J. Food Biochem.*, vol. 44, p. e13402, 2020, doi: 10.1111/jfbc.13402.

[122] H. Xi et al., "Effect of oat consumption on blood pressure: A systematic review and meta-analysis of randomized controlled trials," *J. Acad. Nutr. Diet.*, vol. 123, pp. 809–823, 2023, doi: 10.1016/j.jand.2022.11.010.

[123] Y. Ju et al., "Effect of dietary fiber (oat bran) supplement in heart rate lowering in patients with hypertension: A randomized DASH-diet-controlled clinical trial," *Nutrients.*, vol. 14, p. 3148, 2022, doi: 10.3390/nu14153148.

[124] P. Raj et al., "Oat beta-glucan alone and in combination with hydrochlorothiazide lowers high blood pressure in male but not female spontaneously hypertensive rats," *Nutrients.*, vol. 15, p. 3180, 2023, doi: 10.3390/nu15143180.

[125] R. Mao et al., "Naked oat (Avena nuda L.) oligopeptides: Immunomodulatory effects on innate and adaptive immunity in mice via cytokine secretion, antibody production, and Th cells stimulation," *Nutrients.*, vol. 11, p. 927, 2019, doi: 10.3390/nu11040927.

[126] W. Pan et al., "Oat-derived β-glucans induced trained immunity through metabolic reprogramming," *Inflammation.*, vol. 43, pp. 1323–1336, 2020, doi: 10.1007/s10753-020-01211-2.

[127] F.-L. Liu, C.-L. Chen and C.-H. Huang, "Preparation of fermented oat milk and evaluation of its modulatory effect on antigen-specific immune responses in ovalbumin-sensitized mice," *Food Agric. Immunol.*, vol. 33, pp. 722–735, 2022, doi: 10.1080/09540105.2022.2120851.

[128] R. Akkerman et al., "Endo-1,3(4)-β-glucanase-treatment of oat β-glucan enhances fermentability by infant fecal microbiota, stimulates dectin-1 activation and attenuates inflammatory responses in immature dendritic cells," *Nutrients.*, vol. 12, p. 1660, 2020, doi: 10.3390/nu12061660.

[129] E. Żyła et al., "Anti-inflammatory activity of oat beta-glucans in a Crohn's disease model: Time- and molar mass-dependent effects," *Int. J. Mol. Sci.*, vol. 22, p. 4485, 2021, doi: 10.3390/ijms22094485.

[130] R. Duan et al., "Flavonoids from whole-grain oat alleviated high-fat diet-induced hyperlipidemia via regulating bile acid metabolism and gut microbiota in mice," *J. Agric. Food Chem.*, vol. 69, pp. 7629–7640, 2021, doi: 10.1021/acs.jafc.1c01813.

[131] L. Dong, C. Qin, Y. Li, Z. Wu and L. Liu, "Oat phenolic compounds regulate metabolic syndrome in high fat diet-fed mice via gut microbiota," *Food Biosci.*, vol. 50, p. 101946, 2022, doi: 10.1016/j.fbio.2022.101946.

[132] J. Bai et al., "Oat β-glucan alleviates DSS-induced colitis via regulating gut microbiota metabolism in mice," *Food Funct.*, vol. 12, pp. 8976–8993, 2021, doi: 10.1039/D1FO01446C.

[133] Y. Li et al., "Whole grain benefit: Synergistic effect of oat phenolic compounds and β-glucan on hyperlipidemia via gut microbiota in high-fat-diet mice," *Food Funct.*, vol. 13, pp. 12686–12696, 2022, doi: 10.1039/D2FO01746F.

[134] D. Xu et al., "The prebiotic effects of oats on blood lipids, gut microbiota, and short-chain fatty acids in mildly hypercholesterolemic subjects compared with rice: A randomized, controlled trial," *Front. Immunol.*, vol. 12, 2021, Accessed: Nov. 8, 2023. [Online]. Available: www.frontiersin.org/articles/10.3389/fimmu.2021.787797

[135] H. Guo et al., "Oat β-D-glucan ameliorates type II diabetes through TLR4/PI3K/AKT mediated metabolic axis," *Int. J. Biol. Macromol.*, vol. 249, 2023, p. 126039, doi: 10.1016/j.ijbiomac.2023.126039.

[136] T. Hjorth et al., "Sixteen-week multicentre randomised controlled trial to study the effect of the consumption of an oat beta-glucan-enriched bread versus a whole-grain wheat bread on glycaemic control among persons with pre-diabetes: A study protocol of the CarbHealth study," *BMJ Open.*, vol. 12, p. e062066, 2022, doi: 10.1136/bmjopen-2022-062066.

[137] J. L. Pino, V. Mujica and M. Arredondo, "Effect of dietary supplementation with oat β-glucan for 3 months in subjects with type 2 diabetes: A randomized, double-blind, controlled clinical trial," *J. Funct. Foods.*, vol. 77, p. 104311, 2021, doi: 10.1016/j.jff.2020.104311.

[138] X. L. Shen, T. Zhao, Y. Zhou, X. Shi, Y. Zou and G. Zhao, "Effect of oat β-glucan intake on glycaemic control and insulin sensitivity of diabetic patients: A meta-analysis of randomized controlled trials," *Nutrients.*, vol. 8, p. 39, 2016, doi: 10.3390/nu8010039.

β-Glucan
Role in Health Promotion and Disease Prevention

7

Maharishi Tomar, Prabha Singh, Ishwar Singh,
Rakesh Bhardwaj, Ajeet Singh Dhaka,
Prince Choyal, Archana Sachdev, Anil Dahuja,
Awnindra Kumar Singh, Vijay Kumar Yadav,
and Veda Krishnan

7.1 INTRODUCTION

The mixed-linkage polysaccharide (1→3) (1→4)-β-d-glucan (β-glucan), found in cereals exhibits numerous functions and characteristics that set it apart as both a distinctive component of plant cell walls and a dietary fibre. Oat β-glucan is formed by the bonding of glucose molecules through (1→3) and (1→4) linkages, resulting in a linear structure. Specifically, the β-(1→3, 1→4) glucan found in oats is commonly referred to as oat β-glucan. In this structure, more than 85% of oat β-glucan molecules feature one β-(1→3) glycosidic bond positioned between every 2 and 3 β-(1→4) glycosidic bonds. The remaining 15% of oat β-glucan is made up of long-chain β-(1→4) glycosidic bonds separated by a single β-(1→3) glycosidic bond. These long-chain segments may contain four, five, or eight glucose residues [1]. β-Glucans are large polysaccharide molecules composed of D-glucose units linked through β-glycosidic bonds, found extensively in

DOI: 10.1201/ 9781003263302-7

both microorganisms and plants. The most prevalent β-glucans found in cereals include betafectin (PGG), krestin (PSK), schizophyllan (SPG), lentinan, and zymosan (MG). Various origins of β-glucans result in distinct physicochemical and structural characteristics. The variations in side-chain length and distribution in β-glucans are primarily influenced by the β-glucan source and extraction method employed [2]. Nonetheless, the most suitable extraction method is contingent upon the specific origin and structures of β-glucans. β-Glucans are commonly categorized into insoluble and soluble forms, and this classification is associated with their degree of polymerization (DP). β-Glucans with DPs exceeding 100 are typically entirely insoluble in water [3].

Zhang et al. [4] conducted a study involving hot water extraction, enzymatic purification, membrane separation, and the Douglas method to determine the content of various soluble non-starch polysaccharides in different grains. Their findings revealed that oats had the highest level of soluble non-starch polysaccharides, measuring 35.92 g/kg, followed by barley (35.48 g/kg), rye (32.19 g/kg), wheat (21.85 g/kg), rice (26.41 g/kg), and corn (16.61 g/kg). The β-glucan content in oat grains ranged from 2.3% to 3.2%, with an average molecular weight within the range of 1.73 to 2.02 × 10⁶ g/mol.

Both soluble and insoluble β-glucans find diverse applications in various aspects of daily life. For instance, they are employed in beverages to modify texture by providing a thickening effect. Additionally, they serve as food additives in products like milk, yoghurt, and bread to help lower calorie intake and reduce cholesterol levels [5], [6]. Furthermore, β-glucans are crucial as functional ingredients in the production of nutritious and health-promoting products. They are also incorporated into certain medicinal formulations to investigate new pharmaceuticals with additional functions within the pharmaceutical sector. Moreover, β-glucans are utilized in cosmetics due to their wound-healing, anti-ageing benefits, and moisturizing properties [7]. Oat β-glucan, in particular, has been extensively studied and has demonstrated several health benefits. It has been shown to lower blood lipid and cholesterol levels, regulate blood sugar levels, enhance immune function, exhibit antitumour activity, and help prevent cardiovascular diseases. β-glucan has the capability to target and destroy malignant tumour cells, including sarcoma cells and melanocytes. Importantly, its inhibition rate against liver cancer, breast cancer, and bowel cancer is comparable to that of anticancer drugs, all while not exhibiting any adverse side effects. The potential therapeutic properties of β-glucans have been categorized into two main groups: immune-modulating effects and metabolic and gastrointestinal effects.

The discovery of oat β-glucan in oat kernels was initially documented by Morris et al. [8]. A comparable polysaccharide in barley, with its notable role in malt and beer production, spurred substantial research into barley (1→3) (1→4)-β-d-glucan. However, until the 1980s, no similar impetus existed for comparable research on oats. During the 1980s, clinical studies suggested that incorporating rolled oats and oat bran into one's diet could potentially reduce serum cholesterol levels. This discovery sparked a surge of interest in oat (and barley) β-glucan and foods containing these components. Drawing from research on the capacity of viscous, water-soluble polysaccharides like guar gum to mitigate blood glucose and insulin levels and decrease serum cholesterol, it was proposed that the physiological effects of oats were attributed to β-glucan, a water-soluble viscous polysaccharide akin to guar gum [9]. It is widely acknowledged that for every 1% reduction in serum low-density lipoprotein (LDL) cholesterol levels, the risk of developing coronary heart disease diminishes by 1–2%, and reduced insulin levels decrease the risk of developing metabolic syndrome and insulin resistance.

β-Glucans play pivotal roles, particularly in the development of healthy foods and pharmaceutical products, owing to their well-documented beneficial effects. These effects encompass immunomodulation, antitumour properties, the reduction of serum cholesterol and glucose levels, as well as obesity prevention. In 2014, the Food Marketing Institute (FMI) reported that health and dietary supplement products containing β-glucans accounted for 33.7% of the global β-glucans market share. Numerous sources of this functional polysaccharide have been documented, including fungi, protozoa, bacteria, yeast, algae, and cereals such as oats, barley, rye, and wheat, among others. Cereal-derived β-glucans continue to dominate total production, with yeast being another significant source of β-glucans, followed by β-glucans obtained from mushrooms. β-glucan derived from bacteria, protozoans, and algae typically possesses a linear structure with β-(1,3) glycosidic bonds linking glucose monomers, whereas β-glucan from other sources exhibits a branched structure [10]. Cereal-based β-glucan is characterized by β-(1,3/1,4) glycosidic bonds, whereas fungal-based β-glucan features β-(1,3/1,6) glycosidic bonds [11]. These structural arrangements, involving different glycosidic linkage positions (1,3), (1,4), or (1,6), either in a branched or unbranched (linear) form, determine how β-glucan functions and affects underlying medical conditions through various mechanisms. β-glucans with (1,3)/(1,6) glycosidic linkages are recognized by pattern recognition receptors and play a role in modulating immune functions. In contrast, cereal-based β-glucan containing (1,4) glycosidic linkages does not trigger immune responses but exerts its effects by modulating viscosity [12].

In addition to the various sources of β-glucan, the processing techniques employed during the extraction, purification, and functionalization, including chromatography, mechanical or enzymatic digestion, extrusion, heating, drying and the incorporation of functional moieties, have been observed to influence the physicochemical properties of β-glucans. These properties include molecular weight, solubility, concentration, viscosity, gel formation, branching, and glycosidic linkage, among others [13]. It has been found that these physicochemical properties of β-glucans can significantly determine their physiological effects. Comprehensive information on various aspects of β-glucans has already been compiled and summarized by Zhu et al. [14], including their production and industrial applications, modifications [15], and their characteristics [16].

In the present chapter, we have provided a comprehensive summary of the β-glucan extraction, factors that influence their diverse physicochemical properties and how these properties, in turn, impact the physiological effects of β-glucans in regulating human health. Additionally, we have compiled and presented in-depth details regarding the clinical applications of specific β-glucans in managing aspects such as wound care, metabolic dysbiosis, disorders related to fatty liver, and their role in supporting energy metabolism during endurance training.

7.2 β-GLUCANS AS DIETARY FIBRE

Dietary fibre refers to the components in plants or similar carbohydrates that resist digestion and absorption in the human small intestine, undergoing either complete or partial fermentation in the large intestine (AACC, 2001). In a simplified classification based on digestibility in the gastrointestinal tract, carbohydrates are divided into two groups. The first group, which includes starches, simple sugars, and fructans, is easily broken down through enzymatic reactions and absorbed in the small intestine. These components are categorized as non-structural carbohydrates, non-fibrous polysaccharides, or simple carbohydrates. The second group, consisting of cellulose, hemicellulose, lignin, pectin, and β-glucans, resists digestion in the small intestine and requires bacterial fermentation in the large intestine. These components are often referred to as complex carbohydrates, non-starch polysaccharides, or structural carbohydrates. Non-starch polysaccharides make up the primary constituents of dietary fibre [17]. Dietary fibre can be classified based on solubility in water (soluble vs. insoluble fibre), susceptibility to microbial fermentation in the large intestine (fermentable vs. non-fermentable fibres), and viscosity (viscous or gel-forming vs. nonviscous fibres). These properties influence the therapeutic effects of fibre consumption [18]. Soluble fibres dissolve in water and typically form a gel-like substance. They traverse the small intestine without digestion and are readily fermented by the microflora in the large intestine. Soluble fibres can be further categorized into viscous (gel-forming) and nonviscous types [19]. They can be found in oat and barley products, certain vegetables, fruits, and legumes such as dry beans, peas, and lentils. On the other hand, insoluble fibres like cellulose, hemicellulose, and lignin are a significant part of dietary fibres. They are present in wheat bran, whole grain bread, cereals, and some vegetables like cabbage and Brussels sprouts. Insoluble fibres do not form a gel-like substance, and their fermentation is limited [20]. Maintaining an adequate level of dietary fibre in one's diet is crucial for promoting overall health and protecting against certain diseases. It's important to note that different types of dietary fibre have distinct effects [21]. Soluble fibres are known to be particularly effective in managing conditions such as diabetes, obesity, dyslipidemia, and hypertension, especially when compared to insoluble fibres. Soluble fibres have specific properties that contribute to these benefits. They delay the emptying of the stomach, slow down the processes of digestion and absorption, and encourage the production of short-chain fatty acids by the bacteria in the large intestine due to their high fermentability [22]. These properties of soluble fibres make them valuable for regulating blood sugar levels, managing weight, improving lipid profiles, and controlling blood pressure. Consequently, incorporating soluble fibre-rich foods into one's diet can play a significant role in maintaining and promoting good health.

7.3 ß-GLUCANS AND THEIR CHARACTERISTICS

β-glucans are a diverse group of non-starch polysaccharides made up of D-glucose units linked by β-glycosidic bonds [23]. These β-glucans exist in various forms, comprising short and medium chains with $(1{\rightarrow}3)/(1{\rightarrow}4)$ and $(1{\rightarrow}3)/(1{\rightarrow}6)$ bonds, depending on their source [12]. The macromolecular structures of β-glucans can vary significantly based on their origin and how they are isolated [24]. In grains, β-glucans are characterized by $\beta(1{\rightarrow}3/1{\rightarrow}4)$ bonds, whereas in the cell walls of yeast and fungi, they feature $\beta\,(1{\rightarrow}3/1{\rightarrow}6)$ bonds [25] (Figure 7.1). The type of bonds, branching patterns, degree of branching, helical formations, molecular weights, polymer concentrations, water

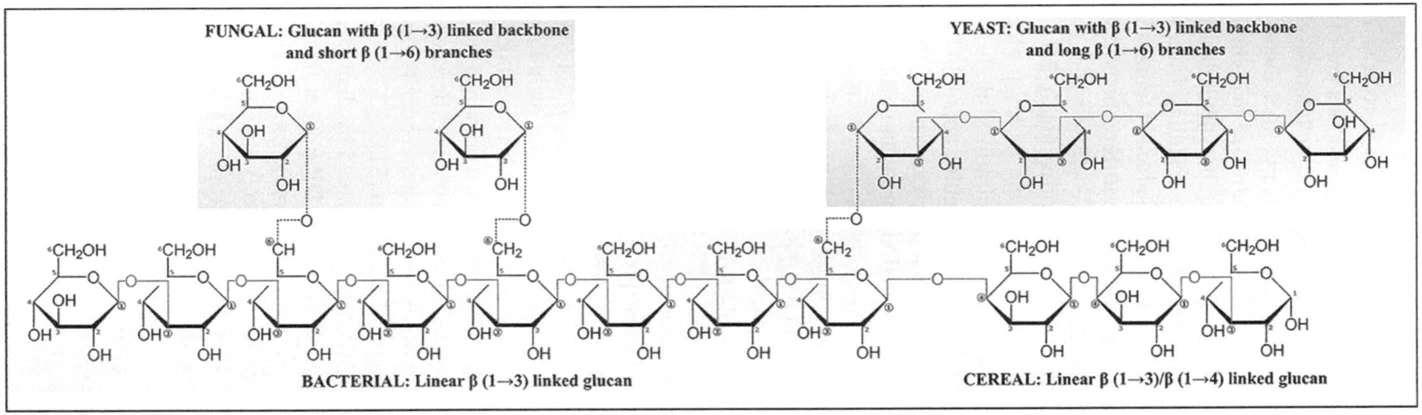

FIGURE 7.1   The structural diversity of β-glucans. This figure presents a comparative overview of β-glucans sourced from fungi, yeast, bacteria, and cereals, highlighting distinctive structural features. Fungal β-glucans exhibit a β (1→3) linked backbone with short β (1→6) branches, while yeast counterparts display a similar β (1→3) linked backbone but with long β (1→6) branches. Bacterial β-glucans present a linear β (1→3) linked structure, and cereal β-glucans showcase a linear β (1→3)/β (1→4) linked arrangement. This structural comparison provides valuable insights into the molecular diversity of β-glucans from different biological origins, contributing to a deeper understanding of their potential functional roles and applications in various fields.

solubility, and ring conformations in a solution can all vary among β-glucans, and these variations impact their biological activities [26].

Cereal (1→3)(1→4)-β-d-glucans, consist of approximately 70% (1→4)-linked and 30% (1→3)-linked β-d-glucopyranosyl residues. These residues are organized predominantly in a sequence of β-(1→3)-linked cellotriosyl and cellotetraosyl units. Structural analysis of β-glucans is made simpler compared to many other dietary fibres by utilizing the specific (1→3)(1→4)-β-d-glucan-4-glucanohydrolase in combination with High-Performance Anion Exchange Chromatography [27]. This method provides a structural fingerprint by analysing the oligosaccharide fragments resulting from the specific cleavage of the (1→4)-linked 3-substituted glucose. The β-glucans found in oats, barley, rye, and wheat, as well as the non-cereal lichenan, can be differentiated by variations in the ratios of the major hydrolysis products, namely 3-*O*-β-cellobiosyl-d-glucose and 3-*O*-β-cellotriosyl-d-glucose [28], [29]. These ratios are approximately 2:1, 3:1, 3:1, 4:1, and 20:1, respectively. Enzymatic digestion of both oat and barley β-glucans produces, in addition to 3-*O*-β-cellobiosyl-d-glucose and 3-O-β-cellotriosyl-d-glucose, soluble oligosaccharides with a DP of up to about 9 or 10. Additionally, about 3–4% of the product is insoluble, with approximately 40% of this insoluble fraction being oligosaccharides with a DP of 9. These oligosaccharides resemble cellodextrins and each one is capped at the reducing end by a single (1→3)-linked glucose. They originate from regions of the molecule that resemble cellulose, characterized by more than three consecutive (1→4)-linkages. Among the major cereal crops in commercial production, oats and barley are the primary sources of significant β-glucan content, typically ranging from 3% to 5% on a dry weight basis. However, certain oat cultivars can contain as much as 6% to 7% β-glucan within the groat, while some barley varieties may have 12% or even higher levels. β-glucan is primarily found in the cell walls of the endosperm [30]. During the milling process, these cell walls exhibit resistance to attrition, and subsequent steps such as sieving or other particle separation methods result in coarser particle fractions that are enriched in β-glucan. These milling techniques can yield fractions with β-glucan contents of approximately 20%. For even greater enrichment of β-glucan, specialized extraction techniques are employed. Fungal and yeast-derived β-glucans consist of β(1→3) glycopyranocile molecules with side branches linked by β(1→6) bonds, which give them a branched structure. In contrast, oat and barley β-glucans lack side branches. These structural differences result in distinct functions for β-glucans. The β-bonds within the polymer render β-glucans indigestible, but they undergo fermentation in the caecum and colon [31].

The solubility of β-glucans is significantly influenced by their structural characteristics. Highly polymerized (1→3) β-glucans, with a DP greater than 100, do not fully dissolve in water. Solubility decreases as the polymerization grade decreases. Additionally, the composition of side branches attached to β-glucan molecules plays a role in determining their solubility [32]. The viscosity properties of β-glucans are dependent on factors such as molecular weight, solubility, and concentration. β-glucans with high molecular weights exhibit greater viscosity compared to those with low molecular weights [33]. Oat β-glucan, for example, has a higher molecular weight than barley β-glucan [34]. The primary mechanism attributed to the cholesterol and blood glucose-lowering effects of β-glucans is the increase in intestinal viscosity. β-glucans stand out in terms of their positive health effects compared to other soluble and fermentable dietary fibres because they can create highly viscous solutions at lower concentrations (1%) and maintain stability across a range of pH levels.

β-glucans naturally occur in the cell walls of plants, grain seeds, and certain fungi, yeasts, algae, and bacteria. Polysaccharides belonging to the β-D-glucan group, which exhibit activities in modifying biological responses, can be sourced from three primary origins: (i) Fungal Mycelia/Cell Wall Materials: These polysaccharides are obtained from fungal sources such as yeasts and mushrooms. The extraction process involves sequential steps, beginning with the use of solvents for the selective removal of lipids. Subsequently, the defatted mycelia are treated with cold and hot water, acid, and alkalis to extract the cell wall polysaccharides. Enzymes are employed to further purify the final polysaccharide products [35]. (ii) Cereal Brans (Oat, Barley): β-glucans can also be extracted from cereal brans, specifically oats and barley, using similar extractive procedures as those applied to fungal sources [36]. (iii) Submerged Fermentation (SmF) of Microorganisms: In this approach, microorganisms like bacteria and fungi are cultivated in submerged fermentation conditions, typically on carbohydrate substrates such as glucose or sucrose [37]. The exopolysaccharides present in the cell-free fermentation broths are then recovered through precipitation with alcohol [12]. These methods enable the isolation and purification of β-D-glucans from different sources, making them available for various applications, including their potential use in modifying biological responses.

Significant quantities of cereal β-glucans can be generated through agricultural processes, and there is a substantial supply of spent brewers' yeasts, primarily *Saccharomyces cerevisiae*, which can be commercially utilized for the extraction of cell wall β-glucans. Regrettably, except for xanthan, only limited commercial volumes of exopolysaccharides are currently derived from submerged fermentation. Nevertheless, it is important to recognize that this biotechnological method holds tremendous potential for the large-scale production of exocellular polysaccharides, including β-glucans, through scaled-up industrial fermentations. Importantly, these industrial-scale fermentation processes can be carried out in an environmentally sustainable manner, making them a promising avenue for increasing the production of these polysaccharides [38].

Various sources can be used to obtain β-glucans, including fungi (*Schizophyllum commune, Lentinus edodes*, and *Coriolus versicolor*), bread yeast (*Saccharomyces cerevisiae*), algae, and some bacteria (*Agrobacterium* sp., *Alcaligenes faecalis*). They are primarily found in the endosperm cell walls of oats and barley (constituting approximately 75%) and in bran (approximately 10.4%). Among grains, barley has the highest reported β-glucan content, ranging from 2 to 20 g/100 g of dry weight, with 65% being soluble. Oats also contain significant β-glucan, ranging from 3 to 8 g/100 g of dry weight, with 82% being soluble. In contrast, other grains generally have much lower β-glucan levels, such as rice (0.13 g), hard wheat (0.5–0.6 g), wheat (0.5–1.0 g), triticale (0.3–1.2 g), corn (0.8–1.7 g), rye (1.3–2.7 g), and sorghum (1.1–6.2 g) [39].

7.4 ß-GLUCAN BIOCHEMISTRY

β-Glucans containing $(1\rightarrow3)(1\rightarrow4)$-linkages are typically found in the outer shell layer, known as bran, of cereal grain kernels such as barley, oats, and wheat. They are also present in the aleurone and starchy endosperm cell walls, typically accounting for 3 to 10% of the composition. These β-glucans are homopolysaccharides characterized by a linear, unbranched structure composed of D-glucose residues connected through (1→4)- and (1→3)- linkages [40]. The molecular structure consists of a block polymer made up of β-1,4-linked D-glucose residues, including cellotriose and cellotetraose, which are linked through β-1,3-linkages. The distribution of these linkages in these polysaccharides is approximately 70% (1→4)-glucose linkages and 30% (1→3)-linkages, and this distribution appears to be random. Studies indicate that oat and barley β-glucans primarily consist of β-(1→3)-linked cellotriosyl and β-(1 → 3)-linked cellotetraosyl units [12]. The molar ratios of these units can vary between oats (2:1) and barley (3:1), respectively. These units, organized in three consecutive block structures of β-(1→4)-linked cellotriosyl units, are believed to associate to form junction zones with a DP of 9. These junction zones may play a role in determining the rheological properties of these β-glucans [41]. The diverse molecular composition of β-glucans results in a wide range of molecular weights (MW), spanning from 10^3 to 10^5 g/mol, as reported by Luo et al. [42] and Varelas et al. [43]. Generally, bacterial β-glucans have MWs ranging from 2 to 30 × 10^5 g/mol, cereal β-glucans fall within the range of 0.5 to 2.5 × 10^5 g/mol, and yeast β-glucans have MWs ranging from 0.5 to 0.8 × 10^5 g/mol (Table 7.1).

The molecular structure composition and MW of β-glucans are closely linked to their physicochemical properties, including solubility and viscosity in solutions. Research, as reviewed by Han et al. [44], has shown that higher Mw β-glucans tend to exhibit increased viscosity, while lower Mw β-glucans tend to have reduced viscosity. In general, β-glucans consisting of d-glucose monomers linked through (1→3)/(1→4)-glycosidic bonds tend to form insoluble fibres. On the other hand, β-glucans composed of high-molecular-weight β-(1→3)/(1→6)-linked glucose monomers tend to create soluble and viscous fibres. This distinction in solubility has implications for various applications, including the stability of formulations, emulsifying properties, and the design of membrane-binding drug delivery systems, as noted by Cummings et al. [45].

In addition to the differences in sources, the methods used for the extraction and purification of β-glucans also lead to variations in their structure. These structural differences likely contribute to the diverse functionalities observed among β-glucans. These variations encompass molecular linkages, branching degree, MW, charge, solubility, and viscosity, as reported by Du et al. [46] and Varelas et al. [43]. It is probable that these variations in molecular structure and physicochemical properties result in different interactions with host systems, giving rise to specific properties of β-glucans and, consequently, diverse biological activities. Indeed, numerous studies have demonstrated various clinically significant and effective biological activities of β-glucans, as discussed in this chapter Daou et al. [47].

As previously discussed, β-glucans exhibit variations in their fine chemical structures, including the degree of branching with substituents. They can also differ in terms of molecular mass and conformation, which play a crucial role in their structure-function relationships [48], [49]. These variations include existing as random coils, single helices, or triple helices, and they significantly impact the biological functions of β-glucans. For instance, linear (1→3)-β-glucans like bacterial curdlan tend to have random coil conformations [50]. In contrast, branched (1→3)-β-glucans such as lentinan

TABLE 7.1 β-Glucan Types and Glycosidic Linkages

COMPONENT	CEREALS	BACTERIA	MUSHROOM	YEAST
Structure	(1→3) (1→4) β-1,4 glucan (linear)	(1→3) β-1,3 glucan (linear)	(1→3) (1→6) β-1,6 branch glucan (short branched)	(1→3) (1→6) β-1,6 branch glucan (long branched)
Source	Oat, barley, rye	*Bacillus* sp., *Aspergillus* sp	*Lentinula edodes, Pleurotus ostreatus, Agaricus Blazei Murill, Agaricus bisporus, Cantharella cibarius, Pleurotus eryngii, Pleurotus djamor*	*Saccharomyces cerevisiae, Candida albicans*
Isolated part	Surface of grain	Exopolysaccharide	Mycelium fruit body	Cell wall of yeast
Health benefits	Metabolic activities (cholesterol lowering, microbiota modulation, blood glucose reduction)	Metabolic activities (cholesterol lowering, microbiota modulation, blood glucose reduction)	Immunomodulatory functions (antimicrobial properties, immunomodulation, anticancer properties)	Immunomodulatmy functions (antimicrobial properties, immuno-modulation, anticancer properties)
Action mechanism	Dietary fibres	Dietary fibres	Pathogen-associated molecular patterns	Pathogen-associated molecular patterns

from *Lentinula edodes*, which feature single β-(1→6)-linked D-glucose substituents along the backbone chain, tend to form helical conformations due to the presence of hydrogen bonding in their side chains. These structural characteristics also influence the solubility of β-glucans in water [13]. Solubility in aqueous solutions is determined by various physical and chemical structural properties, and it is an important characteristic that affects the biological activity of β-glucans.

7.5 β-GLUCANS ISOLATION AND PURIFICATION FROM OATS

The isolation and purification of oat β-glucan can be a challenging process, but it has undergone ongoing development and refinement over the years. β-glucans can be extracted using various methods, with some common ones including hot water extraction, alkali extraction, enzyme extraction, acidic extraction, and other assisted extraction methods like ultrasound and microwave-assisted extraction. The process typically involves separating the dissolved proteins through isoelectric precipitation and then precipitating the β-glucan using substances like ammonium sulphate, 2-propanol, or ethanol. These steps help in obtaining purified β-glucan from oats. It's important to note that acid and alkali extraction methods can disrupt the viscosity of β-glucan, while hot water extraction tends to yield a higher extraction rate of water-soluble β-glucan. Furthermore, the yield and molecular weight of β-glucan obtained through alkali extraction are typically greater than those obtained through hot water extraction with the addition of enzymes like amylase or xylanase. Consequently, alkali and hot water extraction are considered more favourable methods. The extraction rate of β-glucan can be influenced by factors such as the type of grains, environmental conditions, and the specific extraction methods used. The extraction process typically involves several steps, including the use of ethanol to inhibit endogenous enzymes and remove free sugar, protein, and non-polar compounds. Subsequently, starch is treated with thermostable α-amylase for degradation, followed by extraction and concentration using water, alkali, or acid. Finally, ethanol, propanone, or ammonium sulphate is added to facilitate the extraction of β-glucan [36]. The extraction process for β-glucans from cereals often involves isolating proteins and starch. This is achieved by dissolving β-glucans in hot water and alkaline solutions, followed by separating the dissolved proteins through isoelectric precipitation. Residual starch is isolated through repeated precipitation and enzymatic hydrolysis, resulting in high purities of up to 99% (Figure 7.2).

To further purify crude β-glucan extracts, column chromatography and gel-filtration chromatography are commonly employed techniques. These methods help refine and isolate β-glucans for various applications [51]. For research purposes, further purification of oat β-glucan involves several methods. Repeated precipitations and enzymatic hydrolysis of residual starch are commonly used, leading to a purity level of up to 99% [52]. Bhatty et al. [53] employed a method using distilled water with an adjusted pH of 10 using 20% sodium carbonate to extract β-glucan from oat bran. This method yielded a higher extraction rate of 61%, with the separated fraction containing 84% β-glucan. Beer et al. [54] used a similar approach to extract oat β-glucan and further purified the preparations through dialysis, ultrafiltration, or alcohol precipitation. These methods resulted in preparations with β-glucan content ranging from 60% to 65%. Among the methods, dialysis produced a preparation with higher viscosity. Ahmad et al. [55] conducted acid, alkaline, and enzymatic extraction and purification of oat β-glucan. They found that enzymatic extraction was the most effective, as it not only yielded the highest quantity but also removed more starch, fat, and pentosans during the extraction process, along with a fair amount of minerals, without significantly affecting its physicochemical properties.

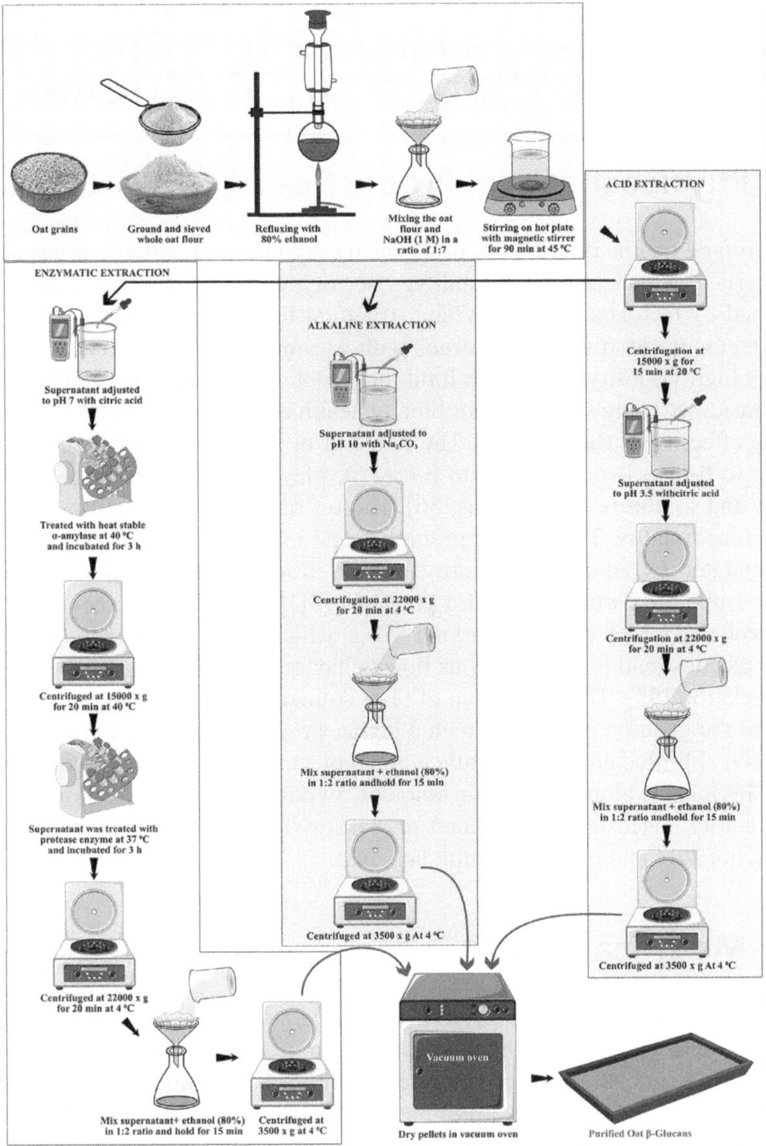

FIGURE 7.2 Comparative extraction methods for β-glucans. This figure illustrates three distinct extraction techniques employed for obtaining β-glucans from various biological sources: enzymatic extraction, alkaline extraction, and acid extraction. The enzymatic extraction method involves the use of specific enzymes to break down cell wall components, releasing β-glucans. In the alkaline extraction approach, an alkaline solution is utilized to solubilize and extract β-glucans. Acid extraction, on the other hand, employs acid treatments to hydrolyse cell wall components, facilitating the isolation of β-glucans. This visual representation highlights the diversity of methods available for extracting β-glucans, each with its unique advantages and considerations, contributing to the understanding of optimal extraction strategies for specific applications.

7.6 PHYSICOCHEMICAL PROPERTIES AND MODIFICATION OF OAT ß-GLUCANS

7.6.1 Physicochemical Properties of Oat ß-Glucans

The nutritional and health benefits of β-glucans are closely tied to their physicochemical properties, which include solubility, viscosity, and gelation. These properties are determined by factors such as MW and structural features. Different sources and processing methods can result in β-glucans with varying MWs. High-MW β-glucans tend to exhibit high viscosity, which can limit their applications. Soluble β-glucans are generally considered more beneficial for human health compared to insoluble ones, as they are more effective as dietary fibre. The ratios of different glycosidic linkages, such as β-(1→3) to β-(1→4) or β-(1→3) to β-(1→6), play a crucial role in determining the viscosity and solubility of β-glucans [56]. These structural characteristics are important for their functionality. The textural properties and melting profiles of β-glucan gels can be manipulated by adjusting the ratios of MW fractions. Rheological properties can help determine the particle sizes of β-glucans [57]. Different β-glucans extracted from oats, wheat, and barley can have varying MWs, which affect their behaviour. High-MW cereal β-glucans tend to show viscous flow behaviours, while lower MW materials can exhibit gelation [58]. The proportion of (1→3)-linked cellotriose units in the structure influences the gelation properties, with a higher proportion leading to more rapid gelation for cereal β-glucans [59]. To suffice, the molecular weight and structural characteristics of β-glucans, along with their ratios of glycosidic linkages, significantly impact their solubility, viscosity, and gelation properties. These properties, in turn, influence their functionality and potential health benefits.

7.6.2 Modification

In general, alterations in water solubility, chain conformation, and the incorporation of suitable ionic groups with the appropriate degree of substitution can lead to modifications in the bioactivities of polysaccharides [60]. β-Glucans, for instance, can undergo physical and chemical crosslinking reactions to enhance their bioavailability, yielding a range of derivatives with potential applications in industry and medicine [61]. Various techniques have been commonly employed to modify β-glucans, encompassing chemical methods like sulphation, carboxymethylation, and oxidation, as well as physical methods such as radiation, microwaves, and heating. These modification methods can be tailored to achieve specific desired outcomes in terms of molecular weight, polymerization, solubility, viscosity, gelation and other properties, making them versatile tools for optimizing the functionality of β-glucans for various applications (Table 7.2).

TABLE 7.2   Impact of β-Glucan Modifications on Biological Functions

MODIFICATION TYPE	MODIFICATION METHOD	SOURCE	BOND	BIOLOGICAL FUNCTION	REFERENCE
Physical	Gamma irradiation	Oat (*Avena sativa*)	(1→3) (1→4)-β-d-glucan	Hypoglycaemic, anti-cancer, antioxidant, anticancer activity	[62]
	Gamma irradiation	Yeast (*Saccharomyces cerevisiae*)	(1→3) (1→6)-β-d-glucan	Plant growth promotion	[63]
	Microwave	Barley (*Hordeum vulgare* L)	(1→3) (1→4)-β-d-glucan	Antioxidant	[64]
	Ultrasound-degradation	*Cordyceps sinensis* Cs-HK1	(1→3) (1→6)-β-d-glucan	Moisturizing	[65]
	Drying	Yeast (*Saccharomyces cerevisiae*)	(1→3) (1→4)-β-d-glucan	Immunomodulatory	[66]
Chemical	Acid degradation	Yeast (*Saccharomyces cerevisiae*)	(1→3) (1→6)-β-d-glucan	Immunomodulatory	[67]
	Sulphation	Yeast (*Saccharomyces cerevisiae*)	(1→3) (1→6)-β-d-glucan	Immunomodulatory	[68]
	Sulphation	Mushroom (*Russula virescens*)	(1→3) (1→6)-β-d-glucan	Antitumour	[69]
	Carboxymethylation	Mushroom (*Pleurotus tuber-regium*)	(1→3) (1→6)-β-d-glucan	Antitumour	[70]
	Carboxymethylation	Fungus (*Lasiodiplodia theobromae*)	(1→3) (1→6)-β-d-glucan	Immunomodulatory	[15]
	Phosphorylation	Yeast (*Saccharomyces cerevisiae*)	(1→3) (1→6)-β-d-glucan	Immunomodulatory	[71]
	Carboxymethylation–sulphation	*Poria cocos*	(1→3) (1→6)-β-d-glucan	Immunomodulatory	[72]
	Acetylation	Oat (*Avena sativa*)	(1→3) (1→4)-β-d-glucan	Increased bile acid binding capacity	[73]

7.6.3 Chemical Modifications

Sulphated polysaccharides are widely distributed in nature. Polysaccharides that are insoluble in water typically exhibit limited bioactivity, whereas their water-soluble sulphated derivatives demonstrate significant antitumour and antiviral properties [74]. The process of sulphation can enhance the water solubility of β-glucans, making them suitable for various applications in the food and pharmaceutical industries to improve texture. Moreover, numerous studies have highlighted the health benefits associated with sulphated β-glucans, including antimicrobial, antithrombotic, antiherpetic [75], anticoagulant [76], and immunomodulatory effects [77]. Sulphated natural glucan derived from *Phellinus ribis* has been shown to possess antiangiogenic activity, which is crucial in controlling the growth, metastasis, and prognosis of malignant solid tumours. Similarly, Tao et al. [60] reported that sulphated derivatives exhibit relatively higher in vitro antitumour activity against the human hepatic cancer cell line HepG2 compared to native water-soluble hyper-branched β-glucan. The introduction of sulphate groups is the primary factor responsible for enhancing this antitumour activity.

The carboxymethylation of β-glucans is recognized as a promising chemical modification due to its potential to enhance health benefits compared to unmodified β-glucans. Research has shown that carboxymethylated β-glucan from yeast (CM-G) has a positive impact on vascular function, particularly in NO-dependent responses. Notably, CM-G exhibits a higher selectivity than native β-glucan when it comes to inhibiting adenosine diphosphate-induced platelet aggregation [78]. Similarly, carboxymethylated glucan extracted from *Saccharomyces cerevisiae* has been found to induce vasodilation through the NOS/NO/SCG pathway and display negative inotropic effects in rats. Studies conducted by Chen et al. [65] have emphasized the crucial role played by the type of substituent and the degree of substitution in determining the bioactivities of β-glucan derivatives. Furthermore, Kogan et al. [79] have reported on the radical scavenging activity of carboxymethylated β-glucan in vivo using an adjuvant arthritis model. This finding suggests the potential medicinal applications of this glucan derivative in the treatment of arthritis.

Modifications of β-glucans, which involve oxidation and chemical degradation, have also been documented. For instance, oat-derived β-glucans underwent chemical modification through a process mediated by 2,2,6,6-tetramethyl-1-piperidine oxoammonium ions, leading to selective oxidation of the C6 primary hydroxyl groups and their conversion into carboxyl groups. This oxidation increased the water solubility of oat β-glucan. The oxidized oat β-glucan has shown potential as an active ingredient for lowering cholesterol levels [80]. Furthermore, low-MW soluble yeast glucan, which has undergone acid degradation (ad-sBBG-low), can modulate immunity by binding to dectin-1, an innate immunity receptor specific to β-glucan. This binding leads to antagonistic effects against reactive oxygen production and cytokine synthesis by macrophages, thereby influencing immune responses [81].

7.6.4 Physical Modifications

In the context of physical modifications applied to β-glucans, gamma irradiation has demonstrated its capacity to induce the formation of low-MW β-glucan from barley.

This modified β-glucan exhibits heightened antioxidant and antiproliferative properties when tested against human cancer cell lines Colo-205, T47D, and MCF7 [82]. Similarly, low-MW oat β-glucan, subjected to gamma irradiation, also displays altered biological effects. Specifically, gamma-irradiated oat β-glucan exhibits greater cytotoxicity against colo-205 and MCF7 cancer cells in comparison to T47D cells. Remarkably, no cytotoxicity is observed when normal cell lines are exposed to this modified β-glucan at all tested concentrations [62]. Additionally, microwave modification can alter the structural and physicochemical properties of β-glucan derived from barley, leading to an enhancement in its antioxidant potential. Structural analysis has revealed that this process involves the cleavage of the polymeric chain and glycosidic linkages within β-glucan [64]. Furthermore, when solubilized yeast β-glucan (hd-sBBG) is heated at 135 °C for several hours, it demonstrates antagonistic activity against reactive oxygen production and cytokine synthesis in macrophages. This procedure holds significance in the production of immunomodulating soluble yeast β-glucan [81].

7.7 BIOLOGICAL FUNCTIONS OF OAT ß-GLUCANS

Typical (1→3) (1→4)-β-glucans found in cereals have garnered significant interest due to their notable effects, such as reducing blood glucose and cholesterol levels, which can be beneficial for individuals dealing with obesity and cardiovascular disease (CVD). On the other hand, (1→3) (1→6)-β-glucans originating from microorganisms tend to exhibit more pronounced antitumour, anti-inflammatory, and antiviral activities, making them particularly valuable in the context of immune system-related diseases (Figure 7.3 and Table 7.3).

7.7.1 Gastrointestinal Effects of Oat ß-Glucan

Both soluble and insoluble oat fibres exert gastrointestinal effects through distinct mechanisms. Soluble fibre primarily acts by virtue of its capacity for high swelling and water-binding. It also serves as a substrate in fermentations within the colon. On the other hand, insoluble fibre exerts its influence through its bulking effect. The gastrointestinal effects of oat β-glucan have been extensively reviewed by Mälkki et al. [91]. In the stomach, oat β-glucan exhibits a smaller hydrodynamic size, and its aggregates appear to be reduced or disrupted. This behaviour change could be attributed to the low pH environment in the stomach, as no significant alteration was observed when pepsin, an enzyme present in the stomach, was absent [92].

Ulmius et al. [93] conducted a study in which they found that the release of oat β-glucan was primarily attributed to gastric digestion. They also observed that the process of milling the oat particles into smaller sizes significantly improved the releasability of β-glucan, increasing it from 20% to 55%. Additionally, this milling process reduced the protein and starch content to 5% and decreased fat content to 45%. Another study by Wang et al. [94] indicated that the rate of β-glucan recovery increased to 90%

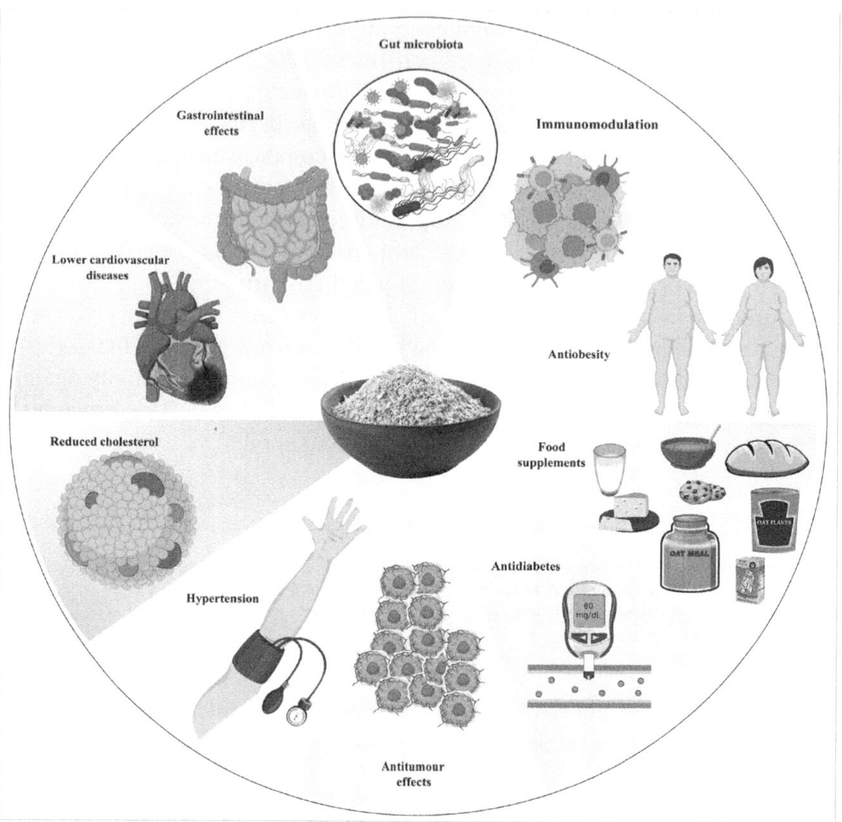

FIGURE 7.3   Multifaceted biological functions of oat β-glucans. This figure encapsulates the diverse range of biological functions associated with oat β-glucans, reflecting their potential health-promoting properties. Oat β-glucans have been implicated in fostering a healthy gut microbiota, influencing gastrointestinal functions, and modulating immune responses. Additionally, they exhibit effects on cardiovascular health by potentially lowering the risk of cardiovascular diseases and reducing cholesterol levels. Their antitumour properties, along with potential antidiabetic effects, underscore their significance in disease prevention. Furthermore, oat β-glucans are explored for their role in food supplements, showcasing versatility in dietary applications. The figure aims to comprehensively illustrate the multifaceted impact of oat β-glucans across various health domains, contributing to their recognition as valuable bioactive compounds with wide-ranging health benefits.

after microwave heating, compared to 75% for samples treated using conventional dissolution methods. This improvement was attributed to the large particle size of β-glucan aggregates in the sample, which was reduced or disrupted after microwave heating, ultimately leading to a higher recovery of β-glucan.

In their study to quantify the viscosity of soluble and insoluble fibres in various concentrations of solution, Dikeman et al. [95] investigated the effects of altering shear rate on the viscosity of these solutions. They also explored the impacts of fibre source, incubation time, and shear rate on the viscosity of solutions using a two-stage in vitro

TABLE 7.3 Oat ß-Glucan in Metabolic Disorders Management

METABOLIC ISSUE	ß-GLUCAN SOURCE	DOSE	MODEL USED	SALIENT FINDINGS	REFERENCES
Obesity, cholesterol levels, diabetes	Oat	3 to 5 g per day	Four groups of human subjects (n = 15 each), 6 weeks	Significant improvements were observed in the following parameters: total cholesterol levels, LDL cholesterol levels, VLDL cholesterol levels, triglyceride levels, alanine aminotransferase levels, aspartate aminotransferase levels, haemoglobin A1c levels, insulin levels, systolic blood pressure (SBP), total body fat percentage (TBF%), visceral fat percentage, as well as waist and hip circumferences	[83]
Obesity, cholesterol levels	Oat	2.5 g per day	29 (T2D) human subjects; 8 weeks	Low-density lipoprotein (VLDL-C) cholesterol and diastolic blood pressure decreased, improving lipid and glucose homeostasis in overweight/obese subjects	[84]
Obesity, cholesterol levels	Oat	1 g/kg body weight	30 male C57BL/6 J mice, 10-week	The serum lipid profile, encompassing triglycerides, total cholesterol, high-density lipoprotein cholesterol, and low-density lipoprotein cholesterol levels, exhibited significant improvements. Additionally, there was a noticeable reduction in the size of epididymal adipocytes. Moreover, water-insoluble ß-glucan played a role in decreasing lipid accumulation and expediting lipid decomposition in the liver	[85]
Obesity, cholesterol levels, cardio-vascular disease (CVD)	Oat	3 g per day	207 human sub-jects; 4 weeks	Incorporating a drink containing 1 g of high-molecular-weight oat ß-glucan three times daily over four weeks resulted in a noteworthy reduction of approximately 6% in LDL cholesterol levels and a corresponding decrease of approximately 8% in CVD risk among healthy adults with LDL cholesterol ranging from 3 to 5 mmol/L	[86]

(Continued)

TABLE 7.2   (Continued) Oat ß-Glucan in Metabolic Disorders Management

METABOLIC ISSUE	ß-GLUCAN SOURCE	DOSE	MODEL USED	SALIENT FINDINGS	REFERENCES
Cognitive behaviour, atherosclerosis, cholesterol levels	Oat	0.8% oat fibre, 14 weeks	Male low-density lipoprotein receptor knock-out (LDLR–/–) mice	Dietary oat fibre containing ß-glucan was found to slow down the advancement of cognitive decline in a mouse model of atherosclerosis. The underlying mechanism behind this neuroprotective effect was associated with oat fibre and its byproducts known as short-chain fatty acids (SCFAs). These compounds influenced the composition and quantity of gut microbiota, leading to the production of anti-inflammatory metabolites. This, in turn, resulted in the suppression of neuroinflammation and a decrease in gut permeability through the microbiome–gut–brain axis	[87]
Hypertension	Oat	305 mg/kg/day, 15 weeks	Male and female spontaneously hypertensive rats (SHR)	Administration of ß-glucan and hydrochlorothiazide (for hypertension treatment) exhibited distinct preventive effects on high blood pressure, and cardiac dysfunction, as well as changes in malondialdehyde, angiotensin II, and norepinephrine levels in 20-week-old male and female SHRs	[88]
Hypertension	Oat	15 weeks	Spontaneously (SHR) hypertensive rats	In addition to measuring oxidative stress and inflammation, the effects of various treatments were assessed. Beta-glucan, when administered alone, effectively prevented the elevation of systolic and diastolic blood pressure in SHR. In comparison to SHR treated solely with ß-glucan (excluding avenanthramide C or the combination), these animals exhibited reduced isovolumetric relaxation time. Furthermore, the combination of ß-glucan and avenanthramide C (phenolic antioxidant in oats) led to a decrease in malondialdehyde levels, which serves as a marker for oxidative stress, in SHR	[89]
Inflammation and oxidative stress	Oat	6 weeks	Sprague–Dawley rats	Increased lactic acid bacteria, glutathione, and lower IL-12 and TNF-α	[90]

digestion simulation model. The authors found that a short exposure time (1 to 2 hours) of oat bran to gastric fluids *in vitro*, as well as in pigs, increased the viscosity of the solution. This viscosity increase was attributed to the hydration of the substrate. However, with a longer exposure time, the viscosity decreased. This decrease could be attributed to the conditions within the gastric environment, which may have led to the breakdown of the polymeric structure of the fibres, resulting in reduced viscosity.

When oat dietary fibre is consumed, it starts to absorb water, swell, and dissolve, with the extent of these changes depending on its size and previous hydrothermal treatments. This increase in volume can lead to stomach distension, which in turn affects the sensation of satiety. However, data regarding the impact of oat fibre on stomach emptying are inconsistent. A common concept is that viscous dietary fibres slow down the rate of gastric emptying, while larger and coarser particles tend to leave the stomach more quickly (M¨alkki and others 2001).

In the small intestine of humans, β-glucan remains intact because mammalian enzymes are unable to hydrolyse it, thus contributing to an increase in viscosity. However, viscosity can also be enhanced by increased mucin production [91]. Some sources of both insoluble and soluble fibre have been shown to stimulate mucin production [96]. In pigs, the molecular weight of β-glucan decreases, especially in the distal portion of the small intestine, due to the action of bacterial enzymes. Despite physical barriers to hydration and enzymatic activity, intact remnants of plant tissues can still be observed. Individual variations in viscosity have been reported, ranging from 2 to 195 mPa·s, with the highest mean value (90 mPa·s) observed in the distal third of the small intestine three hours after a meal [97]. In human ileal effluents, it was found that 88.5% of the ingested β-glucan could be recovered, indicating that a significant portion of β-glucan remains intact throughout the digestive process.

The increase in the viscosity of β-glucans during digestion in the small intestine may indeed result from the formation of reorganized aggregates, as suggested by Grundy et al. [98]. Additionally, Grundy et al. [99] observed that pure β-glucan fractions underwent a significant increase in size during small intestine digestion. This phenomenon may be attributed to the fact that pure β-glucan was partially depolymerized during gastric digestion, and the resulting smaller polymers had a higher tendency to aggregate, leading to the formation of more condensed aggregates and, eventually, gel-like structures when the pH was neutralized, as described by Mäkelä et al. [100]. Several other studies, conducted in both humans and animals, have reported the depolymerization of β-glucan in the gastrointestinal tract, as noted by Karunaratne et al. [101]. However, it's important to acknowledge that Bai et al. [102] and colleagues, in their study in 2021, did not detect any degradation of oat β-glucan polymers under conditions similar to those of the human stomach. The discrepancies in findings across studies may be due to variations in factors such as the source of β-glucan, specific digestive conditions, and individual differences.

Following digestion in the small intestine, the molar mass of β-glucan increases, regardless of the presence or absence of bile acids or digestive enzymes. This suggests that there is no binding of β-glucan to bile acids or pepsin/pancreatin. Instead, the increase in aggregate size is likely a result of the normalization of pH (6.8). The molar mass, expressed in g/mol, for oat bran β-glucans, ranges from 10 to 100×10^6 g/mol. The formation of pure reformed aggregates results in a range of MWs (200 to 700×10^6 g/mol) for β-glucans, indicating that the aggregation of β-glucan can lead to the formation of aggregates with varying sizes.

The behaviour of β-glucan during gastrointestinal digestion highlights that various fibre fractions have distinct optimal acidification levels at which the polymers are released and viscosity increases. Beyond these optimal levels, the polymers can break down and lose their ability to create viscosity. Zhang et al. [103] have confirmed that β-glucan derived from pure fractions and oat bran exhibit different behaviours in the gastrointestinal tract and may operate through distinct mechanisms. The β-glucan aggregate from oat bran contributes to viscosity within the intestinal tract. In contrast, the pure β-glucans may potentially form gels that decrease the viscosity of the surrounding medium. This differentiation in behaviour suggests that the source and composition of β-glucans can influence their impact on the digestive process and viscosity.

In the large intestine, oat dietary fibre undergoes fermentation, similar to other dietary fibre sources. The primary fermentation products are short-chain fatty acids (SCFAs), which include acetic, propionic, and butyric acids. Oat dietary fibre is distinct from other sources due to its high fermentability and its capacity to yield higher amounts of butyric acid [104]. Oat β-glucan acts as a prebiotic, which is a non-digestible food ingredient that has a beneficial impact on the host by selectively stimulating the growth and/or activity of specific bacterial strains in the colon, ultimately contributing to improved host health [23]. β-Glucan itself decomposes in the large intestine. The increase in the dry weight of colon contents is primarily attributed to the growth of microbial cells, as evidenced in several studies. Microbial cell material also retains more water compared to insoluble fibre, leading to an increase in the water content of faeces (Figure 7.4).

To summarize, in the large intestine, β-glucan functions as a substrate that promotes the production of SCFAs. Its oligosaccharides have been shown to act as selective factors, encouraging the growth of specific bacterial strains. The beneficial effect on colon function is attributed to the increased production of microbial mass, which possesses good water retention properties, as well as the bulking effect of the insoluble components of the fibre.

7.7.2 Obesity-Overweight Condition

Obesity, defined as having a body mass index (BMI) exceeding 30 kg/m^2, is a significant risk factor for the development of various health issues, including cardiovascular diseases, type 2 diabetes, dyslipidemia, and several types of cancer. It typically occurs when there is an imbalance between caloric intake, which exceeds the body's energy expenditure. The distribution of body fat, particularly the presence of visceral white adipose tissue, is associated with the risk of metabolic dysfunction in individuals with obesity. In obesity, excess white adipose tissue consists of lipid-filled adipocytes stored in the body as an energy source. Dyslipidemia, characterized by abnormal lipid levels in the blood, is a common feature in overweight and obese individuals and is a crucial risk factor for cardiovascular-related diseases. The connection between obesity and dyslipidemia is closely related to the distribution of body fat, particularly visceral adipose tissue, and its impact on insulin resistance. After a meal, blood glucose levels typically rise as the body absorbs glucose from the intestine. In response, the body produces insulin to regulate blood glucose levels. β-Glucan, which remains undigested in the gut, promotes a gradual and sustained release of glucose derived from the diet into the bloodstream.

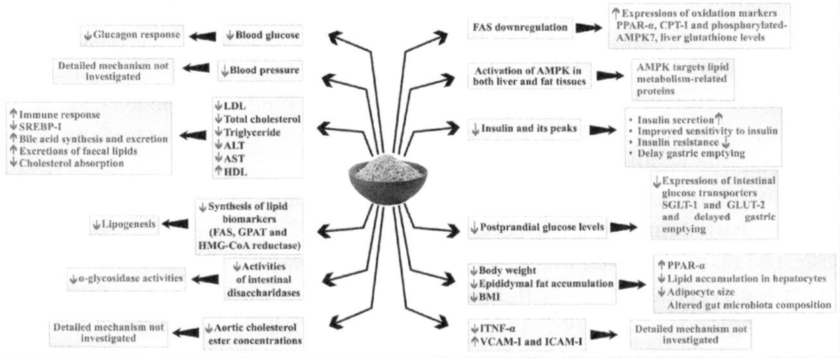

FIGURE 7.4 Bioactivity targets of oat-derived ß-glucans. This schematic representation illustrates the diverse bioactivities of oat-derived ß-glucans and their molecular targets. Oat ß-glucans demonstrate modulation of peroxisome proliferator-activated receptor-alpha (PPAR-α), impacting lipid metabolism through regulation of fatty acid synthase (FAS), glycerol-3-phosphate acyltransferase, and carnitine palmitoyltransferase I. They also influence sterol regulatory element-binding transcription factor 1, linking to lipid homeostasis. Oat ß-glucans exhibit anti-inflammatory effects by affecting vascular cell adhesion molecule, intracellular cell adhesion molecule, and tumour necrosis factor-α (TNF-α). Additionally, they may influence glucose homeostasis through interactions with sodium-glucose co-transporter 1 (SGLT) and glucose transporter 2 (GLUT-2). The figure comprehensively outlines the molecular pathways and targets involved in the bioactive functions of oat-derived ß-glucans, shedding light on their potential therapeutic applications in various health contexts.

This glucose is then available for the body's energy needs over an extended period. Consequently, this process helps control appetite, as low blood glucose levels are one of the hunger signals recognized by the body [105].

Oat grains contain various types of fibres, including β-glucans, which can influence the regulation of satiety by affecting the secretion of gut hormones such as ghrelin, GLP-1 (glucagon-like peptide-1), and leptin by adipocytes. These hormones play crucial roles in regulating energy balance and have the ability to impact multiple organs and tissues [106]. Additionally, the fermentation of dietary fibre in the colon leads to a decrease in pH levels, creating a more acidic environment. This change in pH promotes the growth and diversity of colonic bacteria, including different genera and species. As a result of this fermentation process, short-chain fatty acids (SCFA, including acetate, propionate, and butyrate) are produced. These SCFAs play a significant role in improving metabolic regulation and are critical in the prevention and treatment of CVDs [107].

Research has indeed indicated that β-glucans can contribute to reducing body weight. In a clinical trial, the use of barley β-glucan was found to have notable effects on weight management. Specifically, participants in the trial experienced reduced food intake and absorbed fewer nutrients, including glucose and lipids, from their diet. [108] conducted a study that examined the impact of cereal-based bread consumed during evening meals, varying in glycaemic content and the presence of indigestible carbohydrates, on glucose tolerance and related factors after a subsequent standardized breakfast in healthy individuals. The study's findings revealed that increased levels of indigestible carbohydrates from barley, particularly β-glucan, had a significant and positive effect on enhancing feelings of fullness (satiety), regulating glucose metabolism, and reducing markers of inflammation. These results suggest that including β-glucans, such as those found in barley, in one's diet can play a role in promoting weight control and improving overall metabolic health.

The study conducted by Tapola et al. [109] demonstrated that the consumption of oats had a positive impact on blood glucose levels following a dietary load of 12.5 g of glucose. The results showed that blood glucose levels were lower at 15, 30, and 45 minutes after the glucose load but slightly higher at the 90-minute mark. Importantly, the peak level of glucose was more moderate, and the shape of the plasma glucose response curve was smoother and less pronounced. These changes in glucose levels had the effect of reducing feelings of hunger (increasing satiety) caused by rapid fluctuations in blood glucose. Consequently, oat products that contain β-glucans have the potential to decrease appetite and reduce overall food intake. One possible mechanism for the blood glucose-lowering effect of β-glucans is that they may delay stomach emptying, resulting in a more gradual absorption of dietary glucose. This, in turn, helps stabilize blood glucose levels, promoting a sense of fullness and reducing the urge to eat.

In a related study, by Dong et al. [110] obese male Sprague–Dawley rats were fed three different oat products (meal, flour, and bran) that were rich in β-glucans as part of high-fat diets over eight weeks. The results of this study showed several positive outcomes like reduction in body weight, decreased accumulation of epididymal fat, lowered levels of inflammatory factors in the serum, regulation of serum lipid levels, and increased levels of SCFAs above normal. The oat bran product, which contained 8% β-glucan with a molecular weight of 8.20×10^5 Da, produced the highest levels of SCFAs among the oat products tested. Based on these findings, the authors concluded that oat products rich in β-glucans could have a beneficial impact on attenuating obesity and related metabolic disorders. These effects were attributed to the modulation of the gut microbiota and the elevated levels of SCFAs. Additionally, oat β-glucan intake was associated with a reduction in lipid accumulation in hepatocytes (liver cells) and a decrease in the size of adipocytes (fat cells). Overall, these findings suggest that β-glucans from oats may have anti-obesity effects and contribute to improved metabolic health.

The study by Tian et al. [111] provided evidence that the consumption of foods enriched with oat β-glucan resulted in a reduction in fat mass accumulation while concurrently promoting the production of SCFAs, such as butyrate. It is widely recognized that SCFAs can diminish lipid buildup in adipose tissue and enhance lipid oxidation in both liver and adipose tissues.

The study examined the impact of oat β-glucan on glycaemic control, appetite-regulating hormones, and the microbiota in individuals with type 2 diabetes (T2DM) [112]. In a group of 37 T2DM patients, the addition of 5 g of oat β-glucan to their regular diet for 12 weeks resulted in several significant changes. These changes included a reduction in HbA1c (glycated haemoglobin), insulin, C-peptide, and homeostatic model assessment (HOMA) values. Moreover, there was a decrease in the presence of Lactobacillus spp. and butyrate-producing bacteria in the gut microbiota. Interestingly, the levels of leptin, GLP-1 (glucagon-like peptide 1), and PYY (peptide YY) were also altered, indicating an enhancement in satiety levels.

In a similar vein, another study focused on examining how oats influence feelings of hunger, blood sugar levels, and insulin levels in a group of 33 adults with normal weight (comprising 22 females and 11 males, with a mean age of 26.9 ± 1.0 years and a BMI of 23.5 ± 0.4) [113]. During the study, participants were given an ad libitum meal with 4 g of high-MW oat β-glucan. Researchers evaluated subjective sensations of hunger, as well as glycaemia, insulin levels, and plasma GLP-1 (glucagon-like peptide-1) responses. Throughout the study, blood samples were collected at regular intervals, and participants provided subjective assessments of hunger following their meals. The intake of oat β-glucan led to increased feelings of satiety and fullness, although it did not impact the amount of energy or food consumed during the ad libitum meal. Notably, there was a significant interaction between treatment and time for blood glucose, plasma insulin, and plasma GLP-1 levels. Compared to the control meal, GLP-1 secretion was notably reduced after 90 minutes, blood glucose levels were lower at 30 minutes, and plasma insulin levels were lower at both 30 and 60 minutes, respectively. These findings suggest that the 4 g of high-molecular-weight oat β-glucan helped suppress hunger and improve post-meal blood sugar levels but did not influence the secretion of plasma GLP-1.

In a study involving 106 obese women (with an average BMI of 37.73 kg/m^2) who followed a hypocaloric diet for 8 weeks, the early effects of oat supplementation were investigated as a means to address metabolic issues associated with obesity [114]. The findings showed significant improvements in various anthropometric measurements, including reductions in waist-to-hip ratio, waist circumference, body fat percentage, and systolic blood pressure (SBP). This study provided strong support for the positive impacts of incorporating a dietary oat supplement into the treatment of central obesity, body fat percentage, and various metabolic disorders.

Additionally, another controlled clinical trial involved 62 individuals with hypercholesterolemia, both men and women between the ages of 18 and 65, who were given a daily intake of 80 g of oatmeal [115]. This trial revealed a consistent association between the modification of gut microorganisms and substantial improvements in hypercholesterolemia. These improvements were characterized by reduced levels of total cholesterol (TC), LDL cholesterol (LDL-C), and apolipoprotein B, indicating the potential of oatmeal consumption as an effective strategy for managing high cholesterol levels.

In another study of rats with hyperlipidemia induced by a high-fat diet (HFD), the consumption of oat β-glucan resulted in several positive effects Liu et al. [116]. These effects included a reduction in body weight gain, the inhibition of hepatic adipocyte hyperplasia, and a decrease in the size of the epididymal fat pad. These outcomes were associated with specific molecular changes in both the liver and adipose tissues. The mechanisms underlying these effects were characterized by the downregulation of fatty acid synthase (FAS) and sterol regulatory element-binding protein-1 (SREBP-1), as well as the upregulation of peroxisome proliferator-activated receptor (PPAR) and the activation of AMP-activated protein kinase (AMPK) signalling. Oat β-glucan supplementation partially reduced the process of lipogenesis and activated AMPK, resulting in the reduced production of proteins associated with lipid metabolism, including SREBP-1, Fas cell surface death receptor (FAS), PPAR, carnitine palmitoyltransferase 1 (CPT-1), and activating acetyl-CoA carboxylase, all of which are downstream targets of AMPK. These findings collectively demonstrate that oat β-glucan administration can effectively lower lipid levels in HFD-induced hyperlipidemic rats by modulating the AMPK signalling pathway. This suggests the potential utility of oat β-glucan in both the prevention and treatment of CVD and obesity.

Obesity-associated inflammation is often associated with a compromised intestinal barrier. The supplementation of β-glucan has been shown to have several beneficial effects in countering inflammation linked to obesity. It can increase the thickness of the mucosal lining, enhance the expression of occludin (a protein crucial for maintaining barrier integrity), and inhibit the accumulation of proinflammatory macrophages in the colon. Additionally, β-glucan exhibits the capacity to generate SCFAs through fermentation by gut microbiota. A study by Suzuki et al. [117] demonstrated that a diet rich in β-glucan increased the levels of SCFAs in the cecum of obese mice. Obesity is often accompanied by dysbiosis in the gut microbiota. The supplementation of β-glucan in obese mice led to a shift in the gut microbiota composition. This shift involved an increase in beneficial bacteria such as *Coprobacillus*, *Anaerostipes*, and *Roseburia*, while decreasing harmful bacteria like *Lactococcus* and *Parabacteroides*. Furthermore, β-glucan intake elevated the abundance of Bifidobacterium and Lactobacillus, resulting in higher concentrations of SCFAs, which, in turn, stimulated the immune system (Figure 7.4).

In summary, β-glucan plays a multifaceted role in the treatment of obesity. It contributes to the reduction of energy metabolism, promotes the secretion of satiety hormones, suppresses inflammation, and helps regulate the composition of the gut microbiota. These mechanisms collectively support its potential as a valuable intervention in the management of obesity.

7.7.3 Effect on Cholesterol Level and Cardiovascular-Related Diseases

Dyslipidemia represents a significant risk factor for cardiovascular-related diseases, characterized by the abnormal elevation of cholesterol or lipids in the bloodstream. It stands as the primary underlying cause of atherosclerotic vascular diseases, myocardial infarction (heart attack), and both ischaemic and haemorrhagic strokes. Given its profound impact on health, the prevention and effective management of dyslipidemia are of paramount importance in reducing the alarming rates of morbidity and mortality associated with heart disease [118].

The health advantages associated with dietary fibre, particularly oat β-glucans, encompass a range of benefits. These include the decrease in the time it takes for food to pass through the digestive system, the prevention of constipation, a reduced likelihood of colorectal cancer, decreased levels of blood cholesterol, the control of blood sugar levels for diabetes management, the generation of SCFAs, and the encouragement of the growth of beneficial microorganisms in the colon [119]. Research has shown that β-glucans can decrease cholesterol levels (both total and LDL) in various species, including humans, rats, mice, and hamsters. Moreover, alongside the reduction in total fat, saturated fat, and dietary cholesterol consumption, the incorporation of fibre into one's diet, particularly from sources abundant in β-glucan like oats, can lead to even greater reductions in serum cholesterol levels (Figure 7.4).

7.7.3.1 Mechanism of Cholesterol Reduction by Oat ß-Glucan

The reduction of cholesterol through the consumption of oat β-glucan involves multiple interconnected effects. Nonetheless, it is widely accepted that the primary mechanism responsible for β-glucan's cholesterol lowering involves its capacity to capture complete micelles containing bile acids within the intestinal contents, owing to its viscosity. This action prevents these micelles from engaging with luminal membrane transporters in the intestinal epithelium, consequently reducing the absorption or reabsorption of fats, including cholesterol and bile acids. This, in turn, leads to an increased discharge of these components in faeces. Consequently, the conversion of cholesterol into bile acids in the liver rises, the stores of free cholesterol in the liver diminish, and to restore equilibrium, the body increases its production of endogenous cholesterol. This results in heightened activity of enzymes like 7α-hydroxylase and 3-hydroxy-3-methyl glutaryl-coenzyme A (HMG-CoA) reductase to compensate for the losses of bile acids and cholesterol from liver stores. Additionally, hepatic LDL cholesterol receptors become more active to replenish hepatic cholesterol reserves, leading to a reduction in serum LDL cholesterol levels. This mechanism is corroborated by an observable increase in bile acid excretion in faeces, which can range from 35% to 65%. While there is no direct evidence for the mechanism of reduced absorption, it is likely primarily caused by increased viscosity in the small intestine. This viscosity effect influences diffusion rates and the thickness of the unstirred layer at the absorption site. This concept also applies to β-glucan's effects on glucose absorption. The decreased presence of bile acids in the small intestine reduces fat emulsification, which, combined with viscosity effects, decreases fat absorption and increases fat excretion.

Another suggested mechanism for cholesterol reduction is the action of SCFAs. Oat β-glucans consist of mixed β-(1→3) and β-(1→4) linkages. Humans lack the small intestine enzymes necessary to break down β-glucans, allowing them to pass into the large intestine undigested. Oat β-glucan is a fermentable and viscous fibre that lowers LDL cholesterol by reducing the enterohepatic recirculation of cholesterol and bile acids. Soluble fibre entering the colon is largely fermented, with the main byproducts being acetic, propionic, and butyric acids. Butyrate is metabolized by colonic mucosal cells, while acetate and propionate are absorbed. The production of SCFAs, especially the propionate: acetate ratio, may influence lipid metabolism. Although propionic acid has been shown to inhibit cholesterol synthesis in isolated rat hepatocytes at concentrations of 1.0–2.5 mM, the concentration of propionate in the hepatic portal vein of rats fed oat bran was found to be only 0.35 mmol/L. Therefore, this mechanism appears unlikely or to have only a minor effect, if any, in humans. Researchers have noted significant positive associations between the serum propionate: acetate ratio and total and LDL cholesterol levels in healthy men, but not in women. Oat β-glucan increases intestinal viscosity and reduces the rate of glucose absorption, resulting in lower post-meal insulin levels and reduced insulin-stimulated hepatic HMG-CoA activity, subsequently lowering cholesterol synthesis (Figure 7.4).

7.7.3.2 Research on Cholesterol Reduction by Oat ß-Glucan

In a murine model of hyperlipidemia, researchers compared the physiological effects of a β-glucan, specifically carboxymethylated β-glucan (CMG), with those of a statin/atorvastatin (HMG-CoA reductase inhibitor). While atorvastatin did lead to reductions in triglyceride and total cholesterol levels, they did not quite reach the levels observed in the control group. On the other hand, CMG did induce a decrease in triglyceride levels, but this effect was not as potent as the action of atorvastatin on its own. It's noteworthy that atorvastatin increased the activity of serum matrix metalloproteases, whereas CMG did not have an impact on this parameter. The triglyceride-lowering effect of CMG was suggested to be associated with its ability to stimulate macrophages in the liver [120]. It is crucial to emphasize that the mechanism of action of β-glucan may differ from that of statins. β-glucans work by reestablishing a balance in cholesterol levels by influencing the patient's physiological processes. For instance, in hyperlipidemic hamsters, barley β-glucans were found to lower cholesterol levels and reduce their absorption in the gut. This was achieved by diminishing the activity of HMG-CoA reductase in the liver, which is the enzyme primarily targeted by statins for cholesterol synthesis [121].

In human clinical trials involving individuals with elevated blood cholesterol levels (hypercholesterolemia) or high triglyceride levels (hyperlipidemia), the administration of oat bran β-glucan resulted in noteworthy enhancements in their lipid profiles. It's worth noting that even in healthy human subjects, similar improvements were observed [122]. The initial observation of oats' ability to reduce serum total cholesterol levels dates back to 1963 [123], and subsequent research identified oat β-glucan as the responsible factor for this effect [124]. Studies involving oat bran β-glucan revealed its capacity to facilitate the excretion of bile acids in ileostomy patients, providing a potential explanation for the reduction in serum lipid levels. Other investigations also noted an increase in the excretion of bile acids following oat treatment in both hypercholesterolemic rats and individuals with elevated cholesterol levels, as well as in healthy subjects. This mechanism may be linked to the synthesis of 7α-hydroxy-4-cholesten-3-one (α-HC), a metabolite used as an indicator of heightened bile acid excretion induced by dietary factors [125].

Joyce et al. [126] conducted a comprehensive review of the literature regarding the cholesterol-lowering effects of oat products containing β-glucans. They presented clinical evidence suggesting that the consumption of these products could effectively modulate the risks of CVD. This effect is believed to be primarily attributed to the gel-forming properties of oat β-glucan, which in turn influences the metabolism of bile acids and cholesterol. It's thought that this process may lead to the excretion of intestinal cholesterol in faeces. In another study, a fermented oat-based product enriched with β-glucan was shown to reduce cholesterol levels by 6% in the subjects under investigation. The authors of this study proposed that this effect might be associated with the fact that the treatment also stimulated the growth of bifidobacterial flora in the gastrointestinal tract. An alternative explanation, put forward by Sima et al. [127], suggests that β-glucans create a gel-like layer on the mucosal lining of the intestines. This gel formation prompts the synthesis of biliary salts in the liver and inhibits the reabsorption of these salts. As a result, more biliary salts become active, promoting the utilization of circulating cholesterol and ultimately leading to a decrease in cholesterol levels.

Several studies have presented conflicting evidence regarding the impact of oat β-glucan on plasma cholesterol levels, including LDL and HDL cholesterol. Wood et al. [128] proposed that the MW and solubility of cereal β-glucans play a crucial role in determining the physiological effects of these glucose-containing polysaccharides. The MW profile of β-glucans was found to be influenced by the extraction method used and was also linked to their viscoelastic properties. Consequently, it is important to take into account the MW of β-glucans when extracted from various barley and oat cultivars, as it may influence their behaviour in food systems. Furthermore, Theuwissen et al. [129] emphasized that several factors can impact the cholesterol-lowering properties of cereal β-glucans. These factors include the mode of administration, differences in solubility or MW, the composition of the food matrix, and various food processing methods. All of these variables can contribute to variations in the hypocholesterolemic effects of cereal β-glucans.

An *in vitro* study conducted by Grundy et al. [99] examined the impact of the structures and physicochemical properties of oat β-glucans on lipid and cholesterol metabolism. Their findings indicated that isolated β-glucan had a weaker effect on lipolysis compared to oat flakes and oat flour. They suggested that this variation in effect was related to the oat matrix and the form in which this biopolymer was delivered for ingestion. In contrast, Delaney et al. [130] proposed a mechanism for the reduction of cholesterol levels induced by oat β-glucan that might operate outside of the gut environment. They conducted a study in which hypercholesterolemic hamsters were treated with varying concentrations of oat and barley β-glucans for eight weeks. Following the treatment, the results demonstrated an increase in the total faecal-neutral sterol concentrations. Moreover, they asserted that there was no discernible difference between the β-glucans sourced from oats and barley in this regard.

In a study, oat β-glucan was administered orally to mice following a regimen that spanned seven days before and ten weeks after inducing hypercholesterolemia through an HFD [116]. The treatment resulted in several beneficial effects, including a reduction in body weight, decreased size of the epididymal fat pad, and inhibition of hepatic adipocyte hyperplasia. The authors in this study proposed that these outcomes were linked to the upregulation of PPAR-α and the downregulation of two key factors in lipid metabolism, namely FAS and SREBP-1. This upregulation was attributed to the activation of AMPK signalling in both liver and fat tissues. Subsequent in vitro analyses using oleic acid-induced HepG2 cells, a human liver cancer cell line, produced similar results. These findings indicate that oat β-glucan treatment can inhibit the expression of genes associated with glucose and lipid synthesis, and it may interfere with transcription factors involved in metabolic syndrome.

The dose-response effect of oat products, including oat bran and oatmeal, was examined in a study involving hypercholesterolemic human subjects [131]. Participants were given oatmeal or oat bran at daily doses of 28, 56, and 84 g over six weeks. The results showed that oat bran at doses of 56 and 84 g, as well as oatmeal at a dose of 84 g, significantly reduced both total cholesterol and LDL cholesterol concentrations when compared to a control group that received 28 g of oat flour. The superior efficacy of oat bran was likely due to its higher β-glucan content. The conclusion that β-glucan was the active component was further supported by a study conducted by Braaten et al. [124]. In this study, hypercholesterolemic participants were given a fibre preparation containing oat gum with added oat β-glucans (80%) mixed into a beverage for four weeks. This preparation significantly lowered total and LDL cholesterol levels without affecting HDL cholesterol, as compared to a maltodextrin placebo drink. In another study, oat-based products that were fermented using the non-dairy lactic acid bacterium, *Pediococcus damnosus* 2.6 (now reclassified as *P. parvulus*), which produces a 2-substituted

$(1\rightarrow3)$-β-D-glucan, were found to reduce cholesterol levels and promote the growth of bifidobacterial flora in humans.

The economic impact of daily intake of $\geq$ 3 g of oat β-glucan in primary prevention of coronary heart disease (CHD) in patients receiving statins or no pharmacologic treatment was assessed [132]. This level of β-glucan intake was associated with a potential reduction in the first occurrences of infarction (heart attack) and a decreased risk of coronary heart disease-related mortality, particularly in middle-aged men (45, 55, and 65 years) without a history of CVD. However, it's important to note that the long-term effectiveness of β-glucans in lowering cholesterol levels may diminish over time. Some more extended studies have shown that the cholesterol-lowering effects of β-glucan intake may become less significant. For instance, in one study, significant reductions in cholesterol levels were observed after four weeks of β-glucan consumption, but these effects were not maintained after eight weeks [133]. Additionally, a study conducted by Keogh et al. [134] found that in a group of mildly hypercholesterolemic men who were given 8.1–11.9 g of barley β-glucans per day, no significant changes in total and LDL cholesterol levels were observed.

According to research presented at the First International Congress on Pre-Diabetes and Metabolic Syndrome, barley β-glucan demonstrated the ability to lower serum lipid levels, including cholesterol and triglycerides [135]. During a six-week study involving 76 men and 79 women ranging in age from 25 to 73 years, all of whom had hypercholesterolemia, participants were provided with doses of 3 and 5 g of barley β-glucan with lower high-MW content twice daily. These doses were mixed with cereals and fruit juice. After the six-week treatment period, assessments of blood lipids and other biomarkers related to CVD were conducted. The results showed improvements in levels of LDL cholesterol, total cholesterol, and triglycerides, as well as markers associated with glycaemic control (such as glycosylated haemoglobin and the HOMA model) and inflammation (measured by high-sensitivity C-reactive protein, hs-CRP). As a result of these findings, the researchers concluded that both low- and high-molecular-weight barley β-glucans, when administered at the specified doses, led to improved blood lipid profiles throughout the six-week treatment period. This suggests the potential benefits of incorporating barley β-glucan into the diet for individuals with hypercholesterolemia and highlights its positive impact on cardiovascular health (Figure 7.4).

Much like oat β-glucans, the mechanism through which barley β-glucans reduce cholesterol and other lipid levels appears to be associated with an increase in faecal lipid excretion. Tong et al. [136] conducted a study in hypercholesterolemic hamsters, where a 30-day treatment regimen with barley β-glucan was administered. This treatment resulted in a decrease in the activity of the enzyme HMG-CoA reductase and an increase in cholesterol 7-α-hydroxylase (CYP7A1) activity in the liver. HMG-CoA reductase regulates the synthesis of cholesterol, while CYP7A1 is involved in cholesterol excretion. This led researchers to suggest that barley β-glucan could be a potential hypocholesterolemic agent. Similar results were observed in another study where hypercholesterolemic hamsters were given a 30-day treatment regimen with wheat bran. This regimen also led to a decrease in HMG-CoA reductase activity and an increase in CYP7A1 activity in the liver, suggesting a potential cholesterol-lowering effect. Additionally, both studies found an increase in the concentrations of propionic acid and total SCFAs. This increase suggests that treatment with β-glucan acted as a prebiotic, modulating the microbiota in the colon. These findings highlight the potential role of β-glucans, whether from barley or wheat bran, in influencing cholesterol metabolism and gut microbiota, contributing to their hypocholesterolemic effects.

7.7.3.3 Oat ß-Glucans and Cardiovascular Diseases

Oxidative stress and inflammation are known contributors to the development and progression of various cardiovascular diseases. Elevated levels of reactive oxygen species (ROS) can lead to adverse cardiac remodelling, ultimately resulting in heart failure. ROS can inflict damage on critical components involved in excitation-contraction coupling, including the contractile units, the sodium-calcium exchanger, and sarcoendoplasmic reticulum-calcium ATPase. Additionally, ROS can influence apoptosis processes, activate signalling kinases related to hypertrophy, and impact transcription factors. Zhang et al. [137] have shown an increase in free radical species in patients with ischaemic heart disease. These free radicals have the potential to trigger dysfunction in cardiac myocytes, impairing heart function and creating a detrimental cycle.

Research conducted on rats has identified a correlation between heart failure and subsequent myocardial infarction, with oxidative stress being a contributing factor. This condition may be linked to impaired antioxidant defences, leading to elevated levels of free radicals. Given that heart failure is associated with an excess of free radicals, potential therapeutic strategies to enhance the prognosis of patients may focus on regulating oxidative stress in both skeletal muscle and the heart. However, it's worth noting that studies directly linking the antioxidant activity of β-glucans to cardiovascular diseases are relatively scarce. Most research has been conducted in vitro and has primarily demonstrated the general antioxidant properties of β-glucans without specific disease-related implications [138].

β-glucan has demonstrated potential antioxidant effects in human hepatocytes. In this context, its antioxidant action was observed when ROS production was induced by lipopolysaccharide (LPS), which is an endotoxin component found on the outer membrane of gram-negative bacteria. LPS is known to trigger inflammatory reactions through ROS generation. The β-glucan preparation was found to reduce the expression of proteins associated with the NADPH oxidase homologs NOX1, NOX2, and NOX4. Understanding the biology of NOX enzymes is essential in comprehending their role in generating ROS. In the cardiovascular system, NOX enzymes are primarily expressed in vascular smooth muscle cells but can also be present in endothelial cells, cardiomyocytes, and fibroblasts. They play distinct roles in redox-sensitive signal transduction pathways activated by various stimuli, contributing to processes such as cardiac hypertrophy, endothelial activation, angiogenesis, and atherosclerosis. These results indicate that the antioxidant effect of fungal β-glucan is associated with the suppression of NADPH oxidase activation, which is a critical source of ROS. Furthermore, treatment with β-glucan was found to inhibit several signalling transduction pathways involving protein kinases like Akt (serine/threonine-specific protein kinase), p38 (mitogen-activated protein kinase), and ERK (extracellular signal-regulated kinase) [12] (Figure 7.4).

7.8 CONCLUSION

According to data from FMI surveys, the global β-glucans market had a value of $307.8 million in 2016. Projections from Markets and Markets anticipated that by 2022, this market would grow to reach $476.5 million. This substantial growth potential underscores the increasing application of β-glucans. In this chapter, we have provided a summary of the physiological functions of both regular β-glucans and modified β-glucans. We have also delved into the underlying mechanisms governing the activities of β-glucans. Our goal has been to enhance understanding regarding how β-glucans can be applied clinically, safely, and effectively. While various biological activities of β-glucans have been presented, it's important to note that some proposed mechanisms are still based on assumptions, and further research is needed to fully clarify these mechanisms. Future research efforts should be directed towards investigating the intricate interaction mechanisms between β-glucans and different subjects, as well as establishing links among these various mechanisms. This research would greatly contribute to our comprehension of the changes induced by β-glucans in both humans and animals. Additionally, it would aid in the development and utilization of β-glucans from diverse sources. In the realms of food and pharmaceutical manufacturing, it's often the case that the impact of a single component is limited. Therefore, it's crucial to explore products that exhibit synergistic effects when combined with β-glucans. These complementary products warrant attention as they could potentially enhance the overall benefits of β-glucans in various applications.

REFERENCES

[1] Y. Tang et al., "Bioactive components and health functions of oat," *Food Rev. Int.*, vol. 39, pp. 4545–4564, 2023, doi: 10.1080/87559129.2022.2029477.

[2] S. Peesapati, K. A. Sajeevan, S. K. Patel and D. Roy, "Relation between glycosidic linkage, structure and dynamics of α- and β-glucans in water," *Biopolymers.*, vol. 112, p. e23423, 2021, doi: 10.1002/bip.23423.

[3] J. Bai et al., "Physiological functionalities and mechanisms of β-glucans," *Trends Food Sci. Technol.*, vol. 88, pp. 57–66, 2019, doi: 10.1016/j.tifs.2019.03.023.

[4] J. Zhang, L. Yan, M. Liu, G. Guo and B. Wu, "Analysis of β-d-glucan biosynthetic genes in oat reveals glucan synthesis regulation by light," *Ann. Botany.*, vol. 127, pp. 371–380, 2021, doi: 10.1093/aob/mcaa185.

[5] R. Barone Lumaga, D. Azzali, V. Fogliano, L. Scalfi and P. Vitaglione, "Sugar and dietary fibre composition influence, by different hormonal response, the satiating capacity of a fruit-based and a β-glucan-enriched beverage," *Food Funct.*, vol. 3, pp. 67–75, 2012, doi: 10.1039/c1fo10065c.

[6] N. Sharafbafi, S. M. Tosh, M. Alexander and M. Corredig, "Phase behaviour, rheological properties, and microstructure of oat β-glucan-milk mixtures," *Food Hydrocoll.*, vol. 41, pp. 274–280, 2014, doi: 10.1016/j.foodhyd.2014.03.030.

[7] F. S. Reis, A. Martins, M. H. Vasconcelos, P. Morales and I. C. F. R. Ferreira, "Functional foods based on extracts or compounds derived from mushrooms," *Trends Food Sci. Technol.*, vol. 66, pp. 48–62, 2017, doi: 10.1016/j.tifs.2017.05.010.

[8] D. L. Morris, "Lichenin and Araban in oats. (Avena sativa)," *J. Biol. Chem.*, vol. 142, pp. 881–891, 1942, doi: 10.1016/S0021-9258(18)45086-7.

[9] M. Korčok, J. Calle, M. Veverka and V. Vietoris, "Understanding the health benefits and technological properties of β-glucan for the development of easy-to-swallow gels to guarantee food security among seniors," *Crit. Rev. Food Sci. Nutr.*, pp. 1–18, 2022, doi: 10.1080/10408398.2022.2093325.

[10] R. R. Philippini, S. E. Martiniano, J. C. dos Santos, S. S. da Silva and A. K. Chandel, "Fermentative production of beta-glucan: Properties and potential applications," in *Bioprocessing for Biomolecules Production*, John Wiley & Sons, Ltd, 2019, pp. 303–320, doi: 10.1002/9781119434436.ch15.

[11] K. Muthuramalingam, Y. Kim and M. Cho, "β-glucan, 'the knight of health sector': Critical insights on physiochemical heterogeneities, action mechanisms and health implications," *Crit. Rev. Food Sci. Nutr.*, vol. 62, pp. 6908–6931, 2022, doi: 10.1080/10408398.2021.1908221.

[12] J. Wouk, R. F. H. Dekker, E. A. I. F. Queiroz and A. M. Barbosa-Dekker, "β-glucans as a panacea for a healthy heart? Their roles in preventing and treating cardiovascular diseases," *Int. J. Biol. Macromol.*, vol. 177, pp. 176–203, 2021, doi: 10.1016/j.ijbiomac.2021.02.087.

[13] A. Lante, E. Canazza and P. Tessari, "Beta-glucans of cereals: Functional and technological properties," *Nutrients.*, vol. 15, p. 2124, 2023, doi: 10.3390/nu15092124.

[14] F. Zhu, B. Du and B. Xu, "A critical review on production and industrial applications of beta-glucans," *Food Hydrocoll.*, vol. 52, pp. 275–288, 2016, doi: 10.1016/j.foodhyd.2015.07.003.

[15] F.Y. Kagimura et al., "Carboxymethylation of (1→6)-β-glucan (lasiodiplodan): Preparation, characterization and antioxidant evaluation," *Carbohydr. Polym.*, vol. 127, pp. 390–399, 2015, doi: 10.1016/j.carbpol.2015.03.045.

[16] F. Zhu, B. Du, Z. Bian and B. Xu, "Beta-glucans from edible and medicinal mushrooms: Characteristics, physicochemical and biological activities," *J. Food Compos. Anal.*, vol. 41, pp. 165–173, 2015, doi: 10.1016/j.jfca.2015.01.019.

[17] F. Saeed et al., "Functional and nutraceutical properties of maize bran cell wall non-starch polysaccharides," *Int. J. Food Prop.*, vol. 24, pp. 233–248, 2021, doi: 10.1080/10942912.2020.1858864.

[18] S. K. Gill, M. Rossi, B. Bajka and K. Whelan, "Dietary fibre in gastrointestinal health and disease," *Nat. Rev. Gastroenterol. Hepatol.*, vol. 18, pp. 101–116, 2021, doi: 10.1038/s41575-020-00375-4.

[19] J. W. J. McRorie, R. D. Gibb, K. J. Sloan and N. M. McKeown, "Psyllium: The gel-forming nonfermented isolated fiber that delivers multiple fiber-related health benefits," *Nutr. Today.*, vol. 56, p. 169, 2021, doi: 10.1097/NT.0000000000000489.

[20] M. Antunes-Ricardo, J. Villela-Castrejón, J. A. Gutiérrez-Uribe and S. O. Serna Saldívar, "Dietary fiber and cancer," in *Science and Technology of Fibers in Food Systems*, J. Welti-Chanes, S. O. Serna-Saldívar, O. Campanella and V. Tejada-Ortigoza, Eds. Cham, Germany: Springer International Publishing, 2020, pp. 241–276, doi: 10.1007/978-3-030-38654-2_11.

[21] S. Fuller, E. Beck, H. Salman and L. Tapsell, "New horizons for the study of dietary fiber and health: A review," *Plant Foods Hum. Nutr.*, vol. 71, pp. 1–12, 2016, doi: 10.1007/s11130-016-0529-6.

[22] S. Pathania and N. Kaur, "Utilization of fruits and vegetable by-products for isolation of dietary fibres and its potential application as functional ingredients," *Bioact. Carbohydr. Diet. Fibre.*, vol. 27, p. 100295, 2022, doi: 10.1016/j.bcdf.2021.100295.

[23] K. Sivieri, S. M. de Oliveira, A. de S. Marquez, J. Pérez-Jiménez and S. N. Diniz, "Insights on β-glucan as a prebiotic coadjuvant in the treatment of diabetes mellitus: A review," *Food Hydrocoll. Heal.*, vol. 2, p. 100056, 2022, doi: 10.1016/j.fhfh.2022.100056.

[24] D. El Khoury, C. Cuda, B. L. Luhovyy and G. H. Anderson, "Beta glucan: Health benefits in obesity and metabolic syndrome," *J. Nutr. Metab.*, vol. 2012, p. e851362, 2011, doi: 10.1155/2012/851362.

[25] B. Golisch, Z. Lei, K. Tamura and H. Brumer, "Configured for the human gut microbiota: Molecular mechanisms of dietary β-glucan utilization," *ACS Chem. Biol.*, vol. 16, pp. 2087–2102, 2021, doi: 10.1021/acschembio.1c00563.

[26] Y. Meng, F. Lyu, X. Xu and L. Zhang, "Recent advances in chain conformation and bioactivities of triple-helix polysaccharides," *Biomacromolecules.*, vol. 21, pp. 1653–1677, 2020, doi: 10.1021/acs.biomac.9b01644.

[27] M. Shoukat and A. Sorrentino, "Cereal β-glucan: A promising prebiotic polysaccharide and its impact on the gut health," *Int. J. Food Sci. Technol.*, vol. 56, pp. 2088–2097, 2021, doi: 10.1111/ijfs.14971.

[28] E. De Arcangelis, S. Djurle, A. A. M. Andersson, E. Marconi, M. C. Messia and R. Andersson, "Structure analysis of β-glucan in barley and effects of wheat β-glucanase," *J. Cereal Sci.*, vol. 85, pp. 175–181, 2019, doi: 10.1016/j.jcs.2018.12.002.

[29] S. M. Tosh and N. Bordenave, "Emerging science on benefits of whole grain oat and barley and their soluble dietary fibers for heart health, glycemic response, and gut microbiota," *Nutr. Rev.*, vol. 78, pp. 13–20, 2020, doi: 10.1093/nutrit/nuz085.

[30] Y.-P. Bai, H.-M. Zhou, K.-R. Zhu and Q. Li, "Effect of thermal processing on the molecular, structural, and antioxidant characteristics of highland barley β-glucan," *Carbohydr. Polym.*, vol. 271, p. 118416, 2021, doi: 10.1016/j.carbpol.2021.118416.

[31] J. Gangoiti, S. F. Corwin, L. M. Lamothe, C. Vafiadi, B. R. Hamaker and L. Dijkhuizen, "Synthesis of novel α-glucans with potential health benefits through controlled glucose release in the human gastrointestinal tract," *Crit. Rev. Food Sci. Nutr.*, vol. 60, pp. 123–146, 2020, doi: 10.1080/10408398.2018.1516621.

[32] A. Kheto, Y. Bist, A. Bhati, S. Kaur, Y. Kumar and R. Sehrawat, "Utilization of inulin as a functional ingredient in food: Processing, physicochemical characteristics, food applications, and future research directions," *Food Chem. Adv.*, 2023, p. 100443, doi: 10.1016/j.focha.2023.100443.

[33] H. Liu, Y. Li, M. You and X. Liu, "Comparison of physicochemical properties of β-glucans extracted from hull-less barley bran by different methods," *Int. J. Biol. Macromol.*, vol. 182, pp. 1192–1199, 2021, doi: 10.1016/j.ijbiomac.2021.05.043.

[34] G. Goudar, P. Sharma, S. Janghu and T. Longvah, "Effect of processing on barley β-glucan content, its molecular weight and extractability," *Int. J. Biol. Macromol.*, vol. 162, pp. 1204–1216, 2020, doi: 10.1016/j.ijbiomac.2020.06.208.

[35] A. Sharma, A. Sharma and A. Tripathi, "Biological activities of Pleurotus spp. polysaccharides: A review," *J. Food Biochem.*, vol. 45, p. e13748, 2021, doi: 10.1111/jfbc.13748.

[36] S. M. V. Mejía, A. de Francisco and B. M. Bohrer, "A comprehensive review on cereal β-glucan: Extraction, characterization, causes of degradation, and food application," *Crit. Rev. Food Sci. Nutr.*, vol. 60, pp. 3693–3704, 2020, doi: 10.1080/10408398.2019.1706444.

[37] P. J. Strong et al., "Filamentous fungi for future functional food and feed," *Curr. Opin. Biotechnol.*, vol. 76, p. 102729, 2022, doi: 10.1016/j.copbio.2022.102729.

[38] L. Luft, T. C. Confortin, I. Todero, G. L. Zabot and M. A. Mazutti, "An overview of fungal biopolymers: Bioemulsifiers and biosurfactants compounds production," *Crit. Rev. Biotechnol.*, vol. 40, pp. 1059–1080, 2020, doi: 10.1080/07388551.2020.1805405.

[39] R. Bozbulut and N. Sanlier, "Promising effects of β-glucans on glyceamic control in diabetes," *Trends Food Sci. Technol.*, vol. 83, pp. 159–166, 2019, doi: 10.1016/j.tifs.2018.11.018.

[40] A. Clarke and B. Stone, "Enzymic hydrolysis of barley and other β-glucans by a β-(1→4)-glucan hydrolase," *Biochem. J.*, vol. 99, pp. 582–588, 1966, doi: 10.1042/bj0990582.

[41] S. M. Tosh, Y. Brummer, P. J. Wood, Q. Wang and J. Weisz, "Evaluation of structure in the formation of gels by structurally diverse (1→3)(1→4)-β-d-glucans from four cereal and one lichen species," *Carbohydr. Polym.*, vol. 57, pp. 249–259, 2004, doi: 10.1016/j.carbpol.2004.05.009.

[42] J. Luo et al., "Purified β-glucans of different molecular weights enhance growth performance of LPS-challenged piglets via improved gut barrier function and microbiota," *Animals.*, vol. 9, p. 602, 2019, doi: 10.3390/ani9090602.

[43] V. Varelas, M. Liouni, A. C. Calokerinos and E. T. Nerantzis, "An evaluation study of different methods for the production of β-D-glucan from yeast biomass," *Drug Test. Anal.*, vol. 8, pp. 46–55, 2016, doi: 10.1002/dta.1833.

[44] B. Han, K. Baruah, E. Cox, D. Vanrompay and P. Bossier, "Structure-functional activity relationship of β-glucans from the perspective of immunomodulation: A mini-review," *Front. Immunol.*, vol. 11, 2020. Accessed: Sept. 18, 2023. [Online]. Available: www.frontiersin.org/articles/10.3389/fimmu.2020.00658

[45] J. H. Cummings and A. M. Stephen, "Carbohydrate terminology and classification," *Eur. J. Clin Nutr.*, vol. 61, pp. S5–S18, 2007, doi: 10.1038/sj.ejcn.1602936.

[46] B. Du, M. Meenu, H. Liu and B. Xu, "A concise review on the molecular structure and function relationship of β-glucan," *Int. J. Mol. Sci.*, vol. 20, p. 4032, 2019, doi: 10.3390/ijms20164032.

[47] C. Daou and H. Zhang, "Oat beta-glucan: Its role in health promotion and prevention of diseases," *Compr. Rev. Food Sci. Food Saf.*, vol. 11, pp. 355–365, 2012, doi: 10.1111/j.1541-4337.2012.00189.x.

[48] M. Y. K. Leung, C. Liu, J. C. M. Koon and K.P. Fung, "Polysaccharide biological response modifiers," *Immunol. Lett.*, vol. 105, pp. 101–114, 2006, doi: 10.1016/j.imlet.2006.01.009.

[49] Q. Wang et al., "β-glucans: Relationships between modification, conformation and functional activities," *Molecules.*, vol. 22, p. 257, 2017, doi: 10.3390/molecules 22020257.

[50] G. Fittolani, P. H. Seeberger and M. Delbianco, "Helical polysaccharides," *Pept. Sci.*, vol. 112, p. e24124, 2020, doi: 10.1002/pep2.24124.

[51] C.M. Camelini, M. Maraschin, M. M. de Mendonça, C. Zucco, A. G. Ferreira and L. A. Tavares, "Structural characterization of β-glucans of Agaricus brasiliensis in different stages of fruiting body maturity and their use in nutraceutical products," *Biotechnol. Lett.*, vol. 27, pp. 1295–1299, 2005, doi: 10.1007/s10529-005-0222-6.

[52] E. Westerlund, R. Andersson and P. Åman, "Isolation and chemical characterization of water-soluble mixed-linked β-glucans and arabinoxylans in oat milling fractions," *Carbohydr. Polym.*, vol. 20, pp. 115–123, 1993, doi: 10.1016/0144-8617(93)90086-J.

[53] R. S. Bhatty, "Extraction and enrichment of (1->3), (1->4)-β-D-glucan from barley and oat brans.," *Cereal Chem.*, vol. 70, pp. 73–77, 1993.

[54] M. U. Beer, E. Arrigoni and R. Amado, "Extraction of oat gum from oat bran: Effects of process on yield, molecular weight distribution, viscosity and (1→3)(1→4)-β-D-glucan content of the gum," *Cereal Chem.*, vol. 73, pp. 58–62, 1996.

[55] A. Ahmad, F. M. Anjum, T. Zahoor, H. Nawaz and Z. Ahmed, "Extraction and characterization of β-d-glucan from oat for industrial utilization," *Int. J. Biol. Macromol.*, vol. 46, pp. 304–309, 2010, doi: 10.1016/j.ijbiomac.2010.01.002.

[56] A. Skendi, C. G. Biliaderis, A. Lazaridou and M. S. Izydorczyk, "Structure and rheological properties of water soluble β-glucans from oat cultivars of Avena sativa and Avena bysantina," *J. Cereal Sci.*, vol. 38, pp. 15–31, 2003, doi: 10.1016/S0733-5210(02)00137-6.

[57] Y. Brummer, C. Defelice, Y. Wu, M. Kwong, P. J. Wood and S. M. Tosh, "Textural and rheological properties of oat beta-glucan gels with varying molecular weight composition," *J. Agric. Food Chem.*, vol. 62, pp. 3160–3167, 2014, doi: 10.1021/jf405131d.

[58] Q. Zhao et al., "Physicochemical properties and regulatory effects on db/db diabetic mice of β-glucans extracted from oat, wheat and barley," *Food Hydrocoll.*, vol. 37, pp. 60–68, 2014, doi: 10.1016/j.foodhyd.2013.10.007.

[59] N. Böhm and W.-M. Kulicke, "Rheological studies of barley (1→3)(1→4)-β-glucan in concentrated solution: Mechanistic and kinetic investigation of the gel formation," *Carbohydr. Res.*, vol. 315, pp. 302–311, 1999, doi: 10.1016/S0008-6215(99)00036-1.

[60] Y. Tao, L. Zhang and P. C. K. Cheung, "Physicochemical properties and antitumor activities of water-soluble native and sulfated hyperbranched mushroom polysaccharides," *Carbohydr. Res.*, vol. 341, pp. 2261–2269, 2006, doi: 10.1016/j.carres.2006.05.024.

[61] A. Synytsya and M. Novák, "Structural diversity of fungal glucans," *Carbohydr. Polym.*, vol. 92, pp. 792–809, 2013, doi: 10.1016/j.carbpol.2012.09.077.

[62] P. R. Hussain, S. A. Rather and P. P. Suradkar, "Structural characterization and evaluation of antioxidant, anticancer and hypoglycemic activity of radiation degraded oat (Avena sativa) β- glucan," *Radiat. Phys. Chem.*, vol. 144, pp. 218–230, 2018, doi: 10.1016/j.radphyschem.2017.08.018.

[63] L. Q. Luan and N. H. P. Uyen, "Radiation degradation of (1→3)-β-d-glucan from yeast with a potential application as a plant growth promoter," *Int. J. Biol. Macromol.*, vol. 69, pp. 165–170, 2014, doi: 10.1016/j.ijbiomac.2014.05.041.

[64] M. Ahmad, A. Gani, A. Shah, A. Gani and F. A. Masoodi, "Germination and microwave processing of barley (Hordeum vulgare L) changes the structural and physicochemical properties of β-d-glucan & enhances its antioxidant potential," *Carbohydr. Polym.*, vol. 153, pp. 696–702, 2016, doi: 10.1016/j.carbpol.2016.07.022.

[65] X. Chen, K.-C. Siu, Y.-C. Cheung and J.-Y. Wu, "Structure and properties of a (1→3)-β-d-glucan from ultrasound-degraded exopolysaccharides of a medicinal fungus," *Carbohydr. Polym.*, vol. 106, pp. 270–275, 2014, doi: 10.1016/j.carbpol.2014.02.040.

[66] J. Liepins, E. Kovačova, K. Shvirksts, M. Grube, A. Rapoport and G. Kogan, "Drying enhances immunoactivity of spent brewer's yeast cell wall β-d-glucans," *J. Biotechnol.*, vol. 206, pp. 12–16, 2015, doi: 10.1016/j.jbiotec.2015.03.024.

[67] Y. Ishimoto et al., "Production of low-molecular weight soluble yeast β-glucan by an acid degradation method," *Int. J. Biol. Macromol.*, vol. 107, pp. 2269–2278, 2018, doi: 10.1016/j.ijbiomac.2017.10.094.

[68] M. Wang et al., "Improvement of immune responses to influenza vaccine (H5N1) by sulfated yeast beta-glucan," *Int. J. Biol. Macromol.*, vol. 93, pp. 203–207, 2016, doi: 10.1016/j.ijbiomac.2016.06.057.

[69] Z. Sun, Y. He, Z. Liang, W. Zhou and T. Niu, "Sulfation of (1→3)-β-d-glucan from the fruiting bodies of Russula virescens and antitumor activities of the modifiers," *Carbohydr. Polym.*, vol. 77, pp. 628–633, 2009, doi: 10.1016/j.carbpol.2009.02.001.

[70] M. Zhang, P. C. K. Cheung, L. Zhang, C.-M. Chiu and V. E. C. Ooi, "Carboxymethylated β-glucans from mushroom sclerotium of Pleurotus tuber-regium as novel water-soluble anti-tumor agent," *Carbohydr. Polym.*, vol. 57, pp. 319–325, 2004, doi: 10.1016/j.carbpol.2004.05.008.

[71] F. Shi, J. Shi and Y. Li, "Mechanochemical phosphorylation and solubilisation of β-D-glucan from yeast saccharomyces cerevisiae and its biological activities," *PLoS One.*, vol. 9, p. e103494, 2014, doi: 10.1371/journal.pone.0103494.

[72] H. Wang et al., "In vivo immunological activity of carboxymethylated-sulfated (1→3)-β-d-glucan from sclerotium of Poria cocos," *Int. J. Biol. Macromol.*, vol. 79, pp. 511–517, 2015, doi: 10.1016/j.ijbiomac.2015.05.020.

[73] N. L. de Souza et al., "Functional, thermal and rheological properties of oat β-glucan modified by acetylation," *Food Chem.*, vol. 178, pp. 243–250, 2015, doi: 10.1016/j.foodchem.2015.01.079.

[74] R. Zhang, X. Zhang, Y. Tang and J. Mao, "Composition, isolation, purification and biological activities of Sargassum fusiforme polysaccharides: A review," *Carbohydr. Polym.*, vol. 228, p. 115381, 2020, doi: 10.1016/j.carbpol.2019.115381.

[75] X. Liu, Z. Wan, L. Shi and X. Lu, "Preparation and antiherpetic activities of chemically modified polysaccharides from Polygonatum cyrtonema Hua," *Carbohydr. Polym.*, vol. 83, pp. 737–742, 2011, doi: 10.1016/j.carbpol.2010.08.044.

[76] N. M. Mestechkina and V. D. Shcherbukhin, "Sulfated polysaccharides and their anticoagulant activity: A review," *Appl. Biochem. Microbiol.*, vol. 46, pp. 267–273, 2010, doi: 10.1134/S000368381003004X.

[77] Y. Zhang, X. Lu, Y. Zhang, L. Qin and J. Zhang, "Sulfated modification and immunomodulatory activity of water-soluble polysaccharides derived from fresh Chinese persimmon fruit," *Int. J. Biol. Macromol.*, vol. 46, pp. 67–71, 2010, doi: 10.1016/j.ijbiomac.2009.10.007.

[78] L. S. Bezerra et al., "Modulation of vascular function and anti-aggregation effect induced by (1→3) (1→6)-β-d-glucan of Saccharomyces cerevisiae and its carboxymethylated derivative in rats," *Pharmacol. Rep.*, vol. 69, pp. 448–455, 2017, doi: 10.1016/j.pharep.2017.01.002.

[79] G. Kogan et al., "Antioxidant properties of yeast (1→3)-β-d-glucan studied by electron paramagnetic resonance spectroscopy and its activity in the adjuvant arthritis," *Carbohydr. Polym.*, vol. 61, pp. 18–28, 2005, doi: 10.1016/j.carbpol.2005.02.010.

[80] S.Y. Park, I. Y. Bae, S. Lee and H. G. Lee, "Physicochemical and hypocholesterolemic characterization of oxidized oat β-glucan," *J. Agric. Food Chem.*, vol. 57, pp. 439–443, 2009, doi: 10.1021/jf802811b.

[81] Y. Ishimoto et al., "Modulation of an innate immune response by soluble yeast β-glucan prepared by a heat degradation method," *Int. J. Biol. Macromol.*, vol. 104, pp. 367–376, 2017, doi: 10.1016/j.ijbiomac.2017.06.036.

[82] A. Shah et al., "Effect of γ-irradiation on structure and nutraceutical potential of β-d-glucan from barley (Hordeum vulgare)," *Int. J. Biol. Macromol.*, vol. 72, pp. 1168–1175, 2015, doi: 10.1016/j.ijbiomac.2014.08.056.

[83] R. Mateos, J. García-Cordero, L. Bravo-Clemente and B. Sarriá, "Evaluation of novel nutraceuticals based on the combination of oat beta-glucans and a green coffee phenolic extract to combat obesity and its comorbidities. A randomized, dose–response, parallel trial," *Food Funct.*, vol. 13, pp. 574–586, 2022, doi: 10.1039/D1FO02272E.

[84] J. García-Cordero et al., "Dietary supplements containing oat beta-glucan and/or green coffee (poly)phenols showed limited effect in modulating cardiometabolic risk biomarkers in overweight/obese patients without a lifestyle intervention," *Nutrients.*, vol. 15, p. 2223, 2023, doi: 10.3390/nu15092223.

[85] S. Yu, J. Wang, Y. Li, X. Wang, F. Ren and X. Wang, "Structural studies of water-insoluble β-glucan from oat bran and its effect on improving lipid metabolism in mice fed high-fat diet," *Nutrients.*, vol. 13, p. 3254, 2021, doi: 10.3390/nu13093254.

[86] T. M. S. Wolever et al., "An oat β-glucan beverage reduces LDL cholesterol and cardiovascular disease risk in men and women with borderline high cholesterol: A double-blind, randomized, controlled clinical trial," *J. Nutr.*, vol. 151, pp. 2655–2666, 2021, doi: 10.1093/jn/nxab154.

[87] H. Gao et al., "Effects of oat fiber intervention on cognitive behavior in LDLR–/– mice modeling atherosclerosis by targeting the microbiome–gut–brain axis," *J. Agric. Food Chem.*, 2020, doi: 10.1021/acs.jafc.0c05677.

[88] P. Raj et al., "Oat beta-glucan alone and in combination with hydrochlorothiazide lowers high blood pressure in male but not female spontaneously hypertensive rats," *Nutrients.*, vol. 15, p. 3180, 2023, doi: 10.3390/nu15143180.

[89] P. Raj, N. Ames, S. Joseph Thandapilly, L. Yu and T. Netticadan, "The effects of oat ingredients on blood pressure in spontaneously hypertensive rats," *J. Food Biochem.*, vol. 44, p. e13402, 2020, doi: 10.1111/jfbc.13402.

[90] J. Wilczak et al., "The effect of low or high molecular weight oat beta-glucans on the inflammatory and oxidative stress status in the colon of rats with LPS-induced enteritis," *Food Funct.*, vol. 6, pp. 590–603, 2015, doi: 10.1039/C4FO00638K.

[91] Y. Mälkki and E. Virtanen, "Gastrointestinal effects of oat bran and oat gum: A review," *LWT.*, vol. 34, pp. 337–347, 2001, doi: 10.1006/fstl.2001.0795.

[92] M. Ulmius, S. Adapa, G. Önning and L. Nilsson, "Gastrointestinal conditions influence the solution behaviour of cereal β-glucans in vitro," *Food Chem.*, vol. 130, pp. 536–540, 2012, doi: 10.1016/j.foodchem.2011.07.066.

[93] M. Ulmius, A. Johansson-Persson, T. I. Nordén, B. Bergenståhl and G. Önning, "Gastrointestinal release of β-glucan and pectin using an in vitro method," *Cereal Chem.*, vol. 88, pp. 385–390, 2011, doi: 10.1094/CCHEM-11-10-0169.

[94] Q. Wang, P. J. Wood and W. Cui, "Microwave assisted dissolution of β-glucan in water – Implications for the characterisation of this polymer," *Carbohydr. Polym.*, vol. 47, pp. 35–38, 2002, doi: 10.1016/S0144-8617(00)00340-4.

[95] C. L. Dikeman, M. R. Murphy and G. C. Fahey, "Dietary fibers affect viscosity of solutions and simulated human gastric and small intestinal digesta," *J. Nutr.*, vol. 136, pp. 913–919, 2006, doi: 10.1093/jn/136.4.913.

[96] S. Satchithanandam, M. Vargofcak-Apker, R. J. Calvert, A. R. Leeds and M. M. Cassidy, "Alteration of gastrointestinal mucin by fiber feeding in rats," *J. Nutr.*, vol. 120, pp. 1179–1184, 1990, doi: 10.1093/jn/120.10.1179.

[97] H. N. Johansen, K. E. Bach Knudsen, P. J. Wood and R. G. Fulcher, "Physico-chemical properties and the degradation of oat bran polysaccharides in the gut of pigs," *J. Sci. Food Agric.*, vol. 73, pp. 81–92, 1997, doi: 10.1002/(SICI)1097-0010(199701)73:1<81::AID-JSFA695>3.0.CO;2-Z.

[98] M. M. L. Grundy, A. Fardet, S. M. Tosh, G. T. Rich and P. J. Wilde, "Processing of oat: The impact on oat's cholesterol lowering effect," *Food Funct.*, vol. 9, pp. 1328–1343, 2018, doi: 10.1039/C7FO02006F.

[99] M. M. L. Grundy et al., "The impact of oat structure and β-glucan on in vitro lipid digestion," *J. Funct. Foods.*, vol. 38, pp. 378–388, 2017, doi: 10.1016/j.jff.2017.09.011.

[100] N. Mäkelä, N. Rosa-Sibakov, Y.-J. Wang, O. Mattila, E. Nordlund and T. Sontag-Strohm, 'Role of β-glucan content, molecular weight and phytate in the bile acid binding of oat β-glucan," *Food Chem.*, vol. 358, p. 129917, 2021, doi: 10.1016/j.foodchem.2021.129917.

[101] N. D. Karunaratne, R. W. Newkirk, N. P. Ames, A. G. Van Kessel, M. R. Bedford and H. L. Classen, "Hulless barley and β-glucanase affect ileal digesta soluble β-glucan molecular weight and digestive tract characteristics of coccidiosis-vaccinated broilers," *Anim. Nutr.*, vol. 7, pp. 595–608, 2021, doi: 10.1016/j.aninu.2020.09.006.

[102] J. Bai et al., "Source of gut microbiota determines oat β-glucan degradation and short chain fatty acid-producing pathway," *Food Biosci.*, vol. 41, p. 101010, 2021, doi: 10.1016/j.fbio.2021.101010.

[103] H. Zhang, S. Sun and L. Ai, "Physical barrier effects of dietary fibers on lowering starch digestibility," *Curr. Opin. Food Sci.*, vol. 48, p. 100940, 2022, doi: 10.1016/j.cofs.2022.100940.

[104] Y. Bao et al., "The microbial communities and natural fermentation quality of ensiling oat (Avena sativa L.) harvest from different elevations on the Qinghai-Tibet Plateau," *Front. Microbiol.*, vol. 13, 2023. Accessed: Sept. 18, 2023. [Online]. Available: www.frontiersin.org/articles/10.3389/fmicb.2022.1108890

[105] Q. Luong, J. Huang and K. Y. Lee, "Deciphering white adipose tissue heterogeneity," *Biology.*, vol. 8, p. 23, 2019, doi: 10.3390/biology8020023.

[106] J. M. Makaronidis and R. L. Batterham, "The role of gut hormones in the pathogenesis and management of obesity," *Curr. Opin. Physiol.*, vol. 12, pp. 1–11, 2019, doi: 10.1016/j.cophys.2019.04.007.

[107] E. S. Chambers, T. Preston, G. Frost and D. J. Morrison, "Role of gut microbiota-generated short-chain fatty acids in metabolic and cardiovascular health," *Curr. Nutr. Rep.*, vol. 7, pp. 198–206, 2018, doi: 10.1007/s13668-018-0248-8.

[108] A. C. Nilsson, E. M. Östman, J. J. Holst and I. M.E. BjÖrck, "Including indigestible carbohydrates in the evening meal of healthy subjects improves glucose tolerance, lowers inflammatory markers, and increases satiety after a subsequent standardized breakfast11," *J. Nutr.*, vol. 138, pp. 732–739, 2008, doi: 10.1093/jn/138.4.732.

[109] N. Tapola, H. Karvonen, L. Niskanen, M. Mikola and E. Sarkkinen, "Glycemic responses of oat bran products in type 2 diabetic patients," *Nutr. Metabol. Cardiovasc. Dis.*, vol. 15, pp. 255–261, 2005, doi: 10.1016/j.numecd.2004.09.003.

[110] J. Dong, Y. Zhu, Y. Ma, Q. Xiang, R. Shen and Y. Liu, "Oat products modulate the gut microbiota and produce anti-obesity effects in obese rats," *J. Funct. Foods.*, vol. 25, pp. 408–420, 2016, doi: 10.1016/j.jff.2016.06.025.

[111] L. Tian et al., "Effect of oat and soybean rich in distinct non-starch polysaccharides on fermentation, appetite regulation and fat accumulation in rat," *Int. J. Biol. Macromol.*, vol. 140, pp. 515–521, 2019, doi: 10.1016/j.ijbiomac.2019.08.032.

[112] J. L. Pino, V. Mujica and M. Arredondo, "Effect of dietary supplementation with oat β-glucan for 3 months in subjects with type 2 diabetes: A randomized, double-blind, controlled clinical trial," *J. Funct. Foods.*, vol. 77, p. 104311, 2021, doi: 10.1016/j.jff.2020.104311.

[113] S. M. M. Zaremba, I. F. Gow, S. Drummond, J. T. McCluskey and R. E. Steinert, "Effects of oat β-glucan consumption at breakfast on ad libitum eating, appetite, glycemia, insulinemia and GLP-1 concentrations in healthy subjects," *Appetite.*, vol. 128, pp. 197–204, 2018, doi: 10.1016/j.appet.2018.06.019.

[114] S. M. El Shebini, M. I. A. Moaty, S. Fouad, N. H. Ahmed and S. T. Tapozada, "Obesity related metabolic disorders and risk of renal disease: Impact of hypocaloric diet and Avena sativa supplement," *Open Access Maced J Med Sci.*, vol. 6, pp. 1376–1381, 2018, doi: 10.3889/oamjms.2018.292.

[115] M. Ye et al., "Oatmeal induced gut microbiota alteration and its relationship with improved lipid profiles: A secondary analysis of a randomized clinical trial," *Nutr. Metabol.*, vol. 17, p. 85, 2020, doi: 10.1186/s12986-020-00505-4.

[116] B. Liu et al., "Oat β-glucan inhibits adipogenesis and hepatic steatosis in high fat diet-induced hyperlipidemic mice via AMPK signaling," *J. Funct. Foods.*, vol. 41, pp. 72–82, 2018, doi: 10.1016/j.jff.2017.12.045.

[117] S. Suzuki and S. Aoe, "High β-glucan barley supplementation improves glucose tolerance by increasing GLP-1 secretion in diet-induced obesity mice," *Nutrients.*, vol. 13, p. 527, 2021, doi: 10.3390/nu13020527.

[118] J. Vekic, A. Stefanovic and A. Zeljkovic, "Obesity and dyslipidemia: A review of current evidence," *Curr. Obes. Rep.*, vol. 12, pp. 207–222, 2023, doi: 10.1007/s13679-023-00518-z.

[119] G. F. Alemayehu, S. F. Forsido, Y. B. Tola and E. Amare, "Nutritional and phytochemical composition and associated health benefits of oat (*Avena sativa*) grains and oat-based fermented food products," *Sci. World J.*, vol. 2023, p. e2730175, 2023, doi: 10.1155/2023/2730175.

[120] T. A. Korolenko et al., "Influence of atorvastatin and carboxymethylated glucan on the serum lipoprotein profile and MMP activity of mice with lipemia induced by poloxamer 407," *Can. J. Physiol. Pharmacol.*, vol. 90, pp. 141–153, 2012, doi: 10.1139/y11-118.

[121] A. H. Gora et al., "Microbial oil, alone or paired with β-glucans, can control hypercholesterolemia in a zebrafish model," *Biochim. Biophys. Acta. Mol. Cell Biol. Lipids*, vol. 1868, p. 159383, 2023, doi: 10.1016/j.bbalip.2023.159383.

[122] D. A. Kerckhoffs, G. Hornstra and R. P. Mensink, "Cholesterol-lowering effect of β-glucan from oat bran in mildly hypercholesterolemic subjects may decrease when β-glucan is incorporated into bread and cookies," *Am. J. Clin. Nutr.*, vol. 78, pp. 221–227, 2003, doi: 10.1093/ajcn/78.2.221.

[123] A.P. de Groot, R. Luyken and N. A. Pikaar, "Cholesterol-lowering effect of rolled oats," *Lancet.*, vol. 282, pp. 303–304, 1963, doi: 10.1016/S0140-6736(63)90210-1.

[124] J. T. Braaten et al., "Oat beta-glucan reduces blood cholesterol concentration in hypercholesterolemic subjects," *Eur. J. Clin. Nutr.*, vol. 48, pp. 465–474, 1994.

[125] S. Ötles and S. Ozgoz, "Health effects of dietary fiber," *Acta Sci. Pol. Technol.*, vol. 13, pp. 191–202, 2014, doi: 10.17306/J.AFS.2014.2.8.

[126] S. A. Joyce, A. Kamil, L. Fleige and C. G. M. Gahan, "The cholesterol-lowering effect of oats and oat beta glucan: Modes of action and potential role of bile acids and the microbiome," *Front. Nutr.*, vol. 6, p. 171, 2019, doi: 10.3389/fnut.2019.00171.

[127] P. Sima, L. Vannucci and V. Vetvicka, "β-glucans and cholesterol (review)," *Int. J. Mol. Med.*, vol. 41, pp. 1799–1808, 2018, doi: 10.3892/ijmm.2018.3411.

[128] P.J. Wood, M. U. Beer and G. Butler, "Evaluation of role of concentration and molecular weight of oat β-glucan in determining effect of viscosity on plasma glucose and insulin following an oral glucose load," *Br. J. Nutr.*, vol. 84, pp. 19–23, 2000, doi: 10.1017/S0007114500001185.

[129] E. Theuwissen and R. P. Mensink, "Water-soluble dietary fibers and cardiovascular disease," *Physiol. Behav.*, vol. 94, pp. 285–292, 2008, doi: 10.1016/j.physbeh.2008.01.001.

[130] B. Delaney et al., "β-glucan fractions from barley and oats are similarly antiatherogenic in hypercholesterolemic syrian golden hamsters," *J. Nutr.*, vol. 133, pp. 468–475, 2003, doi: 10.1093/jn/133.2.468.

[131] M. H. Davidson, L. D. Dugan, J. H. Burns, J. Bova, K. Story and K. B. Drennan, "The hypocholesterolemic effects of β-glucan in oatmeal and oat bran: A dose-controlled study," *JAMA.*, vol. 265, pp. 1833–1839, 1991, doi: 10.1001/jama.1991.03460140061027.

[132] S. R. Earnshaw, C. L. McDade, Y. Chu, L. E. Fleige and J. L. Sievenpiper, "Cost-effectiveness of maintaining daily intake of oat β-glucan for coronary heart disease primary prevention," *Clin. Therap.*, vol. 39, pp. 804–818.e3, 2017, doi: 10.1016/j.clinthera.2017.02.012.

[133] M. I. Uusitupa et al., "A controlled study on the effect of beta-glucan-rich oat bran on serum lipids in hypercholesterolemic subjects: Relation to apolipoprotein E phenotype," *J. Am. Coll. Nutr.*, vol. 11, pp. 651–659, 1992, doi: 10.1080/07315724.1992.10718264.

[134] G. F. Keogh et al., "Randomized controlled crossover study of the effect of a highly β-glucan–enriched barley on cardiovascular disease risk factors in mildly hyper-cholesterolemic men," *Am. J. Clin. Nutr.*, vol. 78, pp. 711–718, 2003, doi: 10.1093/ajcn/78.4.711.

[135] P. Segal and P. Zimmet, "The epidemiology of prediabetes and the metabolic syndrome," in *Medscape*. Berlin, Germany, 2005, pp. 1–8. [Online]. Available: www. medscape.com/viewarticle/506474_2

[136] L.-T. Tong, K. Zhong, L. Liu, X. Zhou, J. Qiu and S. Zhou, "Effects of dietary hull-less barley β-glucan on the cholesterol metabolism of hypercholesterolemic hamsters," *Food Chem.*, vol. 169, pp. 344–349, 2015, doi: 10.1016/j.foodchem.2014.07.157.

[137] Z. Zhang et al., "Reactive oxygen species scavenging nanomedicine for the treatment of ischemic heart disease," *Adv. Mater.*, vol. 34, p. 2202169, 2022, doi: 10.1002/adma.202202169.

[138] E. Llanaj et al., "Effect of oat supplementation interventions on cardiovascular disease risk markers: A systematic review and meta-analysis of randomized controlled trials," *Eur. J. Nutr.*, vol. 61, pp. 1749–1778, 2022, doi: 10.1007/s00394-021-02763-1.

Application of Oats and Their Components in Diverse Functional Food Products

Simardeep Kaur, Karishma Seem,
Preetiman Kaur, Sohel Rahaman, Kamlesh Kumar,
Naseeb Singh, and Binay Kumar Singh

8.1 INTRODUCTION

The health benefits of oats are extensively recognized and well-documented. Oats are commonly employed within the food industry, featuring prominently in various food products like oat flakes [1], porridge [2], cereal bars [3], cookies [4], noodles [5], bread [6], yoghurt [7], and oat-based beverages. This extensive use is underpinned by the oat's exceptional attributes: a noteworthy protein content ranging from 12% to 20%, high digestibility at approximately 90–94%, and a significant dietary fibre content, particularly 4–8% in the form of β-glucan [8]. Oats are considered a healthy dietary choice due to their rich β-glucan content, scientifically proven to confer significant health benefits for managing chronic diseases. In 1997, the U.S. Food and Drug Administration (FDA) endorsed health claims on food labels concerning the role of oat β-glucan in promoting heart health and reducing cholesterol levels. Nonetheless, incorporating oats into food production poses challenges, primarily arising from the development of undesirable lipid-derived off-flavours and suboptimal textural quality in oat-based foods like oat bread. Raw oats are rather bland in flavour, and the sought-after cereal-like flavours typically develop during intensive processing, often involving heat treatment. Oat production involves multiple steps, encompassing the cleaning and grading of raw oat seeds, dehulling, and industrial processing. The lipid-rich nature of oats can result in off-flavour formation during these stages and extended storage. Additionally, various processing techniques, such as peeling, milling, and fractionation, have been identified as influencing the flavour of oat-based cereal products [9]. Furthermore, oats possess unique physiochemical properties characterized by the absence of gluten and distinct starch attributes, including low paste clarity, high pasting temperature, and viscosity. These attributes present particular challenges in achieving high-textural quality food products compared to other cereal counterparts like wheat.

Beyond the creation of plain porridge, which can consist entirely of oats, the majority of consumer products incorporate oats as an ingredient, aiming to enhance their value to consumers. Oat ingredients, for instance, are incorporated into a wide range of consumer goods to offer health-promoting properties, adjust flavour and visual appeal, or achieve specific technological objectives, such as water retention [10]. Notably, many of the recent innovations in oat ingredients revolve around oat bran or oat fractions enriched with β-glucan. In addition to their fibre content, which is renowned for its health-promoting and versatile properties, oats are also abundant in beneficial fatty acids and lipid classes. They feature protein with a high content of valuable amino acids and contain distinctive phenolic compounds, including avenanthramides, alongside other minor nutrients. Despite these valuable attributes, only a small fraction of oat crops undergo processing for human food and other valuable products, with the majority being allocated for animal feed. The solubility kinetics of β-glucan and its propensity to form highly viscous, shear-thinning gels differ among various oat products [11]. As a result, modern oat ingredients are suitable for a wide array of food applications, and they do not exhibit the adverse characteristics seen in conventional oat products. These novel oat ingredients are accessible in diverse forms, boasting varying compositions, appearances, tastes, and technological functionalities [12].

The major sectors within the food industry that heavily rely on functional ingredients include baking, beverages, meat processing, dairy, and confectionery [13]. One of the most explored industrial applications involves the incorporation of β-glucan into food products. As a hydrocolloid, β-glucan can effectively modify the rheological and textural properties of numerous food products. This is primarily because β-glucan exhibits promising characteristics as a stabilizing, thickening, gelating, and emulsifying agent, enhancing water and oil holding capacity [14]. These attributes are of significant industrial importance, as they enable the transformation of basic raw materials into novel food products, such as functional beverages, health-oriented bread, ready-to-serve soups, nutritious snack foods, a variety of sauces, and many other food items. The utilization of β-glucan also plays a pivotal role in maintaining and enhancing product quality. In these industrial applications, β-glucan has found an essential role. The demand for this natural substance is rapidly increasing in the industry. Numerous functional food products containing β-glucan are already making their way into the commercial market, and their presence is expected to steadily rise in the global marketplace.

Consequently, the use of β-glucan as a food ingredient is gaining widespread attention for two primary objectives: augmenting the dietary fibre content of food products and enhancing their health-promoting properties. Oats possess the highest fat content among grains, ranging from 4.2 to 11.8 g/100 g, as compared to wheat (2.1 to 3.8 g/100 g), rice (2.0 to 3.1 g/100 g), barley (3.3 to 4.6 g/100 g), and rye (2.0 to 3.5 g/100 g) [15]. Notably, vitamin E, a fat-soluble nutrient, is a component of the total lipid content and is represented by tocopherols and tocotrienols, collectively forming tocols. The most substantial vitamin E activity is attributed to α-tocopherol, followed by β-tocopherol and α-tocotrienol. Alpha-tocopherol serves as a key antioxidant component in unprocessed oat grain and remains unaffected even after lipid refinement.

Similar to other cereal grains, oat is primarily composed of starch, which accounts for over 60% of its grain weight and plays a pivotal role in defining the structural and physicochemical characteristics of oat-based foods [16]. The primary constituent of oats is starch, which accounts for up to 60% of its dry weight and is primarily located in the endosperm. However, due to variations stemming from environmental factors and plant genotype, the starch content in oats can range from 51% to 65%. This starch is composed of amylopectin and amylose, which are closely packed in a semicrystalline granular form. Amylopectin is a branching polymer consisting of short, linear chains (linked through (1→4) bonds) with branching points created by (1→6) linkages, while amylose is a linear polymer of (1→4) linked-d-glucopyranosyl units. The distinctive features of oat starch, such as its high lipid content, small granule size, short amylose chain length, and relative crystallinity, set it apart from other cereal starches [17].

Oat starch, due to its exceptional attributes, such as a clustered granular structure, small granule size, unique rheological behaviour, biodegradability, biocompatibility, renewable sourcing, and non-allergenic properties, exhibits distinct functional features [18]. These include its ability to form films, contribute to texture in reduced-fat products, and facilitate foaming, emulsification, gelation, and water binding, rendering it applicable in a wide range of food and pharmaceutical applications [19]. The physical characteristics of products containing oats are largely influenced by the starch they contain. The molecular properties of starch dictate phenomena like gelatinization, retrogradation, and pasting qualities, which can vary between different sources of starch.

Nonetheless, the extensive use of oat starch in its native form in food applications has been associated with certain issues, including low thermostability, reduced paste clarity, poor shear resistance, and elevated paste viscosity rendering it less favourable for many food applications. To address these challenges, physical and chemical modification methods have been introduced as viable strategies. The chemical modification involves subjecting starch to a small amount of a reactive chemical, resulting in the creation of new starch derivatives, including etherified, grafted, esterified, and cross-linked starches, which possess novel physicochemical properties significantly different from those of the primary native starch [18]. Chemical modification approaches have been well-established for laboratory and industrial applications due to their cost-effectiveness, reduced processing time, and simplicity. However, concerns have arisen regarding the impact of chemical treatment on consumer health.

In contrast to chemical modification, physical modification methods do not alter the D-glucopyranosyl residues of starch molecules but instead, modify the molecular packing arrangement within granules through the reorganization of amylose and amylopectin structures [20]. A notable feature of physically modified starches is that they do not require labelling as "modified starch" since no chemical treatment is involved in their production. In recent studies, a combination of physical and chemical techniques (referred to as dual modifications) or the incorporation of starch with other biopolymers, such as proteins, lipids, and other polysaccharides, has been employed to enhance the physicochemical characteristics of oat starch. Regardless of the type of modification, substantial alterations in the physical, chemical, functional, and nutritional properties of starch occur as a result of these modifications. All of these techniques result in alterations to the physicochemical and structural properties of the starch polymer. Consequently, modified starch finds increased utility in the food industry. When incorporated into food products, modified starch prevents retrogradation, enhances product flavour and consistency, improves freeze-thaw stability, and extends the shelf life of frozen foods by preventing oxidation [21].

The global oat protein market is projected to experience a compound annual growth rate of 1.22% during the forecast period from 2019 to 2024 [22]. Oat proteins have gained significant acceptance among consumers when compared to other plant-based alternatives like soy, pea, and lupine proteins, primarily because they do not raise concerns about undesirable off-flavours. From a sustainability perspective, food products containing oat proteins demonstrate a reduced carbon footprint and lower land use when contrasted with their counterparts made with animal proteins [23]. Replacing 24% of animal-based foods with oat protein concentrate-based products could potentially result in an 8% reduction in greenhouse gas emissions and a 14% reduction in land use.

Oats find common usage in various commercial liquid and semi-solid applications, such as plant-based milk alternatives and yoghurt-like products. However, in products where oats are the sole source of protein, the total protein content tends to be low, typically falling within the range of 0% to 1% [24]. This is primarily attributed to the inherently low protein content in oat flours and flakes, which typically ranges from 10% to 15%. Furthermore, a significant portion of oat protein unintentionally gets removed during the processing of these products, primarily during the physical separation step aimed at extracting insoluble fibre (achieved through processes like centrifugation or decantation). To address this protein deficiency issue in dairy alternatives, oat protein concentrates (OPCs) could serve as an additional source of oat protein [25]. However, currently available commercial OPCs face challenges when used in liquid and semi-solid applications due to the aggregated or denatured state of oat proteins in these ingredients.

Furthermore, oat proteins can function as effective thickeners, emulsifiers, texture modifiers, and stabilizers in food products due to their functional properties, which include gelling ability, emulsification properties, water-holding capacity (WHC), fat-binding capacity (FBC), and foaming properties [26]. However, the functionality of native oat protein is limited in liquid or semi-solid products due to the denatured state of oat protein. To enhance the functionalities of oat proteins, researchers have explored various modifications, including chemical and enzymatic approaches.

The gelation of oat proteins and the establishment of a stable network are essential requirements for many food products. Within this context, the gelling properties of proteins can be classified based on the mechanism of gelation (acid-induced, heat-induced, cooling-induced, enzymatically induced, or induced by the addition of salts), as well as by the resulting gel's morphological characteristics (fine-stranded, mixed, or particulate gels) [27]. In the case of globular proteins, heat-induced gelation involves a sequence of events, beginning with the unfolding of protein molecules, followed by their association and aggregation, culminating in the formation of a three-dimensional network through protein-protein interactions. The morphological features of the gel are influenced by the specific mechanisms of binding between the proteins, including hydrophobic interactions, hydrogen bonds, ionic interactions, and covalent bonds. These binding mechanisms, in turn, impact the microstructure, texture, viscoelasticity, and stability of the gel. All of these attributes serve as indicators of a high-performing ingredient from technological, nutritional, and sensory perspectives [28]. Ultimately, these qualities determine the consumer's willingness to purchase and consume the products.

Studies in the past have been conducted to assess the functional properties of oat proteins [29]. Researchers have examined oat protein fractions to evaluate their solubility, emulsifying abilities, FBC, water hydration characteristics, and foaming properties. The findings suggest that oat protein demonstrates superior emulsifying and fat-binding properties when compared to soy protein [30]. Furthermore, it has been proposed that oat protein isolate (OPI) can serve as a cost-effective gelling ingredient when subjected to enzymatic hydrolysis, addressing the needs of the vegan and vegetarian food processing industry. Oat proteins that have been modified through enzymatic hydrolysis are better suited for creating new food products with enhanced protein functionality, and they are gaining prominence in the functional food market. Additionally, there have been investigations into the potential use of oat protein to supplement proteins in plant-based diets by incorporating them into meat analogues [31].

However, the techno-functionality of oat proteins presents certain challenges. These proteins have low solubility, limited emulsifying capacity, foam-forming properties, and gelation abilities, which can restrict their application in various food products [32]. To address these limitations, a range of chemical, physical, and enzymatic methods have been developed to enhance the techno-functional and nutritional properties of oat proteins. Considering these factors, this review aims to provide an updated and comprehensive compilation of information on oat proteins, covering fundamental aspects of their practical applications [33].

Oat protein is inherently gluten-free, making it a suitable choice for individuals with celiac disease who need to avoid gluten-containing products [34]. However, in solid products (such as bakery items and cereal bars), semi-solid products (like yoghurt), and liquid products (including milk and beverages) that are prepared exclusively with oat flour, the protein content is generally low. This is mainly attributed to the naturally low protein content in oat flour, particularly when oats serve as the sole source of protein in these products. To create oat-based products that can serve as alternatives to meat analogues, dairy products, and bakery items, while achieving similar protein content and texture, additional protein must be introduced. In this context, OPIs and concentrates offer an additional source of oat protein. These isolates and concentrates can be further utilized to develop various value-added products, which can be marketed as excellent sources of plant-based protein. With the growing interest in oats as a protein ingredient, there is a need for research to delve into the relationships between protein structure and functionality, eco-friendly defatting techniques, and versatile applications to increase the utilization of oats in the food industry.

The primary objective of this chapter is to provide a comprehensive overview of different extraction and fractionation methods for oat proteins, starch, β-glucans, fats, and other components. It also explores the techno-functionality of these molecules and outlines how their properties can be enhanced and customized through the use of enzymatic and chemical treatments. In addition, this chapter sheds light on the various applications of oats and their fractions in industrial processes and the development of value-added food products. It delves into the latest advancements in the application of innovative food processing technologies as alternatives to traditional methods for the extraction of bioactive compounds from oats.

8.2 FUNCTIONAL COMPONENTS OF OATS AND THEIR APPLICATION IN THE FOOD INDUSTRY

8.2.1 Starch

The predominant constituent of oats is starch, which accounts for approximately 60% of its dry weight. This starch is predominantly located within the endosperm of the oat grain. It's worth noting that the starch content in oats can vary due to factors like environmental conditions and the genetic makeup of the plant, resulting in a starch content range of 51% to 65% [16]. Starch is primarily concentrated within the endosperm of the oat granule, with minimal quantities found in the embryo and other plant organs. Importantly, oat starch granules are not intertwined in a continuous protein matrix; instead, the protein is localized in distinct structures [32], [35]–[42]. The two primary carbohydrate components of oat starch granules are amylose and amylopectin, constituting around 98% to 99% of the total carbohydrate content [43]. The apparent amylose content, which includes some amylose associated with lipids, typically falls within the range of 16.7% to 22.0%. In contrast, the total amylose content, which excludes any lipid-bound amylose, typically falls within the range of 19.4% to 33.6% [16].

Amylose is a polysaccharide comprised of α-d-glucose units bonded to one another through α(1→4) glycosidic bonds. It exhibits a relatively low degree of polymerization (DP) with an average of around 3000 units, and a minimal frequency of branching, with less than 1% of α-1,6 linkages [32], [35], [36]. In contrast, amylopectin typically has a higher DP, averaging around 5000 units, and a greater occurrence of α-1, 6 linkages, ranging from 3% to 4%. Amylopectin stands out due to its exceptional molecular weight, which ranks among the highest observed in naturally occurring polymers [18]. The proportion of these two polysaccharides varies depending on the botanical source of the starch. The relative ratios of amylose and amylopectin within starch granules, as well as the distribution of chain lengths and the presence and distribution of branch points in the amylopectin molecule, significantly impact the properties of the starch. Oat starch contains minor non-carbohydrate constituents, including protein, lipids, ash, and phosphorus. What distinguishes oat starch from other cereal starches are its unique characteristics, such as a high lipid content, small granule size, shorter amylose chains, and a comparatively higher degree of crystallinity. These attributes contribute to the distinctive nature of oat starch [19].

In the context of cereal starches, most commonly, granules take the form of distinct, solid, and optically transparent bodies. However, oat starch exhibits a distinct granular structure. Oat starch granules tend to congregate in clusters, resulting in irregular or polygonal shapes for the majority of these granules. In some instances, particularly those situated on the outer periphery of these clusters, granules may assume a polygonal shape on one side and an ovoid shape on the other. These clusters typically measure between 20 and 150 μm in diameter, with an average diameter of approximately 60 μm [44], [45]. When oat starch is extracted, the resultant granules typically range in diameter from 2 to 12 μm, and their surfaces appear smooth without visible fissures [20], [46]. Oat starch granules exhibit unique characteristics, as they are only weakly birefringent and are irregular in shape, with a propensity to aggregate in clusters. They do not conform to the discrete size distributions, such as the A and B types observed in wheat and barley starches. Oat starch granules are found in clusters composed of irregularly shaped granules, with some having characteristics reminiscent of both A- and B-type granules. Comparatively, the size of oat starch granules is akin to rice starch but smaller than those of wheat, maize, and potato starch. Specifically, the length range, width range, and mean granule width of native oat starches fall within the respective ranges of 5.85–6.9 μm, 3.0–7.5 μm, and 1.5–9.71 μm [46].

8.2.1.1 Isolation and Purification of Oat Starch

Oat starch extraction from oat groats and flours has been a subject of exploration on both industrial and laboratory fronts. In contrast to the majority of other cereal grains, oat starch poses unique challenges in separation due to the robust protein-starch matrix and the presence of β-glucan. Various methods have been scrutinized for oat starch extraction. The yield of oat starch is primarily influenced by the protein content of the oat cultivar. A higher protein content results in diminished starch production, and conversely, lower protein content enhances starch yield. The isolation process comprises steps such as protein extraction, several mechanical separations to eliminate cell wall residues, water washing and neutralization, and recovery through centrifugation [47].

Starch in oats is primarily situated in the endosperm, ensconced within the β-glucan and protein-rich bran layers. In comparison to other cereals, extracting starch from oats is notably intricate due to the strong affinity between starch and protein, as well as the presence of β-glucan. The removal of proteins is a pivotal step that positively impacts the yield of starch extraction. This process involves protein extraction, multiple mechanical separations to eliminate residual cell wall material, water washing and neutralization, and culminates with starch recovery through centrifugation. To extract starch from oats, three primary methods have been employed: water extraction with high-shear homogenization, alkaline extraction using sodium hydroxide solutions, and protease-assisted extraction to expedite the starch isolation process. The use of sodium hydroxide and proteases for oat starch isolation is illustrated in (Figure 8.1).

A notable historical example from MacMasters et al. [48] outlined a starch isolation method involving three steps: steeping oat groats in distilled water, 0.2% sulphur dioxide, or 0.13% sodium hydroxide; wet milling of the oats; and screening of the resulting

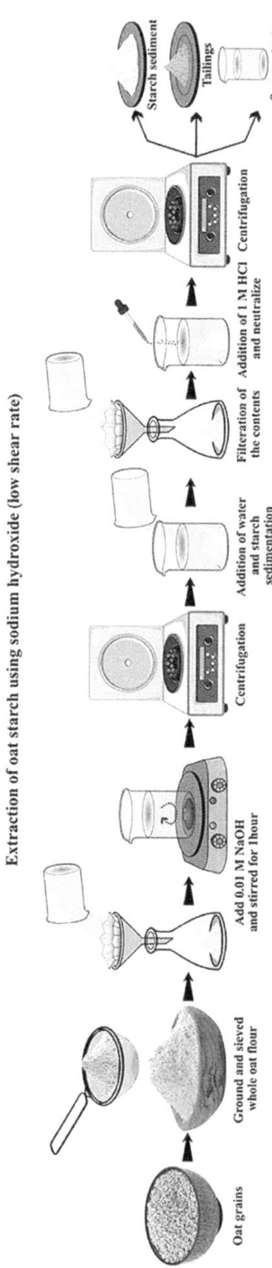

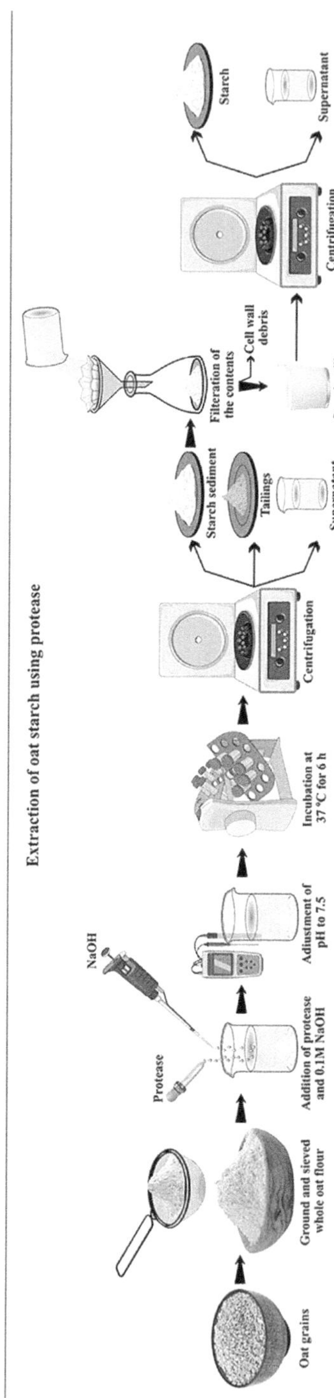

FIGURE 8.1 (Top) Oat starch extraction utilizing sodium hydroxide under low shear rate conditions. This process involves the use of sodium hydroxide to extract oat starch, emphasizing a method characterized by a gentle shear rate. (Bottom) Oat starch extraction employing a protease enzyme. In this scenario, oat starch is extracted through the application of a protease enzyme, highlighting a different approach involving enzymatic action for starch extraction.

pulpy slurry using standard bolting silk screens. Commonly, for the isolation of oat starch, a combination of sodium hydroxide (NaOH) and sodium carbonate (Na_2CO_3) is used. These reagents are applied at low shear rates, while water (H_2O) is utilized at high shear rates. In a related context, [49] employed sodium carbonate as an alkaline solution to facilitate the dissolution of proteins (Figure 8.1).

For industrial-scale oat starch production, the utilization of wet milling is presently limited due to challenges in achieving a complete separation of starch, primarily because of the hydrated bran and protein layers. At this level, dry milling and soaking in cellulase and hemicellulase enzymes are commonly employed to isolate starch, fibre, and protein. Researchers such as Sayar et al. [50] achieved starch isolation by soaking oat groats in distilled water, 0.2% sulphur dioxide, or 0.13% sodium hydroxide, followed by wet milling and screening, resulting in a recovery of 65% to 86% of the starch present in oat groats. Research indicates that the wet milling method is currently of limited practical use for industrial-scale oat starch production, primarily due to challenges associated with separating starch from the hydrated bran and protein layers.

Research by Kasturi et al. [51] indicates that proteases produced the highest oat starch yield, followed by alkaline extraction with either sodium hydroxide (at pH 10.5) or calcium hydroxide (at pH 11.0). Regular water extraction followed by high-shear treatment yielded the least efficient results. In another study by Shah et al. [52] oat starch was isolated using a 0.2 N sodium hydroxide (NaOH) solution, with a pH adjustment to 9. After filtration, centrifugation was employed for starch purification. An alternative method involved the use of 0.1 to 0.01 mol L^{-1} NaOH [53]. Oat starch isolation was also achieved through the addition of wheat gluten to oatmeal in a 3% salt solution [54]. In this process, the dough was kneaded for one hour, forming a gluten network in which oat and gluten proteins interacted. Subsequent washing led to the recovery of the oat starch fraction, converting 60% of the flour weight into starch. This approach resulted in starch with high purity, as lipid and protein content was found to be less than 0.3%. Moreover, neither β-d-glucans nor pentosans were detected in the starch, and the process did not involve the use of any chemicals (Figure 8.1).

Petroleum ether serves as an effective agent for isolating oat starch, primarily due to its ability to expedite the removal of lipids. This lipid removal is particularly advantageous since lipids are interlinked with the starch and protein matrix within oats. By eliminating fats, the separation of the key oat components can be achieved more efficiently through a dry fractionation process. In a specific study, a mixture was created by combining oatmeal with petroleum ether at a ratio of 100 g/500 mL. This mixture was then gently swirled for 4 hours to facilitate the removal of fats. Subsequently, to remove the protein fraction, a 1000-ml solution containing 10 mmol/L of sodium hydroxide (NaOH) at a pH of 11 was utilized. After this step, starch was extracted through a process involving filtration and centrifugation [55].

At the industrial level, processes based on either wet or dry milling, along with the action of various enzymes on oat groats, have demonstrated the capacity to yield starches with remarkable purity levels ranging from 94% to 98%. To enhance the separation of endosperm and bran in the dry milling process, it has been suggested to incorporate a pearling stage [56]. An alternative approach involves lipid extraction utilizing supercritical carbon dioxide (CO_2) before the milling process. This method is proposed to enhance starch separation from cell wall components, possibly by disassembling starch granule clusters. It is worth noting that processes such as steaming and roasting had a similar effect on starch granule clusters as observed in the case of naked oat grains [57]. Evidently, the disruption of granule clusters seems to be an essential step for improving starch extraction efficiency. In a different study, oat flour was immersed in a sodium bisulphite solution with overnight stirring. After this step, the sediment was subjected to centrifugation, and the resulting material was suspended in protease E tricine buffer. This was followed by multiple rounds of centrifugation and washings, ultimately resulting in the isolation of pure oat starch [11].

In the process of extracting oat starch, each method has its own advantages and disadvantages. However, the most substantial yield is achieved through the use of proteases, followed by alkaline extraction methods employing either calcium hydroxide (at pH 11.0) or sodium hydroxide (at pH 10.5). Notably, alkaline and enzymatic extraction techniques stand out as the most effective approaches for oat starch extraction. What sets them apart is their avoidance of high-shear treatments, which, in turn, leads to a reduction in starch damage.

8.2.1.2 Concepts of Starch Swelling and Hydration

Starch granules are inherently water-insoluble compounds, but they possess the ability to undergo hydration at elevated temperatures. This hydration process leads to the swelling of starch granules, accompanied by a disruption of their crystalline structures [32], [58]. Variations in the swelling capacity of starch granules arise from differences in their structural organization and characteristics, which are largely dictated by the botanical source or crop from which they are derived [32], [59]. The structural integrity of starch granules is reinforced by hydrogen bonds that stabilize the double helical structure of amylose and the lateral chains of amylopectin. However, when starch granules are subjected to hydration and exposed to high temperatures, these hydrogen bonds are cleaved and replaced by water molecules [32]. The extent to which starch granules can hydrate and swell hinges on their ability to retain water through hydrogen bonding. Several factors influence this, including the amylose content, the nature of the lateral chains in amylopectin, the presence of phospholipids, granule size, and the existence of cavities and channels within the granules [32], [60]. Hydration and swelling of starch granules lead to changes in starch viscosity. In normal starches, the presence of phospholipids in a complex with amylose inhibits water binding, resulting in lower swelling power and reduced viscosity at high temperatures [32]. Starches with a high amylose content and low amylopectin content exhibit notably low swelling power and viscosity, even at high temperatures. In contrast, starches rich in amylopectin display higher swelling power and viscosity at lower temperatures [32], [61]. The presence of holes and channels within starch granules can weaken their structure, allowing reagents and enzymes to enter, and facilitating starch modifications like hydrolysis [32], [62] Figure 8.2.

The size of starch granules also plays a role in their swelling power. Smaller granules tend to exhibit higher swelling power. Waxy starch granules, rich in amylopectin, particularly with short chains, display a strong positive correlation with swelling power, although the presence of amylose can mitigate this effect. The short chains of amylopectin readily form hydrogen bonds with water molecules, whereas amylose, the amylose–lipid complex, and very long lateral amylopectin chains tend to engage in helical bonds,

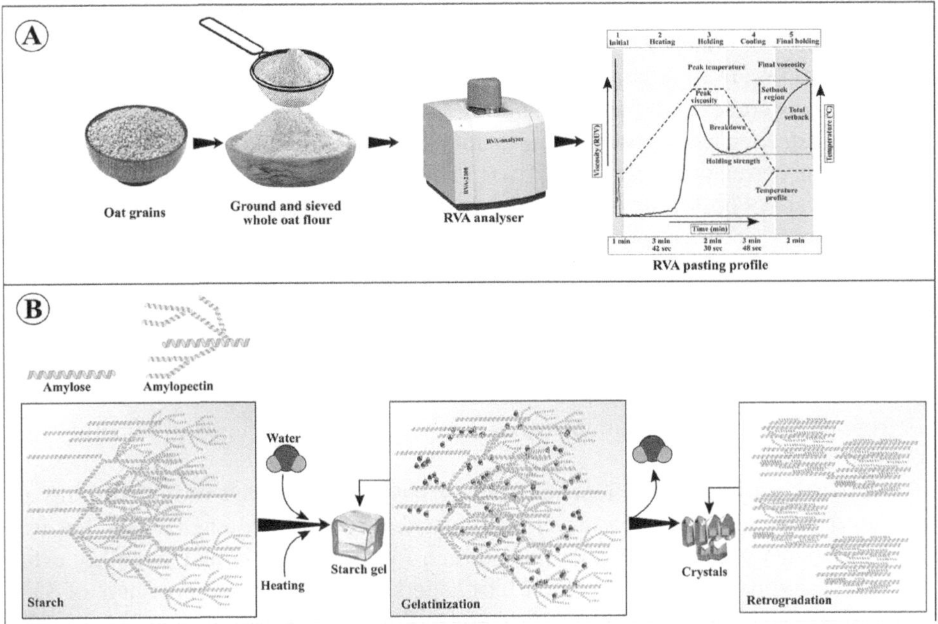

FIGURE 8.2 Typical pasting profiles of oat flour. (A) The characteristic pasting behaviour of oat flour under various conditions. (B) Various functional properties of oat starch, including gelatinization and retrogradation. This part of the figure focuses on highlighting key functional aspects associated with oat starch, such as changes during the heating and cooling processes.

restricting interaction with water molecules [32], [63]. The type of starch granules also matters, with B-type starch granules possessing low amylose content, a high crystallinity percentage, and a large surface area per unit weight, resulting in more efficient hydration and swelling capacities compared to A-type starch granules [64]. The swelling capacity of starch granules is pivotal in enhancing their viscosity and gelling properties [32]. The variations in viscosity and paste properties can be quantitatively assessed using a rapid visco-analyser (RVA). Parameters such as pasting temperature, peak viscosity, pasting time, and setback viscosity are utilized to characterize the behaviour of starch during the heating and cooling process [32], [65]. Shear stress during high-temperature holding periods can further disrupt starch granules and promote amylose leaching, contributing to viscosity breakdown. Upon cooling, viscosity gradually increases until reaching a final viscosity, as reflected in the setback viscosity value [66] Figure 8.2.

8.2.1.3 Hydration Properties of Oat Starch

Swelling power (SP) serves as a metric for assessing the starch's capability to undergo hydration within specific environmental parameters, such as temperature and moisture content. Notably, an inverse relationship exists between the swelling capacity of starch granules and the strength of their internal binding forces [32]. An elevation in temperature was observed to weaken these intragranular binding forces, thus facilitating the ingress of water into the crystalline regions of the starch granules and, consequently, resulting in an augmented SP of the starches. With an increase in temperature, all examined starches exhibited a gradual and anticipated elevation in both their SP and solubility values, a trend observed up to 95°C. A study by Hoover et al. [67] unveiled a significant correlation between SP and the proportion of amylose complexed with lipids; the variety possessing the highest amylose–lipid complexes exhibited the lowest swelling power, and vice versa. Furthermore, Doublier et al. [68] conducted a comparative analysis of the SP of granules and the leaching of amylose in starches from maize, oats, and wheat. Their findings revealed that, under their specified conditions, oats displayed a greater extent of granule swelling and solubilization of glucans compared to other cereal starches. Moreover, in oat starches, amylose was observed to leach out in conjunction with amylopectin. When defatted, oat starches exhibited a reduction in SP from 46.3 to 17.2 while simultaneously experiencing an increase in solubility from 33.3% to 50.7%.

A noteworthy range of genetic diversity has been observed in the swelling and solubility characteristics of oat starch. For instance, when examining oat starches from three different varieties cultivated in the Czech Republic, the SP and solubility exhibited variations spanning from 12.8 to 31.1 g/g and 7% to 35% at a temperature of 85°C, respectively [69]. Moreover, an analysis of swelling volume for oat starches from five different varieties grown across six distinct locations revealed mean values ranging from 5.17 to 6.44 cm³. These findings underscore that the swelling behaviour of oat starch is influenced not only by the genetic makeup of the oat variety but also by the specific conditions of the growth environment [70]. In a comparative study that involved oat and barley starches, each represented by three varieties, it was evident that oat starches exhibited higher SP values. For example, oat starches demonstrated SP values in the range of 24 to 31.5 g/g at 95°C, while barley starches displayed SP values ranging from 20.8 to 21.8 g/g at the same temperature [69]. The factors contributing to the differences in swelling and solubility include amylose content, structural variations within amylose and amylopectin, granular organization, and the presence of minor components such as proteins and lipids [71].

8.2.1.4 Pasting Characteristics of Oat Starch

The assessment of pasting characteristics involves the observation of viscosity changes during the heating of a starch suspension. In the presence of water and at temperatures surpassing the gelatinization point, starch granules undergo swelling, leading to the loss of molecular structure. This results in the leaching of amylose and amylopectin [32]. During this phase, the starch granules become vulnerable to mechanical stress, where shear forces induce granule disruption and the dispersion of amylose and amylopectin, ultimately giving rise to a starch paste. The characteristics of a starch paste are determined by its mechanical and rheological properties [32], [51]. Typically, the pasting process is examined using instruments such as the amylograph, RVA, Brabender amylograph, Ottawa starch viscometer, or dynamic rheometer. These devices monitor the change in viscosity of starch pastes or suspensions under shear stress in relation to temperature. Of these instruments, the RVA is preferred due to its speed and the small sample size it requires, making it a widely employed choice [32]. RVA is a highly versatile and sensitive instrument that is widely preferred for the examination of oat starch's pasting properties. The RVA operates by replicating the cooking process of cereals. It accomplishes this by subjecting a suspension of flour and water to a specific temperature cycle, which involves heating, holding, cooling, and holding again. This meticulous simulation of the cooking procedure provides valuable insights into the behaviour and characteristics of starch under varying temperature conditions Figure 8.2. The viscosity of cereal starches is notably influenced by lipids, which form complexes with amylose, thus retarding or even impeding granule swelling. Consequently, amylose solubility is reduced, leading to a deceleration of the pasting process and limiting gel formation. Such complexes necessitate higher temperatures for dissociation. In comparison to other cereal starches, oat starch exhibits a higher pasting temperature due to its elevated lipid content.

Mukhtar et al. [72] conducted an analysis of pasting parameters for three oat starches, reporting peak viscosity (PV), trough viscosity (TV), breakdown viscosity (BV), and final viscosity (FV) values ranging from 2554 to 3931 cP, 1490 to 2219 cP, 889 to 2369 cP, and 3188 to 3776 cP, respectively. Another study by Dar et al. [73] revealed PV, TV, BV, FV, and setback viscosity (SV) values of 3951 cP, 2634 cP, 1317 cP, 4210 cP, and 1576, respectively, for oat starch. Oat starch, when compared to other starches, is distinguished by its higher pasting temperature, primarily due to its abundant lipid content. SV and FV are attributed to retrogradation and consequently assume significance in the food industry when starch is employed as an ingredient or additive.

8.2.1.5 Gelatinization of Oat Starch

Starch granules undergo a gelatinization process characterized by hydration and swelling at elevated temperatures, resulting in the disordering of crystal structures and the loss of birefringence [32], [74]. This process initiates at the granule's hilum, typically the least organized region. Native starch granules exhibit a distinct hilum with well-defined growth rings formed by the orderly alignment of amylose and amylopectin, giving rise to the "maltese cross" pattern under polarized light [75]. During gelatinization, as starch granules absorb moisture and heat, crystallinity disruption commences at the hilum area, accompanied by partial swelling, a reduction in birefringence, and a slight increase in viscosity [32]. The pattern of disruption is notably influenced by the hilum's position in the granule and its crystalline polymorphism [32], [76]. For granules with an eccentric hilum, crystallinity disruption and swelling commence on the proximal or distal surfaces of the hilum. In contrast, central hilum starches experience disruption and swelling from the central hilum or the entire granule surface [77]. As temperature and time progress, these changes intensify, leading to more extensive disruption of crystallinity, loss of birefringence, and increased swelling and viscosity from the hilum towards the granule's outer regions Figure 8.2. The specific time and temperature requirements for this process are contingent upon the physicochemical characteristics of starch granules from different botanical sources [32]. Differential scanning calorimetry (DSC) is a valuable tool for characterizing the thermal behaviour of starch during heating. Thermal transitions are defined by onset (T_o), peak (T_p), and end-set (T_c) transition temperatures [78]. Enthalpy (ΔH), measured in joules per gram of sample, is calculated from the peak areas in the DSC thermogram. Gelatinization initiates when starch granules can no longer bind additional water molecules, resulting in swelling, partial granule rupture, loss of birefringence, and the leaching of small amylose molecules into the solution. The remaining amylose and amylopectin disperse, forming a sol, accompanied by increased viscosity, reaching its peak value.

T_o marks the start of starch gelatinization, representing the melting of the weakest crystallites. Subsequently, viscosity decreases (medium viscosity) as starch granules break due to agitation, and disrupted granule portions become indistinguishable from the background under polarized light. T_p is achieved when complete birefringence loss occurs [79]. As the temperature continues to rise, a network of swollen starch granules begins to form, transitioning from a sol to a gel, leading to maximum viscosity. T_c corresponds to the final temperature required for complete gelatinization. ΔH provides insight into changes during crystallite melting, serving as a measure of the degree of crystallinity or damage to the starch structure before gelatinization. ΔH is inversely related to amylose content, granule size, and the extent of starch structure damage.

Paton et al. [80] reported that oat starch exhibited a higher melting temperature compared to other cereal starches. Subsequent studies further characterized the thermal properties of oat starches. Mukhtar et al. [72] conducted research on oat starches from three oat cultivars, reporting transition temperatures (T_o), (T_p), and (T_c) within the ranges of 48.5°C to 55.1°C, 79.6°C to 82.5°C, and 100.5°C to 101.2°C, respectively. Pereira et al. [81] found T_o, T_p, and T_c values of 57.42°C, 62.85°C, and 67.71°C, respectively, for oat starch. Rhymer et al. [70] conducted an extensive analysis of oat starches from five Canadian varieties grown in different locations, and they reported varying mean T_p values ranging from 57.72°C to 60.32°C and ΔH values ranging from 8.74 to 9.48 J/g. Notably, these thermal parameters were influenced by both genotype and environmental factors. In a separate study, Šubarić et al. [69] investigated oat starches from three varieties cultivated in the Czech Republic, and they observed enthalpy change (ΔH) values ranging from 7.88 to 10.15 J/g. Comparatively, when oat starches were examined in relation to barley starches, the researchers reported that only the conclusion temperature (T_c) of oat starches was notably higher, while the other DSC parameters, including T_o, T_p, and ΔH, closely resembled those of barley starches. This variation in transition temperatures can be attributed to differences in amylose content.

Vamadevan et al. [82] conducted a comprehensive comparison of the gelatinization profiles of oat starch with 16 other starches from diverse botanical sources. Oat starch, categorized in group 1 based on amylopectin's internal unit chain composition, exhibited one of the lowest gelatinization temperatures and ΔH values. Their analysis indicated a correlation between gelatinization properties and the cluster structure of amylopectin. T_o was negatively correlated with the number of building blocks per cluster and positively correlated with internal building chain length (IB-CL), while ΔH was positively correlated with the external chain length of amylopectin. A structural model of amylopectin was proposed to elucidate the differences in the thermal properties of various starches. Group 1 starches, which include oat starch and other A-type starches, have shorter IB-CL and larger numbers of blocks per cluster, resulting in lower flexibility for conformational packing and an increased likelihood of developing non-parallel double helices during biosynthesis. In contrast, group 4 starches, which include B-type starches, have longer IB-CL and smaller numbers of blocks per cluster, resulting in greater conformational flexibility and an increased likelihood of developing parallel double helices. The significance of amylopectin's internal structure in determining the physicochemical properties of starch has been reviewed extensively.

Furthermore, the effects of developing endosperm and pin-milling on the thermal properties of oat starch were investigated using DSC. Stevenson et al. [83] and Zheng et al. [84] observed that gelatinization temperatures and ΔH values of oat starch increased by approximately 4°C and 2 J/g, respectively, from day 15 to day 33 after anthesis. This increase could be partially attributed to an increase in amylose content and a decrease in the amount of short amylopectin unit chains (DP 6–12). Pin-milling, on the other hand, had minimal impact on starch gelatinization, and starches from milling fractions of different sizes (150–300 μm, <150 μm, and 300–850 μm) exhibited similar gelatinization parameters. It is worth noting that further increases in milling time and energy input might lead to decreased DSC gelatinization parameters.

8.2.1.6 Retrogradation

Starch retrogradation is a phenomenon that occurs subsequent to gelatinization, representing the process by which the amylopectin within gelatinized starch granules transitions from an initial amorphous or disordered state to a more crystalline and ordered state [32], [85]. This transformation is evident in the thickening and stiffening of starch pastes. During retrogradation, the previously dispersed amylopectin and amylose chains reassemble into more organized structures within the gelatinized starch paste [32]. These alterations in starch properties during both gelatinization and retrogradation play a fundamental role in determining its functional characteristics for various food processing and industrial applications [32], [86].

Notably, both amylopectin and amylose contribute to the retrogradation phenomenon. Oat starches exhibit a slower rate of retrogradation compared to starches from other cereals [16]. This can be attributed, at least in part, to the higher lipid content present in oat starch. Several factors, including the amylose content and the formation of amylose–lipid complexes, influence and restrict starch retrogradation [32], [87]. Starches with higher amylose content and lower molecular weight exhibit a greater tendency to undergo retrogradation Figure 8.2. The size of starch granules also plays a crucial role, with larger granules displaying greater stability in retrogradation, while smaller granules are more prone to retrograde [32], [88].

These characteristics not only influence the nutritional profile and quality of food products but also impact their acceptability and shelf-life. The retrogradation of amylose is a relatively swift process owing to its linear structure, which accelerates the re-association process [32]. Conversely, amylopectin retrogradation typically takes several days to develop. However, the influence of starch granule size on retrogradation becomes less pronounced when there is significant variation in granule characteristics [32]. In this context, B-type starch granules characterized by lower amylose content, shorter branched-chain amylopectin, and higher lipid content are less prone to retrograde compared to A-type granules [89]. It's worth noting that the retrogradation properties of small starch granules may not always align with their SP, as starch granule characteristics vary across different types, making it challenging to establish a universal principle that applies to all starches [90].

Numerous researchers [91]–[94] have undertaken comparative analyses of the retrogradation process in cereal starches, consistently noting that oat starches exhibit a notably slower retrogradation rate when compared to wheat and maize starches. Notably, a study by Paton et al. [80] highlighted that oat starches display distinctive characteristics, such as heightened viscosity and the formation of cooled gels that are clearer, less rigid, more elastic, and more adhesive, in addition to displaying a reduced susceptibility to retrogradation when compared to other cereal starches. This phenomenon has been conjectured to be associated with the comparatively higher lipid content found in oat starches, which could potentially serve as a causal factor contributing to the decelerated retrogradation of oat starches. As corroborated by the research, the removal of lipids from oat starch does indeed result in an increased retrogradation rate; however, even under these conditions, the retrogradation process remains less pronounced in oat starches when contrasted with other starches [91]. The researchers also indicated that oat starches exhibited lower rigidity and higher elasticity compared to maize and wheat starches. The oat variety with the highest oil content, Chicauhua, resembled wheat starch in rheological properties. DSC showed consistent gelatinization enthalpy among oat starches but lower compared to maize and wheat. Oat starches had two to three times higher enthalpy for the amylose–lipid complex transition than maize or wheat.

Recent investigations have shed light on the impact of developing endosperm and pin-milling on oat starch retrogradation, as revealed through DSC, as reported by Stevenson et al. [83] and Zheng et al. [84]. In the case of developing endosperm, the retrogradation rate of gelatinized oat starches, stored at 4°C for 1 month, demonstrated an increase of approximately 10–20% between the 15th and 33rd days following anthesis, as observed by Zheng et al. [84]. This increase in retrogradation rate can, at least in part, be ascribed to a reduction in the quantity of short amylopectin unit chains and an augmentation in amylose content. Regarding the influence of pin-milling on oat kernel, it was found to exert a minimal impact on the retrogradation properties of oat starch. Stevenson et al. [83] determined that starches derived from different milling fractions, varying in size from 150–300 μm, <150 μm, and 300–850 μm, exhibited relatively similar retrogradation behaviours when gelatinized starch was stored at 4°C for 7 days. In a comparative assessment involving three varieties of barley starch and three varieties of oat starch, Šubarić et al. [69] found that oat starches consistently displayed lower degrees of retrogradation after 7 and 14 days of gelatinization at 4°C. This was noteworthy, especially given the similarity in melting temperatures between the two starch types. The reduced retrogradation observed in oat starch may, in part, be attributable to a higher concentration of endogenous lipids, a point emphasized in a prior review of oat starch by Autio et al. [95].

8.2.1.7 Rheological Behaviour of Oat Starch

The rheological properties of starch pastes and gels are contingent upon a multitude of factors [32]. These encompass the chemical composition of the starch, the concentration of the starch, the specific pasting conditions (comprising temperature, shear rate, and heating rate), as well as the subsequent storage conditions (including temperature and duration) [32], [96]. T_o explore and analyse the visco-elastic characteristics of starch, the prevailing method employed is the utilization of a dynamic rheometer.

8.2.1.7.1 Steady Shear

As the shear rate increased, there was a rapid initial rise in shear stress, followed by a plateauing effect at higher shear rates. This behaviour is characteristic of shear thinning and is often seen in pseudoplastic fluids [32]. According to Morris et al. [97], this shear-thinning phenomenon can be explained by the disruption of an entangled network of polysaccharide molecules during shearing. As the shear rate increases, the rate of disruption of these intermolecular entanglements becomes greater than the rate of their reformation, resulting in a reduction in apparent viscosity. Singh et al. [98] successfully described the rheological properties of pastes using the Herschel-Bulkley model within a shear rate range of 0 to 1000 s^{-1}, with a high coefficient of determination (R^2 exceeding 0.99). They observed that starch pastes exhibited shear-thinning behaviour, behaving as pseudoplastic fluids, where the storage modulus (G') exceeded the loss modulus (G"), indicating a more elastic than viscous nature. The flow behaviour index (n), which indicates the extent of shear-thinning behaviour as it deviates from 1, fell within the range of 0.42 to 0.50 and 0.59 to 0.94, reflecting the degree of shear thinning. The consistency index (K), a rheological parameter that reflects the viscosity values, ranged from 0.06 to 3.08 Pa·s. Higher K values indicate stronger structural strength and result in less thixotropic behaviour, where the material doesn't regain its viscosity quickly after shearing.

8.2.1.7.2 *Dynamic Shear Properties*

It is essential to document the influence of temperature on the rheological properties of fluids since a wide range of temperatures is encountered during the processing and storage of fluid foods [32]. When examining the rheological properties of starches using a dynamic rheometer, significant variations were observed in peak values for the storage dynamic modulus (G'), the loss modulus (G"), and the tangent delta (tan δ) [99]. Here, G' represents the amount of energy stored in the material and recovered during each cycle of deformation, while G" signifies the amount of energy dissipated or lost during the same deformation cycles. Notably, oat starch displayed a G' that consistently exceeded G" across all starches, indicating its more elastic than viscous behaviour. During a frequency sweep, it became apparent that as the angular frequency (ω) increased, both G' and G" values increased, while the complex viscosity (η*) values decreased, revealing a low-frequency dependency [100]. Complex viscosity (η*) serves as a measure of the overall resistance to flow [16]. Singh et al. [98] conducted an examination of tan δ and η* values for starch pastes from various oat cultivars at an angular frequency of 6.28 rad/s and at a temperature of 25°C. They reported that the values of G" significantly exceeded those of G' at all frequency values, indicating a strong elastic behaviour in the starch samples. The tan δ values fell within the range of 0.04 to 0.22, suggesting that all the samples exhibited a more elastic than viscous nature. Additionally, the complex viscosity values for the starch pastes varied significantly, ranging from 338 to 549 Pa·s.

8.2.1.8 Modifications of Oat Starch for Use as a Functional Food Ingredient

8.2.1.8.1 *Chemical Modification*

Oat starch can undergo several modifications, including oxidation [101], cross-linking [102], phosphorylation [103], and acetylation [104], to yield altered properties. Oxidation introduced carboxyl groups onto the starch and led to a reduction in both molecular size and granule size [105]. This process increased the starch's water-binding capacity and solubility while reducing viscosity during pasting events. It also decreased the yield stress and consistency coefficient of flow properties. For cross-linking oat starch, two methods were employed: one involving sodium trimetaphosphate and sodium tripolyphosphate, and another using $POCl_3$ [106]. Cross-linking resulted in a decrease in granular swelling and made the starch less susceptible to α-amylase, rendering it a type of resistant starch. Research by Woo et al. [107] suggested that cross-linking raised the gelatinization temperatures and reduced the ΔH (enthalpy change) of gelatinization. However, Mirmoghtadaie et al. [106] reported that this modification had little effect on the DSC gelatinization temperatures. Hence, the gelatinization properties of modified starch largely depend on the specific preparation method. Both phosphorylation and acetylation, which are substitution-type modifications of oat starch, had similar outcomes with subtle distinctions as described by Berski et al. [105] and Mirmoghtadaie et al. [106]. These modifications led to a decrease in starch molecular weight, an increase in water solubility and water-binding capacity, and a reduction in DSC gelatinization parameters. During pasting events, acetylation reduced starch viscosity, while phosphorylation increased it. This difference is likely due to the significantly increased ionic interactions between starch chains resulting from phosphorylation, as noted by Berski et al. [105] (Table 8.1).

8.2.1.8.2 Physical Modifications

Various hydrothermal treatments, such as steaming and roasting, are commonly employed to both dry oats and deactivate endogenous enzymes, thereby extending the shelf life. These treatments have notable effects on the properties of oat starch [32]. Specifically, steaming and roasting cause changes in granule shapes and may distort the larger granules within oat kernels. In a study conducted by Ovando-Martínez et al. [108], various hydrothermal treatments, including ethanol boiling, ethanol boiling and roasting, steaming at 106°C, steaming at 106°C followed by roasting, autoclaving with cover at 120°C or 130°C, and autoclaving without cover at 120°C or 130°C, were applied to treat oat flour. These treatments resulted in a reduction in the molecular size of amylopectin, which may be attributed to the action of endogenous amylases [109]. The impact of these treatments on starch properties varied depending on the specific treatment type. For instance, uncovered autoclaving led to a substantial decrease in the enthalpy change (ΔH) of gelatinization while increasing gelatinization temperatures. Covered autoclaving at 120°C and steaming significantly hindered retrogradation. Uncovered autoclaving at 120°C notably reduced starch viscosity during pasting events and reduced the content of resistant starch [108].

Shah et al. [52] found that autoclaving oat starch at 121°C for 30 minutes, followed by storage at 4°C for 24 hours, also led to a decrease in gelatinization temperatures and ΔH, as well as a reduction in resistant starch content by approximately 10–15%. This combined treatment similarly decreased starch viscosity during pasting events. These hydrothermal treatments are believed to impact the interactions between starch chains within the crystalline and amorphous domains of the granules, potentially disrupting the crystalline units [110]. Different treatment conditions can affect the properties and structures of starch to varying degrees. Vamadevan et al. [82] conducted a study comparing the effects of annealing on the DSC gelatinization behaviours of starches from various botanical origins, including oats. Significant correlations were identified between structural parameters, such as the number of building blocks in clusters, the inter-block

TABLE 8.1   Chemical and Physical Modifications of Oat Starch

MODIFICATION TYPE	FINDINGS	REFERENCE
Physical		
Autoclaving-storage	Oat starch, comprising 20% starch content, underwent autoclaving at 121°C for 30 minutes, followed by storage at 4°C for 24 hours. Subsequent enzymatic analysis revealed an approximately 10–15% increase in resistant starch content. The morphological characteristics of oat starches transformed into a continuous network, resulting in increased values for onset temperature (T_o), peak temperature (i_p), and conclusion temperature (T_c). X-ray diffraction (XRD) analysis unveiled an additional peak at 13° and an intensified peak at 20°, encompassing the primary XRD peaks. These findings indicate the formation of an amylose–lipid complex resulting from a dual autoclaving-retrogradation cycle. Peaks at 13° and 20° are characteristic of the V-type pattern in XRD. Rheological analysis indicated that retrograded oat starches exhibited shear-thickening behaviour, as evidenced by the Herschel-Bulkley model and frequency sweep analysis.	[52]
Annealing	Annealing, applied for up to 24 hours, had the effect of raising the temperatures and increasing the enthalpy change (ΔH) associated with gelatinization in oat starch. Additionally, it led to a reduction in the range of melting temperatures during the gelatinization process.	[111]
Hydrothermal treatments	Various hydrothermal treatments were applied to oat flour, encompassing ethanol boiling, ethanol boiling followed by roasting, steaming at 106°C, steaming at 106°C followed by roasting, autoclaving at 120°C or 130°C with a cover, and autoclaving at 120°C or 130°C without a cover. Starch was subsequently isolated from the treated flour for analysis. Autoclaving with a cover was found to increase the granule size without impacting the starch composition. These hydrothermal treatments resulted in a decrease in the molecular weight of the amylopectin component. Uncovered autoclaving notably reduced the enthalpy change (ΔH) associated with gelatinization while elevating the gelatinization temperatures. Steaming and covered autoclaving at 120°C exhibited a pronounced inhibitory effect on retrogradation. Additionally, uncovered autoclaving at 120°C significantly reduced starch viscosity during pasting events. Uncovered autoclaving had a substantial impact on reducing the content of resistant starch.	[108]

(Continued)

TABLE 8.1   (Continued) Chemical and Physical Modifications of Oat Starch

MODIFICATION TYPE	FINDINGS	REFERENCE
Steaming, roasting	Oat kernels were subjected to various treatments, including normal pressure steaming, autoclaving, and hot-air/infrared roasting. These treatments had a significant impact on the granule shapes within the kernels, resulting in the deformation of large granules. Moreover, the treatments reduced the interaction between starch and protein in the kernels.	[57]
Chemical		
Acetylation	The molecular weight of acetylated starch, with a number-based molecular weight of 3.51×10^4 g/mol, was notably lower than that of native starch, which had a number-based molecular weight of 8.8×10^4 g/mol. The process of acetylation significantly increased the starch's water-binding capacity, going from 6 to 38 g/g at 95°C, and its water solubility, increasing from 3 to 48% at 95°C, while reducing the granule size. Acetylation also led to a decrease in gelatinization temperatures, as well as a reduction in the enthalpy change (ΔH) of gelatinization. Furthermore, the pasting temperature and peak viscosity during the pasting event of the starch were lowered by acetylation. Additionally, acetylation increased the retrogradation of the starch paste during cooling, especially in the short term. Notably, acetylated oat starch paste exhibited strong gelling properties at 20°C, and the flow curve for this paste was only obtainable at 50°C.	[105]
	The acetylation of oat starch resulted in increased swelling power and a decrease in both syneresis and differential scanning calorimetry (DSC) gelatinization temperatures.	[106]
Phosphorylation	Phosphorylation of oat starch was carried out using sodium tripolyphosphate and sodium phosphate to produce mono starch phosphates. This phosphorylation process led to a decrease in the weight-based molecular weight, reducing it from 9×10^7 to 5×10^7 g/mol. It also resulted in an increase in the starch's water-binding capacity, which rose from 6 to 95 g/g at 95°C, and an increase in water solubility, from 3% to 12% at 95°C. Additionally, phosphorylation decreased the granule size, as well as the onset temperature (T_o) and the enthalpy change (ΔH) associated with DSC gelatinization parameters, while substantially increasing starch viscosity during pasting events. Furthermore, phosphorylation had the effect of increasing the yield stress, from 1.5 to 2.8 Pa at 20°C, and the consistency coefficient, from 3.2 to 5.7 Pa s/n, in the flow curve of oat starch.	[105]

(Continued)

TABLE 8.1   (Continued) Chemical and Physical Modifications of Oat Starch

MODIFICATION TYPE	FINDINGS	REFERENCE
Cross-linking	Cross-linking of oat starch using a $POCl_3$-based method had several effects. It led to a decrease in the swelling power and an increase in syneresis (the expulsion of liquid from a gel or network), but had no significant impact on the DSC gelatinization temperatures.	[106]
	In comparison to native starch, cross-linked starch produced via a method involving sodium trimetaphosphate and sodium tripolyphosphate exhibited several notable changes. These included an increased phosphorus content, decreased swelling powers, decreased solubility in KOH (1M) and DMSO (95%) solutions, increased temperatures, and decreased enthalpy change (ΔH) of gelatinization as measured by DSC. Additionally, cross-linking resulted in reduced susceptibility to enzymatic degradation by α-amylase. Modifying the conditions of this process allowed for the optimization of the content of resistant starch.	[107]
Oxidation	Oxidation of oat starch using sodium hypochlorite resulted in several noteworthy changes. It introduced carboxyl groups (0.25%), decreased the weight-based molecular weight from 9×10^7 to 4×10^7 g/mol, and increased the starch's water-binding capacity, going from 6 to 29 g/g at 95°C, as well as water solubility, which increased from 3% to 39% at 95°C. Oxidation also reduced the granule size, with minimal impact on the DSC gelatinization parameters. It led to an increase in pasting temperature and a decrease in viscosity during the pasting events. Additionally, oxidation lowered the yield stress and consistency coefficient in the flow curve of oat starch.	[105]

chain length, and the length of external chains, and various gelatinization parameters. The onset gelatinization temperature exhibited a negative correlation with the number of building blocks ($r = -0.952$, $p < 0.01$) and a positive correlation with inter-block chain length ($r = 0.905$, $p < 0.01$). Moreover, the enthalpy of gelatinization demonstrated a positive correlation with the length of external chains ($r = 0.854$, $p < 0.01$). These findings underscore that the internal structure of starch is indicative of trends in its thermal properties. A model has been proposed based on amylopectin's backbone concept to elucidate how the organization of chains within the semicrystalline lamellae of starch granules is linked to its thermal characteristics (Table 8.1).

8.2.1.9 Applications of Oat Starch as a Functional Food and Non-Food Ingredient

Oat starch is a versatile ingredient found in a wide range of both food and non-food products. Starch, with its soluble macromolecules, contributes essential properties such as adhesion, high viscosity, and surface-coating capabilities, all of which are highly valuable in the food industry [32]. Starches serve various functions, including thickening, stabilizing, gelling, fat replacement, bulking, and texturizing in food products [19]. Comparatively, oat starch has received less industrial attention when contrasted with other cereal starches. This can be attributed to its higher cost and limited availability. Nevertheless, oat starch possesses distinctive properties suitable for specific applications. Its soluble macromolecules bestow adhesion, surface-coating attributes, and high viscosity, all of which are highly desirable in the food sector [112]. Additionally, it finds utility in the paper and pulp industry, where it is employed for sizing and coating papers due to its small granule size and elevated lipid content. Oat starch is extensively employed in the processing of oat-based foods, including the preparation of sauces, snacks, noodles, milk products, and baked goods. It also finds applications in non-food products [19]. One notable industrial use of oat starch is in Oatrim, a fat substitute developed by the U.S. Department of Agriculture. Resistant starch from oats has been employed to create health-conscious products such as low-fat, low-calorie, high-fibre granola cereals and bars [113].

In the realm of cosmetics, oat starch serves as a suitable alternative to talcum powder and functions as a dusting powder for medical gloves. Companies like Alpine Gloves Inc. have patented latex gloves powdered with oat starch, asserting that it reduces the risk of latex allergies by not binding to latex proteins as corn starch does [114]. In research, oat starch has been examined as a fat replacer in mayonnaise, revealing improved stability with increasing oat starch content [115]. Moreover, oat starch plays a pivotal role in various products such as fat replacers, soup, gravy, sauce, and dessert ingredients, as well as paper and cardboard applications. Recent studies have predominantly focused on the potential of oat starch in thermoplastic film production due to its relatively high endogenous lipid content, reaching up to 2.5%. These lipids enhance the hydrophobicity of oat starch films and form inclusion complexes with amylose, preventing phase separation [116].

Studies tracking structural changes in oat starch films plasticized with glycerol over time have shown that these films become rough and heterogeneous during storage. Glycerol diffuses onto the film surface, reducing friction and stickiness. In contrast, barley starch films exhibited different behaviour, with oat starch being notably slower to crystallize initially, likely due to its higher endogenous lipid content [117]. The properties of oat starch films are influenced by various factors, including film production method, type of plasticizer, film thickness, and more. For instance, the choice of plasticizer significantly impacts properties like glass transition temperature, water vapour permeability, and stress/strain at the breaking point. Different plasticizers lead to distinct outcomes, affecting film characteristics [118].

Furthermore, acetylated oat starch, deamidated oat proteins, and succinylated oat proteins have been used in oat cake formulation, enhancing batter viscosity, cake crust colour, and cake volume [116]. This is attributed to the increased viscosity of acetylated oat starch compared to native starch. Oat starch offers potential advantages, particularly in its unique lipid content and small granule size, making it suitable for various industrial applications [18]. It may be considered a viable alternative to other starches in brown paper and cardboard products and as a coating agent for pharmaceutical tablets.

8.2.2 ß-Glucan

Oat β-glucan is a linear polysaccharide composed of β-d-glucopyranose units connected through (1→4) and (1→3) glycosidic bonds. From a technological standpoint, the physicochemical properties of β-glucan hold significant importance in the context of food and industrial applications. Molecular structure, size, solubility, and viscosity emerge as the primary parameters influencing product quality, and they are closely intertwined with the physiological attributes of β-glucan [8]. Molar mass stands out as a critical attribute in understanding the origin and properties of oat β-glucan. Existing literature reveals a range of molar mass values for β-glucans derived from various sources: 35 to 3100 g/mol for oats, 31 to 2700 g/mol for barley, 209 to 416 g/mol for wheat, and 21 to 1100 ×103 g/mol for rye [119]. Additionally, several external factors, including environmental conditions, β-glucanase activity, processing and storage conditions, and the methods employed for extraction and purification, have been identified as impacting molar mass [120]. Traditionally, discussions regarding the use of β-glucan for technological or nutraceutical purposes have revolved around its content and molar mass. However, this section aims to shed light on other essential characteristics that warrant consideration.

8.2.2.1 Molar Mass and Molar Ratio

The molar mass of β-glucans plays a crucial role in shaping their viscosity and functional attributes within the realm of food science [121]. Moreover, it bears significance concerning the physiological effects when these compounds are ingested. Notably, the molar mass of cereal β-glucan displays considerable variability. According to the European Food Safety Authority, the molar mass of barley β-glucan can span a wide range from 50 to 2000 kDa [122]. These variations primarily stem from environmental factors but can also be influenced by factors such as extraction methods, purification processes, depolymerization events, and the specific analytical techniques employed, including the choice of detector and standards used. Mejía et al. [123] highlighted several factors that impact the molar mass of β-glucan homopolymers. These include the physical state of β-glucan within the plant material, the activity of β-glucanase enzymes, the conditions employed during processing, and the storage environment.

The molar ratio, defined as the ratio between cellotriosyl and cellotetraosyl units (DP3/DP4), emerges as a unique feature specific to each cereal, essentially serving as a fingerprint of the β-glucan's structural profile. The molar ratio, or DP, specifically the ratio of DP3 to DP4 units, wields a substantial influence over the functional properties of the β-glucan molecule. It is the longer subunits, such as cellotetraosyl and beyond, that primarily account for the gel-forming and highly viscous characteristics. Meanwhile, cellotriosyl units are instrumental in forming stronger bonds between individual β-glucan chains [124].

This ratio varies across sources, for instance, wheat (ranging from 3.0 to 4.5), barley (1.8 to 3.5), rye (1.9 to 3.0), and oat (1.5 to 2.3) (Lazaridou and Biliaderis, 2007). According to Ryu et al. [125], segments characterized by β-(1–4) bonds exhibit a degree of semi-flexibility, enhancing intermolecular connections and thereby resulting in stronger bonds between the glucan chains. This configuration imparts resistance to flow and elevates viscosity. In contrast, β-(1–3) segments introduce twists into the chains. Notably, the cellotetraosyl units and longer segments with β-(1–4) bonds significantly contribute to increased viscosity and gel formation in oat β-glucan.

There exists a relationship between the DP of β-glucans and their molar mass. Longer chains correspond to higher molar mass. Therefore, a lower molar ratio, indicating a greater presence of DP4 units, is expected to yield a higher molar mass, thus establishing an inverse relationship between the molar ratio and molar mass. Comparative studies, employing the same extraction procedure on a high β-glucan barley mutant and its parent variety, have revealed substantial differences in solubility. The reduced solubility of barley β-glucans can be attributed to the high prevalence of DP3 oligomer blocks. Comparative investigations, conducted using the same extraction method on both a high β-glucan barley mutant and its parent variety, have unveiled marked differences in solubility. Notably, the high β-glucan barley mutant exhibited a distinctive block structure characterized by a higher composition of DP3 (78.9%) and a lower proportion of DP4 (16.7%) in contrast to the barley mother (72.1% DP3 and 21.4% DP4) and oat (66.1% DP3 and 29.1% DP4). The diminished solubility of the barley samples can potentially be attributed to the presence of substructures comprising extended and repetitive cellotriosyl sequences [126]. Similar findings were reported by Håkansson et al. [127], who observed that purified oat and barley β-glucan preparations with a high molar ratio exhibit reduced solubility due to the higher proportion of cellotriosyl units, leading to tight packing of the β-glucan chains, limiting water interaction.

Comparing oat β-glucan (molar ratio 1.5–2.3) to barley β-glucan (molar ratio 2.3–3.4), the research data consistently highlights the superior solubility of oat β-glucan [119], [128]. It's crucial to note that the molar ratio is heavily influenced by cultivar and environmental conditions, as demonstrated among Canadian oat varieties. These factors significantly impact the molar ratio and should be carefully considered when selecting grains for specific β-glucan applications [126].

Recent evidence suggests that barley β-glucan with a higher molar ratio (DP3/DP4) exhibits greater resistance to wheat β-glucanase [129]. This insight potentially allows for estimating and controlling the fate of β-glucan during food processing, particularly with respect to enzymatic degradation. The application of β-glucan in products like bread has historically posed challenges due to enzymatic activity in the added flour [130]. The selective use of high molar ratio β-glucan could offer a viable solution, although reduced solubility is a factor to be considered. Current knowledge regarding the relationship between molar ratio and functionality is limited, necessitating further exploration. Studies on the structure-function relationship of cereal β-glucan, particularly concerning the molar ratio, remain scarce. Nevertheless, existing reports underscore the significance of the DP3/DP4 ratio in determining the technological and physiological functionality of β-glucan, demanding more comprehensive research in this domain.

8.2.2.2 Solubility

The solubility of β-glucan is a pivotal physicochemical property, profoundly influencing its extractability and potential applications. Despite the shared general molecular structure among cereal-derived β-glucans, there exist notable differences in their solubility, primarily stemming from variations in the molar ratio. Solubility, in this context, denotes the maximum amount of β-glucan that can be diluted in water to create homogeneous polymer solutions under controlled conditions of temperature and pressure [131].

Notably, even though β-glucans fall under the category of soluble fibres, their water solubility is affected by the molecular irregularity of their structures [121]. Elleuch et al. [132] demonstrated that the presence of carboxyl (COOH) or sulphite (SO_2) groups increases β-glucan solubility. The chemical conformation of the molecule enables significant interactions and associations with water molecules, but excessive polymerization can decrease solubility [133]. Furthermore, β-glucan solubility and extraction into water decrease with time, temperature, pH, and other physical extraction conditions. Additionally, moisture during β-glucan processing has been found to promote depolymerization, and treatments such as microwave treatment or germination before extraction have been shown to improve extractability and nutraceutical properties [134].

Comparing the solubility of oat-derived β-glucans to barley-derived β-glucans, it is generally observed that oat-sourced β-glucans exhibit higher solubility, primarily because solubility decreases as the molar ratio increases [135]. The presence of various biopolymers in the cell wall, along with their spatial arrangement and interactions between cell wall components, can potentially affect mechanical resistance, permeability, and thus compromise compound solubility [136]. Several studies have explored the optimal extraction conditions for barley β-glucan and indicated that maximum solubility is achieved at around 55°C. However, under these conditions, partial solubilization of starch can occur, leading to fibre contamination [134].

Furthermore, the solubility of β-glucan is influenced by its intermolecular aggregation states and high-level structure [137]. Physical treatments, even without modifying the molecular structure, can impact β-glucan solubility and associated physiological properties. Håkansson et al. [127] demonstrated that extracted barley β-glucans dissolve at a molecular level, whereas oat β-glucans dissolve as aggregates. Studies on the aggregation properties of barley and oat β-glucans have shown loosely and highly aggregated structures for both types [138]. Some aggregates formed by barley β-glucans were notably dense and well-defined spheres.

It's essential to note that while solubility was traditionally considered a key factor for the health-endorsing properties of β-glucans, recent research suggests that insoluble β-glucan may also possess nutraceutical traits, albeit through different mechanisms [139]. However, further research is necessary to extend the understanding of these properties and the mechanisms behind them. Additionally, the formation of aggregates and its implications on solubility require further investigation. Beyond its impact on physiological effects, β-glucan solubility plays a crucial role in extraction and food applications. Controlled depolymerization for adjusting technological and physiological properties shows promise for future research, and a better comprehension of β-glucan behaviour in solution can lead to more efficient extraction methods, making cereal β-glucan a valuable ingredient for the food industry.

8.2.2.3 Viscosity

The formation of a highly viscous solution is of paramount significance, both in terms of technological applicability and physiological benefits. The viscosity of a β-glucan solution primarily hinges on two factors: the distribution of molecular weight and the concentration within the solution, constrained by β-glucan solubility [134]. Furthermore, the viscosity of β-glucan preparations can exhibit substantial variability, influenced by factors such as cultivar and environmental conditions [140]. Research conducted by Mikkelsen et al. [141] explored the viscosity of crude and purified β-glucan extracts from oats and barley concerning concentration, shear rate, and temperature. Their findings indicated significant distinctions between barley and oat β-glucan. Barley β-glucan demonstrated low viscosity with Newtonian flow behaviour, while oat β-glucan displayed shear-thinning, high viscosity behaviour, approximately 100 times greater than barley β-glucan at similar concentrations. These observations align with the stronger affinity of oat β-glucan toward the formation of micro-gel structures [142].

Studies investigating the impact of dissolution temperature on the gelling properties of oat and barley β-glucan at low concentrations (1 and 1.5%) revealed that gelation did not occur at 85°C [143]. The viscosity is found to be independent of starch and α-dextrin impurities but can be enhanced by the presence of mucin. The ideal gelation temperature was reported as 37°C for oat β-glucan and 57°C for barley β-glucan. Notably, cooking prior to extraction increased the viscosity of β-glucan extract from pasta [144], but no correlation was found between viscosity and β-glucan content. Oxidative treatment of β-glucan led to gelation at the same temperatures but produced weaker gels due to polymer degradation by oxidizing agents [143]. Oxidation of barley β-glucan, particularly with hydrogen peroxide, emerged as a cost-effective and efficient means to modify β-glucan for industrial food applications [145]. However, it should be noted that, especially under elevated temperatures, oxidation may lead to complete depolymerization, necessitating careful adjustments to maintain the desired functional properties.

Debates persist regarding the influence of molar mass on β-glucan solution viscosity. Some studies have found a direct correlation between molecular weight and apparent viscosity [141], [146], [147]. This explains the lower viscosity of extracts obtained through digestive enzyme use, leading to partially degraded β-glucan, which, according to Mäkelä et al. [147], could compromise its physiological properties. Conversely, other researchers have proposed that the product of molar mass and soluble β-glucan exhibits a direct correlation with viscosity [148]. Thus, a reduction in molar mass due to enzymatic activity or other events does not necessarily cause a decrease in viscosity or related physiological properties. Nonetheless, a reduction in apparent viscosity may enhance the ease of handling and processing for industrial applications. Therefore, further research should focus on understanding the intricate structure-size-function relationship of β-glucan comprehensively. This will enable the development of β-glucan preparations that combine health-endorsing properties with efficient processability, maximizing the utility of cereal β-glucan.

Moreover, aside from the technological considerations, the viscosity of β-glucan solutions during their passage through the gastrointestinal tract warrants attention. It is a pivotal property, primarily responsible for the health-endorsing characteristics. Recent in vivo studies have reported differences in intestinal viscosity between barley and oat β-glucan [149]. Using MRI technology, higher intestinal viscosity was observed following the consumption of a barley β-glucan meal compared to an oat β-glucan meal. These distinctions were attributed to structural differences between barley and oat β-glucan, with impurities in the extract also being considered as potential influencing factors. Both β-glucan samples exhibited significantly higher intestinal viscosity compared to the control glucose solution.

Furthermore, evidence suggests that products containing β-glucan processed in a dry manner result in higher extractability and viscosity during their passage through a gastrointestinal model. Regand et al. [120] reported that increasing the content of soluble β-glucan led to higher in vitro viscosity during gastric system passage, reducing starch digestibility and consequently lowering the glycaemic response. However, a recent study on the incorporation of β-glucan into bread products found that viscosity did not correlate with the reduction in glycaemic response after in vitro digestion [150]. While these results require further validation, they raise questions about the significance of viscosity in the health-endorsing effects of β-glucan, especially given that high viscosity can pose challenges in many industrial applications. Consequently, a β-glucan preparation with low viscosity, yet maintaining health-endorsing properties, would be ideal, expanding the industrial utility of cereal β-glucan within health claim concentrations.

Despite the key role of β-glucan solution viscosity in technological and physiological aspects, the attributes influencing viscosity and its impact on the human gastrointestinal system remain incompletely understood. Approaches like oxidation and modification can be valuable tools for adjusting solubility and resultant viscosity but are underutilized due to knowledge gaps in the structure-size-function relationship of β-glucan.

8.2.2.4 Extraction of ß-Glucan from Cereals

Cereal β-glucans represent distinct glucose polymers, set apart not only by their origin but also by their unique physicochemical characteristics [151]. The extraction of cereal β-glucans poses considerable challenges, rendering them more costly compared to β-glucans derived from alternative sources. Over the years, methodologies for producing cereal β-glucans have continued to evolve. These methods are primarily based on the solubility of β-glucans in hot water and alkaline solutions, followed by the separation of dissolved proteins through isoelectric precipitation, and precipitation of β-glucans using ammonium sulphate, 2-propanol, or ethanol [152]. For research purposes, additional purification steps involve repeated precipitations and enzymatic hydrolysis of residual starch, leading to a purity level of 99% [153], [154] (Figure 8.3).

Du et al. [155] introduced an innovative extraction method for β-glucans from hull-less barley bran, utilizing water in combination with accelerated solvent extraction (ASE) and response surface methodology. When compared with other techniques such as ultrasound-assisted extraction, microwave-assisted extraction, and reflux extraction, the ASE method demonstrated superior extraction yields, specifically at 16.39 ± 0.3%. ASE not only produced higher β-glucan yields but also proved to be an environmentally friendly, efficient, and time-saving extraction method, holding promise for industrial-scale applications. Furthermore, Redmond et al. [151] conducted research on the extraction and purification of oat β-glucans, leading to the production of highly

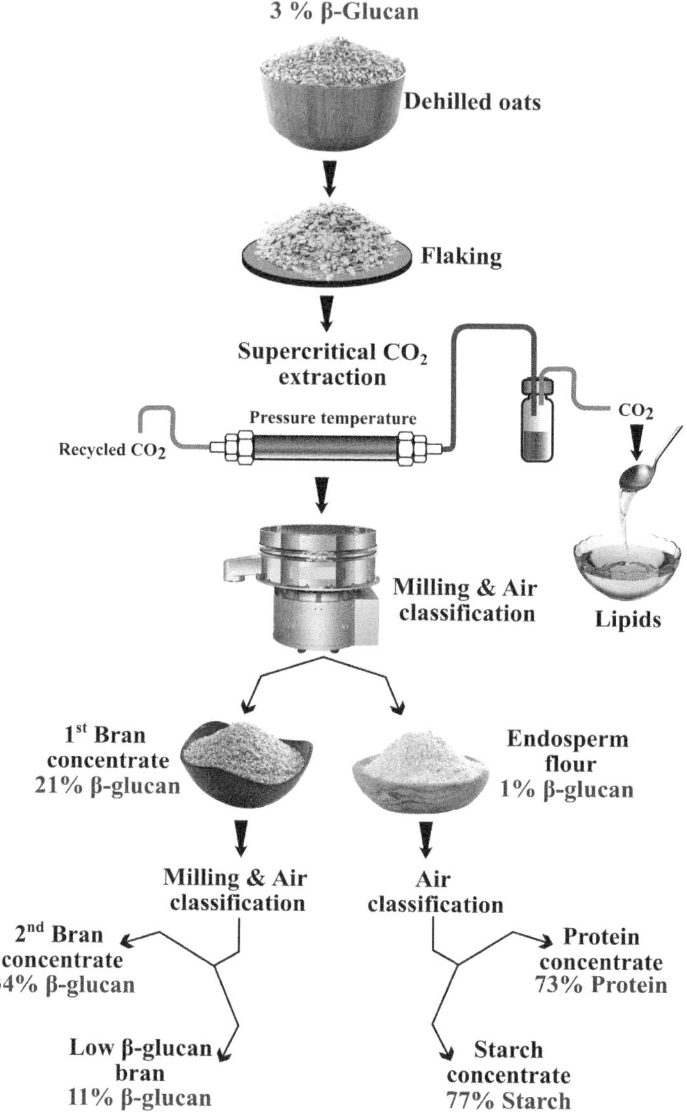

FIGURE 8.3 The steps involved in the extraction and production of oat ß-glucans on an industrial scale.

pure β-glucans. These preparations are distinguished by their clarity, colourlessness, viscosity, and stability, particularly when stored at ambient temperatures with low ash concentrations (Figure 8.3).

In the study by Benito-Roman et al. (2013), various types of cereal β-glucan were successfully extracted using pressurized hot water (20 bar) as a solvent within a fixed bed extractor. The authors achieved impressive yields, with 97% of purified β-glucan, having an approximate molar mass of 500 kDa. This high yield was obtained by utilizing 4 g of water and subjecting it to a temperature of 155°C per minute for a total operation time of 105 minutes. These results underscore the feasibility of this method for effectively extracting soluble fibre (Figure 8.3).

Another promising approach for β-glucan extraction involved the use of supercritical fluids. This method not only facilitated the extraction of β-glucan but also allowed for the creation of β-glucan gels without the damage often associated with conventional drying techniques such as oven or freeze-drying, as observed by Comin et al. [156]. The resulting aerogels exhibited lower densities compared to those obtained through dry air drying, and they possessed a more uniform structure when compared to freeze-drying. The authors highlighted the significant potential of β-glucan aerogels as carriers for medicinal or pharmaceutical products due to their desirable attributes, including biodegradability, biocompatibility, and edibility. In a recent investigation by Yoo et al. [157], the extraction of β-glucan using a subcritical-water extraction method under high-temperature and high-pressure conditions demonstrated optimized β-glucan yields. This finding further supports the notion that this methodology could serve as a viable single-step alternative for β-glucan extraction.

A method for obtaining β-glucans from barley involved freezing the solution, allowing it to thaw, and separating solids, as established by Morgan et al. [158]. Morgan et al. [158] further investigated the process for obtaining β-glucan products from both barley and oats. This process entails creating flour from cereal grains, forming a slurry of an aqueous β-glucan solution and solid residue, separating the aqueous solution from the solid residue, and dehydrating the aqueous solution through evaporation or ultrafiltration, resulting in a β-glucan-containing gel or solid.

Van Lengerich et al. [159] introduced an innovative method for producing high-quality soluble dietary fibre enriched with β-glucan. Their approach involves homogenizing an aqueous extraction slurry of β-glucan-containing grain material, acidifying it, and enzymatically digesting it to reduce viscosity and optimize the separation of insolubles. The extract is then heat-processed to precipitate denatured protein components, culminating in the production of dry products. Bhatty et al. [160] explored a technique for obtaining substantial β-glucan levels from cereals by employing sodium hydroxide as the initial extraction solvent. The resulting extract can be further purified to yield a β-glucan preparation.

Potter et al. [161] developed a process for producing β-glucans from milled cereal bran, grains, and distiller's dried grain. Their method involves creating an alkaline aqueous extract, acidifying or neutralizing the extract, heating it, cooling it to form a flocculate, and ultimately removing the flocculate from the aqueous solution to generate an intermediate solution. Beer et al. [162] successfully produced substantial quantities of high-quality oat gum rich in (1→3) (1→4)-β-d-glucan through various processing technologies. They extracted and isolated oat gums from untreated and enzyme-deactivated oat bran concentrate using aqueous sodium carbonate, yielding products with a β-glucan content of 60–65%. Alcoholic precipitation was identified as the preferred process, though ultrafiltration and dialysis were deemed suitable alternatives for generating significant quantities of oat gum rich in β-d-glucan.

Sharma et al. [163] assessed the impact of extrusion variables, such as temperature and moisture, on hulled barley β-glucan and its physicochemical properties. Extrusion, particularly at high temperatures and moisture levels, led to an increase in β-glucan extractability by up to 8%. The fine structure of β-glucan preparations extracted from milled seeds of two Greek cultivars was examined, revealing that these preparations were primarily composed of β-glucans (>85%) [164]. Irakli et al. [165] isolated β-glucans from six Greek barley cultivars through water extraction, enzymatic starch and protein removal, and subsequent precipitation with ammonium sulphate saturation, resulting in high purity (>93% on a dry weight basis). Zhu et al. [166] utilized a variety of solvents, including organic solvents, acidified water, and aqueous alkali, for slurrying grain flour. This process was especially effective in concentrating β-glucans close to their native form from the endosperm of barley and oat grains.

Following β-glucan extraction, it's important to note that purification processes, specifically the removal of starch and proteins, are not consistently carried out. The presence of these contaminants in the extract can hinder proper characterization and pose substantial challenges when incorporating β-glucan into food products. The primary purification technique for β-glucan involves enzymatic treatment using α-amylase and a protease, as outlined by [167]. To minimize contaminant levels, it is advisable to assess various enzymatic combinations during the β-glucan extraction process, as suggested by Limberger et al. [168].

8.2.2.5 Applications of ß-Glucan

8.2.2.5.1 Food Industry

The application of β-glucan in various food matrices has generated considerable interest due to its technological properties as texture enhancers [169]. A recent study demonstrated that soluble fibre from hull-less barley β-glucan could serve as a thickener and a source of dietary fibre in beverages and liquid products, based on rheological assessments. However, the adoption of β-glucan in the food industry is constrained by its high viscosity and challenges related to handling [123]. When incorporating β-glucan, it's crucial to consider the characteristics it imparts to the final products, especially at higher concentrations. The introduction of barley components into foods significantly increases water absorption, impacting the viscoelastic properties of the products [170].

In recent years, β-glucans have been explored for a range of applications in the food industry. They can serve as thickening agents [171], fat substitutes [172], emulsifiers, and stabilizers for foams and emulsions [173]. This polysaccharide also exhibits potential as a prebiotic in products with high folate content and can be a valuable source of soluble fibre in meat emulsions when combined with other hydrocolloids [10].

The choice of β-glucan extraction techniques depends on the specific objectives for the ingredient and the final product. For products with high carbohydrate content like pasta, flour, and bread, dry extraction methods can be used, resulting in less concentrated extracts that work well alongside other molecules such as proteins and starch [174]. Conversely, for products with low carbohydrate content, such as dairy and meat products, more concentrated β-glucan products obtained through wet extraction methods are recommended. These higher inclusion levels should be approached with caution to avoid negative effects on taste and texture caused by β-glucan's high viscosity [175].

It's worth noting that food applications may involve β-glucan from various sources, some more purified than others. These can still yield acceptable quality in the final products. The β-glucan content in foods varies depending on whether commercial or laboratory extraction is used [176]. The quantity used in food applications is contingent on the specific characteristics of the food matrix. For instance, noodles can typically handle up to 10% β-glucan, while soups might accommodate a maximum of 2%, and meat emulsions vary from 0.3% to 3%. Milk and dairy products can include up to 2.5% β-glucan, and bread can incorporate anywhere from 5.5% to 20% [123]. Despite these guidelines, there isn't a consensus on the maximum and minimum amounts of β-glucan that can be used in different food categories, nor on the specific application procedures for β-glucans in each group.

While there are limited studies focused on the evaluation of soluble fibre when combined with other ingredients to determine optimal levels or assess synergistic or antagonistic actions, it's essential to consider the potential adverse effects of β-glucan incorporation on final product quality. These effects can be attributed to the inherent characteristics of the fibre, including inconsistency due to impurities like proteins and starches [177]. Furthermore, it may not be feasible to add high fibre content to certain foods when their characteristics are significantly different. Recommendations for consuming β-glucan from oats and barley (3 g/day; FDA, 1997) have been established, with no evidence of toxicity [178]. However, there are limitations in terms of the application of β-glucan in certain foods, and the quantities used might not be sufficient to significantly enhance the nutritional value of these products.

Moreover, few sources of β-glucan contain concentrations exceeding 50%, making it challenging to significantly increase the fibre content in the final product. When using amounts greater than 1%, one needs to work with large quantities of low-concentration β-glucan, which can dramatically alter the characteristics of the conventional product [179]. Additionally, when incorporating β-glucan, similar to other functional ingredients, it's crucial to consider how the macromolecule interacts with the food components and how it might change during typical processing and storage. For example, the presence of other ingredients like sucrose or salt can increase the viscosity of β-glucans [180]. However, information on the interactions of β-glucan with other ingredients is still limited. Recent studies have begun to examine the interactions of β-glucan with other barley components in aqueous solutions, indicating electrostatic interactions during aggregation [181]. Nonetheless, more research is needed to understand the interactions when β-glucan ingredients are added to other foods. When evaluating food applications, it's essential to consider the β-glucan content added during formulation, which is imperative for labelling products as significant sources of fibre and assessing the impact of processing on molecule integrity and interactions.

In the past years, β-glucan research has expanded to explore its role as an encapsulation agent for other ingredients, such as fish oil [182]and probiotics [183]. The growing nutraceutical industry, where consumer demand pushes for the use of natural rather than synthetic ingredients in food products [184], positions dietary fibre and β-glucan as pivotal players. The food industry is well-positioned to benefit from this functional ingredient in response to the increasing consumer demand for healthy and nutraceutical food. To maximize the potential of this nutraceutical ingredient, a high level of purity is essential. This ensures specific composition, which in turn allows for specific health benefits and eliminates uncertainty about which components are responsible for these effects [185].

Work on barley or oat flour and β-glucan-enriched cereal flours may not be directly comparable to the use of purified β-glucan fractions [186]. Furthermore, the incorporation of these agents into food systems, including factors like processing parameters, requires optimization. Hence, extraction procedures should aim to produce consistent raw materials. Various extraction and purification techniques have been explored, including hot water extraction, enzymatic extraction, acidic extraction, alkaline extraction, and solvent extraction. Commercial products in the market differ in terms of β-glucan isolation method, concentration, molecular weight, WHC, and viscosity.

While several studies have incorporated β-glucan into cereal-based and baked products, more research is needed to understand the impact of β-glucan molecular weight on dough and bread quality. Higher molecular weight β-glucans appear to enhance bread quality, particularly when used with flours that have poor bread-making characteristics [187]. Additionally, further studies are required to explore the potential effects of incorporating β-glucan in various food matrices and the potential interactions with other food ingredients. Research should focus on optimizing processing techniques and understanding how β-glucans behave during cooking, baking, or other forms of food preparation. Improved knowledge in this area will lead to more successful applications of β-glucans in a variety of food products.

8.2.3 Protein

Oats contain four distinct groups of proteins classified according to the Osborne classification: globulins (constituting 70–80% of the total protein content), prolamins (comprising 4–14%), albumins (ranging from 1–12%), and glutelins (making up less than 10%). The primary protein fraction in oats is represented by globulins, which are soluble in salt solutions and serve as storage proteins [188]. This fraction is predominantly composed of 12S globulins, with a hexameric structure weighing in at 320 kDa. These hexamers consist of subunits, each of approximately 54 kDa, further subdivided into an α-subunit (32 kDa) and a β-subunit (22 kDa), linked together by a disulphide bond. Oat globulins exhibit a high denaturation temperature, approximately 110°C, which is attributed to robust hydrophobic interactions between their subunits, intensifying at higher temperatures. Additionally, other types of globulins found in oats include the 7S and 3S varieties. Prolamins, on the other hand, are proteins that exhibit good solubility in aqueous alcohol solutions. Oat prolamins are characterized by their high sulphur content and significant glutamic acid content [189]. Albumins, comprising water-soluble proteins, primarily consist of enzymes [188]. Finally, the minor fraction of proteins in oats is known as glutelins, which are soluble under either acidic or alkaline conditions.

8.2.3.1 Techno-Functional Properties of Oat Proteins

The suitability of oat proteins for use in food products hinges significantly on their techno-functionality. These techno-functional attributes encompass qualities like solubility, emulsification, foaming properties, FBC, water-holding capability, and gelling properties. Among these techno-functional properties, solubility, emulsification, foaming, and gelling properties stand out as particularly pertinent for applications in liquid and semi-solid food products [40].

8.2.3.1.1 *Solubility*

Oat proteins, in comparison to other plant-derived proteins like soy and pea proteins, are known for their relatively lower solubility. This reduced solubility is partly attributed to the surface properties of oat proteins. Notably, oat globulins exhibit glutamine-rich regions on their surface, exposed to the surrounding solvent, which makes them less hydrophilic than other globulins [189]. Consequently, a comprehensive understanding of how oat raw material composition, environmental factors, and processing conditions impact protein solubility is crucial, particularly when considering the use of oat proteins in liquid and semi-solid food applications [32].

The solubility of oat proteins follows a U-shaped curve, which is a common trend among plant proteins where globulins constitute the predominant protein fraction [190]. For instance, Yung Ma et al. [191] observed that the solubility of oat proteins, whether obtained through salt extraction (using 0.5 M $CaCl_2$) or alkaline extraction followed by isoelectric precipitation, was approximately 5% at pH 5.5, which is close to their isoelectric point. In contrast, solubility values were significantly higher, ranging between 80% and 100%, at pH levels either less than 3 or greater than 9. Moreover, when comparing these two extraction methods, it was observed that salt-extracted oat proteins had higher solubility at lower pH values (pH 1.5–5), whereas oat proteins obtained through alkaline extraction followed by isoelectric precipitation exhibited better solubility at neutral and alkaline pH values (pH 6–11). This pH-dependent solubility trend was further supported by Konak et al. [192], who investigated the protein solubility of oat extracts obtained through acid or alkaline extraction from both non-defatted and CO_2-defatted oat flour. They found that solubility increased with rising pH, peaking at pH 10.5. Additionally, CO_2-defatted oat extracts displayed higher protein solubility compared to non-defatted oat extracts, regardless of the pH, primarily due to the absence of non-polar lipids and the presence of tryptophan-rich proteins.

Notably, defatting oat flours using supercritical CO_2 was shown to be a promising approach for enhancing oat protein solubility. However, it's important to mention that heat treatment, commonly employed to prevent rancidity in oat groats, can negatively affect oat protein solubility. Runyon et al. [193] reported that a heat treatment involving steaming at 102°C for 50 minutes, followed by drying at 110–120°C for another 50 minutes, reduced oat protein solubility from 74.6% to 35.7% at pH 9.5. This reduction in solubility was attributed to protein denaturation and the preferential aggregation of albumin and prolamin fractions, while globulin proteins were found to be less sensitive to heat treatment. Thus, careful control of processing conditions, including temperature, is essential to prevent a loss in oat protein solubility. It should be noted that heat treatment not only impacts oat protein solubility but also influences other oat components, such as β-glucans [194], free fatty acids [195], antioxidants [196], and flavours [193].

Solubility is a critical characteristic when considering the application of proteins as functional ingredients in various food products, particularly in semi-solid and liquid products. Oat globulins, due to their glutamine-rich surface regions, exhibit lower solubility compared to other plant globulins. This is mainly because OPI predominantly consist of globulin fractions, which inherently possess lower solubility [33]. pH is a key parameter influencing protein solubility. Ma et al. [29] noted the varying solubility of different oat protein fractions. Albumins exhibited complete solubility over a broad pH range, while globulins displayed low solubility at pH 6–7 but high solubility (over

90%) at pH 9.5, regardless of whether they were isolated using an alkaline or salt-based process. Yung Ma et al. [191] found that both alkali-extracted and salt-extracted protein isolates had limited solubility at pH 5.5 (about 5%). In contrast, at acidic pH (≤3) and alkaline pH (≥9), solubility was high (ranging from 80% to 100%).

Moreover, the extraction method also had an impact on solubility. Salt-isolated proteins exhibited reasonable solubility at acidic pH (1.5–5), with the lowest solubility at pH 6. In contrast, alkaline-isolated proteins demonstrated higher solubility between pH 7 and 9. Similar findings were reported by Konak et al. [192], where solubility was higher at alkaline pH for both acid- and alkali-extracted proteins, irrespective of defatting. Mohamed et al. [197] demonstrated that acetylation (4.2 mg/100 mg OPI) and succinylation (41.4 mg/100 mg OPI) enhanced solubility in distilled water (at neutral pH) compared to native OPI (with no solubility).

In a different study, the solubility of oat protein (23%) was significantly improved at pH 7 following acetylation (75–82%) and succinylation (74–88%), with intermediate solubility at pH 5 but reduced solubility at pH 3 [198]. The increase in the aqueous solubility of succinylated proteins was attributed to increased net negative charge, replacing short-range attractive forces with short-range repulsive forces, thus reducing protein-protein interactions while enhancing protein-water interactions. Alterations in protein conformation due to acylation were attributed to increased subunit dissociation from the quaternary structure and a shift in the isoelectric point to lower values.

Only a few studies have reported the extraction of oat proteins from oat flour without removing the lipids. The presence of non-polar lipids interferes with protein solubility. Heat treatment is commonly used to prevent the rancidity process resulting from non-polar lipids. However, heat treatment can negatively influence protein solubility, with Runyon et al. [193] reporting a 50% reduction in oat protein solubility due to denaturation and aggregation of albumin and prolamin molecules, primarily at high temperatures. Globulin fractions were found to be less sensitive to heat than albumin and prolamin. Konak et al. [192] observed that protein solubility increased after removing fat using supercritical carbon dioxide (SC-CO$_2$), possibly because of reduced non-polar lipids and the non-thermal treatment. Also, trypsin enzyme could increase oat protein solubility, with the degree of hydrolysis being a critical factor.

Furthermore, Prosekov et al. [199] found that the solubility of oat proteins treated with amyloglucosidase was higher than control samples across all pH values (3–9), with maximum solubility observed at pH 5, approximately 50%. Various factors, including different protein fractions, heat treatment, oat pre-treatment, extraction methods, and modifications like pH adjustments, acetylation, succinylation, and enzymatic hydrolysis, influence the solubility of oat proteins. The studies indicate that oat protein solubility is a complex interplay of multiple factors, including pH, extraction methods, chemical modifications, and processing conditions, which must be carefully considered when utilizing oat proteins as functional ingredients in food products.

8.2.3.1.2 *Emulsifying and Foaming Properties*

The creation of stable foam through the incorporation of gas or air is a fundamental requirement in the production of various food products, especially those reliant on whipping or foaming characteristics, such as cakes and bread. Protein molecules readily adhere to interfaces, where they construct durable films or foams [200]. The ability to generate and maintain foaming properties is significantly contingent on factors like pH and the treatment undergone during processing [200]. Emulsions are encountered in both industrial and domestic settings. These mixtures consist of two immiscible liquids, typically oil and water, with one dispersed as droplets within the other. The primary method for emulsification involves the introduction of mechanical energy into the system, which causes droplet deformation and break-up, resulting in the formation of smaller droplets.

Extensive research within the field of food colloid science has focused on the interfacial properties of proteins and emulsifiers. Emulsions serve as the foundational components for a wide array of food products, and they are typically stabilized by either proteins or emulsifiers [201]. Oat proteins, for instance, have demonstrated their ability to stabilize emulsions by creating a viscoelastic, adsorbed layer on the oil droplets. This layer acts as a physical barrier, preventing the droplets from coalescing. Emulsifiers can be either oil or water-soluble and form a fluid, closely packed layer at the interface with low interfacial tension, contributing to the stability of the emulsion.

The emulsifying properties of oat proteins are closely linked to their solubility, which is highly influenced by pH. This pH-dependent behaviour was highlighted in earlier sections. For example, Konak et al. [192] noted that the emulsifying capabilities of oat proteins were particularly strong at pH 10.5, surpassing their performance at lower pH values like 4.5, 6.5, and 8.5. This finding is a key consideration for various applications. In a concentrated side stream of oat starch production, the emulsifying capacity of oat proteins resembled that of a commercial soy concentrate and exhibited limited sensitivity to pH variations within the range of pH 3–7 [202]. Additionally, the method of oat protein extraction significantly affects their emulsifying properties. Yung Ma et al. [191] compared oat proteins obtained through salt extraction followed by dialysis with water to those obtained via alkaline extraction followed by isoelectric precipitation. The emulsifying activity index for the alkaline extract was notably more than twice as high as for the salt-extracted proteins.

The presence of lipids was also found to impact oat protein surface properties [203]. Removing lipids through CO_2-supercritical extraction was shown to enhance the foaming properties of oat proteins. This improvement was largely attributed to the positive effect on protein solubility, as CO_2-supercritical extraction selectively removed non-polar lipids, which constitute a significant portion of oat lipids and have a detrimental impact on foaming properties. Tryptophanins, the lipid-binding proteins in oats, played a role in maintaining the stability of oat-based foam structures, countering the destabilizing influence of lipids. Furthermore, Konak et al. [192] demonstrated that foaming in CO_2-defatted oats was pH-dependent and particularly robust at pH 10.5 when compared to lower pH values such as 4.5, 6.5, and 8.5. The addition of NaCl and sucrose to oat protein systems did not significantly influence their foaming properties, although sugar did contribute to improved foaming stability by limiting liquid drainage in the foam, thus enhancing overall stability due to increased viscosity of the continuous phase.

Emulsification properties are typically evaluated using two indices: the emulsifying activity index (EAI) and the emulsion stability index (ESI). EAI measures the capacity of surface-active proteins to cover the oil at the interface that can be emulsified per unit of protein. The higher the EAI, the more it assists in reducing interfacial tension. ESI, on the other hand, indicates the emulsion's ability to resist changes such as flocculation, creaming, and coalescence over a specific period. Oat protein emulsifying properties are notably influenced by solubility, which varies with pH [24]. Ma et al. [29] found that albumins displayed higher EAI at both acidic and alkaline pH compared to neutral pH, though they exhibited lower EAI values under extremely acidic conditions. Oat alkaline isolates outperformed gluten and soy isolates in terms of EAI, while oat salt isolate had a lower EAI.

Konak et al. [192] reported that the maximum EAI and ESI for oat protein occurred at pH 10.5. EAI gradually increased from 1.7 m²/g to 15.4 m²/g as the pH increased from 4.5 to 10.5. However, ESI remained unchanged across this pH range, with a sudden increase observed at pH 10.5. Mirmoghtadaie et al. [204] investigated the impact of deamidation and succinylation on the EAI of OPI and found that succinylation led to the highest emulsification activity, followed by deamidation and native OPI. The increased EAI after succinylation was due to the exposure of functional groups within the protein matrix. Similarly, Mohamed et al. [197] reported that both succinylation and acetylation increased EAI of OPI, with succinylation being more effective. Ponnampalam et al. [205] observed a similar trend regarding the increased EAI of acetylated and succinylated oat proteins. They attributed this improvement to the formation of a soluble protein layer around fat globules, which enhanced the oil-water association.

Moreover, Guan et al. [206] reported an enhancement in EAI of oat protein after enzymatic hydrolysis, with EAI increasing from 7.3 m²/g (native protein) to 39.5 m²/g (degree of hydrolysis, DH, 8.3%) at pH 5. Ponnampalam et al. [198] noted that succinylated oat proteins had higher ESI than acetylated oat proteins, followed by native OPC. However, the emulsion stability of OPI decreased after deamidation and succinylation, primarily due to excessive increases in net charge, reducing protein interactions and, consequently, the formation of a stable protein layer at the oil-liquid interface. Mohamed et al. [197] reported that acetylation and succinylation resulted in a significant decrease in the ESI of OPI, while cross-linking alone improved the ESI. A decrease in ESI at higher DH of oat protein was reported by Guan et al. [206], as shorter and less globular peptides formed at higher DH, resulting in a less stable protein layer around fat/oil droplets.

Improving emulsifying properties via protein-polysaccharide conjugates around the isoelectric pH and heat stability has also been explored. Zhang et al. [207] produced oat protein dextran conjugates through glycation reactions and noted that these conjugates formed superior emulsions. These conjugates exhibited better emulsion stability under various homogenization pressures compared to native OPI and heated OPI. Assessments under different pH and ionic strength conditions demonstrated the excellent emulsion stability of these conjugates under various environmental stresses. To suffice, the emulsification properties of oat proteins are intricately tied to factors like solubility, pH, and extraction methods. Modifying native proteins offers a promising avenue for improving emulsifying properties, particularly at neutral pH.

8.2.3.1.3 Water-Holding Capacity

WHC is a critical property of proteins, signifying their ability to retain water within their structure under specific conditions. It is especially vital in solid products, where low WHC can lead to dryness and texture issues, ultimately affecting the product's palatability. Oat proteins have shown promise in terms of WHC. OPI exhibited higher WHC compared to wheat gluten and was on par with soy protein isolate [26]. Modifications like acetylation, succinylation, and deamidation have been explored for their impact on WHC. These modifications improved WHC, with succinylation having the most significant effect. Deamidation enhanced protein-water interaction due to an increase in net charge and the exposure of ionic and polar groups to the aqueous medium [204].

Partially hydrolysed oat protein displayed excellent WHC (82.8–95.5%) at pH 7–9, similar to animal proteins (egg white). However, it exhibited significant differences at pH 5, where gel formation resulted in more substantial water loss. In a study, gels incorporating different inulin concentrations showed varying WHC, with higher values (85.09–93.29%) at pH 7 and lower (60%) at pH 5 [30]. Polysaccharides like chitosan, dextrin, and carrageenan were examined for their influence on gelling properties. Their addition enhanced WHC by increasing the viscosity of the serum phase, making it less prone to syneresis. However, particulate presence led to protein aggregation and reduced protein-water interactions, resulting in decreased WHC. In summary, chemical modifications and enzymatic hydrolysis of oat proteins positively affected WHC, especially at pH values of 3 and 7. The addition of polysaccharides improved WHC, but its impact varied depending on the pH values.

8.2.3.1.4 Gelling Properties

Gel formation by proteins involves the reorganization of protein matrices through sufficient unfolding of compact protein molecules, which can be induced by various factors, such as heat and enzymes. These treatments expose reactive groups, particularly hydrophobic amino acids, leading to intra- and intermolecular covalent bonding between amino acid chains. These exposed reactive groups, through irreversible interactions and intermolecular bonds, contribute to the formation of a self-supporting three-dimensional structure [208]. Oats primarily contain globulin as their major storage protein, characterized by a heat-stable hexameric structure comprising six monomer protein units. However, even in the context of oat proteins, heat plays a significant role in the gelation process. Short-term heating at 100°C can lead to the dissociation of globulin hexamers into monomers and denaturation of proteins, resulting in the aggregation of globulin and the formation of soluble globulin aggregates. Prolonged heating at 100°C for 60 minutes further leads to the formation of insoluble aggregates [209].

Heat treatment can influence the gelation of oat-soluble protein fractions by altering the distribution of potential aggregate structures. The unfolding of reactive groups under heat can lead to the aggregation of oat proteins, forming a self-supporting three-dimensional network. Studies indicate that short-term heating at 100°C caused globulin hexamer dissociation and aggregation. Runyon et al. [193] reported alterations in total soluble protein amount and the monomeric to globulin hexamer ratio due to heat treatment, which affects potential aggregate structures. In addition to heat, the cold-set gelation behaviour of oat proteins was investigated by Yang et al. [210] through the addition of glucono-δ-lactone (GDL). The incorporation of GDL resulted in an increase in storage modulus (G'), indicating the transformation of the fluid into a viscoelastic solid. Notably, the GDL content influenced the gel's shear strength, with 10% OPI-GDL gels exhibiting greater shear strength compared to 7% and 5% variants.

The impact of partial hydrolysis on the gelling properties of oat proteins was examined by Nieto-Nieto et al. [30] using enzymes such as flavorzyme, alcalase, pepsin, and trypsin. Significant improvements in gel strength were observed after partial hydrolysis with flavorzyme and trypsin at pH 8–9, resulting in gels with mechanical strength comparable to or better than soy protein and egg white protein gels at the same pH conditions. The appropriate peptide size obtained through partial hydrolysis allowed for the association of proteins to form a robust three-dimensional network. Modifying oat proteins through acetylation increased gel strength, while succinylation had the opposite effect. According to Mohamed et al. [197], G' was highest for acetylated oat protein suspension, followed by native OPI, whereas succinylation decreased the elasticity modulus.

Nieto-Nieto et al. [211] investigated the use of inulin to enhance oat protein gelling properties. The addition of a small amount of inulin significantly increased the gel strength, creating a stronger gel at neutral pH. Inulin filled void spaces in the protein network, promoting localized interactions like hydrogen and hydrophobic bonds. Rheological studies showed that elastic behaviour dominated the system, with inulin increasing G' at neutral pH and accelerating gel networking at a lower temperature compared to OPI alone. However, at pH 5, hydrogen and hydrophobic bonds were the primary active bonds, and the gels exhibited lower G' in a sodium dodecyl sulphate solution due to the compact protein structure near its isoelectric point (pH 5). The textural studies indicated increased springiness and gumminess with the addition of inulin, resulting in comparable mechanical strength to egg white gels.

The microstructure and gelling properties of oat protein gels with different polysaccharides were studied by Nieto-Nieto et al. [212]. Carrageenan, dextrin, and chitosan were added, and microscopic analysis revealed distinct structures. Carrageenan transformed gels into a dense, well-packed structure, while dextrin and carrageenan formed gels with thick walls and highly interconnected percolating networks at neutral pH. Oat protein–chitosan exhibited a particulate structure with spherical aggregates distributed among the gel network. Rheological studies showed differences in gel strength, with oat protein-carrageenan exhibiting a higher G' value at higher temperatures. Firm gels with a smooth texture and good WHC can be obtained by heating oat proteins at alkaline conditions (pH 9.7) and temperatures of 90–100°C. A minimum oat protein concentration of 5% was required to form a gel, with higher concentrations resulting in increased gel hardness. Weak gels were formed at lower pH values (pH 2–8) due to low oat protein solubility. Partial hydrolysis and the addition of inulin were found to enhance the hardness of heat-induced oat protein gels. The gelation process involves the dissociation of hexamers and the formation of hydrogen and hydrophobic bonds by highly reactive monomers.

Mäkinen et al. [213] investigated the acid gelation of a commercial ultra-high-temperature-treated oat drink using GDL and found that the oat drink did not form an acid gel. Bacterial acidification also failed to create a protein gel network in a commercial liquid oat base or oat bran concentrate. However, a yoghurt-like structure was obtained with oat bran concentrate due to the presence of starch and non-starch polysaccharides, while studies conducted by Loponen et al. [214] and Mårtensson et al. [215] showed that low protein concentrations hindered the formation of yoghurt-like structures. Brückner-Gühmann et al. [216] produced a non-dairy yoghurt-like product with a higher oat protein content using gelation of starch at 90°C, followed by fermentation. The final product had a pH of 4.2 and consisted of gelatinized starch and aggregated oat protein. In another study, the enrichment of a cow's milk-based yoghurt with oat protein ingredients OPC and OPI resulted in limited syneresis and improved mouthfeel, with oat protein showing no interactions with caseins. The incorporation of OPC proved to be a suitable replacement for skimmed milk powder in hybrid yoghurt production.

In conclusion, the research sheds light on the complex gelling properties of oat proteins, emphasizing their response to various factors and treatments. Heat, enzymatic modifications, and the addition of substances like inulin play pivotal roles in enhancing the gelation of oat proteins. These findings offer valuable insights for the food industry, enabling the development of products with improved texture, WHC, and sensory attributes. Furthermore, the interaction of oat proteins with different polysaccharides, as highlighted in this text, provides a deeper understanding of the intricate dynamics within protein gel networks. These insights open up possibilities for tailoring the properties of oat protein-based gels in food formulations. The findings also underscore the potential of oat proteins in non-dairy product applications, specifically in creating yoghurt-like structures. The successful incorporation of oat protein ingredients in these products demonstrates their versatility and ability to provide improved mouthfeel and reduced syneresis.

8.2.3.2 Modification of Oat Proteins

Previous studies have noted that native OPI demonstrates commendable solubility in alkaline conditions and very low pH ranges, along with proficient emulsifying properties. However, it exhibits poor solubility at neutral pH and slightly acidic pH (4–7), which limits its utility in various food applications [204], [207]. To fully exploit oat protein's potential as an ingredient in diverse food products, there is a need to enhance its solubility and further improve emulsification properties at neutral and slightly acidic pH levels.

The influence of modifications, including chemical alterations (acetylation, succinylation, and deamidation) [192], [204], [217], enzymatic hydrolysis [218], heat treatments [193], and glycation [207], on the functional attributes of oat protein has been documented. Protein succinylation involves the binding of a succinyl group to proteins, leading to changes in positive charges to negative charges, and resulting in the dissociation of succinyl group globulin dimers due to the repulsion of negative charges. Acetylation entails the addition of an acetyl group to a specific amino acid in a protein through an esterification reaction with acetic acid, leading to changes from basic groups to neutral groups. Deamidation, on the other hand, involves the removal of the amide group from the side chains of glutamine or asparagine amino acids. These chemical modifications and protein hydrolysis are known to alter the surface properties of the protein, thus broadening its potential applications (Table 8.2).

8.2.3.3 Extraction of Oat Proteins

Oat protein extraction and isolation can be accomplished through various methods, including wet methods (such as alkaline isolation and saline isolation), dry fractionation, and enzymatic extraction. Each of these methods adds substantial commercial

TABLE 8.2   The Impact of Modification on the Functional Properties of Oat Proteins

MODIFICATION/ TREATMENT	EFFECT OF TREATMENT	REFERENCE
GDL (glucon-d-lactone) acidification of OPI (cold-set OPI)	Enhanced the cold-set gel of oat protein, characterized by a percolating structure and robust mechanical properties.	[210]
Inulin addition to OPI	Enhanced gels have exhibited superior textural profiles and more favourable rheological properties.	[211]
Enzymatic extraction	Enhanced oat protein extraction yields were achieved through the utilization of viscozyme L. Additionally, partial hydrolysis, facilitated by enzymes such as flavourzyme and trypsin, has resulted in improved gelling characteristics, including heightened gel strength and enhanced texture of oat protein isolates, all while maintaining excellent water-holding capacity. Furthermore, these enzymatic processes have led to increased protein solubility, improved foaming properties, heightened emulsification capabilities, and enhanced gelling properties in the resulting oat protein products.	[218] [30]
OPI dextrin conjugation by glycation reaction	Emulsification properties have been enhanced.	[207]
Addition of dextrin and carrageenan	Thermal gelation has been improved.	[212]
Acetylation, succinylation, and cross-linking	Acetylation and succinylation, as chemical modifications, have yielded notable improvements in specific functional attributes, namely foaming and emulsification, while simultaneously introducing a negative impact on rheological properties due to excessive cross-linking. These chemical modifications have been observed to reduce water-holding capacity and concurrently elevate the emulsion activity index.	[197]
Supercritical carbon dioxide (SC-CO$_2$) extraction	The protein extraction yield has been enhanced, resulting in improved foaming and emulsion activity.	[192]

value to oat protein production. In the wet extraction process, proteins are extracted using solvents, and separation is achieved through centrifugation, followed by isoelectric precipitation. Several studies have reported the use of the alkaline method for protein isolation. In this process, a suspension of oat flour (at a ratio of 1:8–10 w/v) is extracted under alkaline conditions (pH 9.2–11.5 with 1 M NaOH solution). This is followed by incubation at temperatures ranging from 20 to 55°C with stirring (100–200 rpm) for 60 minutes. Subsequently, proteins are precipitated at a lower pH (4–5.5) and separated through centrifugation. The recovery of protein from ground oat groats and the protein content of OPIs were found to be in the range of 60.4–72.1% and 72.4–92.6%, respectively, using the alkali extraction method [167] (Figure 8.4).

Salt-soluble OPIs, on the other hand, can be prepared by mixing ground groats with a solution of 1M NaCl/0.5M CaCl$_2$ at a ratio of 1:10 (w/v), followed by centrifugation. This process precipitates OPIs soluble in salt, which can be further processed through dialysis against cold running tap water or simply dilution with water. In the alkaline extraction method (0.015 M NaOH, solid: solvent ratio of 1:10, pH 7.83), oat flour resulted in OPC with 72% oat protein. Lower pH values, such as 6.25 and 7.00, yielded 19% and 57% protein content, respectively, while an alkaline pH (7.83) resulted in a higher protein recovery of 88% [219].

Several studies have emphasized the advantages of alkaline isolation over acid and salt extraction methods due to its higher protein recovery. However, it is essential to note that these studies may have employed different variables, including sample varieties, purity, defatting, solid-to-solvent ratios, temperature, time, pH, and centrifugation conditions. Enzymatic extraction of oat protein from oat bran using enzymes such as viscozyme and amyloglucosidase has also been explored. This method involves blending defatted oat bran with deionized water, followed by pH adjustment, enzyme addition, incubation, and subsequent centrifugation. It has been found that the enzymatic approach can yield higher protein content compared to conventional alkali extraction methods.

Wet methods, particularly the alkaline isolation method, are commonly used for oat protein extraction due to their higher recovery rates. Nonetheless, these methods require substantial amounts of solvents in the process. An alternative approach is dry fractionation, which involves milling oat grains to produce finer particles separated by air, resulting in a concentrated protein fraction. This method retains some lipids, starch, and β-glucans, which may impact the physicochemical and functional properties of the final product.

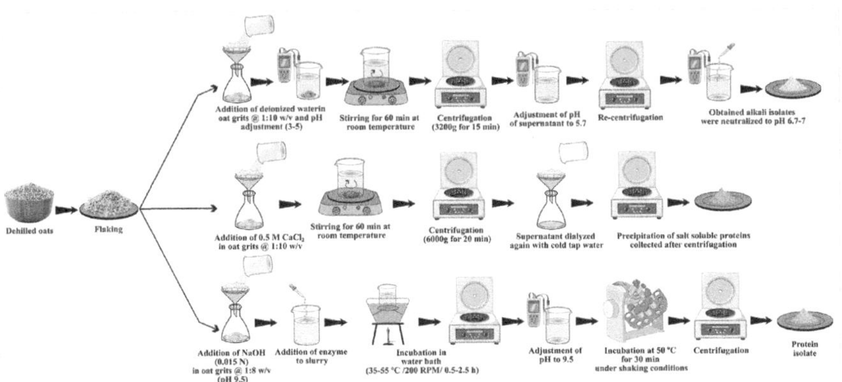

FIGURE 8.4   Various approaches for the isolation of oat proteins.

8.2.3.4 Application of Oat Protein in Food

Oat proteins have yet to see widespread use in the realm of foods and beverages, but an emphasis on enhancing their techno-functionality holds the potential to facilitate their incorporation into industrial food production. A recent study explored the treatment of a pea-oat protein blend with phytase and fermentation, followed by extrusion cooking to create a meat analogue [220]. This process resulted in an improved nutritional profile, marked by a reduction in antinutrients, an increase in protein content, and enhanced essential amino acid levels. Additionally, the physicochemical attributes, including colour and water/oil holding capacity, and the textural properties, such as chewiness and resilience, were enhanced. Moreover, the flavour of the resulting meat analogue was notably improved.

OPCs were integrated at varying levels (1.1%, 1.7%, and 2.5%) in a fermented yoghurt product [25], [28]. The proteolytic enzymes inherent in the yoghurt culture effectively cleaved oat proteins, liberating bioactive peptides that boosted the nutritional value of the yoghurt. Furthermore, OPCs with specific compositions yielded increased viscosity through starch gelatinization, ultimately resulting in a yoghurt that combined nutritional advantages, sustainability, and improved sensory quality. However, when OPIs (90% oat protein with less than 1% starch) were used to make yoghurt, they exhibited low functionality under acidic conditions, leading to substantial sedimentation and high syneresis. This situation necessitates further investigation into the interplay between starch and protein in yoghurt made with fermented oat protein concentrate.

The utilization of oat protein for encapsulation purposes presents a promising avenue for strengthening its presence in the food and nutraceutical product markets. Glycosylated oat protein, conjugated with β-glucan, displayed enhanced solubility, emulsifying capacity, and thermostability compared to untreated oat protein [221]. To address the limited bioavailability of β-carotene, which restricts its utilization, researchers encapsulated β-carotene using a conjugate formed by OPI and *Pleurotus ostreatus* β-glucan. This conjugate effectively protected and stabilized β-carotene, resulting in increased bioavailability and enhanced antioxidant activity. Oat protein-shellac combination gels also improved the bioavailability of resveratrol, safeguarding the compound as it passed through the gastrointestinal tract of rats and facilitating its release in the intestinal environment, in contrast to free resveratrol. These studies suggest that oat proteins could serve as a promising natural biopolymer delivery system for bioactive compounds in both food and biomedical applications. Looking ahead, future experiments should explore the development of stable systems based on oat proteins under neutral pH conditions.

8.2.4 Lipids

Oats are unique among cereals due to their high lipid content, primarily concentrated in the grain's germ. These lipids play a pivotal role in determining the cereal's energy content and significantly impact its nutritional quality, especially through their fatty acid composition. Additionally, in the context of oats, lipids are also known to influence the cereal's flavour attributes [9]. Moreover, these lipids are instrumental in shaping the pasting properties of oat starch and, consequently, the functionality of oat-based products. Specifically, oat stands out with the highest oil content, ranging from 2% to 12%, when compared to other cereal grains [222]. Within oat lipids, approximately 50% to 60% consists of neutral lipids, with triacylglycerols being the predominant component. Furthermore, oat oil is rich in polar lipids, such as phospholipids and glycolipids.

8.2.4.1 Techno-Functional Properties of Oat Lipids

As already discussed in section 8.2, one notable impact of oat lipids is their influence on the pasting properties of oat starch. When studying isolated oat starch, it becomes evident that oat starch possesses a high pasting temperature, primarily due to the presence of substantial lipid content. For instance, research indicated that the pasting properties of oat and corn starches isolated from groats with varying lipid content, ranging from 6.2% to 11.2%. Their findings revealed that the onset of gelatinization and gel stickiness of oat starches was positively correlated with starch-lipid content. Conversely, gel firmness, starch granule size, and clarity exhibited negative correlations with starch-lipid content.

Additionally, lipid removal from oat starch resulted in noteworthy changes in various properties, including decreased swelling factor, PV, setback, gelatinization temperature, and freeze-thaw stability, particularly in solutions with a pH above 4.0 [18]. Conversely, it increased thermal stability, amylose leaching, enthalpy of gelatinization, susceptibility toward α-amylase, and paste clarity, especially in solutions with a pH below 4.0. In oat starch, there is also a small amount of endogenous lipids, ranging from 0.7% to 2.5%. These lipids can complex with amylose to form inclusion complexes. The peak temperature of melting amylose–lipid complexes from oats typically falls in the range of 101.48 to 104.71°C. The physical characteristics and behaviour of oat starch granules are primarily attributed to the crystalline regions created by chains of amylopectin packed as double helices. During gelatinization, the uncoiling of amylopectin chains within these crystalline regions takes place. The influence of the lipid fraction in oat starch is largely due to starch-lipid complexation, impacting starch crystallinity. It's important to note that while lipid-lipid complexation plays a significant role, other factors are likely operative as well.

8.2.4.2 Extraction of Lipids from Oats

8.2.4.2.1 Solvent Extraction Methods

Various methods are employed for the analysis of oat lipids, catering to the determination of both the total lipid fraction and specific lipid groups. The complexity of these methods varies depending on the type of lipid fraction under investigation, namely, whether it is the total lipid content, free lipids, or bound lipids. Furthermore, the method chosen can be influenced by whether the analysis is conducted directly on whole, intact oat grains or after an initial extraction from grains, groats, or oat flour. The selection of a specific method hinges on the intended purpose of the analysis. When determining the total amount of oat lipids, equivalent to oil or fat, several methods come into play. Extraction methods, spectroscopy, or the analysis of the fatty acid profile through chromatography, as outlined by Zhou et al. [223], are commonly employed. Notably, the choice of solvent systems for extraction can significantly impact the results obtained. These variations underscore the importance of selecting an appropriate extraction method to accurately capture the lipid composition within oat-based samples. The determination of lipid content is commonly achieved through solvent extraction [224]–[226].

Traditional methods for isolating fats from solid samples, such as ground oat groats, involve gravimetric measurements using apparatus like the Soxhlet system or Goldfish systems [227]. Extractors employ a wide array of solvent systems, ranging from single-phase non-polar solvents to multiphase polar mixtures, exemplified by water-saturated n-butanol, which facilitates the selective separation of the fat fraction. However, it is noteworthy that only a limited number of solvent systems effectively extract fats. Non-polar solvents like hexane and ether are efficient for isolating so-called inert fats from cereal grains, whereas they exhibit limited effectiveness in extracting polar lipids, particularly phospholipids bound to cell membranes. Polar solvents are more effective for this purpose. An investigation by Sahasrabudhe et al. [226] encompassed seven solvent extraction systems, revealing substantial variations in total lipid content among different lipid groups.

8.2.4.2.2 *Supercritical Carbon Dioxide Based Extraction*

Recent breakthroughs support the viability of utilizing supercritical carbon dioxide (SC-CO$_2$) for the extraction of non-polar oat lipids in future applications [228]. Andersson et al. [229] demonstrated the effectiveness of this extraction method in isolating specific components of oat oil, particularly digalactosyldiacylglycerols (DGDG) from oats. This innovative process involves optimizing fractionation at the nozzle, where a coaxial combination of an oat oil solution and supercritical carbon dioxide generates a spray jet for improved contact with the extractor. Triacylglycerols are dissolved in the CO$_2$ phase during extraction, while the desired product, DGDG, remains within the system. In addition to the aforementioned method, the isolation of the polar fraction of lipids can be achieved by exercising control over the extraction process through the introduction of a co-solvent, such as ethanol or isopropanol [230]. Aro et al. [231] also developed a technique for obtaining the polar oat lipid fraction by incorporating polar ethanol into the process, thereby enhancing the extraction of polar components from grains and oat flakes.

8.2.4.2.3 *Chromatographic and Spectroscopic Methods for Analysing Oat Lipids*

Planar chromatography techniques were employed to conveniently fractionate the total fat content into its individual components, including triacylglycerols, phospholipids, glycolipids, free fatty acids, and sterols. Sahasrabudhe elucidated the lipid composition of oat oil using column chromatography and thin-layer chromatography. Nevertheless, the utility of these methods for characterizing oat lipids was often limited due to the distinct properties of these components and certain inherent analytical constraints. Challenges included the variability of results, modifications in the composition of the mobile phase during analysis, and band dispersion on chromatograms due to the gradual deceleration of the mobile phase with distance travelled.

For more accurate and reliable determinations of oat oil composition, contemporary chromatographic techniques are preferred, bifurcated based on the type of eluent into liquid chromatography (HPLC) and gas chromatography (GC). GC is well-suited for detecting and identifying individual compounds within mixtures. This method is akin to fractional distillation, segregating mixture components based on differences in their boiling points when in gaseous form. Subsequently, a carrier gas (mobile phase) transports the vaporized components to the column for further separation. GC offers dependable separation and facilitates precise quantitative analysis of fatty acids in oat oil. Methanolysis, a process generating methyl esters of fatty acids with relatively high volatility, expedites their analysis via GC.

By employing acid methanolysis in sample preparation for chromatographic examinations, Welch achieved an accurate quantification of fatty acids in oat oil. This approach has proven to be more convenient, rapid, and suitable for small quantities of oil samples for routine composition analyses compared to previous chromatographic methods [232]. Oat oil constituents with polar characteristics, such as glycolipids and phospholipids, demand a more selective and precise approach, namely HPLC [233]. In this technique, the mobile phase (eluent) comprises single solvents or solvent mixtures. The eluent introduced into the column also contains the constituents of the mixture being separated. The choice of mobile phase must align with the composition of the mixture, detector type, and column packing. Moreau et al. effectively employed this method to ascertain the polar lipid fraction within oat oil [234]. Both liquid chromatography and GC are characterized by swiftness, reproducibility, and precision in compound separation, mainly attributed to automation. However, they come at a higher cost due to the need for sophisticated apparatus, including detectors and columns, as well as the consumption of substantial quantities of hazardous solvents and expensive reference standards for the analyses.

Spectroscopic techniques offer rapid and direct lipid content measurement in various samples, including grain, flour, and chopped grain, without the need for prior preparation [235]. For example, Li et al. [236] employed nuclear magnetic resonance (NMR) to determine lipid content in cut grain samples, yielding results comparable to traditional non-polar solvent extraction methods. This method can also directly analyse the lipid composition of previously extracted oat oil samples. Manolache et al. [237] used ^{1}H-NMR to determine fatty acid content in oat oil, allowing for quick sample differentiation and qualitative assessment, which can be valuable for cereal authenticity testing. Other spectroscopic methods include near, medium, and far-infrared spectroscopy. Far-infrared (NIR) spectroscopy, can determine protein moisture and fat content in grain, making it a widely used method for continuous quality control in the food industry. It offers advantages such as non-invasive analysis, low cost, and no use of harmful organic solvents. However, interpreting raw spectra can be challenging [35]. In NIR-based oil determination, specific bands at 1722, 2306, and 2346 nm are examined, corresponding to CH_2 vibrations, and have been used successfully for fat and protein content determination in oats [35]. Although NIR has potential, its application in routine oat analysis remains limited. In the mid-infrared (MIR) and Raman scattering range (400–4000/cm), these techniques allow lipid testing and identification by assigning reference bands. They also enable quantitative analyses, helping determine parameters such as lipid unsaturation, trans-C=C isomers, and fat types present. Manolache et al. [237] utilized MIR to analyse oat oil samples, identifying characteristic bands within specific spectral ranges.

8.2.4.3 Application of Oat-Derived Lipids

Oat lipids, derived from oats, have garnered significant recognition and popularity in the food industry due to their notable nutritional benefits and exceptional versatility. These lipid extracts from oats are increasingly being integrated into a diverse range of food products, offering a wide array of advantages. One prominent application involves their use as a source of healthy fats in food production. They are commonly incorporated into dairy alternatives, such as oat milk, providing a dual benefit of creaminess and enhanced nutritional value to meet the growing demand for plant-based options. In the realm of baked goods, oat lipids are gaining traction for not only imparting a delightful, mild, nutty flavour but also for enhancing the overall nutritional composition. This improvement is achieved through an increased content of heart-healthy monounsaturated and polyunsaturated fats. Beyond sweet applications, savoury culinary creations also benefit from oat lipids, finding their way into dressings and sauces, offering a wholesome and nutty essence. What truly distinguishes oat lipids is their inherent emulsification capabilities, contributing to the creation of stable emulsions and enhancing the mouthfeel of a variety of products. In summary, oat lipids are valued not only for their exceptional health-promoting properties but also for their pivotal role in enhancing the taste and texture of a wide spectrum of food items, firmly establishing them as cherished and versatile ingredients in the continually evolving landscape of food production.

8.3 CONCLUSION

This chapter highlights the diverse and significant role of oats and their derived constituents in the food industry. Oats, renowned for their health benefits, are widely used in various food products due to their exceptional qualities, including substantial protein content, high digestibility, and a significant dietary fibre content in the form of β-glucan. However, the integration of oats in food processing poses challenges related to the development of off-flavours and textural issues, particularly during storage and processing. The unique physicochemical characteristics of oats, such as their lack of gluten and distinct starch properties, add to the intricacies of oat-based food production. In response to these challenges, there has been a drive to harness the potential of oats in the food industry, resulting in the creation of novel oat ingredients, especially those enriched with glucan. These ingredients not only offer health benefits but also enhance the technological aspects of food production. These innovations find applications across a wide spectrum of food sectors, including baking, beverages, meat processing, dairy, and confectionery, where β-glucan plays a pivotal role in improving rheological and textural properties. The demand for oat ingredients is on the rise as they align with the growing consumer preference for functional and health-oriented food products. Oat proteins, cherished for their sustainability and consumer appeal, are particularly relevant for plant-based diets. Their functional attributes, including emulsification, gelation, and water-binding capacities, make them versatile in the food industry. Nonetheless, these proteins present challenges such as low solubility and limited functionality, leading to the development of various modification methods, both chemical and enzymatic, to enhance their utility in food products. Oat proteins, oat starch, and β-glucan play a crucial role in addressing the dietary and nutritional needs of individuals with specific health considerations, such as celiac disease and those seeking plant-based protein alternatives. This review emphasizes the ongoing research efforts to enhance the techno-functionality of oat ingredients, providing a sustainable and health-focused approach to food production. The insights provided in this review encompass the extraction and fractionation methods of oat components, their improved functionality through enzymatic and chemical treatments, and their applications in the development of value-added food products. The utilization of innovative food processing technologies is set to transform the extraction of bioactive compounds from oats, opening the door to a broader and more diverse range of oat-based products in the global market.

REFERENCES

[1] I. Jokinen, P. Silventoinen-Veijalainen, M. Lille, E. Nordlund, U. Holopainen-Mantila, "Variability of carbohydrate composition and pasting properties of oat flakes and oat flours produced by industrial oat milling process – Comparison to non-heat-treated oat flours," *Food Chem.*, vol. 405, p. 134902, 2023, doi: 10.1016/j.foodchem.2022.134902.

[2] R. Mathews and Y. Chu, "The effect of whole-grain oats, oat bran, and isolated beta-glucan on indices of satiety and short-term energy intake," *Food Rev. Int.*, pp. 1–21, 2023, doi: 10.1080/87559129.2023.2214807.

[3] G. L. R. R. de Barros Vinhal, M. A. Ribeiro Sanches, M. T. Barcia, D. Rodrigues and P. B. Pertuzatti, "Murici (Byrsonima verbascifolia): A high bioactive potential fruit for application in cereal bars," *LWT.*, vol. 160, p. 113279, 2022, doi: 10.1016/j.lwt.2022.113279.

[4] D. Dziki, K. Lisiecka, U. Gawlik-Dziki, R. Różyło, A. Krajewska and G. Cacak-Pietrzak, "Shortbread cookies enriched with micronized oat husk: Physicochemical and sensory properties," *Appl. Sci.*, vol. 12, p. 12512, 2022, doi: 10.3390/app122412512.

[5] X. Zou, X. Wang, M. Zhang, P. Peng, Q. Ma and X. Hu, "Pre-baking-steaming of oat induces stronger macromolecular interactions and more resistant starch in oat-buckwheat noodle," *Food Chem.*, vol. 400, p. 134045, 2023, doi: 10.1016/j.foodchem.2022.134045.

[6] X. He, X. Li, D. Chen, S. Huang and N. Tao, "Effect on bread properties of partial substitution of wheat flour with oat flour and flour from oat grain germinated in the light or dark," *Int. J. Food Sci. Technol.*, vol. 58, pp. 1979–1986, 2023, doi: 10.1111/ijfs.16352.

[7] X. Wang, X. Kong, C. Zhang, Y. Hua, Y. Chen and X. Li, "Comparison of physicochemical properties and volatile flavor compounds of plant-based yoghurt and dairy yoghurt," *Food Res. J.*, vol. 164, p. 112375, 2023, doi: 10.1016/j.foodres.2022.112375.

[8] J. C. Noronha, A. Zurbau and T. M. S. Wolever, "The importance of molecular weight in determining the minimum dose of oat β-glucan required to reduce the glycaemic response in healthy subjects without diabetes: A systematic review and meta-regression analysis," *Eur. J. Clin. Nutr.*, vol. 77, pp. 308–315, 2023, doi: 10.1038/s41430-022-01176-5.

[9]   Z. Yang, C. Xie, Y. Bao, F. Liu, H. Wang and Y. Wang, "Oat: Current state and challenges in plant-based food applications," *Trends Food Sci. Technol.*, vol. 134, pp. 56–71, 2023, doi: 10.1016/j.tifs.2023.02.017.

[10] H. Mao et al., "The utilization of oat for the production of wholegrain foods: Processing technology and products," *Food Front.*, vol. 3, pp. 28–45, 2022, doi: 10.1002/fft2.120.

[11] T. T. L. Nguyen et al., "Effect of processing on the solubility and molecular size of oat β-glucan and consequences for starch digestibility of oat-fortified noodles," *Food Chem.*, vol. 372, p. 131291, 2022, doi: 10.1016/j.foodchem.2021.131291.

[12] Y. Yu, X. Li, J. Zhang, X. Li, J. Wang and B. Sun, "Oat milk analogue versus traditional milk: Comprehensive evaluation of scientific evidence for processing techniques and health effects," *Food Chem. X.*, vol. 19, p. 100859, 2023, doi: 10.1016/j.fochx.2023.100859.

[13] J. Muthukumar, P. Selvasekaran, M. Lokanadham and R. Chidambaram, "Food and food products associated with food allergy and food intolerance – An overview," *Food Res. J.*, vol. 138, p. 109780, 2020, doi: 10.1016/j.foodres.2020.109780.

[14] L. Sun et al., "Molecular characteristics, synthase, and food application of cereal β-glucan," *J. Food Qual.*, vol. 2021, p. e6682014, 2021, doi: 10.1155/2021/6682014.

[15] V. Sterna, S. Zute, I. Jansone, L. Brunava and I. Kantane, "Oat grain functional ingredient characterization," *Int. J. Agric. Biosys. Eng.*, vol. 9, pp. 791–794, 2015. Accessed: Oct. 11, 2023. [Online]. Available: https://publications.waset.org/10002148/oat-grain-functional-ingredient-characterization

[16] S. Punia et al., "Oat starch: Physico-chemical, morphological, rheological characteristics and its applications – A review," *Int. J. Biol. Macromol.*, vol. 154, pp. 493–498, 2020, doi: 10.1016/j.ijbiomac.2020.03.083.

[17] J. Zhang, M. Zhang, X. Bai, Y. Zhang and C. Wang, "The impact of high hydrostatic pressure treatment time on the structure, gelatinization and thermal properties and in vitro digestibility of oat starch," *Grain Oil Sci. Technol.*, vol. 5, pp. 1–12, 2022, doi: 10.1016/j.gaost.2022.01.002.

[18] H. Rostamabadi et al., "Oat starch – How physical and chemical modifications affect the physicochemical attributes and digestibility?," *Carbohydr. Polym.*, vol. 296, p. 119931, 2022, doi: 10.1016/j.carbpol.2022.119931.

[19] P. Kaur, K. Kaur, S. J. Basha and J. F. Kennedy, "Current trends in the preparation, characterization and applications of oat starch – A review," *Int. J. Biol. Macromol.*, vol. 212, pp. 172–181, 2022, doi: 10.1016/j.ijbiomac.2022.05.117.

[20] S. R. Falsafi, Y. Maghsoudlou, H. Rostamabadi, M. M. Rostamabadi, H. Hamedi and S. M. H. Hosseini, "Preparation of physically modified oat starch with different sonication treatments," *Food Hydrocoll.*, vol. 89, pp. 311–320, 2019, doi: 10.1016/j.foodhyd.2018.10.046.

[21] H. Shen et al., "A new pre-gelatinized starch preparing by spray drying and electron beam irradiation of oat starch," *Food Chem.*, vol. 398, p. 133938, 2023, doi: 10.1016/j.foodchem.2022.133938.

[22] R. and M. ltd, "Oat protein market – Growth, trends and forecasts (2019–2024)," 2019. Accessed: Oct. 11, 2023. [Online]. Available: www.researchandmarkets.com/reports/4622348/oat-protein-market-growth-trends-and

[23] F. Boukid, "Oat proteins as emerging ingredients for food formulation: Where we stand?," *Eur. Food Res. Technol.*, vol. 247, 535–544, 2021, doi: 10.1007/s00217-020-03661-2.

[24] J. Spaen and J. V. C. Silva, "Oat proteins: Review of extraction methods and techno-functionality for liquid and semi-solid applications," *LWT.*, vol. 147, 111478, 2021, doi: 10.1016/j.lwt.2021.111478.

[25] M. Brückner-Gühmann, E. Vasil'eva, A. Culetu, D. Duta, N. Sozer and S. Drusch, "Oat protein concentrate as alternative ingredient for non-dairy yoghurt-type product," *J. Sci. Food Agric.*, vol. 99, 5852–5857, 2019, doi: 10.1002/jsfa.9858.

[26] L. Kumar, R. Sehrawat and Y. Kong, "Oat proteins: A perspective on functional properties," *LWT.*, vol. 152, p. 112307, 2021, doi: 10.1016/j.lwt.2021.112307.

[27] M. Brückner-Gühmann, A. Kratzsch, N. Sozer and S. Drusch, "Oat protein as plant-derived gelling agent: Properties and potential of modification," *Future Foods.*, vol. 4, p. 100053, 2021, doi: 10.1016/j.fufo.2021.100053.

[28] M. Brückner-Gühmann, M. Banovic and S. Drusch, "Towards an increased plant protein intake: Rheological properties, sensory perception and consumer acceptability of lactic acid fermented, oat-based gels," *Food Hydrocoll.*, vol. 96, pp. 201–208, 2019, doi: 10.1016/j.foodhyd.2019.05.016.

[29] C. Y. Ma and V. R. Harwalkar, "Chemical characterization and functionality assessment of oat protein fractions," *J. Agric. Food Chem.*, vol. 32, 144–149, 1984, doi: 10.1021/jf00121a035.

[30] T. V. Nieto-Nieto, Y. X. Wang, L. Ozimek and L. Chen, "Effects of partial hydrolysis on structure and gelling properties of oat globular proteins, *Food Res. J.*, vol. 55, pp. 418–425, 2014, doi: 10.1016/j.foodres.2013.11.038.

[31] O. P. Malav, S. Talukder, P. Gokulakrishnan and S. Chand, "Meat analog: A review," *Crit. Rev. Food Sci. Nutr.*, vol. 55, pp. 1241–1245, 2015, doi: 10.1080/10408398.2012.689381.

[32] M. Tomar et al., "Interactome of millet-based food matrices: A review," *Food Chem.*, vol. 385, p. 132636, 2022, doi: 10.1016/j.foodchem.2022.132636.

[33] R. Mel and M. Malalgoda, "Oat protein as a novel protein ingredient: Structure, functionality, and factors impacting utilization," *Cereal Chem.*, vol. 99, pp. 21–36, 2022, doi: 10.1002/cche.10488.

[34] K. Garsed and B. B. Scott, "Can oats be taken in a gluten-free diet? A systematic review," *Scand. J. Gastroenterol.*, vol. 42, pp. 171–178, 2007, doi: 10.1080/00365520600863944.

[35] M. Tomar et al., "Development of NIR spectroscopy based prediction models for nutritional profiling of pearl millet (*Pennisetum glaucum* (L.)) R.Br: A chemometrics approach," *LWT.*, vol. 149, p. 111813, 2021, doi: 10.1016/j.lwt.2021.111813.

[36] M. Tomar et al., "Nutritional composition patterns and application of multivariate analysis to evaluate indigenous Pearl millet ((*Pennisetum glaucum* (L.) R. Br.) germplasm," *J. Food Compos. Anal.*, vol. 103, p. 104086, 2021, doi: 10.1016/j.jfca.2021.104086.

[37] V. Krishnan, M. Tomar, L. N. Malunga and S. J. Thandapilly, "Food matrix: Implications for nutritional quality," in *Conceptualizing Plant-Based Nutrition: Bioresources, Nutrients Repertoire and Bioavailability*, S. V. Ramesh and S. Praveen, Eds. Singapore, Singapore: Springer Nature, 2022, pp. 43–60, doi: 10.1007/978-981-19-4590-8_3.

[38] M. Kumar et al., "Cottonseed feedstock as a source of plant-based protein and bioactive peptides: Evidence based on biofunctionalities and industrial applications," *Food Hydrocoll.*, vol. 131, p. 107776, 2022, doi: 10.1016/j.foodhyd.2022.107776.

[39] M. Kumar et al., "Advances in the plant protein extraction: Mechanism and recommendations," *Food Hydrocoll.*, vol. 115, p. 106595, 2021, doi: 10.1016/j.foodhyd.2021.106595.

[40] M. Kumar et al., "Functional characterization of plant-based protein to determine its quality for food applications," *Food Hydrocoll.*, 2021, p. 106986, doi: 10.1016/j.foodhyd.2021.106986.

[41] M. Kumar et al., "Cottonseed: A sustainable contributor to global protein requirements," *Trends Food Sci. Technol.*, vol. 111, pp. 100–113, 2021, doi: 10.1016/j.tifs.2021.02.058.

[42] M. Kumar et al., "Plant-based proteins and their multifaceted industrial applications," *LWT.*, vol. 154, 112620, 2022, doi: 10.1016/j.lwt.2021.112620.

[43] K. Mahmood, H. Kamilah, P. L. Shang, S. Sulaiman, F. Ariffin and A.K. Alias, "A review: Interaction of starch/non-starch hydrocolloid blending and the recent food applications," *Food Biosci.*, vol. 19, pp. 110–120, 2017, doi: 10.1016/j.fbio.2017.05.006.

[44] D. B. Bechtel and Y. Pomeranz, "Ultrastructure and cytochemistry of mature oat (Avena sativa L.) endosperm." *AL and SE.*, vol. 58, pp. 61–69, 1981. Accessed: Oct. 11, 2023. [Online]. Available: http://pascal-francis.inist.fr/vibad/index.php?action=getRecordDetail&idt=PASCAL8110272793

[45] S. A. Matz, *Chemistry and Technology of Cereals as Food and Feed*, 2nd ed., New York, NY, USA: Springer, 1991. Accessed: Oct. 11, 2023. [Online]. Available: https://link. springer.com/book/9780442308308

[46] A. Shah, F. A. Masoodi, A. Gani and B. Ashwar, "Dual enzyme modified oat starch: Structural characterisation, rheological properties, and digestibility in simulated GI tract," *Int. J. Biol. Macromol.*, vol. 106, pp. 140–147, 2018, doi: 10.1016/j.ijbiomac.2017.08.013.

[47] S. L. M. El Halal, D. H. Kringel, E. da R. Zavareze and A. R. G. Dias, "Methods for extracting cereal starches from different sources: A review," *Starch – Stärke.*, vol. 71, p. 1900128, 2019, doi: 10.1002/star.201900128.

[48] M. M. MacMasters, R. L. Slotter and C. M. Jaeger, "The possible use of oats and other small grains for starch production," *Am. Miller.*, vol. 75, pp. 82–83, 1947.

[49] D. Paton, "Oat starch part 1. Extraction, purification and pasting properties," *Starch – Stärke.*, vol. 29, pp. 149–153, 1977, doi: 10.1002/star.19770290502.

[50] S. Sayar and P. J. White, "Oat starch: Physicochemical properties and function," in *Oats: Chemistry and Technology*, American Association of Cereal Chemists, Inc (AACC), 2011, pp. 109–122. Accessed: Oct. 11, 2023. [Online]. Available: www.cabdirect.org/ cabdirect/abstract/20113242305

[51] P. Kasturi and N. Bordenave, "Oat starch," in *Oats Nutrition and Technology*, John Wiley & Sons, Ltd., 2013, pp. 95–121, doi: 10.1002/9781118354100.ch5.

[52] A. Shah, F. A. Masoodi, A. Gani and B. A. Ashwar, "In-vitro digestibility, rheology, structure, and functionality of RS3 from oat starch," *Food Chem.*, vol. 212, pp. 749–758, 2016, doi: 10.1016/j.foodchem.2016.06.019.

[53] J. Xu et al., "Insights into molecular structure and digestion rate of oat starch," *Food Chem.*, vol. 220, pp. 25–30, 2017, doi: 10.1016/j.foodchem.2016.09.191.

[54] J. Al-Hakkak and F. Al-Hakkak, "New non-destructive method using gluten to isolate starch from plant materials other than wheat," *Starch – Stärke.*, vol. 59, pp. 117–124, 2007, doi: 10.1002/star.200600564.

[55] J. Zhang, K. Luo and G. Zhang, "Impact of native form oat β-glucan on starch digestion and postprandial glycemia," *J. Cereal Sci.*, vol. 73, pp. 84–90, 2017, doi: 10.1016/j. jcs.2016.11.013.

[56] R. Wang, A. A. Koutinas and G. M. Campbell, "Dry processing of oats – Application of dry milling," *J. Food Eng.*, vol. 82, pp. 559–567, 2007, doi: 10.1016/j. jfoodeng.2007.03.011.

[57] X. Hu, X. Xing and C. Ren, "The effects of steaming and roasting treatments on β-glucan, lipid and starch in the kernels of naked oat (Avena nuda)," *J. Sci. Food Agric.*, vol. 90, pp. 690–695, 2010, doi: 10.1002/jsfa.3870.

[58] H. Ma et al., "Research progress on properties of pre-gelatinized starch and its application in wheat flour products," *Grain Oil Sci. Technol.*, vol. 5, pp. 87–97, 2022, doi: 10.1016/j.gaost.2022.01.001.

[59] B. Pan et al., "Quantitative study of starch swelling capacity during gelatinization with an efficient automatic segmentation methodology," *Carbohydr. Polym.*, vol. 255, p. 117372, 2021, doi: 10.1016/j.carbpol.2020.117372.

[60] Q. Xie et al., "Insight into the effect of garlic peptides on the physicochemical and anti-staling properties of wheat starch," *Int. J. Biol. Macromol.*, vol. 229, pp. 363–371, 2023, doi: 10.1016/j.ijbiomac.2022.12.253.

[61] F. Zhu and R. Cui, "Comparison of physicochemical properties of oca (Oxalis tuberosa), potato, and maize starches," *Int. J. Biol. Macromol.*, vol. 148, pp. 601–607, 2020, doi: 10.1016/j.ijbiomac.2020.01.028.

[62] E. Abedi, S. Maleki, K. Pourmohammadi and M. R. Kazemi, "Which one is important to achieve maximum degree of hydrolysis, starch pre-treatment or activated α-amylase: Kinetics and mathematical modeling for liquefaction," *Food Measure.*, vol. 17, pp. 4938–4953, 2023, doi: 10.1007/s11694-023-01995-5.

[63] Z. Fu, J. Chen, S.-J. Luo, C.-M. Liu and W. Liu, "Effect of food additives on starch retrogradation: A review," *Starch – Stärke.*, vol. 67, pp. 69–78, 2015, doi: 10.1002/star.201300278.

[64] C. Cai and C. Wei, "In situ observation of crystallinity disruption patterns during starch gelatinization," *Carbohydr. Polym.*, vol. 92, pp. 469–478, 2013, doi: 10.1016/j.carbpol.2012.09.073.

[65] S. Balet, A. Guelpa, G. Fox and M. Manley, "Rapid visco analyser (RVA) as a tool for measuring starch-related physiochemical properties in cereals: A review," *Food Anal. Methods.*, vol. 12, pp. 2344–2360, 2019, doi: 10.1007/s12161-019-01581-w.

[66] H.-T. Li, E. D. Kerr, B. L. Schulz, M. J. Gidley and S. Dhital, "Pasting properties of high-amylose wheat in conventional and high-temperature rapid visco analyzer: Molecular contribution of starch and gluten proteins," *Food Hydrocoll.*, vol. 131, p. 107840, 2022, doi: 10.1016/j.foodhyd.2022.107840.

[67] R. Hoover, C. Smith, Y. Zhou and R. M. W. S. Ratnayake, "Physicochemical properties of Canadian oat starches," *Carbohydr. Polym.*, vol. 52, pp. 253–261, 2003, doi: 10.1016/S0144-8617(02)00271-0.

[68] J. L. Doublier, D. Paton, G. Llamas, "A rheological investigation of oat starch pastes," *Cereal Chem.*, vol. 64, pp. 21–26, 1987. Accessed: Oct. 12, 2023. [Online]. Available: http://pascal-francis.inist.fr/vibad/index.php?action=getRecordDetail&idt=8032683

[69] D. Šubarić, J. Babić, A. Lalić, Đ. Ačkar and M. Kopjar, "Isolation and characterisation of starch from different barley and oat varieties," *Czech J. Food Sci.*, vol. 29, pp. 354–360, 2011, doi: 10.17221/297/2010-CJFS.

[70] C. Rhymer, N. Ames, L. Malcolmson, D. Brown and S. Duguid, "Effects of genotype and environment on the starch properties and end-product quality of oats," *Cereal Chem.*, vol. 82, pp. 197–203, 2005, doi: 10.1094/CC-82-0197.

[71] S. Srichuwong and J.-I. Jane, "Physicochemical properties of starch affected by molecular composition and structures: A review," *Food Sci. Biotechnol.*, vol. 16, pp. 663–674, 2007. Accessed: Oct. 12, 2023. [Online]. Available: https://koreascience.kr/article/JAKO200735822355808.page

[72] R. Mukhtar et al., "γ-irradiation of oat grain – Effect on physico-chemical, structural, thermal, and antioxidant properties of extracted starch," *Int. J. Biol. Macromol.*, vol. 104, pp. 1313–1320, 2017, doi: 10.1016/j.ijbiomac.2017.05.092.

[73] M. Z. Dar et al., "Modification of structure and physicochemical properties of buckwheat and oat starch by γ-irradiation," *Int. J. Biol. Macromol.*, vol. 108, pp. 1348–1356, 2018, doi: 10.1016/j.ijbiomac.2017.11.067.

[74] S. Han et al., "Changes in morphological and structural characteristics of high amylose maize starch in alkaline solution at different temperatures," *Int. J. Biol. Macromol.*, vol. 244, p. 125397, 2023, doi: 10.1016/j.ijbiomac.2023.125397.

[75] S. Wang, H. Xu and H. Luan, "Multiscale structures of starch granules," in *Starch Structure, Functionality and Application in Foods*, S. Wang, Ed. Springer, 2020, pp. 41–55, doi: 10.1007/978-981-15-0622-2_4.

[76] Y. I. Cornejo-Ramírez, O. Martínez-Cruz, C. L. Del Toro-Sánchez, F. J. Wong-Corral, J. Borboa-Flores and F. J. Cinco-Moroyoqui, "The structural characteristics of starches and their functional properties," *CyTA J. Food.*, vol. 16, pp. 1003–1017, 2018, doi: 10.1080/19476337.2018.1518343.

[77] I. A. Duceac, M.-C. Stanciu, M. Nechifor, F. Tanasă and C.-A. Teacă, "Insights on some polysaccharide gel type materials and their structural peculiarities," *Gels.*, 8, p. 771, 2022, doi: 10.3390/gels8120771.

[78] B. Dereje, "Composition, morphology and physicochemical properties of starches derived from indigenous Ethiopian tuber crops: A review," *Int. J. Biol. Macromol.*, vol. 187, pp. 911–921, 2021, doi: 10.1016/j.ijbiomac.2021.07.188.

[79] H. Rostamabadi et al., "How non-thermal processing treatments affect physicochemical and structural attributes of tuber and root starches?," *Trends Food Sci. Technol.*, vol. 128, pp. 217–237, 2022, doi: 10.1016/j.tifs.2022.08.009.

[80] D. Paton, "Differential scanning calorimetry of oat starch pastes," *Cereal Chem.*, vol. 64, pp. 394–399, 1987. Accessed: Oct. 12, 2023. [Online]. Available: http://pascal-francis.inist.fr/vibad/index.php?action=getRecordDetail&idt=7420797

[81] J. M. Pereira, J. A. Evangelho, F. A. Moura, L. C. Gutkoski, E. R. Zavareze, A. R. G. Dias, "Crystallinity, thermal and gel properties of oat starch oxidized using hydrogen peroxide," *Int. Food Res. J.*, vol. 24, pp. 1545–1552, 2017. Accessed: Oct. 12, 2023. [Online]. Available: www.cabdirect.org/cabdirect/abstract/20173358199

[82] V. Vamadevan, E. Bertoft and K. Seetharaman, "On the importance of organization of glucan chains on thermal properties of starch," *Carbohydr. Polym.*, vol. 92, pp. 1653–1659, 2013, doi: 10.1016/j.carbpol.2012.11.003.

[83] D. G. Stevenson, J. Jane and G. E. Inglett, "Structure and physicochemical properties of starches from sieve fractions of oat flour compared with whole and pin-milled flour," *Cereal Chem.*, vol. 84, pp. 533–539, 2007, doi: 10.1094/CCHEM-84-6-0533.

[84] K. Zheng et al., "Characterization of starch morphology, composition, physicochemical properties and gene expressions in oat," *J. Integr. Agric.*, vol. 14, pp. 20–28, 2015, doi: 10.1016/S2095-3119(14)60765-6.

[85] Q. Chang, B. Zheng, Y. Zhang and H. Zeng, "A comprehensive review of the factors influencing the formation of retrograded starch," *Int. J. Biol. Macromol.*, vol. 186, pp. 163–173, 2021, doi: 10.1016/j.ijbiomac.2021.07.050.

[86] A. Ranathunga, P. Suwannaporn, W. Kiatponglarp, R. Wansuksri and L. M. C. Sagis, "Molecular structure and linear-non linear rheology relation of rice starch during milky, dough, and mature stages," *Carbohydr. Polym.*, vol. 312, p. 120812, 2023, doi: 10.1016/j.carbpol.2023.120812.

[87] A. Stevnebø, S. Sahlström and B. Svihus, "Starch structure and degree of starch hydrolysis of small and large starch granules from barley varieties with varying amylose content," *Anim. Feed Sci. Technol.*, vol. 130, pp. 23–38, 2006, doi: 10.1016/j.anifeedsci.2006.01.015.

[88] Q. Huang, X. Chen, S. Wang and J. Zhu, "Amylose–lipid complex," in *Starch Structure, Functionality and Application in Foods*, S. Wang, Ed. Singapore, Singapore: Springer, 2020, pp. 57–76, doi: 10.1007/978-981-15-0622-2_5.

[89] Z. Ao and J. Jane, "Characterization and modeling of the A- and B-granule starches of wheat, triticale, and barley," *Carbohydr. Polym.*, vol. 67, pp. 46–55, 2007, doi: 10.1016/j.carbpol.2006.04.013.

[90] H. Tang, T. Mitsunaga and Y. Kawamura, "Relationship between functionality and structure in barley starches," *Carbohydr. Polym.*, vol. 57, pp. 145–152, 2004, doi: 10.1016/j.carbpol.2004.03.023.

[91] M. Gudmundsson and A. C. Eliasson, "Some physico-chemical properties of oat starches extracted from varieties with different oil content," *Acta Agric. Scand.*, vol. 39, pp. 101–111, 1989, doi: 10.1080/00015128909438502.

[92] S. M. Hartunian Sowa and P. J. White, "Characterization of starch isolated from oat groats with different amounts of lipid," *Cereal Chem.*, vol. 69, pp. 521–527, 1992. Accessed: Oct. 13, 2023. [Online]. Available: www.cerealsgrains.org/publications/cc/backissues/1992/Documents/CC1992a133.html

[93] R. Hoover, T. Vasanthan, N. J. Senanayake and A. M. Martin, "The effects of defatting and heat-moisture treatment on the retrogradation of starch gels from wheat, oat, potato, and lentil," *Carbohydr. Res.*, vol. 261, pp. 13–24, 1994, doi: 10.1016/0008-6215(94)80002-2.

[94] M. Zhou, K. Robards, M. Glennie-Holmes and S. Helliwell, "Structure and pasting properties of oat starch," *Cereal Chem.*, vol. 75, pp. 273–281, 1998, doi: 10.1094/CCHEM.1998.75.3.273.

[95] K. Autio and A.-C. Eliasson, "Oat starch," in *Starch (Third Edition)*, J. BeMiller and R. Whistler, Eds. San Diego, CA, USA: Academic Press, 2009, pp. 589–599, doi: 10.1016/B978-0-12-746275-2.00015-X.

[96] W. Yan, L. Yin, M. Zhang, M. Zhang and X. Jia, "Gelatinization, retrogradation and gel properties of wheat starch–wheat bran arabinoxylan complexes," *Gels.*, vol. 7, p. 200, 2021, doi: 10.3390/gels7040200.

[97] E. R. Morris, "Shear-thinning of 'random coil' polysaccharides: Characterisation by two parameters from a simple linear plot," *Carbohydr. Polym.*, vol. 13, pp. 85–96, 1990, doi: 10.1016/0144-8617(90)90053-U.

[98] S. Singh and M. Kaur, "Steady and dynamic shear rheology of starches from different oat cultivars in relation to their physicochemical and structural properties," *Int. J. Food Prop.*, vol. 20, pp. 3282–3294, 2017, doi: 10.1080/10942912.2017.1286504.

[99] N. Liu, S. Ma, L. Li and X. Wang, "Study on the effect of wheat bran dietary fiber on the rheological properties of dough," *Grain Oil Sci. Technol.*, vol. 2, pp. 1–5, 2019, doi: 10.1016/j.gaost.2019.04.005.

[100] X. Qian, B. Sun, C. Zhu, Z. Zhang, X. Tian and X. Wang, "Effect of stir-frying on oat milling and pasting properties and rheological properties of oat flour," *J. Cereal Sci.*, vol. 92, p. 102908, 2020, doi: 10.1016/j.jcs.2020.102908.

[101] M. Kurdziel, M. Łabanowska, S. Pietrzyk, J. Sobolewska-Zielińska and M. Michalec, "Changes in the physicochemical properties of barley and oat starches upon the use of environmentally friendly oxidation methods," *Carbohydr. Polym.*, vol. 210, pp. 339–349, 2019, doi: 10.1016/j.carbpol.2019.01.088.

[102] R. Shukri, S. Alavi, H. Dogan and Y.-C. Shi, "Properties of extruded cross-linked waxy maize starches and their effects on extruded oat flour," *Carbohydr. Polym.*, vol. 253, p. 117259, 2021, doi: 10.1016/j.carbpol.2020.117259.

[103] G. P. Bruni, J. P. de Oliveira, L. M. Fonseca, F. T. da Silva, A. R. G. Dias and E. da Rosa Zavareze, "Biocomposite films based on phosphorylated wheat starch and cellulose nanocrystals from rice, oat, and eucalyptus husks," *Starch – Stärke.*, vol. 72, p. 1900051, 2020, doi: 10.1002/star.201900051.

[104] E. Subroto, Y. Cahyana, R. Indiarto and T. A. Rahmah, "Modification of starches and flours by acetylation and its dual modifications: A review of impact on physicochemical properties and their applications," *Polymers.*, vol. 15, p. 2990, 2023, doi: 10.3390/polym15142990.

[105] W. Berski et al., "Pasting and rheological properties of oat starch and its derivatives," *Carbohydr. Polym.*, vol. 83, pp. 665–671, 2011, doi: 10.1016/j.carbpol.2010.08.036.

[106] L. Mirmoghtadaie, M. Kadivar and M. Shahedi, "Effect of modified oat starch and protein on batter properties and quality of cake," *Cereal Chem.*, vol. 86, 685–691, 2009, doi: 10.1094/CCHEM-86-6-0685.

[107] K. S. Woo and P. A. Seib, "Cross-linked resistant starch: Preparation and properties," *Cereal Chem.*, vol. 79, pp. 819–825, 2002, doi: 10.1094/CCHEM.2002.79.6.819.

[108] M. Ovando-Martínez, K. Whitney, B. L. Reuhs, Douglas. C. Doehlert, S. Simsek, "Effect of hydrothermal treatment on physicochemical and digestibility properties of oat starch," *Food Res. J.*, vol. 52, pp. 17–25, 2013, doi: 10.1016/j.foodres.2013.02.035.

[109] J. B. Smith and M. D. Bennett, "Amylase isozymes of oats (Avena sativa L.)," *J. Sci. Food Agric.*, vol. 25, pp. 67–71, 1974, doi: 10.1002/jsfa.2740250108.

[110] R. Hoover, "The impact of heat-moisture treatment on molecular structures and properties of starches isolated from different botanical sources," *Crit. Rev. Food Sci. Nutr.*, vol. 50, pp. 835–847, 2010, doi: 10.1080/10408390903001735.

[111] V. Vamadevan, E. Bertoft, D. V. Soldatov and K. Seetharaman, "Impact on molecular organization of amylopectin in starch granules upon annealing," *Carbohydr. Polym.*, vol. 98, pp. 1045–1055, 2013, doi: 10.1016/j.carbpol.2013.07.006.

[112] B. Olawoye et al., "Modification of starch," in *Starch: Advances in Modifications, Technologies and Applications*, V. S. Sharanagat, D. C. Saxena, K. Kumar and Y. Kumar, Eds. Cham, Germany: Springer International Publishing, 2023, pp. 11–54, doi: 10.1007/978-3-031-35843-2_2.

[113] A. Jędrusek-Golińska, D. Górecka, M. Buchowski, K. Wieczorowska-Tobis, A. Gramza-Michałowska and K. Szymandera-Buszka, "Recent progress in the use of functional foods for older adults: A narrative review," *Compr. Rev. Food Sci. Food Saf.*, vol. 19, pp. 835–856, 2020, doi: 10.1111/1541-4337.12530.

[114] K. Janda, A. Orłowska, K. Watychowicz and K. Jakubczyk, "The role of oat products in the prevention and therapy of type 2 diabetes, hypercholesterolemia and obesity*," *Pomeranian J. Life Sci.*, vol. 65, 2019, doi: 10.21164/pomjlifesci.630.

[115] S. Werlang, C. Bonfante, T. Oro, B. Biduski, T. E. Bertolin and L. C. Gutkoski, "Native and annealed oat starches as a fat replacer in mayonnaise," *J. Food Process. Preserv.*, vol. 45, p. e15211, 2021, doi: 10.1111/jfpp.15211.

[116] F. Zhu, "Structures, properties, modifications, and uses of oat starch," *Food Chem.*, vol. 229, pp. 329–340, 2017, doi: 10.1016/j.foodchem.2017.02.064.

[117] N. M. Thani, M. M. Mazlan, N. I. N. Haris and M. H. Wondi, "Oat thermoplastic starch nanocomposite films reinforced with nanocellulose," *Phys. Sci. Rev.*, 2023, doi: 10.1515/psr-2022-0036.

[118] M. C. Galdeano, M. V. E. Grossmann, S. Mali, L. A. Bello-Perez, M. A. Garcia and P. B. Zamudio-Flores, "Effects of production process and plasticizers on stability of films and sheets of oat starch," *Mater. Sci. Eng. C.*, vol. 29, pp. 492–498, 2009, doi: 10.1016/j.msec.2008.08.031.

[119] A. Lazaridou and C. G. Biliaderis, "Molecular aspects of cereal β-glucan functionality: Physical properties, technological applications and physiological effects," *J. Cereal Sci.*, vol. 46, pp. 101–118, 2007, doi: 10.1016/j.jcs.2007.05.003.

[120] A. Regand, Z. Chowdhury, S. M. Tosh, T. M. S. Wolever and P. Wood, "The molecular weight, solubility and viscosity of oat beta-glucan affect human glycemic response by modifying starch digestibility," *Food Chem.*, vol. 129, pp. 297–304, 2011, doi: 10.1016/j.foodchem.2011.04.053.

[121] M. Manzoor and S. P. Bangar, "The functionality of β-glucans and fibers in cereals," in *Functional Cereals and Cereal Foods: Properties, Functionality and Applications*, S. Punia Bangar and A. Kumar Siroha, Eds. Cham, Germany: Springer International Publishing, 2022, pp. 139–160, doi: 10.1007/978-3-031-05611-6_6.

[122] EFSA Panel on Dietetic Products, "Nutrition and Allergies (NDA), Scientific Opinion on the substantiation of health claims related to beta-glucans from oats and barley and maintenance of normal blood LDL-cholesterol concentrations (ID 1236, 1299), increase in satiety leading to a reduction in energy intake (ID 851, 852), reduction of post-prandial glycaemic responses (ID 821, 824), and "digestive function" (ID 850) pursuant to Article 13(1) of Regulation (EC) No 1924/2006," *EFSA J.*, vol. 9, p. 2207, 2011, doi: 10.2903/j.efsa.2011.2207.

[123] S. M. V. Mejía, A. de Francisco and Benjamin M. Bohrer, "A comprehensive review on cereal β-glucan: Extraction, characterization, causes of degradation, and food application," *Crit. Rev. Food Sci. Nutr.*, vol. 60, pp. 3693–3704, 2020, doi: 10.1080/10408398.2019.1706444.

[124] M. Laitinen, N. Mäkelä-Salmi and N. H. Maina, "Gelation of cereal β-glucan after partial dissolution at physiological temperature: Effect of molecular structure," *Food Hydrocoll.*, vol. 141, p. 108722, 2023, doi: 10.1016/j.foodhyd.2023.108722.

[125] J.-H. Ryu, S. Lee, S. You, J.-H. Shim and S.-H. Yoo, "Effects of barley and oat β-glucan structures on their rheological and thermal characteristics," *Carbohydr. Polym.*, vol. 89, pp. 1238–1243, 2012, doi: 10.1016/j.carbpol.2012.04.025.

[126] M. S. Mikkelsen, B. M. Jespersen, F. H. Larsen, A. Blennow and S. B. Engelsen, "Molecular structure of large-scale extracted β-glucan from barley and oat: Identification of a significantly changed block structure in a high β-glucan barley mutant," *Food Chem.*, vol. 136, pp. 130–138, 2013, doi: 10.1016/j.foodchem.2012.07.097.

[127] A. Håkansson, M. Ulmius and L. Nilsson, "Asymmetrical flow field-flow fractionation enables the characterization of molecular and supramolecular properties of cereal β-glucan dispersions," *Carbohydr. Polym.*, vol. 87, pp. 518–523, 2012, doi: 10.1016/j.carbpol.2011.08.014.

[128] M. S. Izydorczyk and J. E. Dexter, "Barley β-glucans and arabinoxylans: Molecular structure, physicochemical properties, and uses in food products–a review," *Food Res. J.*, vol. 41, pp. 850–868, 2008, doi: 10.1016/j.foodres.2008.04.001.

[129] E. De Arcangelis, S. Djurle, A. A. M. Andersson, E. Marconi, M. C. Messia and R. Andersson, "Structure analysis of β-glucan in barley and effects of wheat β-glucanase," *J. Cereal Sci.*, vol. 85, pp. 175–181, 2019, doi: 10.1016/j.jcs.2018.12.002.

[130] K. M. Andrzej, M. Małgorzata, K. Sabina, O. K. Horbańczuk and E. Rodak, "Application of rich in β-glucan flours and preparations in bread baked from frozen dough," *Food Sci. Technol. Int.*, vol. 26, pp. 53–64, 2020, doi: 10.1177/1082013219865379.

[131] F. Chaari, S. Zouari-Ellouzi, L. Belguith-Fendri, M. Yosra, S. Ellouz-Chaabouni and R. Ellouz-Ghorbel, "Valorization of cereal by products extracted fibre and potential use in breadmaking," *Chem. Africa.*, vol. 5, pp. 2011–2019, 2022, doi: 10.1007/s42250-022-00454-w.

[132] M. Elleuch, D. Bedigian, O. Roiseux, S. Besbes, C. Blecker and H. Attia, "Dietary fibre and fibre-rich by-products of food processing: Characterisation, technological functionality and commercial applications: A review," *Food Chem.*, vol. 124, pp. 411–421, 2011, doi: 10.1016/j.foodchem.2010.06.077.

[133] H. Chen, N. Liu, F. He, Q. Liu and X. Xu, "Specific β-glucans in chain conformations and their biological functions," *Polym. J.*, vol. 54, pp. 427–453, 2022, doi: 10.1038/s41428-021-00587-8.

[134] A. Lante and E. Canazza, "Insight on extraction and preservation of biological activity of cereal β-D-glucans," *Appl. Sci.*, vol. 13, p. 11080, 2023, doi: 10.3390/app131911080.

[135] S. Machmudah, Wahyudiono, T. Adschiri and M. Goto, "Hydrothermal extraction and micronization in a one-step process for enhancement of β–glucan concentrate at subcritical water conditions," *S. Afr. J. Chem. Eng.*, vol. 46, pp. 72–87, 2023, doi: 10.1016/j.sajce.2023.07.009.

[136] J. R. da Silva Alves, A. F. Magalhães dos Santos, W. Cantanhêde and J. L. Magalhães, "Uses of natural biopolymers in food and biomedical applications," in *Studies in Natural Products Chemistry*, A.-Rahman, Ed. Elsevier, 2023, pp. 1–40, doi: 10.1016/B978-0-323-91296-9.00005-8.

[137] Z. Li et al., "Mechanism underlying the weakening effect of β-glucan on the gluten system," *Food Chem.*, vol. 420, p. 136002, 2023, doi: 10.1016/j.foodchem.2023.136002.

[138] Q. Li et al., "Extraction and characterization of waxy and normal barley β-glucans and their effects on waxy and normal barley starch pasting and degradation properties and mash filtration rate," *Carbohydr. Polym.*, vol. 302, p. 120405, 2023, doi: 10.1016/j.carbpol.2022.120405.

[139] Z. Sinangil, Ö. Taştan and T. Baysal, "Beta-glucan as a novel functional fiber: Functional properties, health benefits and food applications," *Turkish JAF Sci. Tech.*, vol. 10, pp. 1957–1965, 2022, doi: 10.24925/turjaf.v10i10.1957-1965.5430.

[140] S. Leković, S. Marković, Đ. Minić, J. Todosijević, A. Torbica and N. Đukić, "B-glucan content variability in seed of barley cultivars," *Kragujevac J. Sci.*, pp. 111–120, 2023, doi: 10.5937/KgJSci2345111L.

[141] M. S. Mikkelsen, B. M. Jespersen, B. L. Møller, H. N. Lærke, F. H. Larsen and S. B. Engelsen, "Comparative spectroscopic and rheological studies on crude and purified soluble barley and oat β-glucan preparations," *Food Res. J.*, vol. 43, pp. 2417–2424, 2010, doi: 10.1016/j.foodres.2010.09.016.

[142] C. Zielke, A. Stradner and L. Nilsson, "Characterization of cereal β-glucan extracts: Conformation and structural aspects," *Food Hydrocoll.*, vol. 79, pp. 218–227, 2018, doi: 10.1016/j.foodhyd.2017.12.036.

[143] N. Mäkelä, N. H. Maina, P. Vikgren and T. Sontag-Strohm, "Gelation of cereal β-glucan at low concentrations," *Food Hydrocoll.*, vol. 73, pp. 60–66, 2017, doi: 10.1016/j.foodhyd.2017.06.026.

[144] R. De Paula, E.-S. M. Abdel-Aal, M. C. Messia, I. Rabalski and E. Marconi, "Effect of processing on the beta-glucan physicochemical properties in barley and semolina pasta," *J. Cereal Sci.*, vol. 75, pp 124–131, 2017, doi: 10.1016/j.jcs.2017.03.030.

[145] S. H. Lee et al., "Physicochemical and in vitro binding properties of barley β-glucan treated with hydrogen peroxide," *Food Chem.*, vol. 192, pp. 729–735, 2016, doi: 10.1016/j.foodchem.2015.07.063.

[146] T. H. Gamel, E.-S. M. Abdel-Aal, N. P. Ames, R. Duss and S. M. Tosh, "Enzymatic extraction of beta-glucan from oat bran cereals and oat crackers and optimization of viscosity measurement," *J. Cereal Sci.*, vol. 59, pp. 33–40, 2014, doi: 10.1016/j.jcs.2013.10.011.

[147] N. Mäkelä, O. Brinck and T. Sontag-Strohm, "Viscosity of β-glucan from oat products at the intestinal phase of the gastrointestinal model," *Food Hydrocoll.*, vol. 100, p. 105422, 2020, doi: 10.1016/j.foodhyd.2019.105422.

[148] Y. Brummer, R. Duss, T. M. S. Wolever and S. M. Tosh, "Glycemic response to extruded oat bran cereals processed to vary in molecular weight," *Cereal Chem.*, vol. 89, pp. 255–261, 2012, doi: 10.1094/CCHEM-03-12-0031-R.

[149] S. Leuzinger, A. Steingötter and L. Nyström, "Viscosity of cereal ?-glucan in the gastrointestinal tract: Swiss Society for Food Chemistry Young Scientist Awards 2019," *CHIMIA.*, vol. 72, pp. 733–733, 2018, doi: 10.2533/chimia.2018.733.

[150] A. Rieder, S. H. Knutsen, A. S. Fernandez and S. Ballance, "At a high dose even partially degraded beta-glucan with decreased solubility significantly reduced the glycaemic response to bread," *Food Funct.*, vol. 10, pp. 1529–1539, 2019, doi: 10.1039/C8FO02098A.

[151] M. J. Redmond and D. A. Fielder, "Extraction and purification method for cereal beta-glucan, 20060122149, 2006. Accessed: Oct. 16, 2023. [Online]. Available: www.freepatentsonline.com/y2006/0122149.html

[152] P. J. Wood, I. R. Siddiqui and D. Paton, "Extraction of high-viscosity gums from oats," *Cereal Chem.*, vol. 55, pp. 1038–1049, 1978.

[153] E. Westerlund, R. Andersson and P. Åman, "Isolation and chemical characterization of water-soluble mixed-linked β-glucans and arabinoxylans in oat milling fractions," *Carbohydr. Polym.*, vol. 20, pp. 115–123, 1993, doi: 10.1016/0144-8617(93)90086-J.

[154] P. J. Wood, J. Weisz and B. A. Blackwell, "Molecular characterization of cereal β-D-glucans. Structural analysis of oat β-D-glucan and rapid structural evaluation of β-D-glucans from different sources by high-performance liquid chromatography of oligosaccharides released by lichenase," *Cereal Chem.*, vol. 68, pp. 31–39, 1991. Accessed: Oct. 16, 2023. [Online]. Available: https://cir.nii.ac.jp/crid/1573105976498573824

[155] B. Du, F. Zhu and B. Xu, "β-glucan extraction from bran of hull-less barley by accelerated solvent extraction combined with response surface methodology," *J. Cereal Sci.*, vol. 59, pp. 95–100, 2014, doi: 10.1016/j.jcs.2013.11.004.

[156] L. M. Comin, F. Temelli and M. D. A. Saldaña, "Barley beta-glucan aerogels via supercritical CO_2 drying," *Food Res. J.*, vol. 48, pp. 442–448, 2012, doi: 10.1016/j.foodres.2012.05.002.

[157] H.-U. Yoo, M.-J. Ko and M.-S. Chung, "Hydrolysis of beta-glucan in oat flour during subcritical-water extraction," *Food Chem.*, vol. 308, p. 125670, 2020, doi: 10.1016/j.foodchem.2019.125670.

[158] K. R. Morgan, "β-glucan products and extraction processes from cereals," 6426201, 2002. Accessed: Oct. 16, 2023. [Online]. Available: www.freepatentsonline.com/6426201.html

[159] B. H. Van Lengerich, O. Gruess and F. P. Meuser, "Beta-glucan compositions and process therefore," 6835558, 2004. Accessed: Oct. 16, 2023. [Online]. Available: www.freepatentsonline.com/6835558.html

[160] R. S. Bhatty, "Methods for extracting cereal β-glucans," 5518710, 1996. Accessed: Oct. 16, 2023. [Online]. Available: www.freepatentsonline.com/5518710.html

[161] R. C. Potter, P. A. Fisher, K. R. Hash Sr. and J. D. Neidt, "Method for concentrating β-glucan," 6323338, 2001. Accessed: Oct. 16, 2023. [Online]. Available: www.freepatentsonline.com/6323338.html

[162] M. U. Beer, E. Arrigoni and R. Amado, "Extraction of oat gum from oat bran: Effects of process on yield, molecular weight distribution, viscosity and (1→3)(1→4)-β-D-glucan content of the gum," *Cereal Chem.*, vol. 73, pp. 58–62, 1996.

[163] P. Sharma and H. S. Gujral, "Extrusion of hulled barley affecting β-glucan and properties of extrudates," *Food Bioprocess Technol.*, vol. 6, pp. 1374–1389, 2013, doi: 10.1007/s11947-011-0777-2.

[164] A. Skendi, C. G. Biliaderis, A. Lazaridou and M. S. Izydorczyk, "Structure and rheological properties of water soluble β-glucans from oat cultivars of Avena sativa and Avena bysantina," *J. Cereal Sci.*, vol. 38, pp. 15–31, 2003, doi: 10.1016/S0733-5210(02)00137-6.

[165] M. Irakli, C. G. Biliaderis, M. S. Izydorczyk and I. N. Papadoyannis, "Isolation, structural features and rheological properties of water-extractable β-glucans from different Greek barley cultivars," *J. Sci. Food Agric.*, vol. 84, pp. 1170–1178, 2004, doi: 10.1002/jsfa.1787.

[166] F. Zhu, B. Du and B. Xu, "A critical review on production and industrial applications of beta-glucans," *Food Hydrocoll.*, vol. 52, pp. 275–288, 2016, doi: 10.1016/j.foodhyd.2015.07.003.

[167] K. Liu, "Fractionation of oats into products enriched with protein, beta-glucan, starch, or other carbohydrates," *J. Cereal Sci.*, vol. 60, pp. 317–322, 2014, doi: 10.1016/j.jcs.2014.06.002.

[168] V. M. Limberger et al., "Extração de β-glucanas de cevada e caracterização parcial do amido residual," *Cienc. Rural.*, vol. 41, pp. 2217–2223, 2011, doi: 10.1590/S0103-84782011001200028.

[169] M. Korčok, J. Calle, M. Veverka and V. Vietoris, "Understanding the health benefits and technological properties of β-glucan for the development of easy-to-swallow gels to guarantee food security among seniors," *Crit. Rev. Food Sci. Nutr.*, vol. 2022, pp. 1–18, doi: 10.1080/10408398.2022.2093325.

[170] F. Ronda, S. Perez-Quirce, A. Lazaridou and C. G. Biliaderis, "Effect of barley and oat β-glucan concentrates on gluten-free rice-based doughs and bread characteristics," *Food Hydrocoll.*, vol. 48, pp. 197–207, 2015, doi: 10.1016/j.foodhyd.2015.02.031.

[171] G. Venkatachalam, S. Arumugam and M. Doble, "Industrial production and applications of α/β linear and branched glucans," *Indian Chem. Eng.*, vol. 63, pp. 533–547, 2021, doi: 10.1080/00194506.2020.1798820.

[172] I. Avramia and S. Amariei, "Spent Brewer's Yeast as a source of insoluble β-glucans," *Int. J. Mol. Sci.*, vol. 22, p. 825, 2021, doi: 10.3390/ijms22020825.

[173] M. Jian, S. Li, Z. Zhu, N. Zhang, Q. Deng and G. Cravotto, "Combination modes impact on the stability of β-carotene-loaded emulsion constructed by soy protein isolate, β-glucan and myricetin ternary complex," *Food Res. J.*, vol. 172, p. 113173, 2023, doi: 10.1016/j.foodres.2023.113173.

[174] A. Ahmad and M. Kaleem, "β-glucan as a food ingredient," in *Biopolymers for Food Design*, A. M. Grumezescu and A. M. Holban, Eds. Academic Press, 2018, pp. 351–381, doi: 10.1016/B978-0-12-811449-0.00011-6.

[175] D. Bhaskar, S. K. Khatkar, R. Chawla, H. Panwar and S. Kapoor, "Effect of β-glucan fortification on physico-chemical, rheological, textural, colour and organoleptic characteristics of low fat dahi," *J. Food Sci. Technol.*, vol. 54, pp. 2684–2693, 2017, doi: 10.1007/s13197-017-2705-6.

[176] A. Ahmad, F. M. Anjum, T. Zahoor, H. Nawaz and S. M. R. Dilshad, "Beta glucan: A valuable functional ingredient in foods," *Crit. Rev. Food Sci. Nutr.*, vol. 52, pp. 201–212, 2012, doi: 10.1080/10408398.2010.499806.

[177] S. Karp, J. Wyrwisz and M. A. Kurek, "The impact of different levels of oat β-glucan and water on gluten-free cake rheology and physicochemical characterisation," *J. Food Sci. Technol.*, vol. 57, pp. 3628–3638, 2020, doi: 10.1007/s13197-020-04395-5.

[178] U. Tiwari and E. Cummins, "Dietary exposure assessment of β-glucan in a barley and oat based bread," *LWT.*, vol. 47, pp. 413–420, 2012, doi: 10.1016/j.lwt.2012.02.002.

[179] A. Prins, P. Shewry and A. Lovegrove, "Analysis of mixed linkage β-glucan content and structure in different wheat flour milling fractions," *J. Cereal Sci.*, vol. 113, p. 103753, 2023, doi: 10.1016/j.jcs.2023.103753.

[180] Z. Burkus and F. Temelli, "Stabilization of emulsions and foams using barley β-glucan," *Food Res. J.*, vol. 33, pp. 27–33, 2000, doi: 10.1016/S0963-9969(00)00020-X.

[181] C. Zielke, Y. Lu and L. Nilsson, "Aggregation and microstructure of cereal β-glucan and its association with other biomolecules," *Colloids Surf. A: Physicochem. Eng. Asp.*, vol. 560, pp. 402–409, 2019, doi: 10.1016/j.colsurfa.2018.10.042.

[182] M. Kurek, I. E. Garofulić, M. T. Bakić, M. Ščetar, V. D. Uzelac and K. Galić, "Development and evaluation of a novel antioxidant and pH indicator film based on chitosan and food waste sources of antioxidants," *Food Hydrocoll.*, vol. 84, pp. 238–246, 2018, doi: 10.1016/j.foodhyd.2018.05.050.

[183] V. Nehmi-Filho et al., "Novel Nutraceutical (silymarin, yeast β-glucan, prebiotics, and minerals) shifts gut microbiota and restores large intestine histology of diet-induced metabolic syndrome mice," *J. Funct. Foods.*, vol. 107, p. 105671, 2023, doi: 10.1016/j.jff.2023.105671.

[184] M. Kozarski et al., "Mushroom β-glucan and polyphenol formulations as natural immunity boosters and balancers: Nature of the application," *Food Sci. Hum. Wellness.*, vol. 12, pp. 378–396, 2023, doi: 10.1016/j.fshw.2022.07.040.

[185] N. Mishra, "Cereal β glucan as a functional ingredient," in *Innovations in Food Technology: Current Perspectives and Future Goals*, P. Mishra, R. R. Mishra and C. O. Adetunji, Eds. Singapore, Singapore: Springer, 2020, pp. 109–122, doi: 10.1007/978-981-15-6121-4_8.

[186] A. Montalbano et al., "Quality characteristics and in vitro digestibility study of barley flour enriched ditalini pasta," *LWT.*, vol. 72, pp. 223–228, 2016, doi: 10.1016/j.lwt.2016.04.042.

[187] Z. Li, Y. Dong, X. Xiao and X. Zhou, "Mechanism by which β-glucanase improves the quality of fermented barley flour-based food products," *Food Chem.*, vol. 311, p. 126026, 2020, doi: 10.1016/j.foodchem.2019.126026.

[188] C. Klose and E. K. Arendt, "Proteins in oats; their synthesis and changes during germination: A review," *Crit. Rev. Food Sci. Nutr.*, vol. 52, pp. 629–639, 2012, doi: 10.1080/10408398.2010.504902.

[189] O. E. Mäkinen, N. Sozer, D. Ercili-Cura and K. Poutanen, "Protein from oat: Structure, processes, functionality, and nutrition," in *Sustainable Protein Sources*, S. R. Nadathur, J. P. D. Wanasundara and L. Scanlin, Eds. San Diego, CA, USA: Academic Press, 2017, pp. 105–119, doi: 10.1016/B978-0-12-802778-3.00006-8.

[190] R. Li and Y. L. Xiong, "Sensitivity of oat protein solubility to changing ionic strength and pH," *J. Food Sci.*, vol. 86, pp. 78–85, 2021, doi: 10.1111/1750-3841.15544.

[191] C. Yung Ma, "Preparation, Composition and Functional Properties of Oat Protein Isolates[1] 1 Contribution No. 509. Food Research Institute, Agriculture Canada," *Can. Inst. Food Technol. J.*, vol. 16, pp. 201–205, 1983, doi: 10.1016/S0315-5463(83)72208-X.

[192] Ü. İ. Konak, D. Ercili-Cura, J. Sibakov, T. Sontag-Strohm, M. Certel, J. Loponen, "CO_2-defatted oats: Solubility, emulsification and foaming properties," *J. Cereal Sci.*, vol. 60, pp. 37–41, 2014, doi: 10.1016/j.jcs.2014.01.013.

[193] J. R. Runyon, B. A. Sunilkumar, L. Nilsson, A. Rascon and B. Bergenståhl, "The effect of heat treatment on the soluble protein content of oats," *J. Cereal Sci.*, vol. 65, pp. 119–124, 2015, doi: 10.1016/j.jcs.2015.06.008.

[194] D. Zhang, D. C. Doehlert and W. R. Moore, "Rheological properties of (1→3),(1→4)-β-d-glucans from raw, roasted, and steamed oat groats," *Cereal Chem.*, vol. 75, pp. 433–438, 1998, doi: 10.1094/CCHEM.1998.75.4.433.

[195] E. L. Molteberg, G. Vogt, A. Nilsson and W. Frolich, "Effects of storage and heat processing on the content and composition of free fatty acids in oats," *Cereal Chem.*, vol. 72, pp. 88–93, 1995.

[196] S. Bryngelsson, L. H. Dimberg and A. Kamal-Eldin, "Effects of commercial processing on levels of antioxidants in oats (Avena sativa L.)," *J. Agric. Food Chem.*, vol. 50, pp. 1890–1896, 2002, doi: 10.1021/jf011222z.

[197] A. Mohamed, G. Biresaw, J. Xu, M. P. Hojilla-Evangelista and P. Rayas-Duarte, "Oats protein isolate: Thermal, rheological, surface and functional properties," *Food Res. J.*, vol. 42, pp. 107–114, 2009, doi: 10.1016/j.foodres.2008.10.011.

[198] R. Ponnampalam, G. Goulet, J. Amiot, B. Chamberland and G. J. Brisson, "Some functional properties of acetylated and succinylated oat protein concentrates and a blend of succinylated oat protein and whey protein concentrates," *Food Chem.*, vol. 29, pp. 109–118, 1988, doi: 10.1016/0308-8146(88)90093-3.

[199] A. Prosekov, O. Babich, O. Kriger, S. Ivanova, V. Pavsky, S. Sukhikh, Y. Yang and E. Kashirskih, "Functional properties of the enzyme-modified protein from oat bran," *Food Biosci.*, vol. 24, pp. 46–49, 2018, doi: 10.1016/j.fbio.2018.05.003.

[200] L. Amagliani, J. V. C. Silva, M. Saffon and J. Dombrowski, "On the foaming properties of plant proteins: Current status and future opportunities," *Trends Food Sci. Technol.*, vol. 118, pp. 261–272, 2021, doi: 10.1016/j.tifs.2021.10.001.

[201] E. F. Ribeiro, P. Morell, V. R. Nicoletti, A. Quiles and I. Hernando, "Protein- and polysaccharide-based particles used for Pickering emulsion stabilisation," *Food Hydrocoll.*, vol. 119, p. 106839, 2021, doi: 10.1016/j.foodhyd.2021.106839.

[202] A. Lapveteläinen and T. Aro, "Protein composition and functionality of high-protein oat flour derived from integrated starch-ethanol process," *Cereal Chem.*, vol. 71, pp. 133–139, 1994.

[203] O. Kaukonen, T. Sontag-Strohm, H. Salovaara, A.-M. Lampi, J. Sibakov and J. Loponen, "Foaming of differently processed oats: Role of nonpolar lipids and tryptophanin proteins," *Cereal Chem.*, vol. 88, pp. 239–244, 2011, doi: 10.1094/CCHEM-11-10-0154.

[204] L. Mirmoghtadaie, M. Kadivar and M. Shahedi, "Effects of succinylation and deamidation on functional properties of oat protein isolate," *Food Chem.*, vol. 114, pp. 127–131, 2009, doi: 10.1016/j.foodchem.2008.09.025.

[205] R. Ponnampalam, G. Goulet, J. Amiot and G. J. Brisson, "Some functional and nutritional properties of oat flours as affected by proteolysis," *J. Agric. Food Chem.*, vol. 35, pp. 279–285, 1987, doi: 10.1021/jf00074a028.

[206] X. Guan, H. Yao, Z. Chen, L. Shan and M. Zhang, "Some functional properties of oat bran protein concentrate modified by trypsin," *Food Chem.*, vol. 101, pp. 163–170, 2007, doi: 10.1016/j.foodchem.2006.01.011.

[207] B. Zhang, X. Guo, K. Zhu, W. Peng and H. Zhou, "Improvement of emulsifying properties of oat protein isolate–dextran conjugates by glycation," *Carbohydr. Polym.*, vol. 127, pp. 168–175, 2015, doi: 10.1016/j.carbpol.2015.03.072.

[208] X. He et al., "Effect of oat β-glucan on gel properties and protein conformation of silver carp surimi," *J. Sci. Food Agric.*, vol. 103, pp. 3367–3375, 2023, doi: 10.1002/jsfa.12525.

[209] X. Yin, J. Li, L. Zhu and H. Zhang, "Advances in the formation mechanism of set-type plant-based yogurt gel: A review," *Crit. Rev. Food Sci. Nutr.*, 2023, pp. 1–20, doi: 10.1080/10408398.2023.2212764.

[210] C. Yang, Y. Wang and L. Chen, "Fabrication, characterization and controlled release properties of oat protein gels with percolating structure induced by cold gelation," *Food Hydrocoll.*, vol. 62, pp. 21–34, 2017, doi: 10.1016/j.foodhyd.2016.07.023.

[211] T. V. Nieto-Nieto, Y. X. Wang, L. Ozimek and L. Chen, "Inulin at low concentrations significantly improves the gelling properties of oat protein – A molecular mechanism study," *Food Hydrocoll.*, vol. 50, pp. 116–127, 2015, doi: 10.1016/j.foodhyd.2015.03.031.

[212] T. V. Nieto Nieto, Y. Wang, L. Ozimek and L. Chen, "Improved thermal gelation of oat protein with the formation of controlled phase-separated networks using dextrin and carrageenan polysaccharides," *Food Res. J.*, vol. 82, pp. 95–103, 2016, doi: 10.1016/j.foodres.2016.01.027.

[213] O. E. Mäkinen, T. Uniacke-Lowe, J. A. O'Mahony and E. K. Arendt, "Physicochemical and acid gelation properties of commercial UHT-treated plant-based milk substitutes and lactose free bovine milk," *Food Chem.*, vol. 168, pp. 630–638, 2015, doi: 10.1016/j.foodchem.2014.07.036.

[214] J. Loponen, P. Laine, T. Sontag-Strohm and H. Salovaara, "Behaviour of oat globulins in lactic acid fermentation of oat bran," *Eur. Food Res Technol.*, vol. 225, pp. 105–110, 2007, doi: 10.1007/s00217-006-0387-9.

[215] O. Mårtensson, R. Öste and O. Holst, "Lactic acid bacteria in an oat-based non-dairy milk substitute: Fermentation characteristics and exopolysaccharide formation," *LWT.*, vol. 33, pp. 525–530, 2000, doi: 10.1006/fstl.2000.0718.

[216] M. Brückner-Gühmann, A. Benthin and S. Drusch, "Enrichment of yoghurt with oat protein fractions: Structure formation, textural properties and sensory evaluation," *Food Hydrocoll.*, vol. 86, pp. 146–153, 2019, doi: 10.1016/j.foodhyd.2018.03.019.

[217] P. Laine et al., "Emulsion preparation with modified oat bran: Optimization of the emulsification process for microencapsulation purposes," *J. Food Eng.*, vol. 104, pp. 538–547, 2011, doi: 10.1016/j.jfoodeng.2011.01.014.

[218] X. Guan and H. Yao, "Optimization of viscozyme L-assisted extraction of oat bran protein using response surface methodology," *Food Chem.*, vol. 106, pp. 345–351, 2008, doi: 10.1016/j.foodchem.2007.05.041.

[219] J. E. Cluskey, Y. V. Wu, J. S. Wall and G. E. Inglett, "Oat protein concentrates from a wet-milling process: Preparation," *Cereal Chem.*, vol. 50, pp. 475–481, 1973.

[220] A. Kaleda et al., "Impact of fermentation and phytase treatment of pea-oat protein blend on physicochemical, sensory, and nutritional properties of extruded meat analogs," *Foods.*, vol. 9, p. 1059, 2020, doi: 10.3390/foods9081059.

[221] L. Zhong et al., "Characterization and functional evaluation of oat protein isolate-Pleurotus ostreatus β-glucan conjugates formed via Maillard reaction," *Food Hydrocoll.*, vol. 87, pp. 459–469, 2019, doi: 10.1016/j.foodhyd.2018.08.034.

[222] G. A. Batalova, V. N. Krasilnikov, V. S. Popov and E. E. Safonova, "Characteristics of the fatty acid composition of naked oats of Russian selection," *IOP Conf. Ser. Earth Environ. Sci.*, vol. 337, p. 012039, 2019, doi: 10.1088/1755-1315/337/1/012039.

[223] M. Zhou, K. Robards, M. Glennie-Holmes and S. Helliwell, "Oat lipids," *J. Am. Oil Chem. Soc.*, vol. 76, pp. 159–169, 1999, doi: 10.1007/s11746-999-0213-1.

[224] K. J. Frey and E. G. Hammond, "Genetics, characteristics, and utilization of oil in caryopses of oat species," *J. Am. Oil Chem. Soc.*, vol. 52, pp. 358–362, 1975, doi: 10.1007/BF02639196.

[225] P. B. Price and J. G. Parsons, "Lipids of seven cereal grains," *J. Am. Oil Chem. Soc.*, vol. 52, pp. 490–493, 1975, doi: 10.1007/BF02640738.

[226] M. R. Sahasrabudhe, "Lipid composition of oats (Avena sativa L.)," *J. Am. Oil Chem. Soc.*, vol. 56, pp. 80–84, 1979, doi: 10.1007/BF02914274.

[227] K. Banaś and J. Harasym, "Current knowledge of content and composition of oat oil – Future perspectives of oat as oil source," *Food Bioprocess Technol.*, vol. 14, pp. 232–247, 2021, doi: 10.1007/s11947-020-02535-5.

[228] Y. I. Delgado-García, S. Luna-Suárez, A. López-Malo and J. I. Morales-Camacho, "Effect of supercritical carbon dioxide on physicochemical and techno-functional properties of amaranth flour," *Chem. Eng. Process.: Process Intensif.*, vol. 178, p. 109031, 2022, doi: 10.1016/j.cep.2022.109031.

[229] M. B. O. Andersson, M. Demirbüker and L. G. Blomberg, "Semi-continuous extraction/purification of lipids by means of supercritical fluids," *J. Chromatogr. A.*, vol. 785, pp. 337–343, 1997, doi: 10.1016/S0021-9673(97)00083-6.

[230] P. Forssell, R. Kervinen, M. Alkio and K. Poutanen, "Comparison of methods for separating polar lipids from oat oil," *Lipid/Fett.*, vol. 94, pp. 355–358, 1992, doi: 10.1002/lipi.19920940909.

[231] H. Aro, E. Järvenpää, K. Könkö, R. Huopalahti and V. Hietaniemi, "The characterisation of oat lipids produced by supercritical fluid technologies," *J. Cereal Sci.*, vol. 45, pp. 116–119, 2007, doi: 10.1016/j.jcs.2006.09.001.

[232] R. W. Welch, "A micro-method for the estimation of oil content and composition in seed crops," *J. Sci. Food Agric.*, vol. 28, pp. 635–638, 1977, doi: 10.1002/jsfa.2740280710.

[233] S. Schneider, S. Hammann and H. Hayen, "Determination of polar lipids in wheat and oat by a complementary approach of hydrophilic interaction liquid chromatography and reversed-phase high-performance liquid chromatography hyphenated with high-resolution mass spectrometry," *J. Agric. Food Chem.*, vol. 71, pp. 11263–11275, 2023, doi: 10.1021/acs.jafc.3c02073.

[234] R. A. Moreau et al., "The identification of mono-, di-, tri-, and tetragalactosyl-diacylglycerols and their natural estolides in oat kernels," *Lipids.*, vol. 43, pp. 533–548, 2008, doi: 10.1007/s11745-008-3181-6.

[235] R. Pandiselvam et al., "Recent applications of vibrational spectroscopic techniques in the grain industry," *Food Rev. Int.*, vol. 39, pp. 209–239, 2023, doi: 10.1080/87559129.2021.1904253.

[236] Y. Li, M. Obadi, J. Shi, J. Sun, Z. Chen and B. Xu, "Determination of moisture, total lipid, and bound lipid contents in oats using low-field nuclear magnetic resonance," *J. Food Compos. Anal.*, vol. 87, p. 103401, 2020, doi: 10.1016/j.jfca.2019.103401.

[237] F.-A. Manolache, A. Hanganu, D. E. Duta, N. Belc, D. I. Marin, "The physico-chemical and spectroscopic composition characterization of oat grains and oat oil samples," *Revista de Chimie.*, vol. 64, pp. 45–48, 2013.

Biotechnological, Molecular, and Processing Strategies for Improving Nutritional and Functional Properties of Oats

9

Chirag Maheshwari, Muzaffar Hasan,
Arti Kumari, Prathap V., Brijesh Lekhak,
Nitin Kumar Garg, Nand Lal Meena,
Aruna Tyagi, Ravi Prakash Saini, and Ishwar Singh

9.1 INTRODUCTION

Cultivated oats belong to the hexaploid species *Avena sativa* ($2n = 6x = 42$, with AACCDD genomes), comprising 21 pairs of chromosomes originating from two or three ancestral diploid genomes. Oats are a widely cultivated cool-season annual forage species, serving as a major source of high-quality forage for livestock globally.

DOI: 10.1201/9781003263302-9

Within the genus *Avena*, a polyploid series of wild, weedy, and cultivated species exists across six continents. Diploid species have either the AA or CC genomes, tetraploids predominantly feature AABB or CCDD (previously AACC) genomes, and all hexaploid species, including common oats, share the AACCDD genomic constitution [1]. The phylogenetic history and divergence time among the A, C, and D genomic lineages remain unclear due to the absence of genome sequences from hexaploid oats and their close diploid and tetraploid relatives [2]. Polyploid plants often exhibit advantageous traits, such as increased biomass production, vigour, and adaptability to environmental changes, contributing to the development of important agronomic traits in food crops [3]. Oats' adaptability to a wide range of climatic conditions allows them to thrive in harsh environments, making oat polyploidization a critical factor in enhancing next-generation crop improvement to address food security challenges. Several commercially important crop genomes have been sequenced and assembled, improving our understanding of crop evolutionary history and facilitating the selection of vital traits.

Genetics plays a central role in maintaining quality by mitigating fluctuations resulting from environmental influences, primarily through genetic mechanisms related to disease and stress resistance. A more profound understanding of the genetics underpinning oat quality components opens up opportunities for more efficient manipulation of these traits to achieve the desired quality profile for various end users [4]. Classical genetic studies have revealed that most traits are controlled by one or more genes located along the DNA strands forming the chromosomes within plant cell nuclei. Recent advances in molecular genetic techniques have significantly expanded our knowledge of oat genetics. Recombination mapping and physical mapping unveil the chromosomal locations of genes, while quantitative trait locus (QTL) analysis, utilizing these maps, identifies chromosomal regions with significant genetic effects on specific traits [5]. Comparative mapping allows for inferences in oats based on information acquired from related plant species regarding genes, QTLs, or genomic maps. Various types of molecular markers exist, all designed to identify DNA differences or polymorphisms between individuals. Molecular markers are stable, follow Mendelian inheritance, and typically do not affect phenotype. Moreover, they are numerous and distributed throughout the plant's genome, making them ideal for mapping and QTL analysis. Notably, when a breeder seeks to select a particular QTL or gene, one or more linked molecular markers can serve as diagnostic indicators [6]. These molecular marker "tags" can be assessed more quickly and efficiently in a large number of plants compared to biological or phenotypic assays. This concept forms the foundation of molecular marker-assisted selection (MAS) or breeding.

In theory, a trait governed by a single gene in a diploid organism could be controlled by three homoeologous genes in a hexaploid species. In practice, this is not always the case due to factors like mutations and gene silencing [7]–[11]. Furthermore, most traits of interest in oats are quantitative and influenced by multiple genes [12]. Fortunately, QTL analysis and related techniques enable the dissection of this genetic complexity into more manageable components [7]–[11]. The use of doubled haploids, which are homozygous at all loci, provides a simplifying strategy. Doubled haploids offer genetic stability, allowing the production of numerous genetically identical plants for consistent comparisons across different years, environments, or experiments [13]. Besides cultivated hexaploid oats, there exist related wild diploid, tetraploid, and hexaploid oat species, which serve as a valuable source of additional genetic variation. This variation can be introduced into cultivated oats through a combination of wide sexual crossing, tissue culture, and molecular assays. The potential also exists to introduce genes from an even broader genetic pool through genetic transformation strategies, expanding the genetic repertoire of cultivated oats [14].

Research in oat grain quality has seen substantial growth in both the public and private sectors. Oats are known for their superior nutritional profile compared to other cereals, featuring various storage proteins like avenalin and avenin, a significant level of lipase enzyme, β-glucan, favourable fatty acid composition, as well as flavonoids, micronutrients, and avenanthramides, including dihydroxyphenylalanine, apigenin, luteolin, and tricin [15]. Additionally, oats exhibit high green forage production in conjunction with grain, making them an excellent source of livestock feed due to their desirable crude protein content, neutral detergent fibre, ash content, in vitro dry matter digestibility, crude fat, digestible organic matter, acid detergent lignin, acid detergent fibre, metabolizable energy, dry matter intake, total digestible nutrient, and crude fibre, alongside high palatability [16]. Experimental and human intervention studies have demonstrated that oat consumption reduces the risk of several non-communicable human diseases, including celiac disease, cardiovascular disease, diabetes, obesity, high cholesterol, and hypertension.

Despite the myriad health and nutritional advantages of oats, they have not received commensurate attention compared to other cereals like wheat, corn, and rice. This relative lack of focus has resulted in underfunding of oat research, leading to a scarcity of genomic resources for genetic and genomic studies. The oat genome, spanning approximately 11.3 gigabase pairs (Gbp), is characterized by numerous chromosomal rearrangements, particularly major translocations [17]. These rearrangements, often specific to certain populations, hinder seamless data transfer between different research groups and impede the development of universally applicable genomic tools. However, recent advancements have introduced new tools and genomic resources for oats. Various marker systems, such as the Oat 6 K single-nucleotide polymorphism (SNP) chip and diversity array (DArT) markers, have been developed [18]. The DArT marker system operates on a microarray platform, where reduced representation genomic libraries are created and then hybridized into microarrays. The current DArT platform includes 2,349 polymorphic markers. Simultaneously, the Oat 6 K custom Infinium iSelect Bead-Chip (Illumina, San Diego, California) incorporates 4,975 SNP markers [19]. This SNP chip facilitates the generation of high-density marker data for genome-scale projects. Furthermore, genotyping by sequencing (GBS) has been employed to genotype several oat populations, providing an additional source of genetic markers. The integration of these technologies and marker systems has created a substantial reservoir of genetic markers, streamlining the execution of large-scale genome projects [20].

This chapter aims to highlight recent advances in oat molecular genetics, genomics, and biotechnology, illustrating how they contribute to genetic knowledge and provide molecular tools that assist plant breeders in continuously enhancing the quality of oats.

9.2 DECODING THE GENETIC BLUEPRINT: INSIGHTS INTO THE STRUCTURE AND EVOLUTION OF THE OAT GENOME

9.2.1 Structure and Evolutionary Dynamics of Oat Genome

The genomes of *Avena* species, a genus encompassing oat plants, exhibit a remarkable expanse and intricacy, spanning from 4.12 Gb in the case of *Avena damascena*, the most modest diploid representative, to a substantial 12.6 Gb in *Avena sterilis*, the most extensive hexaploid variant [21]. Noteworthy is the parallelism with the genomic magnitudes of wheat, barley, and their untamed counterparts, which diverged from the *Avena* lineage approximately 25–50 million years ago. Recent analyses lean towards the older end of this temporal spectrum. As of the current composition, no publicly accessible genome references are procurable for *Avena* species [22]. However, several diploid genomes have been conclusively characterized, while endeavours to assemble reference sequences for hexaploid counterparts are actively underway (https://avenagenome.org/).

An initial scrutiny of repetitive sequences within diploid and hexaploid genomes has been documented, affirming the anticipated prevalence of repeat elements, constituting a substantial 72% of *Avena* genomes [23]. Furthermore, this examination identifies specific families that exhibit sub-genomic specificity within the hexaploid configuration. Notably, the C sub-genome manifests as larger than its A and D lineage counterparts, harbouring a higher proportion of heterochromatic regions and sharing repetitive families with the most closely related diploids. This characteristic permits the direct utilization of diploid-derived probes for the identification of the C sub-genome through in situ hybridization [21].

In contrast, distinguishing between the A and D sub-genomes has proven to be a cytogenetic challenge due to their substantial similarity. However, a study by Liu et al. [23] elucidates the preferential amplification of a retrotransposon in the D sub-genome, complementing an earlier discovery of a retrotransposon fragment that underwent preferential amplification in the A sub-genome (Linares et al. 1998). This limited discordance in identified repeats aligns with molecular phylogeny and high-throughput marker analyses, indicating that the hexaploid D sub-genome represents a relatively recent variant of the A (Peng et al. 2008, 2010, 2018; Yan et al. 2016a). Consequently, it can be inferred that the D sub-genome likely shares akin sequence content and organization with its progenitor. Despite the overarching genomic homogeneity, various karyotype variants have been identified, with the most noteworthy hexaploid polymorphism associated with the growth habit in progenitor *A. sterilis* lineages and their potential domesticates [24]. The ancestral karyotype typically adheres to a winter type, while the derived A/C genome translocation exhibits a spring type. Additional rearrangements between sub-genomes are perceptible within the hexaploid configuration. Intriguingly, the D sub-genome appears to have constituted the hexaploid progenitor tetraploid before the subsequent incorporation of the A sub-genome [25]. Consequently, it might be anticipated to be further advanced in the process of diploidization.

Numerous distinctions in inflorescence architecture and grain composition between oat and *Triticeae* species, as outlined by Kellogg et al. [26], suggest divergent gene content and expression. A compelling example lies in the realm of seed storage proteins, where wheat boasts approximately 105 gluten genes contributing to 80% of the protein, while oat, in stark contrast, features a singular family known as avenins, encompassing a mere 10–11 members and contributing 10–15% of the seed storage protein [27]. The juxtaposition of gluten genes and avenins in sizeable clusters implies that substantial changes in copy number may necessitate localized gene amplification rather than genome-wide alterations.

Moreover, the synthesis of oat-specific metabolites, exemplified by the anti-inflammatory avenanthramides, may hinge on relatively minor adjustments in the specificity of common structural genes, potentially requiring the introduction of only two novel enzyme activities [28]. Despite these variances, fundamental biological processes such as the regulation of flowering time exhibit notable conservation between *Avena* and *Triticeae* species [29]. However, a surprising revelation surfaced concerning the genomic arrangement of the avenacin biosynthetic cluster. Avenacins, endowed with antifungal properties and unique to *Avena* species, undergo production in the roots. This biosynthetic cluster experiences an unusual restructuring, with multiple structural genes recruited through duplication and diversification from other pathways, coalescing in a singular chromosomal locale.

Subsequent discoveries of functionally related gene clusters for metabolic pathways in plants underscore the significance of gene functional clustering. While the adaptive advantages are evident, the mechanisms orchestrating such profound genome reorganization in plants remain elusive [30], [31]. The impending comparison of forthcoming *Avena* genomes with their *Triticeae* counterparts holds promise in unravelling the intricacies of these processes, shedding light on the evolutionary dynamics that underpin the functional divergence of plant genomes.

9.2.2 Intra-Species Diversity in Oats

The *Avena* genus, boasting a diverse array of species ranging from diploids and tetraploids to hexaploids, finds its epicentre of diversity in the Western Mediterranean. With the exception of the singular *Avena macrostachya*, which has been deemed an "intermediate" taxon between *Avena* and *Helictotrichon* [32], all members of this genus are annuals. Distinct lineages, notably the A and C branches, have been clearly demarcated [33], with extant diploids unequivocally assigned to either the A or the C lineage. The divergence of these A and C lineages is estimated to have occurred between 4 and 20 million years ago [34], [35]. The origin of sub-genomes within extant polyploids presents a nuanced narrative, albeit with growing consensus. The D lineage, identified as a variant lineage of the A genomes, is prevalent in conjunction with C genome lineages in most existing tetraploids. One of these DC species subsequently gave rise to contemporary ADC hexaploids, encompassing the domesticated *A. sativa* (white oat) and *Avena byzantina* (red oat), along with relatives such as the widespread *A. sterilis* and the weedy *Avena fatua*. Notably, *Avena insularis*, the closest relative to the hexaploid progenitor, *A. insularis*, is situated at the eastern end of their distribution, initially discovered in Sicily [36]. Intriguingly, no extant D genome diploid has been identified.

Another variant of the A genome, designated as B, characterizes the common and widespread tetraploid *Avena barbata*, recognized for its success in North America and utilized as a model for invasive species [37]. Related tetraploids, such as *Avena abyssinica* and *Avena vaviloviana*, are found in Ethiopia, while a distinct A genome configuration is observed in the Moroccan species *Avena agadiriana*. Both genomes of *A. agadiriana* appear to align with A lineage variants. A likely component of *A. agadiriana*, *A. damascena*, seems to have had a more extensive historical distribution, being located at both ends of the Mediterranean, albeit now scarce in the west and potentially extinct in the east [38]. Adding to the genomic tapestry, the A genome diploid *Avena canariensis*, an endemic island species, exhibits notable intraspecific variation, hinting at incipient speciation based on karyotype differences [39]. The precise nature of the B, D, and other A variants, including components of *A. agadiriana*, remains a subject of ongoing discussion and uncertainty, awaiting resolution through meticulous genomic analyses.

9.3 ANALYSING OAT GENOMES: GENETIC MAPPING AND QTL ANALYSIS

The utilization of molecular markers stands as a pivotal instrument in unravelling the intricate genetic landscape governing the quality and adaptability of numerous crop species, while concurrently facilitating the delineation and exploitation of genetic diversity [9]. Historically, the application of such markers in oat breeding has been hindered by the scarcity of polymorphic DNA markers and the formidable dimensions and intricacies inherent in the oat genome, as elucidated by Govindaraj et al. [40]. The advent of technological breakthroughs in DNA sequencing has, however, catalysed a paradigm shift in genomic research for oats. SNPs have emerged as the preeminent choice for molecular markers due to their facile utilization, straightforward scoring, and the relative ease with which they can be automated [41]. The advent of transformative technologies, such as next-generation sequencing (NGS), has revolutionized marker development strategies, especially in plant genomes characterized by complexity, such as oats. The pioneering development of an Illumina 6 K oat chip, housing highly informative SNP markers, and its application across 12 distinct bi-parental populations, led to the inauguration of the inaugural physically-anchored consensus map of oats, as delineated by Oliver et al. [42].

The integration of NGS with a reduction in genome complexity has paved the way for GBS approaches. This innovative approach amalgamates marker discovery and genotyping, culminating in the generation of high-density markers at a notably economical sample cost, as underscored by Rayaprolu et al. [43]. The expansion of the oat consensus map was further facilitated by the augmentation of marker density through the inclusion of additional populations and the incorporation of over 70,000 loci, achieved through the utilization of the GBS programme "Haplotag," as elucidated by Canales et al. [44] and Tinker et al. [45]. This evolution in marker development surmounts erstwhile challenges encountered in the breeding of complex traits, effectively addressing impediments such as the identification of individual genes, the confounding influence of the environment, and the co-occurrence of undesirable linked genes [9].

Yet, the deployment of high-throughput multiplex markers alone is insufficient; the establishment of associations between these markers and phenotypic traits of interest represents a nontrivial undertaking. This necessitates the availability of suitable mapping populations and the implementation of accurate phenotyping methodologies within contextually appropriate environments, particularly for the evaluation of intricate or challenging characters. The adoption of molecular-assisted breeding stands poised as an instrumental strategy to augment the genetic comprehension of pivotal quality attributes and groat-phytochemical compounds in oats. This innovative approach not only refines precision and operational efficiency in oat breeding but also expedites the biofortification process [46]. The synergistic integration of omics resources with speed breeding heralds novel prospects for refining selection methodologies, optimizing genetic yield, and expediting cultivar development in the realm of oat cultivation. QTLs, typically unearthed in experimental mapping populations, mandate subsequent validation in the breeding germplasm, thereby constraining their utility in MAS [47]. To enhance the direct applicability of marker associations for selection, it is imperative to involve at least one parent currently or recently engaged in breeding programmes. The inherent limitations of bi-parental populations, characterized by restricted recombination, result in the mapping of QTLs at a diminished resolution. In a quest to surmount these limitations, novel mapping populations have been conceived, encompassing a more expansive spectrum of genetic and phenotypic variation than their bi-parental counterparts. These innovative models, including association mapping, multi-parent advanced generation inter-cross, and nested association mapping populations, as delineated by Tello et al. [48], Kumar et al. [49] and Kitony et al. [50], respectively, represent a pioneering leap towards enhanced efficiency and precision in unravelling the intricate tapestry of genetic architecture governing complex traits in oats.

Molecular markers, encompassing diverse types such as restriction fragment length polymorphism (RFLP), amplified fragment length polymorphism (AFLP), simple sequence repeat (SSR), SNP, and DArT markers, emerge as invaluable tools in quality enhancement programmes (Figure 9.1). These markers, adeptly employed in evaluating oat germplasm, mapping major and minor quality genes, and facilitating MAS, exemplify the transformative potential outlined by Grover et al. [51]. Notably, the complete sequencing of the hexaploid oat genome (*A. sativa* cv. Sang) represents a significant milestone in genomic exploration. With a vast genome exceeding 11 Gb, comprising two species of distinct ploidy (*Avena longiglumis* with 3.7 Gb, denoted as AA, and *A. insularis* with 7.3 Gb, denoted as CCDD), the recent collaborative efforts showcased in the work of Kamal et al. [1] have culminated in a publicly available draft version. The forthcoming elucidation of the hexaploid *A. sativa* genome promises to be a game-changer, offering avenues for both applied and fundamental research. Applications range from MAS and genomic selection in breeding programmes to comparative genomics, genome-wide association studies (GWAS), QTL mapping, accelerated discovery of new

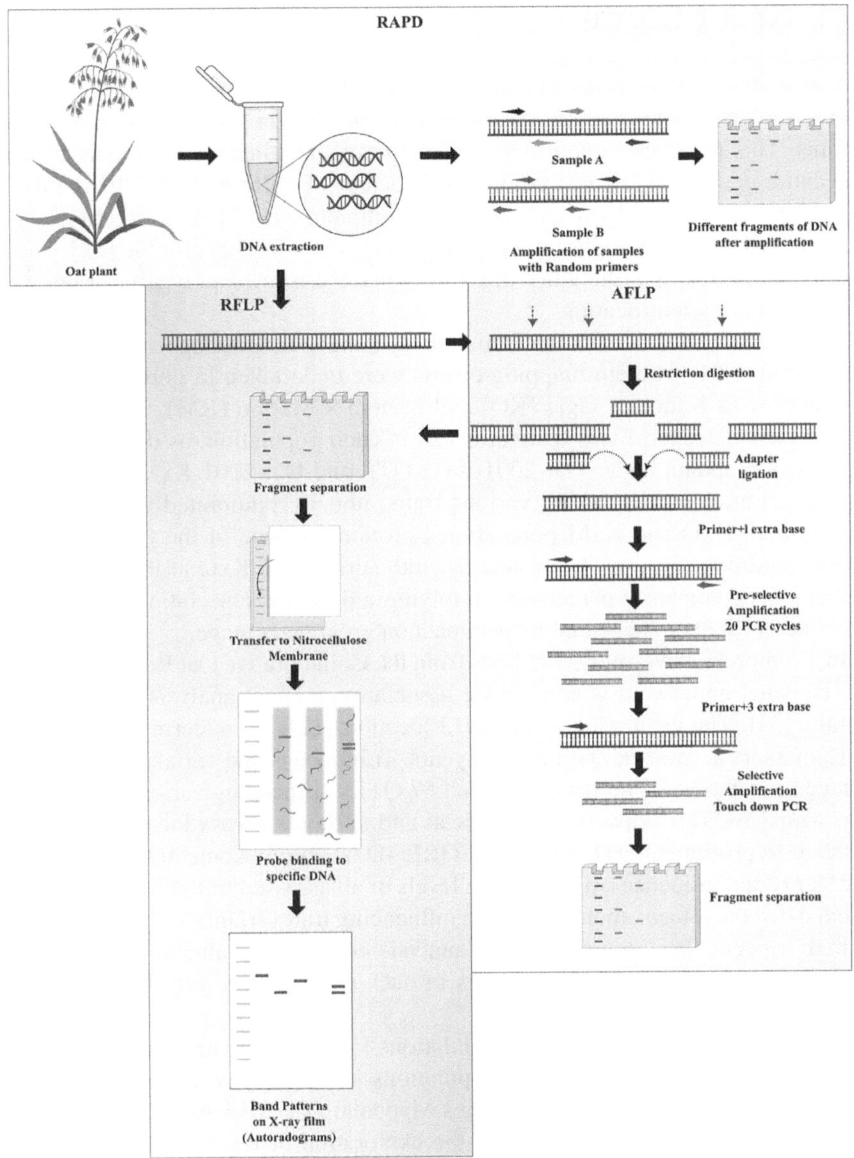

FIGURE 9.1 Molecular markers play a crucial role in oat research, employing diverse types such as restriction fragment length polymorphism (RFLP), amplified fragment length polymorphism (AFLP), and random amplified polymorphic DNA (RAPD). This figure illustrates the application of these molecular techniques, providing insights into the genetic diversity and variability within the oat genome.

genes, detection of natural variation, and advanced exploration through next-generation mutagenesis techniques, genetic engineering, and clustered regularly interspaced short palindromic repeats (CRISPR)-associated protein 9 (CRISPR/Cas9), the latest iteration in genome-editing platforms.

9.3.1 Groat Content

The metric denoted as "groat percentage," variably labelled as "milling yield," "hull content," or "groat content (GC)," assumes a pivotal role in gauging the milling quality of grains. This parameter quantifies the fraction of dehulled whole groats in relation to the entire grain, serving as a prominent indicator of milling quality. Its regulation is predominantly governed by a principal gene complemented by three modifying genes, although the influence of environmental factors is not entirely negligible [52]. The intricacies of the transcripts dictating this trait, characteristic of polygenic traits, remain elusive to precise identification.

A pivotal advancement in elucidating the genetic underpinnings of groat percentage transpired in 2001, wherein mapping efforts were undertaken in populations resulting from the crosses Kanota × Ogle (KO) and Kanota × Marion (KM). These endeavours revealed the existence of two distinct QTLs in each population, as documented in the GrainGenes Mapdata under Oat-2001-KxO-QTL and Oat-2001-KxM-QTL [53]. This mapping venture, encompassing various traits, notably pinpointed a QTL for kernel length in both KxO and KxM populations, proximal to one of the GC QTLs in each instance. Additionally, a QTL for kernel width surfaced in KxO at the precise genetic locus as a QTL for groat percentage, implying a potential correlation between alterations in kernel size or shape and their impact on groat percentage.

In a comprehensive study, 501 lines from the Collaborative Oat Research Enterprise (CORE) panel underwent genome-wide association (GWA) analysis for six key milling traits [54]. The evaluation spanned 13 location years, considering associations for 36,315 markers across and within these years. Trait means and variances were assessed to gauge trait stability. The study unveiled 57 QTLs influencing various milling quality traits, with 14 QTLs impacting both mean and variance across location years. Notably, the most prominent QTL, Qkernel.CORE.4D on chromosome 4D at approximately 212 cM, exerted influence over the mean levels of all assessed traits. The identified QTL exhibited diverse effects, including those influencing trait variance only, trait mean only, and both aspects. This comprehensive analysis contributes valuable insights into the genetic factors influencing milling traits in oats, aiding future breeding strategies for enhanced milling quality.

In the Iltis advanced backcross populations [55], the convergence of one QTL on the same linkage group across both populations is noteworthy. In Population "B," an additional QTL is delineated (GrainGenes Mapdata: Oat-2014-AB_QTL_PopnA, Oat-2014-AB_QTL_PopnB). Analogous to the exploration of test weight (TWT), GWAS conducted on the CORE Collection [54] uncovered QTL associated with the mean and variance of GC. Multiple QTLs were identified, including two for GC variance, one for both GC mean and variance, and a multi-trait QTL governing GC mean, plump mean, thin kernels mean, and variance. These findings, spanning diverse location years, are accompanied by known genetic map locations for significant markers. Of particular note are four QTLs for GC variance, one of which shares a significant marker with mean TWT, and another QTL exercising control over both mean TWT and mean GC, yet eluding precise mapping of its significant markers.

9.3.2 Protein

Oat seed storage proteins consist mainly of two classes: globulins and avenins, with globulins being a significant component in rice and oats [56]. Oats, due to their higher protein content and the presence of these protein classes, exhibit superior nutritional value compared to other cereals. Using expressed sequence tag (EST) resources from a hexaploid oat cultivar, researchers examined avenin and globulin sequences at both gene and protein levels. The study identified nine distinct avenin sequences, suggesting their classification into three to four subclasses across the hexaploid genome. Globulins, on the other hand, displayed greater diversity, with 24 distinct sequences. Variations in globulin size were attributed to a glutamine-rich domain, akin to avenins, and differences in the C-terminal sequence. Notably, two globulin genes had premature stop codons, resulting in truncated polypeptides, and eight sequences formed a previously unreported branch of globulins. This detailed exploration enhances our understanding of oat protein composition and genomic diversity, positioning oats as a captivating subject in plant molecular biology.

In a thorough investigation conducted by Yan et al. [57], the groat protein content (GPC) of 174 diverse oat accessions was meticulously assessed in three distinct field trials. The study revealed a wide spectrum of GPC, ranging from 6.97% to 22.24% within the diverse panel. Notably, hulless oats exhibited significantly higher GPC compared to their hulled counterparts across all environmental contexts, emphasizing the potential impact of hulling status on oat protein content. Through a GWAS involving the scrutiny of 38,313 high-quality single SNPs, the research unveiled 27 non-redundant QTLs intricately linked to GPC. A striking discovery was the identification of 41 SNPs with significant associations with the modulation of GPC. Among the recognized QTLs, QTL16 on chromosome 6C and QTL11 on chromosome 4D consistently manifested across multiple environmental conditions. Notably, QTL16 emerged as the most influential contributor to phenotypic variance across diverse environments, with its dominance only slightly diminished in the CZ20 context (Table 9.1).

9.3.3 Oil

Oat is characterized by a notable abundance of oils, principally comprising healthful unsaturated oleic and linoleic fatty acids. The concentration of lipids in oat grains can reach up to 18%, with a predominant composition of unsaturated fatty acids. This composition renders oats a wholesome energy source for both human and animal consumption. A key facet of breeding efforts involves the preservation and optimization of lipid composition in oats. As lipids constitute a substantial proportion of the oat grain, the identification of genetic loci influencing fatty acid composition not only enhances our understanding of oat metabolism but also provides a strategic roadmap for breeding programmes aimed at cultivating oats with superior nutritional profiles. This endeavour aligns with the broader goal of harnessing the inherent health benefits of oats and fortifying their position as a valuable dietary resource for both human and animal nutrition.

TABLE 9.1 Comprehensive Overview of Quantitative Trait Loci (QTL) Studies in Oat, Investigating Traits Such as ß-Glucan, Protein, and Lipid Content

TRAIT	FINDINGS	REFERENCE
ß-glucan and oil QTLs	• Found strong links between candidate genes and QTLs for heading date, oil, and ß-glucan • Confirmed a significant translocation from 1 C to 1 A and a potential inversion on 7D through genome-wide recombination profiles • GBS-based SNPs • 3 QTLs • 5 RIL populations	[68]
ß-glucan QTLs	• Studied two oat populations (137 lines each) for ß-glucan content • Kanota × Ogle RILs • 4 or 5 QTLs • Identified consistent genomic influence on ß-glucan levels in regions 11 and 14 • Marion, higher in ß-glucan, contributed all positive alleles in Kanota × Marion cross	[72]
ß-glucan QTLs	• Conducted population structure, linkage disequilibrium, and genome-wide association analyses (GWA) • GBS-based SNPs • Utilized the UFRGS Oat Panel, revealing weak population structure and high potential for understanding agronomic traits in subtropical environments • 413 oat genotypes • Identified seven ß-glucan content-associated QTL on Mrg02, Mrg06, Mrg11, Mrg12, Mrg19, and Mrg20, with some regions showing synteny with barley	[65]
ß-glucan QTLs	• Explored *cellulose synthase-like* (*Csl*) genes, especially CslF6, in oat ß-glucan production • Used GWAS on elite oat panels across North America • Viable SNPs, GBS-based SNPs • 56 significant associations • 3 diverse panels of oat • Identified four key genomic regions, pinpointing CslF, CslH, UGPase (UDP-glucose pyrophosphorylase), and AGPase (ADP-glucose pyrophosphorylase) as candidate genes. Subgenome-specific expression highlighted AsCslF6_C, least expressed in low-ß-glucan varieties. Linkage mapping located AsCslF6_D on Mrg02 overlapping with QTL 2.2, and AsCslF6_A on Mrg12 near QTL 12.2.	[69]
ß-glucan QTLs	• Examined 406 inbred lines in Southern Brazil • Performed genome-wide association analyses separately and across environments • Uncovered genomic regions (Mrg06, Mrg21, Mrg24) influencing kernel length • Identified a common quantitative trait locus on Mrg13 of the oat consensus map for genetically linked kernel width and thickness	[73]

(Continued)

TABLE 9.1   (Continued) Comprehensive Overview of Quantitative Trait Loci (QTL) Studies in Oat, Investigating Traits Such as ß-Glucan, Protein, and Lipid Content

TRAIT	FINDINGS	REFERENCE
Protein	• Assessed groat protein content (GPC) in 174 diverse oat accessions across three trials • GWAS identified 27 QTLs with 41 significant SNPs • Chromosomes 6C (QTL16) and 4D (QTL11) consistently influenced GPC • QTL16 was the most significant, explaining the highest phenotypic variation in most environments, except in CZ20	[57]
Lipid content	• Genotyped 500 oat cultivars using GBS and measured concentrations of ten fatty acids in two environments • Noted high correlations among individual fatty acids, indicating shared biosynthetic pathways • Applied two multivariate genome-wide association study (GWAS) approaches: a multivariate linear mixed model and principal component (PC) analysis • The multivariate mixed model identified 148 genome-wide significant SNPs, surpassing the PC and univariate analyses (129 and 73 significant SNPs, respectively) • Explicitly considering correlation structures between fatty acids unveiled loci associated with seed fatty acid variation not detected in univariate analyses	[59]
Lipid content	• Investigated traits in 146 recombinant inbred lines from a cross between "Dal" (high oil) and "Exeter" (low oil) • Constructed a linkage map with 475 DArT markers spanning 1,271.8 cM across 40 linkage groups • Conducted QTL analysis for groat oil content and composition using grain samples from Aberdeen, Idaho, in 1997 • Identified QTLs for oil content and various fatty acids (palmitic acid, stearic acid, oleic acid, linoleic acid, and linolenic acid) • Found two loci associated with oil content influencing all examined fatty acids, with most oil-related QTLs displaying similar effects on the fatty acid profile	[60]

A pivotal locus exerting a major influence on oat groat oil content was pinpointed in linkage group 11 through a comprehensive analysis encompassing single-factor analysis of variance, simple interval mapping, and simplified composite interval mapping [58]. This influential locus was further elucidated through the identification of a polymorphism associated with the plastidic acetyl-CoA carboxylase (ACCase), a critical enzyme catalysing the initial step in *de novo* fatty acid synthesis. The linkage between this major QTL and the ACCase locus was corroborated across two distinct recombinant inbred populations, namely KO and KM, each comprising 137 and 139 individual lines, respectively. Notably, the utilization of these populations, which share a common parent, offers a form of biological replication, thereby reinforcing the robustness of the results. The KO population, mapped with 150 RFLP loci spanning the genome, underwent cultivation in five diverse environments for the measurement of groat oil content.

Similarly, the KM population, mapped with 60 RFLP loci, underwent cultivation in three distinct environments. The QTL linked to *AccaseA* on linkage group 11 exhibited a substantial impact, accounting for up to 48% of the phenotypic variance in groat oil content. This compelling evidence strongly supports the hypothesis that ACCase plays a pivotal role in determining oat groat oil content. Additionally, other QTLs were identified in both populations, collectively contributing to an additional 10–20% of the phenotypic variance, further underscoring the polygenic nature of groat oil content regulation in oats (Table 9.1).

Expanding the scope of genomic-assisted techniques, [59] harnessed a multivariate-GWAS methodology, leveraging SNPs in a natural population. This approach successfully unveiled four seed fatty acid QTLs, holding promise for enhancing the nutritional profile of oats. To assess groat oil content within a population comprising 146 recombinant inbred lines (RILs) resulting from a cross between "Dal" (high oil) and "Exeter" (low oil), a comprehensive linkage map was meticulously assembled [60]. This map, encompassing 475 DArT markers, spanned 1,271.8 cM across 40 linkage groups. The investigation included a QTL analysis conducted on grain samples cultivated at Aberdeen, Idaho, in 1997, focusing on groat oil content and composition. Furthermore, QTL analysis extended to multiple agronomic traits, with data collected from hill plots and field plots in Ottawa, Ontario, in 2010. Through the application of simple and composite interval mapping methods, discernible QTLs were identified for various traits, including oil content, as well as the composition of palmitic acid (16:0), stearic acid (18:0), oleic acid (18:1), linoleic acid (18:2), and linolenic acid (18:3). Notably, certain loci associated with oil content exhibited correlations with all examined fatty acids, indicating a pleiotropic influence on the fatty acid profile. This observation implies the existence of shared genetic mechanisms affecting multiple facets of oil-related traits, particularly at specific nodes within the oil synthesis pathway.

9.3.4 Starch and ß-Glucan

In the realm of starch metabolism, significant strides have been made in genetic elucidation. Portyanko et al. [61] mapped the α-amylase gene in RILs derived from the cross between Ogle and TAM O-301, while Wight et al. [62] mapped the starch synthase gene in RILs resulting from the KO union. Additionally, Wight et al. [62] identified a candidate gene for the β-glucanase enzyme in KO RILs, and Ritala et al. [63] successfully cloned a second candidate gene for β-glucan synthase from oat. A parallel investigative strategy Chawade et al. [64] unearthed key enzymes crucial for blocking the lignin and β-glucan biosynthesis pathway within the oat TILLING (Targeting Induced Local Lesions In Genomes) population. Six distinct mutations were discerned in the phenylalanine ammonia-lyase (*AsPAL1*) gene, offering a nuanced glimpse into the intricate molecular variations shaping this crucial pathway. Simultaneously, the cellulose synthase-like (*AsCslF6*) β-glucan biosynthesis gene bore witness to the emergence of ten diverse mutations, each potentially carrying profound implications for the regulation of β-glucan biosynthesis.

In the study involving a panel of 413 oat genotypes, β-glucan content was evaluated under subtropical conditions across multiple years [65]. GBS was employed, and analyses revealed a Federal University of Rio Grande do Sul (UFRGS) Oat Panel with weak population structure, indicating its potential for investigating various agronomic traits in subtropical environments. GWA mapping identified seven QTLs associated with β-glucan content, located on Mrg02, Mrg06, Mrg11, Mrg12, Mrg19, and Mrg20. Notably, QTLs on Mrg02, Mrg06, and Mrg11 exhibited genomic regions syntenic with barley, suggesting shared genetic factors. These findings provide valuable insights for oat breeding in subtropical regions, offering genetic markers to accelerate the improvement of β-glucan content in oats. The multi-environmental approach enhances the robustness of the results, aiding informed breeding strategies for oat enhancement in subtropical conditions.

Linkage mapping studies pertaining to starch content in oats are relatively scarce, but notable breakthroughs have been achieved. Verhoeven et al. [66] identified three starch mutants within *Avena strigosa*, presenting a promising avenue for the development of new cultivars. In this investigation, a triad of mutant lines, namely *lam-1*, *lam-2*, and *sga-1*, emerged as focal points for discerning alterations within the biochemical landscape. Notably, *lam-1* and *lam-2* mutants exhibited granules that manifested a distinct red hue upon iodine solution application. Concomitantly, a deficiency or substantial reduction in granule-bound starch synthase activity, granule-bound starch synthase I protein, and the amylose constituent of starch in the endosperm characterized these lines, unequivocally designating them as mutations of the waxy phenotype. In stark contrast, the *sga-1* mutant showcased a nuanced profile. Its endosperm harboured soluble material, manifesting a red stain upon iodine treatment, alongside the intriguing presence of blue-staining starch granules. Closer scrutiny unveiled a red-staining, soluble material akin in appearance and chain-length profile to the phytoglycogen observed in the endosperms of *sugary-1* mutants in cereals. Notably, *sugary-1* mutants typically exhibit deficiencies or diminished levels of isoamylase activity. Remarkably, native gel assays conducted on the developing endosperms of *sga-1* disclosed a normal isoamylase activity, deviating from the canonical sugary-1 mutant paradigm. This incongruity challenges conventional expectations, suggesting a unique and divergent mechanism at play in the biochemical orchestration of *sga-1*. The precise location of the starch binding enzyme gene (SBE III) on diploid oat linkage group G was discerned through the utilization of a rice ortholog [67].

Tinker et al. [68] validated QTLs in diverse mapping populations, employing GBS and developing Kompetitive allele-specific PCR markers. Their findings encompassed six, three, and five major QTLs for oil content, β-glucan content, and the number of days to 50% heading, respectively. The study focused on examining genome-wide recombination profiles in oats, confirming the common occurrence of significant chromosomal rearrangements. Specifically, a large, unbalanced translocation from chromosome 1C to 1A and a potential inversion on chromosome 7D were identified. These rearrangements were found to cause pseudo-linkage and recombination suppression in oats, with implications for the segregation, localization, and deployment of QTLs in breeding programmes. Recognizing and understanding these structural alterations is crucial for accurate genetic analysis and the effective use of QTLs in oat breeding efforts.

Another study investigated the genetic factors influencing β-glucan production in hexaploid oats [69]. Emphasizing cellulose synthase-like (Csl) genes, particularly CslF6, GWAS was conducted on three elite oat panels grown in multiple North American locations. The analysis identified 58 significantly associated markers, and synteny with the barley genome pointed to four key regions of interest, implicating CslF and CslH gene families, *UGPase*, and *AGPase* as potential candidate genes. Subgenome-specific expression analysis highlighted the role of AsCslF6_C, the least expressed homoeolog across various tissue types and time points. Linkage mapping of homoeologs placed AsCslF6_D on consensus linkage group Mrg02, overlapping with QTL 2.2, and AsCslF6_A on Mrg12, flanked by markers associated with QTL 12.2. The study identified homoeologous QTLs, suggesting the contribution of duplicated gene copies to β-glucan biosynthesis. These findings provide valuable insights into the genetic basis of β-glucan production in oats, informing future breeding efforts to enhance this health-promoting component. Newell et al. [70] undertook a comprehensive analysis involving 431 oat lines of global origin over two years, employing DArT markers for genotyping. Their GWA study discerned three significant markers (oPt.0133, oPt.6825/oPt.0112, and oPt.17174/oPt.8715) influencing β-glucan content, each contributing to the tune of 0.37%, 0.26%, and 0.25%, respectively. Intriguingly, these markers exhibited homology with the rice genome, substantiating a syntenic relationship and affirming the association of the CslF gene family with β-glucan content.

Building upon this foundation, Asoro et al. [71] explored β-glucan content across diverse environments, identifying 24 and 37 significant DArT markers at Ames and the Oat Performance Nursery in North America. Notably, two of these markers were proximal to a β-glucan candidate gene (CslF gene family) in the rice genome, underscoring the evolutionary conservation of genetic determinants. Employing the advanced backcross QTL (AB-QTL) strategy, Herrmann et al. [55] achieved success in transferring and mapping valuable quality traits in the elite oat cultivar Iltis. Through the formation of two advanced backcross populations (BC2F2–6 populations A and B), comprising 98 and 72 F2 individuals, they unveiled 33 QTLs, elucidating 14–80% of phenotypic variation for various quality and agronomic traits. Noteworthy among these were QTLs for β-glucan content on three linkage groups, explaining >37% of phenotypic variation and 57% of genotypic variation (Table 9.1).

9.3.5 Optimizing Oat Resilience through Genomic Breeding

Biotic and abiotic stresses emerge as pivotal determinants significantly influencing oat yield, notably contributing to yield gaps in rainfed crops. The intricate relationship between these stressors is underscored by their interdependence, wherein environmental conditions play a pivotal role in the development and dissemination of fungi. Consequently, both biotic and abiotic factors intricately shape the distinctive distribution patterns of oat crops across diverse environments [74]. Compounding this intricate web of influences is the global phenomenon of climate change, which amplifies the impact of abiotic stressors. This escalation manifests as heightened irregularity and unpredictability in stress episodes on a planetary scale. In response to this burgeoning challenge, an imperative arises: the urgent need to formulate adaptation strategies tailored to align oat cultivation with the specific exigencies of diverse environments [75].

The exploration of bi-parental populations has yielded a rich tapestry of information, unravelling an expansive array of QTLs intimately associated with pivotal agronomic traits such as height, heading date, yield, and grain quality. In the Terra × Marion population, De Koeyer et al. [76] discerned three QTLs influencing grain yield, notably one on Mrg02 concurrently linked with plant height. Multiple studies have independently pinpointed QTLs associated with plant height on Mrg01, Mrg02, Mrg12, Mrg20, Mrg21, and Mrg28, highlighting a comprehensive exploration by various researchers [76]–[82]. Additionally, QTLs related to lodging susceptibility have been identified on Mrg01 and Mrg21, elucidating the intricate genetic architecture underlying oat phenotypes [76]. It is noteworthy that certain height QTLs were found to be independent of lodging susceptibility QTLs. The oat dwarfing gene dw6, a genetic locus of significance, has been precisely mapped to Mrg04, with closely linked PCR markers recently developed for effective delineation [83]. Heading date, a critical determinant of oat variety adaptation to diverse environments, has garnered substantial attention in QTL analysis. Comparative mapping has illuminated select genomic regions, namely Mrg02, Mrg12, Mrg20, and Mrg21, where multiple QTLs associated with heading date have been consistently mapped across various bi-parental populations [76], [84]. This observation has been corroborated by Klos et al. [85], who, through association analysis across multiple locations and years, confirmed the stability of these QTLs. Remarkably, QTLs for heading date on Mrg02 and Mrg12 were found to coincide with homeologues of the vernalization response gene As-vrn3 [29]. Notably, Mrg20 and Mrg21, considered homologous chromosomes, exhibit QTLs associated with vernalization response, as well as the vernalization gene vrn1 [25], [29]. Additionally, the major day-length response gene, Di1, has been implicated in this region of Mrg02, further unravelling the intricate genetic determinants influencing heading date in oats.

Crown rust, stands as a formidable adversary in the realm of oat diseases, inflicting substantial yield losses across diverse growing regions. The landscape of oat disease resistance has been a focal point of extensive genetic scrutiny, particularly regarding single-gene resistance to major pathogens. Noteworthy among these are the race-specific crown rust (*Puccinia coronate* f. *spavenea*) resistance genes, including but not limited to Pc38, Pc39, Pc48, Pc54, Pc59, Pc58, Pc68, Pc71, Pc91, Pc92, Pc94, and Pcq2, each meticulously mapped [82], [86]–[93]. Association analysis, as undertaken by Klos et al. [85], has corroborated and extended the applicability of these resistance genes across a wider germplasm range, culminating in the development of PCR-based markers for efficient deployment in high-throughput MAS within oat breeding programmes [94]. The genomic disposition of some of these race-specific genes reveals clustering in the oat genome, where markers developed for one gene within a cluster exhibit potential utility in selecting linked genes. However, caution is warranted, as certain resistance genes may not operate independently, and there is suggestive evidence of interference between some genes. For instance, the suppression of Pc62 and Pc94 by Pc38, as elucidated by Chong et al. [95] and Wilson et al. [96], underscores the complexity of these interactions. The precision afforded by markers holds promise for the deliberate selection of allelic combinations, providing a nuanced approach to fortifying resistance in oat varieties. Moreover, a significant advancement in understanding adult plant partial resistance (APR) to crown rust has been achieved through the identification of a major QTL on Mrg06. This discovery, corroborated across three recombinant inbred line populations, has spurred the development of PCR assays for selected SNPs, verifying the QTL [97]. Remarkably, the synteny with wheat suggests that this QTL is orthologous with the stripe rust APR gene *Yr16* in wheat, hinting at broader implications for rust resistance mechanisms across cereals.

A recent breakthrough in the ongoing saga of oat resistance is the identification of a novel crown rust resistance gene in the diploid oat *Avena strigosa*, successfully transferred into hexaploid cultivated oat germplasm by Rines et al. [98]. The closely linked markers to this resistance, situated on linkage group Mrg20, have been adeptly converted into PCR assays, showcasing a promising avenue for precise molecular breeding interventions in the ongoing battle against crown rust. This revelation augments the genetic toolbox available for oat breeders, fostering resilience against the relentless onslaught of crown rust and signalling a paradigm shift in the quest for durable oat disease resistance.

Oat stem rust, induced by *Puccinia graminis* Pers. f. sp. *Avenae* Eriks. and E. Henn., stands as a significant malady in specific environments. Despite the cataloguing of 17 numbered oat stem rust resistance (*Pg*) genes and the *Pg-a* complex, only a subset finds active application in contemporary oat breeding endeavours [99]. Several of these resistance genes have been meticulously mapped, including *Pg3*, *Pg9*, and *Pg11*, and more recently, *Pg13* [100]. Intriguingly, *Pg13* has been discerned to be closely linked with the crown rust resistance gene *Pc91*, revealing a genetic intersection that enriches our understanding of multifaceted disease resistances within oat genomes.

Turning our attention to powdery mildew resistance, a suite of major genes has been identified through monosomic analysis. These include *Pm8* on chromosome 4C, *Pm7* on chromosome 13A, *Pm6* on chromosome 10D, *Pm3* on chromosome 17A, *Pm1* on chromosome 1D [101], [102]. *Pm5*, originating from *A. macrostachya* and introgressed into hexaploid oat, has been genetically mapped to the Mrg20 region [103]. The recently mapped Pm4, derived from the diploid oat species *A. barbata*, showcases the power of modern techniques such as DArTseq in elucidating genetic markers suitable for MAS [104]. Beyond powdery mildew, QTLs associated with barley yellow dwarf virus resistance [82] and Fusarium head blight resistance [105] have also been strategically mapped, further enriching the genetic arsenal available for oat improvement.

In the pursuit of effective MAS, the practicality and cost-effectiveness of identified markers are paramount. Early studies in oats often reported QTLs associated with markers, such as RAPD, AFLP, and DArT, which were not readily applicable for high-throughput genotyping or the detection of heterozygous individuals required for Marker-Assisted Backcrossing (MABC). However, recent strides have seen the conversion of identified markers into user-friendly PCR-based assays, and the advent of sequencing technologies has facilitated the development of custom multiplex SNP assays, aligning with the demands of contemporary breeding programmes.

The path to sustainable crop productivity involves harnessing the genetic diversity harboured in plant genetic resources, including wild relatives and exotic materials. This supplementation of genetic diversity, beyond domesticated crops, has the potential to revolutionize plant breeding. The incorporation of wild *Avena* species, exemplified in the use of wild germplasm for disease-resistance genes, epitomizes the success of this strategy. The preservation, exploration, and application of genetic diversity within both cultivated oats and their wild relatives emerge as indispensable strategies to broaden the genetic base of cultivars and ensure sustained improvement in oat crops. This holistic approach to genetic resources promises a resilient and adaptable future for oat cultivation in the face of evolving challenges.

9.4 OAT TRANSFORMATION TECHNIQUES

Genetic engineering emerges as a powerful tool for delving into the intricate realms of gene function, expression, and manipulation, particularly concerning pivotal traits influencing oat grain quality. In consonance with analogous endeavours in other cereal crops, the genesis of oat genetic transformation systems necessitated the antecedent establishment of regenerable cell culture protocols, methodologies for DNA delivery into totipotent cells, and the provision of marker genes facilitating the discernment and selection of transgenic cells [106]. The initial reports heralding the successful production of fertile, transgenic plants surfaced subsequent to the development of these transformation system components, with oats among the cereal crops entering this transformative era.

The inaugural foray into oat genetic transformation employed microprojectile bombardment, colloquially known as "biolistics," to introduce microscopic, transgene-coated tungsten particles into callus and suspension-culture cells. Subsequently, these cultures were cultivated in the presence of the herbicide phosphinothricin, affecting the selection of transgenic cells endowed with herbicide resistance (*bar*) [107]. The ensuing regeneration of fertile, herbicide-resistant plants from these cultures substantiated the integration and expression of transgene DNA in primary regenerates. Importantly, the heritable expression of transgenes was manifested in the progeny of the original transgenic oat plants [108]. Nevertheless, the nascent stages of oat genetic engineering investigations encountered relatively low transformation efficiencies, while the technical and labour prerequisites of the associated tissue culture systems posed limiting constraints.

To ameliorate these challenges, explorations into alternative target tissues for transgene delivery ensued. These endeavours aimed to alleviate the issues associated with the growth, dissection, manipulation, and response of the primary target tissue, i.e., callus from immature oat embryos. Noteworthy successes were achieved with competent target tissues such as callus from mature embryos, leaf base segments, and shoot meristematic cells, each contributing to the production of fertile transgenic oat plants [109]. The evolution of additional selection systems, featuring paromomycin resistance encoded by the neomycin phosphotransferase gene, *NPTII*, and visual selection employing green fluorescent protein, *gfp*, further bolstered the efficiency and flexibility of oat transformation [110].

Somers et al. [111] achieved a milestone in the realm of oat genetic engineering through the successful generation of transgenic oat plants utilizing the biolistic gene transfer method. The selection markers employed were the *BAR (Phosphinothricin)* and *Escherichia coli uidA (GUS)* genes, with the former conferring herbicide resistance to the plants. Among the 111 transgenic tissue cultures, 38 exhibited the potential to give rise to regenerated plants. Notably, a majority of these plants displayed male sterility, while a commendable portion, numbering over 30, exhibited full fertility. The stable inheritance of the transgenes in the seeds of the fertile plants was substantiated by *GUS* activity and resistance to *PPT*, affirming the resilience and heritability of the introduced genetic modifications. Subsequently, Gless et al. [112] expanded the repertoire of oat transformation techniques by utilizing freshly isolated leaf base segments bombarded with plasmids containing the *UIDA* and *PAT* genes. A discernible success rate of 5%

was observed, culminating in the recovery of transgenic plantlets. The confirmation of foreign gene integration was accomplished through Southern blot analysis. Impressively, the resultant transgenic plants exhibited normal phenotypes and, for the most part, demonstrated fertility, thereby attesting to the Mendelian inheritance of the introduced genes in subsequent generations.

Building upon these foundations, Zhang et al. [113] ventured into the transformation of oat using shoot meristematic cultures. Following a rigorous selection process, seven independent transgenic lines were obtained, five of which exhibited self-fertility. Noteworthy observations included both Mendelian and non-Mendelian segregation ratios of transgene expression in the T1 and T2 progeny. Additionally, a spectrum of physical transmission patterns of the transgenes, encompassing both normal and low transmission rates, underscored the intricacies of transgene inheritance in the transgenic oat lines.

In tandem with these advancements, the identification and cloning of promoter and enhancer sequences garnered significance, propelling the attainment of high-level, constitutive expression of transgenes. The initial utilization of relatively weak promoters, such as the *Cauliflower mosaic virus 35S* (*CaMV35S*) and maize *Adh1* promoters, prompted subsequent refinements [114]. Integration of the maize Adh1 first intron, housing expression-enhancer sequences, augmented expression in the early studies. Subsequent implementations leveraged highly expressing promoter-intron combinations sourced from the rice *actin1* and maize *ubiquitin1* genes, resulting in increased expression and efficient transformation across diverse selection systems [115]. However, it is crucial to note that while strong, constitutive expression of transgenes finds utility in certain contexts, endeavours directed towards enhancing oat quality through altered groat characteristics or metabolic pathways may necessitate tissue-specific expression for optimal outcomes.

To this end, tissue-specific expression patterns were explored using promoters derived from *Commelina yellow mottle virus* (CoYMV) and *Sugarcane bacilliform virus* (SCBV) in transgenic oat lines [116]. The CoYMV promoter exhibited robust transgene expression in the vascular tissues of oats, whereas the SCBV promoter demonstrated high expression in endosperms, leaves, stem, and anther filaments. Notwithstanding these advancements, further refinement in the specificity of expression remains imperative for future initiatives aimed at enhancing grain quality through metabolic engineering. The availability of promoters characterized by precise tissue and timing specificity or inducibility will undoubtedly facilitate the meticulous study and manipulation of genes influencing kernel quality.

Despite marked progress in oat transformation frequency, genotype diversity, and transgene expression level and specificity, challenges persist in ensuring the stability of transgene expression. The inherent complexity and multicopy nature of transgene integration, particularly through biolistics, have engendered issues of instability in transgene expression. Analogous challenges have been documented in other cereal transformation systems, instigating concerted research into the broader phenomenon of transgene silencing in plants [7]–[11], [41], [117]–[120]. Although the production of multiple, independent transgenic lines affords the opportunity to select lines featuring low-copy, simple transgene integration, this necessitates a substantial investment of time and resources, thereby complicating cereal transformation efforts.

The realization that relatively high-frequency, simple, single, and low-copy transgene integration occurs in dicotyledonous plant species transformed using *Agrobacterium tumefaciens* has prompted investigations into developing *Agrobacterium*-based transformation systems for cereal crops. Until the mid-1990s, the application of *Agrobacterium*-mediated transformation was confined to dicot plant species, the natural hosts of the bacterium. Nevertheless, breakthroughs in optimizing infection, co-cultivation, and selection parameters ultimately paved the way for *Agrobacterium*-based transformation in rice, maize, and other cereals [121]. Notably, an *Agrobacterium*-based transformation system for oats has been recently reported, albeit with the determination of its consistency pending further investigation.

Dattgonde et al. [122] further enriched the repertoire of *Agrobacterium*-mediated transformation systems for oats, experimenting with various co-cultivation treatments featuring different incubation periods. The pinnacle of efficacy was achieved through vacuum infiltration coupled with a 72-hour dark incubation, providing a valuable optimization in the transformation process. This nuanced approach not only exemplifies the dedication to refining and enhancing transformation methodologies but also underscores the multifaceted nature of achieving successful genetic modifications in oats.

9.5 GENOME EDITING FOR PRECISION OAT IMPROVEMENT

Site-directed mutagenesis stands as a pivotal biotechnological approach, strategically altering the DNA sequence at predetermined positions within the host genome through nucleotide insertion, deletion, or replacement. This highly efficient, flexible, and reliable technique serves as a powerful tool for swiftly generating novel plant varieties harbouring improved gene variants and traits. Beyond its applications in crop improvement, these methodologies open avenues for investigating gene function and regulation, exerting a profound impact on fundamental scientific inquiry. The arsenal of site-specific nucleases (SSNs) comprises four primary classes: meganucleases, zinc finger nucleases, transcription activator-like effector nucleases, and CRISPR/Cas [123]. Notably, these versatile endonucleases can be precisely customized to target specific DNA sequence motifs within living cells. Subsequently, the cellular DNA repair machinery comes into play, processing the cleaved DNA. The mechanisms governing cellular DNA repair encompass non-homologous end-joining (NHEJ) and homology-directed repair (HDR). In essence, site-directed mutagenesis not only emerges as a transformative tool for crop enhancement but also stands at the forefront of advancing our understanding of the intricate landscape of gene function and regulation. This convergence of applied and basic science underscores the far-reaching implications of site-directed mutagenesis in shaping the future of biotechnology and genetic research.

The revolutionary CRISPR genome-editing technology presents unparalleled opportunities for precisely engineering desirable traits in plants, circumventing the need for transgene integration. Anchored in RNA-guided Cas endonucleases derived from microbial adaptive immune systems, the CRISPR/Cas platform employs a synthetic guide RNA (gRNA) and the Cas protein. The intricately designed gRNA binds specifically to a user-defined DNA sequence, directing the Cas9 endonuclease to the target site for cleavage. A protospacer motif, approximately 20 nucleotides in length, is recognized through complementary base pairing, with a protospacer-adjacent motif (PAM) binding to the Cas9 protein. The ensuing double-strand break occurs between the third and fourth nucleotides in the 5'-direction from the PAM. Subsequent to DNA cleavage, the cell's intrinsic DNA repair mechanisms, namely NHEJ or HDR, are engaged to initiate the repair process.

CRISPR/Cas technology has demonstrated success in both mono- and dicotyledonous plants, employing single guide RNA (gRNA) expression systems. This success spans various plant species, including maize, barley, wheat, rice, tobacco, carrot, and chicory. Targeting a single cleavage site typically results in short deletions and/or insertions, while simultaneous targeting of pairs of motifs can lead to larger and precisely predictable deletions. Moreover, multiplex genome editing has been achieved, enabling the deletion of substantial genomic fragments, including entire genes and chromosomal regions. However, the predominant application of Cas endonuclease technology in plants remains limited to random mutagenesis via NHEJ-based repair mechanisms. Targeted insertion or exchange of genes using HDR has been demonstrated in select cases, primarily in model plants like *Arabidopsis* and *Nicotiana benthamiana*, as well as crops such as soybean and rice.

Despite these advancements, the integration of CRISPR cassettes into genomes poses challenges, potentially causing regulatory and safety concerns. To circumvent these issues, ribonucleoproteins (RNPs) are formed by preassembling the Cas protein and gRNA(s) of the CRISPR system and introducing them into plants. This approach, termed RNP-based CRISPR technology, ensures that edited plants are transgene-free, eliminating recombinant DNA involvement and simplifying the commercialization process. This method, being universally applicable without delivery barriers, offers a promising avenue for generating improved germplasm.

While the engineering of oats using SSNs has not been extensively explored, a pioneering study by Barber et al. [124] delves into the CRISPR/Cas9-mediated editing of Thaumatin-like protein 8 (TLP8) in oats. This study targeted specific homeologues (AsTLP8 A, C, and D), revealing successful editing with transformation frequencies of 5.23%, 0.47%, and 2.86%, respectively. The investigation explored the inverse correlation between TLP8 expression and β-glucan content in germinating barley seeds, prompting further exploration of TLP8's regulatory role in β-glucan synthesis in oats. While the study showcases successful CRISPR/Cas9-mediated editing of AsTLP8 homeologues, the precise impact of these mutations on β-glucan content warrants additional scrutiny.

9.6 CONCLUSION

The escalating utilization of oats for human consumption mirrors a growing recognition of their dietary and health benefits, primarily attributed to their rich content of dietary fibre and β-glucan. Clinical evidence substantiates that a daily intake of 3 g or more of β-glucan from oats, as part of a diet low in saturated fat and cholesterol, may mitigate the risk of coronary heart diseases. This revelation has propelled oats into the spotlight, with consumers increasingly acknowledging the cholesterol-lowering properties of oat-soluble fibre and the holistic advantages of whole grains. The burgeoning market for whole-grain oat products and oat bran in human foods attests to the expanding awareness of the heart-health benefits associated with oat consumption. In tandem with the surge in popularity, preliminary research delves into the potential health implications of minor oat constituents, such as antioxidants known as avenanthramides. These investigations establish links between specific oat components and various health aspects, including allergenic responses, asthma, and the proliferation of cancer cells.

The inherent morphological and genetic diversity of oats renders them invaluable in the realms of plant breeding and agriculture. The convergence of plant breeding capabilities and emerging biological techniques has facilitated significant progress in developing oats with heightened levels of health components. Notably, there is a concerted effort to enhance resistance to prevalent diseases like crown rust, BYDV, and powdery mildew, with particular attention to resistance against mycotoxin-producing organisms due to the poorly defined risks associated with mycotoxins. As our understanding of the agronomic, resistant, and health benefits of oats deepens, the prospect of augmenting oat attributes, particularly in the realms of health and functional traits, becomes increasingly apparent.

While molecular marker-based linkage maps, marker-trait associations, QTL, MAS, and genomic selection have been pivotal in advancing oat research, challenges persist. The enormity of the oat hexaploid genome and the diminishing global oat hectarage pose limitations, impeding the competitiveness of oats with other cereals for research funding. However, the trajectory of oat biotechnology continues to advance, leveraging technological breakthroughs for more rapid, cost-effective marker development, DNA sequencing, and bioinformatic analyses. The imperative need for the complete sequencing of an oat genome remains a pivotal milestone, propelling molecular and breeding laboratories to explore innovative avenues in oat biotechnology research to overcome future challenges and expedite genome investigations.

The advent of emerging functional genomics further accelerates contributions to oat research. ESTs serve as a swift avenue for discovering and sequencing thousands of oat genes, while microarrays efficiently illuminate the conditions influencing gene expression in oats. The synergy of robotics and bioinformatics augments the cost-effectiveness and expediency of data acquisition. This wealth of information enriches existing chromosomal, marker, and QTL maps, forging connections between structural genomic studies and disciplines such as biochemistry and plant physiology.

Anticipating the future, ongoing investments in research and development tools will augment the oat breeder's arsenal. New strategies, including site-directed mutagenesis to tailor the DNA sequence of target genes for enhanced effects, are on the horizon. This evolution, however, demands meticulous knowledge and caution to avoid unintended consequences. Collaborations between oat breeders and professionals in diverse disciplines are indispensable to harnessing the full potential of molecular genetics in oats. As advancements in oat molecular genetics converge with parallel developments in other cereal crops, the prospect of higher-quality oats becomes an exciting reality, underscoring the interdisciplinary nature of progress in oat research.

REFERENCES

[1] N. Kamal et al., "The mosaic oat genome gives insights into a uniquely healthy cereal crop," *Nature.*, vol. 606, pp. 113–119, 2022, doi: 10.1038/s41586-022-04732-y.

[2] H. Yan et al., "High-density marker profiling confirms ancestral genomes of Avena species and identifies D-genome chromosomes of hexaploid oat," *Theor. Appl. Genet.*, vol. 129, pp. 2133–2149, 2016, doi: 10.1007/s00122-016-2762-7.

[3] Y. Van de Peer, E. Mizrachi and K. Marchal, "The evolutionary significance of polyploidy," *Nat. Rev. Genet.*, vol. 18, pp. 411–424, 2017, doi: 10.1038/nrg.2017.26.

[4] D. Marone et al., "Specialized metabolites: Physiological and biochemical role in stress resistance, strategies to improve their accumulation, and new applications in crop breeding and management," *Plant Physiol. Biochem.*, vol. 172, pp. 48–55, 2022, doi: 10.1016/j.plaphy.2021.12.037.

[5] R. Dhariwal and H. S. Randhawa, "Mapping quantitative trait loci in wheat: Historic perspective, tools, and methods for analysis," in *Accelerated Breeding of Cereal Crops*, A. Bilichak and J. D. Laurie, Eds. New York, NY, USA: Springer, 2022, pp. 31–75, doi: 10.1007/978-1-0716-1526-3_2.

[6] V. Kumari et al., "Concepts and employment of molecular markers in crop breeding," in *Molecular Marker Techniques: A Potential Approach of Crop Improvement*, N. Kumar, Ed. Singapore, Singapore: Springer Nature, 2023, pp. 69–79, doi: 10.1007/978-981-99-1612-2_4.

[7] S. Sundaresha et al., "Spraying of dsRNA molecules derived from Phytophthora infestans, along with nanoclay carriers as a proof of concept for developing novel protection strategy for potato late blight," *Pest Manag. Sci.*, vol. 78, pp. 1–10, 2022, doi: 10.1002/ps.6949.

[8] S. Sundaresha et al., "Spraying of dsRNA molecules derived from phytophthora infestans, as a plant protection strategies for the management of potato late blight," 2021, doi: 10.20944/preprints202102.0280.v1.

[9] N. Salaria et al., "Solanum tuberosum (CYCLING DOF FACTOR) CDF1.2 allele: A candidate gene for developing earliness in potato," *S. Afr. J. Bot.*, vol. 132, pp. 242–248, 2020, doi: 10.1016/j.sajb.2020.05.008.

[10] S. Sundaresha et al., "In vitro method for synthesis of large-scale dsRNA molecule as a novel plant protection strategy," in *Plant Gene Silencing: Methods and Protocols*, K. S. Mysore and M. Senthil-Kumar, Eds. New York, NY, USA: Springer, 2022, pp. 211–226, doi: 10.1007/978-1-0716-1875-2_14.

[11] M. Tomar et al., "Validation of molecular response of tuberization in response to elevated temperature by using a transient Virus Induced Gene Silencing (VIGS) in potato," *Funct. Integr. Genomics.*, vol. 21, pp. 215–229, 2021, doi: 10.1007/s10142-021-00771-2.

[12] Z. J. Chen and Z. Ni, "Mechanisms of genomic rearrangements and gene expression changes in plant polyploids," *BioEssays.*, vol. 28, pp. 240–252, 2006, doi: 10.1002/bies.20374.

[13] N. C. Manrique-Carpintero et al., "Genome reduction in tetraploid potato reveals genetic load, haplotype variation, and loci associated with agronomic traits," *Front. Plant Sci.*, vol. 9, 2018. Accessed: Nov. 15, 2023. [Online]. Available: www.frontiersin.org/articles/10.3389/fpls.2018.00944

[14] V. Mohler, E. Paczos-Grzęda and S. Sowa, "Loving the alien: The contribution of the wild in securing the breeding of cultivated hexaploid wheat and oats," *Agriculture.*, vol. 13, p. 2060, 2023, doi: 10.3390/agriculture13112060.

[15] G. F. Alemayehu, S. F. Forsido, Y. B. Tola and E. Amare, "Nutritional and phytochemical composition and associated health benefits of oat (*Avena sativa*) grains and oat-based fermented food products," *Sci. World J.*, 2023, p. e2730175, 2023, doi: 10.1155/2023/2730175.

[16] S. Singh, B. P. Kushwaha, S. K. Nag, A. K. Mishra, A. Singh and U. Y. Anele, "In vitro ruminal fermentation, protein and carbohydrate fractionation, methane production and prediction of twelve commonly used Indian green forages," *Anim. Feed Sci. Technol.*, vol. 178, pp. 2–11, 2012, doi: 10.1016/j.anifeedsci.2012.08.019.

[17] J. M. Leggett and E. Jellen, "Cytogenetic manipulation in oat improvement," in *Genetic Resources, Chromosome Engineering, and Crop Improvement*, R. J. Singh and P. P. Jauhar, Eds. Singapore: Taylor & Francis, 2006, pp. 199–231.

[18] S. Sinha, S. Singh, M. Kumar, R. S. Singh, Satyendra and D. Thakur, "Recent advancements in molecular marker technologies and their applications in crop improvement," in *Molecular Marker Techniques: A Potential Approach of Crop Improvement*, N. Kumar, Ed. Singapore, Singapore: Springer Nature, 2023, pp. 319–337, doi: 10.1007/978-981-99-1612-2_15.

[19] D. Deres and T. Feyissa, "Concepts and applications of diversity array technology (DArT) markers for crop improvement," *J. Crop Improv.*, vol. 37, pp. 913–933, 2023, doi: 10.1080/15427528.2022.2159908.

[20] Y.-F. Huang, J. A. Poland, C. P. Wight, E. W. Jackson and N. A. Tinker, "Using genotyping-by-sequencing (GBS) for genomic discovery in cultivated oat," *PLoS One.*, vol. 9, p. e102448, 2014, doi: 10.1371/journal.pone.0102448.

[21] H. Yan et al., "Genome size variation in the genus Avena," *Genome.*, vol. 59, pp. 209–220, 2016, doi: 10.1139/gen-2015-0132.

[22] M. Schubert, T. Marcussen, A. S. Meseguer and S. Fjellheim, "The grass subfamily Pooideae: Cretaceous–Palaeocene origin and climate-driven Cenozoic diversification," *Global Ecol. Biogeogr.*, vol. 28, pp. 1168–1182, 2019, doi: 10.1111/geb.12923.

[23] Q. Liu et al., "The repetitive DNA landscape in Avena (Poaceae): Chromosome and genome evolution defined by major repeat classes in whole-genome sequence reads," *BMC Plant Biol.*, vol. 19, p. 226, 2019, doi: 10.1186/s12870-019-1769-z.

[24] X. Zhou, E. N. Jellen and J. P. Murphy, "Progenitor germplasm of domisticated hexaploid oat," *Crop Sci.*, vol. 39, p. cropsci1999.0011183X003900040042x, 1999, doi: 10.2135/cropsci1999.0011183X003900040042x.

[25] A.S. Chaffin et al., "A consensus map in cultivated hexaploid oat reveals conserved grass synteny with substantial subgenome rearrangement," *Plant Genome.*, vol. 9, p. plantgenome2015.10.0102, 2016, doi: 10.3835/plantgenome2015.10.0102.

[26] E. Kellogg et al., "Early inflorescence development in the grasses (Poaceae)," *Front. Plant Sci.*, vol. 4, 2013. Accessed: Nov. 15, 2023. [Online]. Available: www.frontiersin.org/articles/10.3389/fpls.2013.00250

[27] B. J. Clavijo et al., "An improved assembly and annotation of the allohexaploid wheat genome identifies complete families of agronomic genes and provides genomic evidence for chromosomal translocations," *Genome Res.*, vol. 27, pp. 885–896, 2017, doi: 10.1101/gr.217117.116.

[28] Z. Li, Y. Chen, D. Meesapyodsuk and X. Qiu, "The biosynthetic pathway of major avenanthramides in oat," *Metabolites.*, vol. 9, p. 163, 2019, doi: 10.3390/metabo9080163.

[29] I. C. Nava, C. P. Wight, M. T. Pacheco, L. C. Federizzi and N. A. Tinker, "Tagging and mapping candidate loci for vernalization and flower initiation in hexaploid oat," *Mol. Breed.*, vol. 30, pp. 1295–1312, 2012, doi: 10.1007/s11032-012-9715-x.

[30] H.-W. Nützmann, C. Scazzocchio and A. Osbourn, "Metabolic gene clusters in eukaryotes," *Annu. Rev. Genet.*, vol. 52, pp. 159–183, 2018, doi: 10.1146/annurev-genet-120417-031237.

[31] H.-W. Nützmann, A. Huang and A. Osbourn, "Plant metabolic clusters – From genetics to genomics," *New Phytol.*, vol. 211, pp. 771–789, 2016, doi: 10.1111/nph.13981.

[32] G. Winterfeld, E. Döring and M. Röser, "Chromosome evolution in wild oat grasses (Aveneae) revealed by molecular phylogeny," *Genome.*, vol. 52, pp. 361–380, 2009, doi: 10.1139/G09-012.

[33] Y.-B. Fu and D. J. Williams, "AFLP variation in 25 Avena species," *Theor. Appl. Genet.*, vol. 117, pp. 333–342, 2008, doi: 10.1007/s00122-008-0778-3.

[34] Y.-B. Fu, "Oat evolution revealed in the maternal lineages of 25 Avena species," *Sci Rep.*, vol. 8, p. 4252, 2018, doi: 10.1038/s41598-018-22478-4.

[35] H. Liu and G.-B. Chen, "A fast genomic selection approach for large genomic data," *Theor. Appl. Genet.*, vol. 130, pp. 1277–1284, 2017, doi: 10.1007/s00122-017-2887-3.

[36] G. Ladizinsky, "A new species of Avena from Sicily, possibly the tetraploid progenitor of hexaploid oats," *Genet. Resour. Crop Evol.*, vol. 45, pp. 263–269, 1998, doi: 10.1023/A:1008657530466.

[37] K. Crosby, T. O. Stokes and R. G. Latta, "Evolving California genotypes of Avena barbata are derived from multiple introductions but still maintain substantial population structure," *PeerJ.*, vol. 2, p. e633, 2014, doi: 10.7717/peerj.633.

[38] E. D. Badaeva, O. Y. Shelukhina, S. V. Goryunova, I. G. Loskutov and V. A. Pukhalskiy, "Phylogenetic relationships of tetraploid AB-genome *Avena* species evaluated by means of cytogenetic (C-banding and FISH) and RAPD analyses," *J. Bot.*, vol. 2010, p. e742307, 2010, doi: 10.1155/2010/742307.

[39] T. Morikawa and J. M. Leggett, "Isozyme polymorphism and genetic differentiation in natural populations of an endemic tetraploid species Avena maroccana in Morocco," *Genet. Resour. Crop Evol.*, vol. 55, pp. 1313–1321, 2008, doi: 10.1007/s10722-008-9330-1.

[40] M. Govindaraj, M. Vetriventhan and M. Srinivasan, "Importance of genetic diversity assessment in crop plants and its recent advances: An overview of its analytical perspectives," *Genet. Res. Int.*, vol. 2015, p. e431487, 2015, doi: 10.1155/2015/431487.

[41] P. Singh et al., "Global gene expression profiling under nitrogen stress identifies key genes involved in nitrogen stress adaptation in maize (Zea mays L.)," *Sci Rep.*, 12, p. 4211, 2022, doi: 10.1038/s41598-022-07709-z.

[42] R.E. Oliver et al., "SNP discovery and chromosome anchoring provide the first physically-anchored hexaploid oat map and reveal synteny with model species," *PLoS One.*, vol. 8, p. e58068, 2013, doi: 10.1371/journal.pone.0058068.

[43] L. Rayaprolu, S. P. Deshpande and R. Gupta, "Genotyping-by-sequencing (GBS) method for accelerating marker-assisted selection (MAS) program," in *Genomics of Cereal Crops*, S. H. Wani and A. Kumar, Eds. New York, NY, USA: Springer, 2022, pp. 245–257, doi: 10.1007/978-1-0716-2533-0_12.

[44] F. J. Canales et al., "Population genomics of Mediterranean oat (A. sativa) reveals high genetic diversity and three loci for heading date," *Theor. Appl. Genet.*, vol. 134, pp. 2063–2077, 2021, doi: 10.1007/s00122-021-03805-2.

[45] N. A. Tinker, W. A. Bekele and J. Hattori, "Haplotag: Software for haplotype-based genotyping-by-sequencing analysis," *G3 Genes|Genomes|Genetics.*, vol. 6, pp. 857–863, 2016, doi: 10.1534/g3.115.024596.

[46] S. Ahmar et al., "Conventional and molecular techniques from simple breeding to speed breeding in crop plants: Recent advances and future outlook," *Int. J. Mol. Sci.*, vol. 21, p. 2590, 2020, doi: 10.3390/ijms21072590.

[47] J. A. Bhat and D. Yu, "High-throughput NGS-based genotyping and phenotyping: Role in genomics-assisted breeding for soybean improvement," *Legume Sci.*, vol. 3, p. e81, 2021, doi: 10.1002/leg3.81.

[48] J. Tello and J. Ibáñez, "Review: Status and prospects of association mapping in grapevine," *Plant Sci.*, vol. 327, p. 111539, 2023, doi: 10.1016/j.plantsci.2022.111539.

[49] N. Kumar et al., "Development and characterization of a sorghum multi-parent advanced generation intercross (MAGIC) population for capturing diversity among seed parent gene pool," *G3 Genes|Genomes|Genetics.*, vol. 13, p. jkad037, 2023, doi: 10.1093/g3journal/jkad037.

[50] J.K. Kitony, "Nested association mapping population in crops: Current status and future prospects," *J. Crop Sci. Biotechnol.*, vol. 26, pp. 1–12, 2023, doi: 10.1007/s12892-022-00158-0.

[51] A. Grover and P. C. Sharma, "Development and use of molecular markers: Past and present," *Crit. Rev. Biotechnol.*, vol. 36, pp. 290–302, 2016, doi: 10.3109/07388551.2014.959891.

[52] A. Gorash, R. Armonienė, J. Mitchell Fetch, Ž. Liatukas, V. Danytė, "Aspects in oat breeding: Nutrition quality, nakedness and disease resistance, challenges and perspectives," *Ann. Appl. Biol.*, vol. 171, pp. 281–302, 2017, doi: 10.1111/aab.12375.

[53] S. Groh et al., "Analysis of factors influencing milling yield and their association to other traits by QTL analysis in two hexaploid oat populations," *Theor. Appl. Genet.*, vol. 103, pp. 9–18, 2001, doi: 10.1007/s001220100579.

[54] K. Esvelt Klos et al., "The genetic architecture of milling quality in spring oat lines of the collaborative oat research enterprise," *Foods.*, vol. 10, p. 2479, 2021, doi: 10.3390/foods10102479.

[55] M. H. Herrmann, J. Yu, S. Beuch, W. E. Weber, "Quantitative trait loci for quality and agronomic traits in two advanced backcross populations in oat (Avena sativa L.)," *Plant Breed.*, vol. 133, pp. 588–601, 2014, doi: 10.1111/pbr.12188.

[56] O. D. Anderson, "The spectrum of major seed storage genes and proteins in oats (Avena sativa)," *PLoS One*, vol. 9, p. e83569, 2014, doi: 10.1371/journal.pone.0083569.

[57] H. Yan, H. Zhang, P. Zhou, C. Ren and Y. Peng, "Genome-wide association mapping of QTL underlying groat protein content of a diverse panel of oat accessions," *Int. J. Mol. Sci.*, vol. 24, p. 5581, 2023, doi: 10.3390/ijms24065581.

[58] S. F. Kianian et al., "Association of a major groat oil content QTL and an acetyl-CoA carboxylase gene in oat," *Theor. Appl. Genet.*, vol. 98, pp. 884–894, 1999, doi: 10.1007/s001220051147.

[59] M. O. Carlson et al., "Multivariate genome-wide association analyses reveal the genetic basis of seed fatty acid composition in oat (Avena sativa L.)," *G3 Genes|Genomes|Genetics.*, vol. 9, pp. 2963–2975, 2019, doi: 10.1534/g3.119.400228.

[60] B. T. Hizbai et al., "Quantitative trait loci affecting oil content, oil composition, and other agronomically important traits in oat," *Plant Genome.*, vol. 5, 2012, doi: 10.3835/plantgenome2012.07.0015.

[61] V. A. Portyanko, D. L. Hoffman, M. Lee and J. B. Holland, "A linkage map of hexaploid oat based on grass anchor DNA clones and its relationship to other oat maps," *Genome.*, vol. 44, pp. 249–265, 2001, doi: 10.1139/g01-003.

[62] C. P. Wight et al., "A molecular marker map in "Kanota" × "Ogle" hexaploid oat (Avena spp.) enhanced by additional markers and a robust framework," *Genome.*, vol. 46, pp. 28–47, 2003, doi: 10.1139/g02-099.

[63] A. Singla et al., "Beta-Glucan as a soluble dietary fiber source: Origins, biosynthesis, extraction, purification, structural characteristics, bioavailability, biofunctional attributes, industrial utilization, and global trade," *Nutrients*, vol. 16, p. 6, 2024, doi: 10.3390/nu16060900.

[64] A. Chawade et al., "Development and characterization of an oat TILLING-population and identification of mutations in lignin and β-glucan biosynthesis genes," *BMC Plant Biol.*, vol. 10, p. 86, 2010, doi: 10.1186/1471-2229-10-86.

[65] C. M. Zimmer et al., "Genome-wide association for β-glucan content, population structure, and linkage disequilibrium in elite oat germplasm adapted to subtropical environments," *Mol. Breed.*, vol. 40, p. 103, 2020, doi: 10.1007/s11032-020-01182-0.

[66] T. Verhoeven, B. Fahy, M. Leggett, G. Moates and K. Denyer, "Isolation and characterisation of novel starch mutants of oats," *J. Cereal Sci.*, vol. 40, pp. 69–79, 2004, doi: 10.1016/j.jcs.2004.04.004.

[67]   S. E. Harrington, H. F. J. Bligh, W. D. Park, C. A. Jones and S. R. McCouch, "Linkage mapping of starch branching enzyme III in rice (Oryza sativa L.) and prediction of location of orthologous genes in other grasses," *Theor. Appl. Genet.*, vol. 94, pp. 564–568, 1997, doi: 10.1007/s001220050452.

[68]   N. A. Tinker et al., "Genome analysis in Avena sativa reveals hidden breeding barriers and opportunities for oat improvement," *Commun Biol.*, vol. 5, pp. 1–11, 2022, doi: 10.1038/s42003-022-03256-5.

[69]   M. C. Fogarty et al., "Identification of mixed linkage β-glucan quantitative trait loci and evaluation of AsCslF6 homoeologs in hexaploid oat," *Crop Sci.*, 60, pp. 914–933, 2020, doi: 10.1002/csc2.20015.

[70]   M. A. Newell, F. G. Asoro, M. P. Scott, P. J. White, W. D. Beavis and J.-L. Jannink, "Genome-wide association study for oat (Avena sativa L.) beta-glucan concentration using germplasm of worldwide origin," *Theor. Appl. Genet.*, vol. 125, pp. 1687–1696, 2012, doi: 10.1007/s00122-012-1945-0.

[71]   F. G. Asoro, M. A. Newell, M. P. Scott, W. D. Beavis and J.-L. Jannink, "Genome-wide association study for beta-glucan concentration in elite North American oat," *Crop Sci.*, vol. 53, pp. 542–553, 2013, doi: 10.2135/cropsci2012.01.0039.

[72]   S. F. Kianian, R. L. Phillips, H. W. Rines, R. G. Fulcher, F. H. Webster and D. D. Stuthman, "Quantitative trait loci influencing β-glucan content in oat (Avena sativa, 2n=6x=42)," *Theor. Appl. Genet.*, vol. 101, pp. 1039–1048, 2000, doi: 10.1007/s001220051578.

[73]   C. M. Zimmer et al., "Genome-wide association mapping for kernel shape and its association with β-glucan content in oats," *Crop Sci.*, vol. 61, pp. 3986–3999, 2021, doi: 10.1002/csc2.20605.

[74]   R. Kapoor and H. J. Hilli, "Amandeep, oats: Role and responses under abiotic stress," in *Sustainable Remedies for Abiotic Stress in Cereals*, A. A. H. Abdel Latef, Ed. Singapore, Singapore: Springer Nature, 2022, pp. 149–169, doi: 10.1007/978-981-19-5121-3_7.

[75]   Z. Fatima et al., "The fingerprints of climate warming on cereal crops phenology and adaptation options," *Sci Rep.*, vol. 10, p. 18013, 2020, doi: 10.1038/s41598-020-74740-3.

[76]   D. L. De Koeyer et al., "A molecular linkage map with associated QTLs from a hulless × covered spring oat population," *Theor. Appl. Genet.*, vol. 108, pp. 1285–1298, 2004, doi: 10.1007/s00122-003-1556-x.

[77]   K. Esvelt Klos et al., "Population genomics related to adaptation in elite oat germplasm," *Plant Genome.*, vol. 9, p. plantgenome2015.10.0103, 2016, doi: 10.3835/plantgenome2015.10.0103.

[78]   P. J. Maughan et al., "Genomic insights from the first chromosome-scale assemblies of oat (Avena spp.) diploid species," *BMC Biology.*, vol. 17, p. 92, 2019, doi: 10.1186/s12915-019-0712-y.

[79]   F. G. Sunstrum, W. A. Bekele, C. P. Wight, W. Yan, Y. Chen and N. A. Tinker, "A genetic linkage map in southern-by-spring oat identifies multiple quantitative trait loci for adaptation and rust resistance," *Plant Breed.*, vol. 138, pp. 82–94, 2019, doi: 10.1111/pbr.12666.

[80]   D. R. Wooten et al., "Quantitative trait loci and epistasis for oat winter-hardiness component traits," *Crop Sci.*, vol. 49, pp. 1989–1998, 2009, doi: 10.2135/cropsci2008.10.0612.

[81]   H. Yan et al., "Genetic diversity and genome-wide association analysis in Chinese hulless oat germplasm," *Theor. Appl. Genet.*, vol. 133, pp. 3365–3380, 2020, doi: 10.1007/s00122-020-03674-1.

[82]   S. Zhu and H. F. Kaeppler, "A genetic linkage map for hexaploid, cultivated oat (Avena sativa L.) based on an intraspecific cross "Ogle/MAM17–5," *Theor. Appl. Genet.*, vol. 107, pp. 26–35, 2003, doi: 10.1007/s00122-003-1191-6.

[83]   H. Yan et al., "Position validation of the dwarfing gene Dw6 in oat (Avena sativa L.) and its correlated effects on agronomic traits," *Front. Plant Sci.*, vol. 12, 2021. Accessed: Nov. 16, 2023. [Online]. Available: www.frontiersin.org/articles/10.3389/fpls.2021.668847

[84] A. B. Locatelli et al., "Loci affecting flowering time in oat under short-day conditions," *Genome.*, vol. 49, pp. 1528–1538, 2006, doi: 10.1139/g06-108.

[85] K. E. Klos et al., "Genome-wide association mapping of crown rust resistance in oat elite germplasm," *Plant Genome.*, vol. 10, p. plantgenome2016.10.0107, 2017, doi: 10.3835/plantgenome2016.10.0107.

[86] J. Chong, E. Reimer, D. Somers, T. Aung and G. A. Penner, "Development of sequence-characterized amplified region (SCAR) markers for resistance gene Pc94 to crown rust in oat," *Can. J. Plant Pathol.*, vol. 26, pp. 89–96, 2004, doi: 10.1080/07060660409507118.

[87] E. W. Jackson et al., "Characterization and mapping of oat crown rust resistance genes using three assessment methods," *Phytopathology®.*, vol. 97, pp. 1063–1070, 2007, doi: 10.1094/PHYTO-97-9-1063.

[88] F. R. Kulcheski, F. A. S. Graichen, J. A. Martinelli, A. B. Locatelli, L. C. Federizzi and C. A. Delatorre, "Molecular mapping of Pc68, a crown rust resistance gene in Avenasativa," *Euphytica.*, vol. 175, pp. 423–432, 2010, doi: 10.1007/s10681-010-0198-8.

[89] C. A. McCartney et al., "Mapping of the oat crown rust resistance gene Pc91," *Theor. Appl. Genet.*, vol. 122, pp. 317–325, 2011, doi: 10.1007/s00122-010-1448-9.

[90] G. A. Penner, J. Chong, C. P. Wight, S. J. Molnar and G. Fedak, "Identification of an RAPD marker for the crown rust resistance gene Pc68 in oats," *Genome.*, vol. 36, pp. 818–820, 1993, doi: 10.1139/g93-108.

[91] W. L. Rooney, H. W. Rines and R. L. Phillips, "Identification of RFLP markers linked to crown rust resistance genes Pc 91 and Pc 92 in oat," *Crop Sci.*, vol. 34, p. cropsci1 994.0011183X003400040019x, 1994, doi: 10.2135/cropsci1994.0011183X00340004 0019x.

[92] S. Satheeskumar, P. J. Sharp, E. S. Lagudah, R. A. McIntosh and S. J. Molnar, "Genetic association of crown rust resistance gene Pc68, storage protein loci, and resistance gene analogues in oats," *Genome.*, vol. 54, pp. 484–497, 2011, doi: 10.1139/g11-014.

[93] C. P. Wight, L. S. O'Donoughue, J. Chong, N. A. Tinker, S. J. Molnar, "Discovery, local-ization, and sequence characterization of molecular markers for the crown rust resis-tance genes Pc38, Pc39, and Pc48 in cultivated oat (Avena sativa L.)," *Mol. Breed.*, vol. 14, pp. 349–361, 2004, doi: 10.1007/s11032-004-0148-z.

[94] B. N. Gnanesh, J. Mitchell Fetch, J. G. Menzies, A. D. Beattie, P. E. Eckstein and C. A. McCartney, "Chromosome location and allele-specific PCR markers for marker-assisted selection of the oat crown rust resistance gene Pc91," *Mol. Breed.*, vol. 32, pp. 679–686, 2013, doi: 10.1007/s11032-013-9900-6.

[95] J. Chong and W. L. Seaman, "Incidence and virulence of Puccinia coronata f. sp. avenae in Canada in 1993," *Can. J. Plant Pathol.*, vol. 16, pp. 335–340, 1994, doi: 10.1080/07060669409500740.

[96] W. A. Wilson and M. S. McMullen, "Dosage dependent genetic suppression of oat crown rust resistance gene Pc-62," *Crop Sci.*, vol. 37, p. cropsci1997.0011183X003700 060004x, 1997, doi: 10.2135/cropsci1997.0011183X003700060004x.

[97] Y. Lin et al., "A major quantitative trait locus conferring adult plant partial resis-tance to crown rust in oat," *BMC Plant Biol.*, vol. 14, p. 250, 2014, doi: 10.1186/ s12870-014-0250-2.

[98] H. W. Rines et al., "Identification, introgression, and molecular marker genetic anal-ysis and selection of a highly effective novel oat crown rust resistance from diploid oat, Avena strigosa," *Theor. Appl. Genet.*, vol. 131, pp. 721–733, 2018, doi: 10.1007/ s00122-017-3031-0.

[99] T. C. Gordon et al., "Comparative sequencing and SNP marker validation for oat stem rust resistance gene Pg6 in a diverse collection of Avena accessions," *Theor. Appl. Genet.*, vol. 135, pp. 1307–1318, 2022, doi: 10.1007/s00122-022-04032-z.

[100] A. Z. Kebede et al., "Mapping of the stem rust resistance gene Pg13 in cultivated oat," *Theor. Appl. Genet.*, vol. 133, pp. 259–270, 2020, doi: 10.1007/s00122-019-03455-5.

[101]   S. L. K. Hsam, V. Mohler and F. J. Zeller, "The genetics of resistance to powdery mildew in cultivated oats (Avena sativa L.): Current status of major genes," *J Appl Genetics.*, vol. 55, pp. 155–162, 2014, doi: 10.1007/s13353-014-0196-y.

[102]   M. J. Sanz, E. N. Jellen, Y. Loarce, M. L. Irigoyen, E. Ferrer and A. Fominaya, "A new chromosome nomenclature system for oat (Avena sativa L. and A. byzantina C. Koch) based on FISH analysis of monosomic lines," *Theor. Appl. Genet.*, vol. 121, pp. 1541–1552, 2010, doi: 10.1007/s00122-010-1409-3.

[103]   J. Yu and M. Herrmann, "Inheritance and mapping of a powdery mildew resistance gene introgressed from Avena macrostachya in cultivated oat," *Theor. Appl. Genet.*, vol. 113, pp. 429–437, 2006, doi: 10.1007/s00122-006-0308-0.

[104]   S. M. Okoń and T. Ociepa, "Effectiveness of new sources of resistance against oat powdery mildew identified in A. sterilis," *J. Plant Dis. Prot.*, vol. 125, pp. 505–510, 2018, doi: 10.1007/s41348-018-0171-7.

[105]   X. He, H. Skinnes, R.E. Oliver, E. W. Jackson and Å. Bjørnstad, "Linkage mapping and identification of QTL affecting deoxynivalenol (DON) content (Fusarium resistance) in oats (Avena sativa L.)," *Theor. Appl. Genet.*, vol. 126, pp. 2655–2670, 2013, doi: 10.1007/s00122-013-2163-0.

[106]   K. M. Pathi and T. Sprink, "From petri dish to field: Plant tissue culture and genetic engineering of oats for improved agricultural outcomes," *Plants.*, vol. 12, p. 3782, 2023, doi: 10.3390/plants12213782.

[107]   S. Maqbool et al., "Competence of oat (Avena sativa L.) shoot apical meristems for integrative transformation, inherited expression, and osmotic tolerance of transgenic lines containing hva1," *Theor. Appl. Genet.*, vol. 105, pp. 201–208, 2002, doi: 10.1007/s00122-002-0984-3.

[108]   Y. Ishida, Y. Hiei and T. Komari, "High-efficiency transformation techniques," in *Applications of Genetic and Genomic Research in Cereals*, T. Miedaner and V. Korzun, Eds. Woodhead Publishing, 2019, pp. 97–120, doi: 10.1016/B978-0-08-102163-7.00005-3.

[109]   P. A. Lazzeri and H. D. Jones, "Transgenic wheat, barley and oats: Production and characterization," in *Transgenic Wheat, Barley and Oats: Production and Characterization Protocols*, H. D. Jones and P. R. Shewry, Eds. Totowa, NJ, USA: Humana Press, 2009, pp. 3–20, doi: 10.1007/978-1-59745-379-0_1.

[110]   H. D. Jones and C. A. Sparks, "Selection of transformed plants," in *Transgenic Wheat, Barley and Oats: Production and Characterization Protocols*, H. D. Jones and P.R. Shewry, Eds. Totowa, NJ, USA: Humana Press, 2009, pp. 23–37, doi: 10.1007/978-1-59745-379-0_2.

[111]   D. A. Somers, H. W. Rines, W. Gu, H. F. Kaeppler, W. R. Bushnell, "Fertile, transgenic oat plants," *Nat. Biotechnol.*, vol. 10, pp. 1589–1594, 1992, doi: 10.1038/nbt1292-1589.

[112]   C. Gless, H. Lörz and A. Jähne-Gärtner, "Transgenic oat plants obtained at high efficiency by microprojectile bombardment of leaf base segments," *J. Plant Physiol.*, vol. 152, pp. 151–157, 1998, doi: 10.1016/S0176-1617(98)80126-0.

[113]   S. Zhang, M.-J. Cho, T. Koprek, R. Yun, P. Bregitzer and P. G. Lemaux, "Genetic transformation of commercial cultivars of oat (Avena sativa L.) and barley (Hordeum vulgare L.) using in vitro shoot meristematic cultures derived from germinated seedlings," *Plant Cell Rep.*, vol. 18, pp. 959–966, 1999, doi: 10.1007/s002990050691.

[114]   D. Kummari et al., "An update and perspectives on the use of promoters in plant genetic engineering," *J. Biosci.*, vol. 45, p. 119, 2020, doi: 10.1007/s12038-020-00087-6.

[115]   A. Nadolska-Orczyk, A. Przetakiewicz, K. Kopera, A. Binka and W. Orczyk, Efficient method of agrobacterium-mediated transformation for triticale (x triticosecale wittmack)," *J. Plant Growth Regul.*, vol. 24, pp. 2–10, 2005, doi: 10.1007/s00344-004-0046-y.

[116]   D. A. Somers, "Transgenic cereals: Avena sativa (oat)," in *Molecular Improvement of Cereal Crops*, I. K. Vasil, Ed. Dordrecht, Netherlands: Springer, 1999, pp. 317–339, doi: 10.1007/978-94-011-4802-3_10.

[117] A. Kumar et al., "Genomics-assisted improvement of grain quality and nutraceutical properties in millets," in *Millets and Millet Technology*, A. Kumar, M. K. Tripathi, D. Joshi and V. Kumar, Eds. Singapore, Singapore: Springer, 2021, pp. 333–343, doi: 10.1007/978-981-16-0676-2_17.

[118] R. S. S. T. Kumar, S. Tiwari, P. Singh, K. B. Naik, and Anil Kumar, "Genome editing for improvement of wheat and millets," in *Genome Editing in Plants (First Edition)*, Boca Raton, Florida: CRC Press, 2021, pp. 1–12.

[119] I. Singh, K. Kumar, P. Singh, P. Yadava and S. Rakshit, "Physiological and molecular interventions for improving nitrogen-use efficiency in maize," in *Molecular Breeding in Wheat, Maize and Sorghum: Strategies for Improving Abiotic Stress Tolerance and Yield*, M. A. Hossain, M. Alam, S. Seneweera, S. Rakshit, R. Henry, Eds. Wallingford: CABI, 2021, pp. 325–339.

[120] R. S. Tomar et al., "Genomics approaches for restoration and conservation of agro-biodiversity," in *Agro-Biodiversity and Agri-Ecosystem Management*, P. Kumar, R. S. Tomar, J. A. Bhat, M. Dobriyal and M. Rani, Eds. Singapore, Singapore: Springer Nature, 2022, pp. 273–283, doi: 10.1007/978-981-19-0928-3_14.

[121] A. K. Shrawat and H. Lörz, "Agrobacterium-mediated transformation of cereals: A promising approach crossing barriers," *Plant Biotechnol. J.*, vol. 4, pp. 575–603, 2006, doi: 10.1111/j.1467-7652.2006.00209.x.

[122] N. Dattgonde, S. Tiwari, S. Sapre and I. Gontia-Mishra, "Genetic transformation of oat mediated by agrobacterium is enhanced with sonication and vacuum infiltration," *Iran. J. Biotechnol.*, vol. 17, pp. 68–73, 2019. Accessed: Nov. 16, 2023. [Online]. Available: www.ijbiotech.com/article_85121.html

[123] T. Sprink, J. Metje and F. Hartung, "Plant genome editing by novel tools: TALEN and other sequence specific nucleases, Current Opinion in Biotechnology. 32, pp. 47–53, 2015, doi: 10.1016/j.copbio.2014.11.010.

[124] T. Barber, *Standardizing the CRISPR-Cas9 System in Oat to Understand Beta-Glucan Regulation*. McGill University, 2021. [Online]. Available: https://escholarship.mcgill.ca/concern/theses/7p88cn79j

Future Prospectives and Development of Novel Value-Added Oat-Based Superfoods

Prabha Singh, Maharishi Tomar,
Awnindra Kumar Singh, Vijay Kumar Yadav,
Meenakshi Arya, Prashant P. Jambhulkar,
Rakesh Bhardwaj, and Deepmala Jain

10.1 INTRODUCTION

Throughout history, food has played a pivotal role in shaping human civilization, primarily serving two fundamental purposes: addressing hunger and supplying essential energy. However, in recent times, food has evolved to encompass functions beyond mere sustenance, extending to the realm of promoting overall health and offering additional benefits [1]. Recent research has shed light on a robust connection between the consumption of phytochemicals found in fruits and the prevention of various chronic diseases, largely attributed to the potent anticancer and antioxidant properties of these fruits.

DOI: 10.1201/ 9781003263302-10

These findings have paved the way for the development of foods specifically designed to target distinct health issues, and over the past decade, the concept of "functional foods" has emerged, with its origins traced back to Japan. Functional foods can be defined as food products that contribute to health by enhancing both physical and mental well-being. They achieve this by reducing the risk of certain diseases and may even be used for therapeutic purposes, all while satisfying hunger and providing essential nutrients. This evolution in our understanding of food highlights its expanding role in promoting not only nutrition but also holistic well-being and health maintenance [2], [3].

In general, functional foods are not initially consumed for their health benefits; instead, they are deliberately modified, fortified, enriched, or otherwise adjusted to enhance their nutritional profiles and are often marketed as industrial products [4]. These foods have proven to be advantageous for human health and have received official support. However, as trends have recently shifted towards a preference for more natural and traditional lifestyles, functional foods have raised concerns for some individuals [3]. Among Western consumers who are often considered well-informed about their health, there is a growing perception that functional foods are heavily processed to incorporate specific functional components [5]. This evolving perspective suggests that while functional foods may offer health benefits, they are increasingly seen as products that have undergone significant processing to include these beneficial elements.

A significant shift in the trajectory of functional food consumption trends has been driven primarily by recent research findings that have linked the consumption of ultra-processed foods to a surge in obesity rates [6]. As a result, consumer perceptions have increasingly favoured freshness over heavy processing. This shift in perception has given rise to novel concepts, notably the emergence of minimally processed functional foods. Minimally processed functional foods can be defined as functional food products that undergo only mild processing and are packaged using simple unit operations. These operations may include actions like washing, trimming, peeling, size reduction, pasteurization, packaging, storage, refrigeration, or freezing, all while ensuring that temperatures remain below 100°C [7]. This approach aligns with the contemporary consumer preference for foods that are less heavily processed and closer to their natural state.

Another category of foods referred to as "superfoods" has emerged, and while they share similarities with functional foods in terms of offering health benefits beyond basic nutrition, they also exhibit some distinctive characteristics. Superfoods can be described as traditional and minimally processed functional foods with a unique attribute: they have a history of "traditional use." What sets superfoods apart is their longstanding presence in certain culinary and medicinal practices, often in distant or specific regions. Superfoods are not only recognized for their remarkable and naturally occurring health benefits, but they also stand out due to their association with remote, authentic, or exotic communities [8]. This dual distinction, rooted in both their health-enhancing properties and their cultural significance, places superfoods in a unique spotlight within the realm of dietary choices.

In response to the pressing need to address the complex interplay between diet, the environment, and health on a global scale, the term "superfoods" has gained significant attention as a potential solution in recent years [9]. It is important to note that "superfood" lacks an official definition, meaning there is no scientifically, legally, or regulatory defined description provided by food safety authorities. Instead, it is informally used to describe foods that offer high quantities of essential nutrients and play a pivotal role in one's diet, contributing to the proper functioning of the body [10]. A wealth of research suggests that superfoods offer significant potential to enhance overall health. They are believed to boost the immune system, stimulate the production of serotonin and other vital hormones, and support the efficient functioning of the body's metabolic systems [1], [11].

Furthermore, there has been criticism surrounding the term "superfood," with some researchers suggesting that it is primarily employed for advertising and marketing purposes rather than being rooted in scientific evidence [12]. Conversely, for certain researchers, it has been regarded as a more accessible replacement for the term "functional food" within the general population [2]. Alternatively, some researchers have proposed that "superfood" serves as a valuable tool for introducing unfamiliar or lesser-known food items to Western consumers who are interested in enhancing their quality of life through better dietary choices. In this context, it is seen as a way to bridge the gap between novel or exotic foods and consumers seeking to improve their overall well-being. Some researchers state that superfoods are often compared to functional foods that offer health benefits by reducing the risk of diseases and positively influencing specific bodily functions beyond basic nutritional requirements [8].

Superfoods are also associated with "nutraceuticals," which is a fusion of "nutrient" and "pharmaceutical," was first introduced by Stephen DeFelice. He defined nutraceuticals as "food or components of food that offer medical or health advantages, encompassing disease prevention and/or treatment" [13]. This concept represents a contemporary perspective within the field of food science and is situated in a realm that extends beyond typical dietary items but precedes pharmaceutical drugs in terms of their potential applications [14]. However, some experts argue that superfoods differ in their conceptualization from functional foods by emphasizing their "natural" nutrient density and "traditional" or "exotic" qualities. In contrast, functional foods are often enriched with bioactive compounds known for their immune-boosting and functional properties, thus warranting distinct analysis [15]. Conceptually, a superfood must be a singular food item, not a multi-component product, and it should be "natural," meaning it has not undergone human intervention to add ingredients, supplements, or additional nutrients.

Oats unquestionably qualify as superfoods and a potent nutraceutical source is celebrated for their exceptional nutritional composition and the multitude of health advantages they provide. Oats are abundant in various beneficial nutrients including protein, fibre, calcium, vitamins (such as B, C, E, and K), amino acids, and antioxidants (like β-carotene, polyphenols, chlorophyll, and flavonoids). Among these, β-glucan and avenanthramides play a crucial role in enhancing the immune system, facilitating the removal of harmful substances from the body, reducing blood cholesterol levels, and aiding in weight loss through improved lipid profiles and fat breakdown. β-Glucan also plays a role in regulating insulin secretion, which can help in preventing diabetes. Progladins are another essential component of oats, known for their ability to lower cholesterol levels, inhibit triglyceride accumulation, reduce blood sugar levels, alleviate inflammation, and promote healthier skin. Saponin-based avanacosidase and flavone glycoside, which are found in oats, contribute to improved immune function, inflammation control, and skin protection. Additionally, lignin and phytoestrogens found in oats can assist in preventing hormone-related cancers and enhance the quality of life for postmenopausal women. Sprouted oats, in particular, are rich in saponarin, which aids in detoxifying the liver. Their adaptability makes them a convenient addition to a wide range of dishes, and their diverse array of macronutrients makes them a well-rounded dietary option. The capacity of oats to nourish the body while contributing to overall health firmly establishes their position as a superfood that deserves inclusion in a nutritious diet. This chapter primarily focuses on the latest trends in oat-based superfoods and the potential of oats and their active components for the future development of healthy and functional resources for human well-being.

10.2 OATS AS A SUPERFOOD AND NUTRACEUTICAL SOURCE

Superfood benefits often stem from their close association with phytochemicals (plant chemicals) and nutraceuticals. These essential elements are abundant in oats, and the "super" designation is typically linked to their remarkably elevated levels of health-improving components like antioxidants, fibres, vitamins, minerals, and more. In a broader context, the common attributes of superfoods can be summarized as their supportive role in bolstering the immune system and their exceptional nutritional value. They are characterized by significant concentrations of vitamins, valuable trace minerals, essential amino acids, phytosterols, dietary fibre, monounsaturated fats, and antioxidants [16].

Oat-based dietary phytochemicals are linked to health benefits and include glucosinolates, sulphur-containing compounds found in the Alliaceae family, terpenoids (such as phytosterols, monoterpenes, and carotenoids) as well as various categories of polyphenols (including ellagic acid, stilbenoids, isoflavones, flavones, and anthocyanins). This diverse range of compounds cannot be strictly classified as "food," leading to the creation of a hybrid term that combines elements of both nutrients and pharmaceuticals: "nutraceuticals" [17]. Nutraceuticals have garnered significant attention in recent years from the scientific community, consumers, and food manufacturers. The list of nutraceutical compounds, including vitamins, probiotics, bioactive peptides, antioxidants, and more, is extensive, and the scientific evidence supporting the idea of food ingredients that promote health continues to grow steadily. Functional foods, on the other hand, are those that, when consumed regularly, produce specific health-related benefits beyond their basic nutritional properties. These benefits can include contributing to a healthier state or reducing the risk of disease, and they must be substantiated through scientific research and evidence. On the other hand, functional foods share similarities with conventional foods in that they are typically consumed as part of a regular diet. However, what sets them apart is their recognized ability to enhance health beyond fulfilling basic nutritional functions.

A nutraceutical is a dietary supplement designed to provide a concentrated form of a presumed bioactive substance found in food. It is presented in a non-food matrix and is intended to enhance health when taken in doses exceeding what can be obtained from regular foods. These products are typically available in formats similar to drugs, such as pills, extracts, and tablets. Functional foods, on the other hand, are foods or dietary components whose consumption may offer health benefits beyond their basic nutritional properties. Health Canada defines functional foods as products resembling traditional foods but with demonstrated physiological benefits. In South Korea, functional foods are defined as dietary supplements meant to supplement a regular diet, usually marketed in measured doses like pills or tablets. Functional foods should resemble conventional foods in appearance (e.g., beverages or food matrices), be part of a typical diet, contain biologically active components with proven physiological benefits, and have the potential to reduce the risk of chronic diseases beyond basic nutrition [18].

The distinction between nutraceuticals and functional foods is often blurred, with many consumers and industries using these terms interchangeably. In a broad sense, functional foods are typically regarded as those foods meant to be part of a regular diet but contain biologically active components that have the potential to improve health or reduce the risk of diseases. Examples of functional foods include items that provide specific minerals, vitamins, fatty acids, or dietary fibre, as well as foods enriched with biologically active substances like phytochemicals, antioxidants, and probiotics. Under this definition, unmodified whole foods such as fruits and vegetables represent the simplest form of functional foods. For instance, broccoli, carrots, or tomatoes are considered functional foods because they are naturally rich in physiologically active components like sulforaphane, β-carotene, and lycopene, respectively.

Food fraud has increased as a result of disruptions in the food supply chain, and finding convincing evidence about the true health benefits of nutraceuticals and functional foods has become an area of artificial intelligence (AI) to support the real-time needs of the food industry, smart agriculture, the supply chain, and food security (e.g., remote monitoring and management decision tools). Furthermore, the proliferation of new technologies aided in the digitization of the food supply chain and increased investments in traceability systems to mitigate risk, improve efficiency, and support sustainability initiatives. Overall, it is challenging to predict the holistic consequences of this COVID-19 pandemic, at what point we will emerge from it, and which innovations and technologies will disrupt the food sector.

Ensuring the authenticity of food and detecting adulterants in a wide range of food products is paramount to safeguarding consumers against fraudulent practices. To address this challenge, the integration of science and engineering methods that link tangible food items to their digital representations, often through means like barcodes and QR codes, has proven to be highly effective, particularly when combined with the power of AI. AI technology has emerged as a cutting-edge tool within the food industry, enhancing its capabilities in this regard. Leveraging provenance information, which encompasses the history and origin of a food product, can play a crucial role in identifying food fraud, including adulteration. Adulteration occurs when an element of the final food product is deceitful or substandard. It's essential to note that the risk of food fraud arises due to the potential disconnect between the physical food item and its digital representation. Thus, utilizing advanced technologies and data-driven approaches, including AI, can significantly bolster efforts to combat food fraud and ensure the integrity of the food supply chain. Figure 10.1 illustrates distinct boundaries defining various food categories. Each category represents a unique classification based on its characteristics and intended purpose in the context of human consumption.

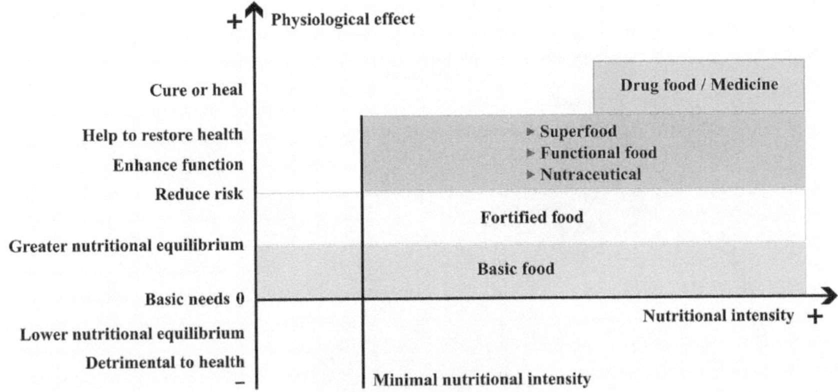

FIGURE 10.1 Visual representation of distinct boundaries defining various food categories. Each category is distinctly classified based on its unique characteristics and intended purpose in the context of human consumption. The featured categories encompass Drug Food/Medicine, Superfood, Functional Food, Nutraceutical, Fortified Food, and Basic Food. These classifications represent a spectrum of foods that go beyond typical dietary items but precede pharmaceutical drugs in their intended effects on health and well-being.

10.3 NUTRACEUTICAL POTENTIAL OF OATS

Oats are renowned for their reputation as both a wholesome and nutritious food, as well as a versatile nutraceutical and functional food. They boast a higher content of well-balanced protein and soluble fibre, providing a valuable source of energy-producing carbohydrates and fats (Figure 10.2; Table 10.1). Oats are also rich in phytic acid, antioxidants, and various phenolic compounds. Their ample fibre content contributes to the presence of polyphenols, which play a role in reducing cholesterol levels and mitigating the risk of cancer and cardiovascular disease (CVD) [19]. The fibre derived from oats offers particular benefits to individuals with diabetes by effectively lowering low-density lipoprotein (LDL) cholesterol levels [20]. Oats have garnered considerable research and commercial interest due to their elevated levels of β-glucan and other antioxidant-active compounds. To harness the health benefits of β-glucan, such as cholesterol reduction, improved gastrointestinal function, and enhanced glucose metabolism, a daily intake of 10 g of oats is recommended. β-Glucan accomplishes these effects by increasing gastrointestinal transit time, enhancing luminal viscosity, and delaying stomach emptying [21]. Additionally, soluble oat fibres play significant roles in the digestive tract as they are available for fermentation by probiotics. This fermentation process leads to prebiotic effects, which are crucial for maintaining a healthy colon wall and creating a favourable colonic environment. Thus, oats offer a wide range of nutritional and health benefits, making them a valuable addition to a balanced diet.

In general, incorporating oats into your diet is a preferable option for reducing blood pressure when compared to relying solely on antihypertensive medications. Oat

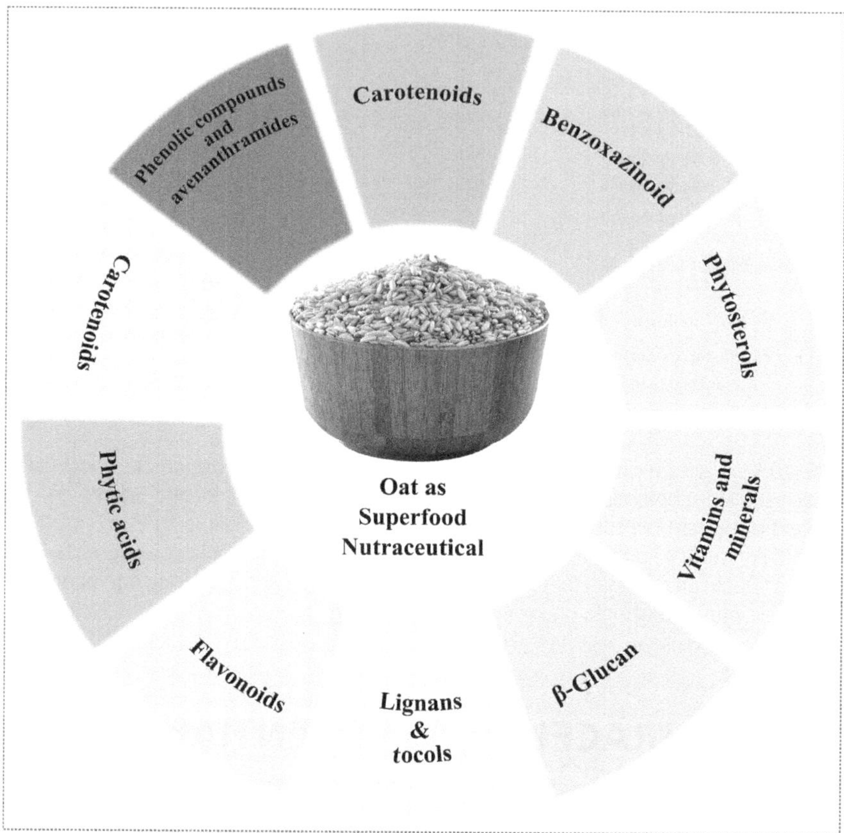

FIGURE 10.2 Oats as a dual-classified entity, embodying the characteristics of both a superfood and a nutraceutical. Oats, celebrated for their nutrient-rich composition, are recognized as a superfood due to their exceptional nutritional profile and potential health benefits. Additionally, their role as a nutraceutical signifies their capacity to contribute not only to basic nutrition but also to overall health and well-being through their potential therapeutic and medicinal properties.

kernels contain polyphenols and phenolic acids and possess antioxidant properties, which collectively help maintain and stabilize blood cholesterol levels, regulate blood sugar, and facilitate nutrient absorption after the stomach has emptied. Additionally, the antioxidants in oats play a crucial role in preserving the stability of processed oat products. Oats also contribute to preventing rancidity by stabilizing oils and lipids. Oat fibre is particularly effective in reducing both total plasma cholesterol and LDL cholesterol. Recent research has unveiled that oat polyphenols offer additional health benefits, such as anti-inflammatory, antiproliferative, and anti-itching properties [22]. These properties may provide added protection against conditions like skin irritation, colon cancer, and coronary heart disease. Hence, oats serve as a versatile and health-enhancing addition to one's dietary regimen.

TABLE 10.1 Various Health Benefits Associated with Nutraceutical Compounds Found in Oats

NUTRACEUTICAL TYPE	NUTRACEUTICAL	ACTION
Amino acids	N-Acetylcysteine	Elevation in glycine, cysteine, and glutathione levels in red blood cells; reduction in oxidative stress and indicators of damage caused by oxidants in plasma
Carotenoids	ß-Carotene	Suppresses the activity of free radicals and singlet oxygen-induced lipid peroxidation while also reducing the activity of matrix metallopeptidase-9
	Zeaxanthin and Lutein	Prevents harm caused by blue wavelengths and safeguards against free radical-induced damage
	Lycopene	Acts as a quencher for singlet oxygen, reduces Matrix metalloproteinase-1 activity, triggers cell cycle arrest, and promotes apoptosis
Fatty acids	Docosahexaenoic acid, eicosapen-taenoic acid, α-linolenic acid (ALA)	Restrains the generation of proinflammatory cytokines, such as prostaglandins and leukotrienes, while also reducing prostaglandin-E_2 production
Minerals	Copper	Serves as a cofactor in enzymatic reactions involved in collagen crosslinking through lysyl oxidase and in the process of skin pigmentation via tyrosinase; additionally, stimulates the proliferation of keratinocytes and fibroblasts
	Selenium	Assists glutathione peroxidases and thioredoxin reductases in eliminating harmful lipid hydroperoxides, hydrogen peroxide, and peroxynitrites
	Zinc	Safeguards against lipid peroxidation, shields from cytotoxicity induced by ultraviolet radiation (UVR), and mitigates oxidative stress; essential for epidermal proliferation and the differentiation of keratinocytes; additionally, impedes intracellular adhesion molecule 1 and reduces nitric oxide production
Polyphenols	Curcumin	Inhibits the generation of cancer cells, fosters apoptosis, facilitates cell death by modulating p53 expression, and reduces NF-κB production; also dampens the production of proinflammatory cytokines, curbs reactive oxygen species (ROS) production by scavenging free oxygen radicals, and hinders lipid peroxidation; furthermore, leads to a decrease in C-reactive protein levels

(Continued)

TABLE 10.1 (Continued) Various Health Benefits Associated with Nutraceutical Compounds Found in Oats

NUTRACEUTICAL TYPE	NUTRACEUTICAL	*ACTION*
	Epigallocatechin gallate (EGCG)	Restrains lipid peroxidation, restricts DNA damage caused by UVR, diminishes the production of ROS and free radicals; additionally, suppresses proinflammatory factors like cyclooxygenase-2 and matrix metalloproteinases (MMPs) and encourages cell cycle arrest and apoptosis
Vitamins – water soluble	Vitamin C	Acts as a scavenger for free radicals, serving as a crucial cofactor and electron donor during collagen hydroxylation; mitigates oxidative damage induced by UVB radiation and safeguards against UVA-induced lipid peroxidation; additionally, leads to a reduction in malondialdehyde levels
Vitamins – fat soluble	Vitamin E; alpha-tocopherol (αT)	Halts the creation of ROS, scavenges free radicals, stabilizes cell membranes, decreases apoptotic cell count, and minimizes the activation of nuclear factor kappa B (NF-κB)
Organosulphur compounds	Sulphoranes, glucosinloates	Asserted to possess potent antioxidant properties; furthermore, believed to exhibit various other beneficial activities, including anti-platelet effects, immunomodulation, fibrinolysis promotion, anti-ageing properties, anti-inflammatory actions, antimicrobial and antiparasitic activity, as well as the ability to lower blood pressure, reduce lipid levels, mitigate atherosclerosis, and combat viral infections
Phytosterol	Stigmosterol	Reported to possess cholesterol-lowering capabilities and exhibit a range of health-promoting properties, including antioxidant, anti-inflammatory, anticancer, and antiosteoarthritis effects; has demonstrated anti-tumour activity in several types of cancers, including breast, lung, liver, and ovarian cancers, by facilitating apoptosis (cell death), suppressing proliferation, inhibiting metastasis and invasion, and inducing autophagy within tumour cells

A combination of various compounds in oats solidifies their status as both a nutraceutical and a superfood, highlighting their exceptional value in a balanced diet and overall health (Figure 10.3). Some of these compounds are as follows.

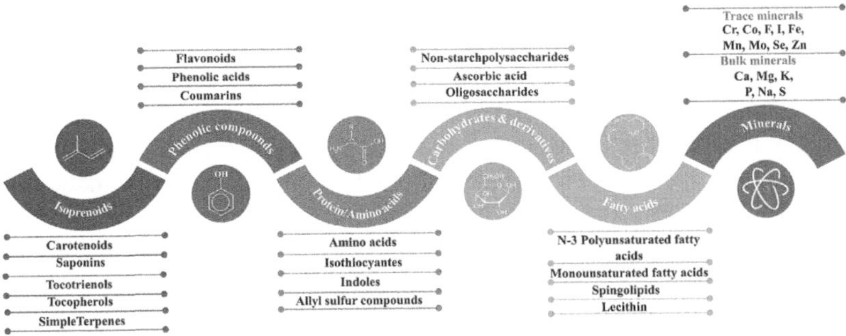

FIGURE 10.3   The diverse array of bioactive and therapeutic compounds present in oats. The depicted compounds encompass a wide range of nutritional and health-promoting elements, including carotenoids, saponins, tocotrienols, tocopherols, simple terpenes, flavonoids, phenolic acids, coumarins, amino acids, isothiocyanates, indoles, allyl sulphur compounds, non-starch polysaccharides, ascorbic acid, oligosaccharides, N-3 polyunsaturated fatty acids, monounsaturated fatty acids, sphingolipids, lecithin, trace minerals (Cr, Co, F, I, Fe, Mn, Mo, Se, Zn), and bulk minerals (Ca, Mg, K). This comprehensive depiction underscores the rich and diverse composition of bioactive and nutritive components found in oats, contributing to their potential health benefits.

10.3.1 Oat Proteins

Oat peptides, which possess bioactive qualities, are typically derived through the enzymatic breakdown of oat proteins and are recognized for their diverse regulatory functions [23]. Several studies indicate the valuable nutraceutical attributes of oat proteins and peptides, while also discussing the utilization of oat protein as a functional ingredient [3], [24]–[28]. The findings also indicate that oat protein and peptides exhibit a wide range of therapeutic properties, including the ability to address conditions such as diabetes, provide antioxidant benefits, combat hypoxia, manage hypertension, prevent thrombosis, reduce fatigue, modulate the immune system, and lower cholesterol levels [29]. However, it's worth noting that the majority of these studies have been conducted in vitro, and there is limited data available on the effectiveness of oat peptides in vivo. To further advance the development of functional food products and nutraceutical and therapeutic applications, future research should focus on comprehensive animal studies and, ultimately, clinical trials.

10.3.2 Carotenoids

Carotenoids are essential phytochemicals found in cereals, imparting the characteristic yellow hue to the endosperm and serving as critical visual and nutritional indicators of grain quality. Cereals like wheat, maize, rice, and sorghum predominantly contain xanthophylls in their carotenoid profiles, with lutein being the most abundant, followed by β-cryptoxanthin and zeaxanthin, along with smaller quantities of carotenes such as β- and α-carotene [30]. In oat grains, the total carotenoid content amounts to 1.8 µg/g, comprising 0.10 µg/g of lutein and 0.35 µg/g of zeaxanthin. Carotenoids are lipophilic pigments composed of C40 isoprenoids featuring extended conjugated polyene chains. These crucial natural compounds can be categorized into two classes: carotenes (hydrocarbons, including lycopene and β-carotene) and xanthophylls (oxygenated derivatives of carotenes, including astaxanthin, lutein, and zeaxanthin) [31]. They are present in various types of plastids.

Oat-based carotenoids have gained widespread recognition as superfoods and nutraceuticals, owing to their impressive health benefits. Carotenoids, including β-carotene, lutein, and zeaxanthin, which are naturally found in oats, serve as potent antioxidants that shield cells from oxidative stress and help lower the risk of chronic illnesses such as heart disease and age-related macular degeneration. These compounds also contribute to maintaining healthy skin and promoting a vibrant complexion. It's important to note that both humans and animals are incapable of producing carotenoids on their own, necessitating the consumption of plant-based foods to meet their daily health and physiological requirements [32]. Provitamins like β-cryptoxanthin, β-carotene, and α-carotene play a crucial role in the formation of light-sensing retinal molecules. Additionally, β-carotene and β-cryptoxanthin contain unsubstituted β-rings that, upon ingestion, are converted into retinol (i.e., vitamin A), effectively preventing detrimental eye conditions such as Bitot's spots, xerophthalmia, night blindness, corneal ulcers, and lesions. Xanthophyll carotenoids like zeaxanthin and lutein may also help in preventing age-related macular degeneration [33].

Moreover, carotenoids play a pivotal role in regulating various intracellular signalling pathways, gap-junction communication, growth factors, and the immune system. They influence cell differentiation, cell cycles, and apoptosis. Carotenoids offer photoprotection against the damaging effects of UV radiation and reduce the risk of chronic diseases and specific forms of cancer development. Regularly incorporating a carotenoid-rich diet, particularly with the inclusion of oat-based carotenoids, can provide a delectable and versatile way to enhance overall well-being while enjoying the numerous health benefits associated with these natural compounds. Consequently, a consistent intake of a diet rich in carotenoids can effectively lower the risk of non-communicable diseases. Therefore, including oat-based carotenoids in one's diet can serve as a delightful and adaptable approach to improving overall well-being, all while indulging in a wholesome, plant-based nutritional enhancement.

10.3.3 Benzoxazinoid

Benzoxazinoids, which are present in oat grains, constitute a group of natural chemical compounds believed to possess pharmacological and health-protective properties. These compounds are primarily found in young plants of the monocotyledonous family, Gramineae [34]. Chemically, benzoxazinoids can be classified into benzoxazolinones, lactams, and hydroxamic acids. Various studies, including in vitro experiments and a limited number of investigations involving humans and animal models, have explored the potential health effects and pharmacological responses of different benzoxazinoid compounds. These studies have revealed several noteworthy findings, such as the antimicrobial, anticancer, and stimulatory effects on the reproductive and central nervous systems, immunoregulatory properties, as well as appetite and weight-reducing effects associated with benzoxazinoids and their derivatives [35]. The health benefits attributed to the consumption of whole grains may be linked to the diverse and sometimes overlapping biological effects of components like fibres, lignans, phenolic acids, alkylresorcinols, benzoxazinoids, and other bioactive compounds. Regarding benzoxazinoids as dietary constituents, there is a pressing need for more comprehensive research. This research should aim to better understand their biological functions, elucidate the underlying mechanisms of their actions, explore their potential contributions to the health benefits associated with whole-grain consumption, and assess their suitability as components of oat-based nutraceuticals and superfoods.

10.3.4 Phytic Acids

Myo-inositol-1,2,3,4,5,6-hexakisphosphoric acid, commonly referred to as phytic acid or IP6, is a prevalent component found in plants, particularly in grains and plant seeds, where it accumulates during the maturation process [1], [3], [36]. Phytic acid possesses a unique structure characterized by 12 ionizable protons, which gives it distinct properties, notably the ability to form chelates with polyvalent metal ions like calcium, zinc, and iron. These interactions result in the formation of insoluble salts known as phytates. Additionally, other compounds such as pentaphosphate (IP5), tetraphosphate (IP4), and inositol triphosphate (IP3) are also commonly referred to as phytates [1], [3], [36]. Phytic acid is often described as an "anti-nutrient" due to its capacity to chelate micronutrients in food, rendering them unabsorbable and, consequently, reducing their bioavailability. However, this effect is primarily associated with diets that are simultaneously deficient in trace elements and high in phytic acid intake. It's worth noting that bioavailability can also be influenced by the binding of micronutrients with other components in the diet, and the molar ratio of metal ions to phytic acid should be considered [37]. On the other hand, numerous studies, both in vitro (lab experiments) and in vivo (studies involving living organisms), have provided compelling evidence of the potent anticancer properties of phytic acid.

Phytic acid content in oats typically ranges from 0.5 to 1.2 g/100 g. Phytic acid derived from oats has garnered attention both as a "nutraceutical" and as a superfood ingredient. Various studies investigating its potential health and physiological benefits suggest that phytic acid may have positive effects in addressing several diseases, including diabetes, preventing vascular calcifications, reducing the risk of cardiovascular events, coronary heart disease, Parkinson's disease, and treating kidney stones. What makes phytic acid particularly appealing is its non-toxic and non-reactive nature, making it suitable for a range of applications [38]. It has long been employed as a versatile and unique food preservative, often added to various food products to extend shelf life and prevent discolouration. Additionally, different studies indicate that phytic acid may possess antimicrobial properties against foodborne pathogens and natural spoilage fungi. Beyond its role in the food industry, phytic acid finds application in various industrial sectors. It is used in treating heavy-metal-contaminated waste, as a coating to prevent rusting and corrosion on metals, and more recently, it has been incorporated as a bio-based component in fabrics to provide flame-retardant properties [39]. Phytic acid derived from oats exhibits a wide range of potential applications, from promoting health and preserving food to addressing environmental and industrial challenges.

10.3.5 Phenolic Compounds and Avenanthramides

Phenolic compounds are a class of organic compounds characterized by the presence of at least one aromatic ring with one or more hydroxyl groups [1], [3], [36]. They are typically classified into various groups, including phenolic acids, flavonoids, stilbenes, coumarins, and tannins. These compounds serve as optional metabolites in plants, playing crucial roles in their growth, development, and acting as a defence mechanism [40], [41]. Oats contain a range of phenolic compounds, including phenolic acids, flavonoids, avenanthramides, and lignans.

Phenolic acids, particularly ferulic acid, are the predominant phenolic compounds in oats, with ferulic acid being present at a concentration of approximately 250 mg/kg. Ferulic acid is primarily bound to cell wall components through ester or ether linkages but can also be found in free forms within the oats [38]. Oats also contain other phenolic acids, including *p*-coumaric acid, vanillin, caffeic acid, vanillic acid, and *p*-hydroxybenzoic acid. The oat phenolic extracts demonstrated increased antimicrobial effectiveness against *Aspergillus flavus* and *Bacillus cereus*. Total phenolic content in the phenolic extracts of oats exhibited a significantly positive correlation with antioxidant activity. Phenolic compounds in oats are predominantly found in the outer layer (bran) of the grains, where they are concentrated. In addition to phenolic acids, oats contain a unique class of compounds called avenanthramides, which are specific *N*-cinnamoylanthranilate alkaloids exclusive to oats that have displayed antioxidant properties in an in vitro linoleic acid oxidation system. Researchers have identified a total of 25 different avenanthramides (AVAs) in oats [42]. Among these, AVA-A (2p), AVA-B (2f), and AVA-C (2c) are the most abundant. Avenanthramides are notable for their documented antioxidant, anti-inflammatory, and anti-proliferative properties, which contribute to the health benefits associated with oat consumption.

These phenolic compounds make oats a valuable dietary choice for promoting overall well-being. In pigmented whole-grain cereals, you can find additional compounds like anthocyanins, proanthocyanidins, and their derivatives, which contribute to their potent antioxidant properties. Flavonoids, which are part of the phenolic mix, have been associated with potentially halting the progression of certain chronic diseases. Significant grain crops, such as wheat, sorghum, rice, rye, corn, oats, barley, and millet, contain an abundance of specific phenolic compounds like ferulic acid, *p*-hydroxybenzoic acid, and diadzene. The presence of these phenolic compounds underscores the health benefits associated with consuming whole grains. These compounds contribute to the nutritional value and potential health-promoting effects of whole cereals.

10.3.6 Phytosterols

In grains, plant sterols manifest in various forms, including free sterols, steryl esters linked to unsaturated fats or phenolic acids, steryl glycosides, and acylated steryl glycosides. They play a pivotal role as structural components that stabilize plant cell membranes. These sterols can exist in either a "free" unbound state or covalently bound through ester or glycosidic bonds. Phytosterol glucosides, notably found in the lipid rafts of plant cell plasma membranes, are considered essential for the proper function of plasma membrane enzymes and potentially other proteins [43]. Phytosterols also serve as precursors for the synthesis of vital bioactive compounds such as steroidal saponins, steroidal glycoalkaloids, phytoecdysteroids, and brassinosteroids [44].

Oat phytosterols have gained acclaim as both a superfood and nutraceutical due to their remarkable health advantages. Various types of oat phytosterols have been identified, including sitosterol, sitostanol, campesterol, campestanol, and stigmasterol. Numerous studies have suggested that phytosterols may offer health-promoting benefits, including potential anticancer properties. Prior research has indicated that dietary phytosterols can reduce the absorption of cholesterol in the gastrointestinal tract, leading to lower levels of serum LDL and total cholesterol [45]. Furthermore, oat phytosterols have been demonstrated to possess antioxidant, antiatherosclerotic, anti-inflammatory, antidiabetic, and chemopreventive activities.

10.3.7 ß-Glucan

β-Glucan is typically composed of d-glucose monomers linked by a combination of β-(1→3) and β-(1→4) glycosidic linkages, forming a backbone of β-(1→3)-linked-dglucopyranosyl units with β-(1→6)-linked side chains of varying distribution and size [46]. These compounds are predominantly found in cereals like barley and oats, yeast, and mushrooms, and their versatility has led to growing interest in their applications across biomedical, pharmaceutical, food, and cosmetic industries. The popularity of foods and dietary supplements containing β-glucans has surged, with significant contributions to reducing insulin resistance and improving glycaemic control. β-Glucan intake has been shown to lower glycaemia and insulin levels, although the treatment effect varies with dosage and physicochemical characteristics. Higher molecular weight β-glucans exhibit more pronounced effects in reducing oxidative stress and hyperlipidemia in diabetic mice. Viscous β-glucans also influence the expression of key intestinal glucose transporters [47].

Studies have demonstrated that β-glucan can aid in weight management by inducing satiety and reducing body weight, serum cholesterol levels, and lipoprotein profiles in mice. It also shows promise in controlling adipogenesis. β-Glucan plays a crucial role in modulating gut microbiota, particularly increasing the production of short-chain fatty acids, which are fermented by gut microbiota. These changes in microbiota composition contribute to cardiovascular health, as high-molecular-weight β-glucan has been shown to increase the relative abundance of *Bacteroidetes* while decreasing *Firmicutes*. Furthermore, β-glucan has been linked to lower blood pressure, with its viscosity properties playing a significant role in its antihypertensive effects. The viscosity-induced weight loss effect is associated with reduced blood pressure, suggesting strong interconnections between β-glucan viscosity, body weight, blood glucose levels, serum cholesterol, and blood pressure.

These multifaceted attributes position oat β-glucan as an ideal candidate for superfood and nutraceutical applications, given its potential to positively impact various aspects of health, including glycaemic control, cardiovascular health, and weight management.

10.3.8 Tocols

Increasing evidence indicates that oats and oat-based products contain significant levels of bioactive compounds with potential health benefits, including natural antioxidants known as tocols. Tocols encompass both tocopherols and tocotrienols and are naturally occurring antioxidants found in oat grains, renowned for their bioactivity. Vitamin E serves as a broad term encompassing a group of structurally related compounds consisting of two vitamers, namely tocopherols and tocotrienols. Tocols exist in eight distinct forms: α-tocopherol (αTP), β-tocopherol (βTP), γ-tocopherol (γTP), δ-tocopherol (δTP), α-tocotrienol (αTT), β-tocotrienol (βTT), γ-tocotrienol (γTT), and δ-tocotrienol (δTT) [48]. Generally, tocols comprise a polar chromanol ring linked to an isoprenoid-derived hydrocarbon chain, differing primarily in the saturation state of the isoprenoid side chain. The fundamental structure of tocopherols consists of 2-methyl 2-(4, 8,12-trimethyltridecyl) chroman-6-ol, while tocotrienols consist of 2-methyl-2-(4,8,12-trimethyltrideca-3, 7, 11-trienyl) chroman-6-ol. The presence of the phenolic hydroxyl group in tocopherols and tocotrienols plays a pivotal role in their antioxidant activity, as it enables the donation of a phenolic hydroxyl group from the chromanol ring to free radicals, thereby stabilizing them and interrupting the propagation phase of oxidative chain reactions [49].

The tocol content in oats typically ranges from 10.2 to 74.7 mg/kg. Beyond their antioxidant properties, the presence of tocols in oats can offer significant health advantages to humans, including the modulation of degenerative diseases such as cancer and CVD, as well as the reduction of blood cholesterol levels. Several reports suggest that the vitamin E activity of tocols depends on their chemical structure and various physiological factors. For instance, different tocol isomers exhibit varying levels of vitamin E activity, with the order of activity being α-tocopherol (αTP) > β-tocopherol (βTP) > α-tocotrienol (αTT) > γ-tocopherol (γTP) > β-tocotrienol (βTT) > δ-tocopherol (δTP), while γ-tocotrienol (γTT) and δ-tocotrienol (δTT) may not exhibit significant activity [50]. Among these, α-tocopherol has the highest vitamin E activity, while α-tocotrienol contributes to the nutritive value of oats due to its excellent antioxidant properties. Tocotrienols, on the other hand, offer a range of unique and beneficial functions. For example, they may have a protective effect by reducing LDL cholesterol levels through the inhibition of cholesterol biosynthesis. Recent studies have also highlighted the positive impact of tocols on coronary artery disease, with evidence indicating that high α-tocopherol intake can decrease lipid peroxidation, platelet aggregation, and function as a potent anti-inflammatory agent [51]. Epidemiological research has further demonstrated that individual tocotrienols and tocopherols exhibit varying potencies in terms of their anticancer activity.

10.3.9 Vitamins and Minerals

Cereals harbour a diverse array of bioactive substances categorized according to their actions, including antibacterial, antioxidant, immunomodulatory, anti-inflammatory, and antithrombotic effects [52]. They are also evaluated for their binding affinity with micronutrients like minerals. Oat bran, in particular, contains trace elements and minerals such as calcium, phosphorus, iron, zinc, manganese, and chromium, which are readily absorbed by the body. Recent research underscores the significant contribution of oat grains and oat products to daily dietary intake, with 64.1% of manganese, followed by copper (31.3%) and iron (34.1%). Additionally, oats provide 20–30% of zinc and phosphorus, and 10–20% of sodium, potassium, and calcium. These elements and substances hold promise in preventing conditions like osteoporosis and anaemia while promoting wound healing. Among various grains, including rice, wheat, and corn, oats stand out as the richest source of selenium, known for enhancing immunity and offering protection against cancer and ageing.

Furthermore, oats are a treasure trove of vitamins and minerals with significant health benefits. They are particularly rich in B vitamins, including vitamin B_1, B_2, B_3, B_6, and B_{12}, as well as vitamin C, vitamin A, and vitamin E. These nutrients underpin the well-deserved reputation of oats as both a superfood and a nutraceutical. Oats are celebrated for their ability to support heart health by lowering LDL cholesterol levels, aid in weight management due to their satiating fibre content, help regulate blood sugar levels owing to their low glycaemic index, promote digestive health through their blend of soluble and insoluble fibre, and offer overall nutrient density. Moreover, oat extracts and derivatives are harnessed in nutraceutical products like oat bran and oat β-glucan supplements, which are marketed for their potential health benefits, encompassing cholesterol management and overall well-being. The versatility and nutritional richness of oats make them a valuable and wholesome addition to a balanced diet.

10.3.10 Lignans

Lignans are polyphenolic bioactive compounds classified as dietary phytoestrogen enhancers and are found in various plant-based food sources, including oats. Some of the most well-known plant lignans in human diets include secoisolariciresinol, matairesinol, lariciresinol, pinoresinol, and syringaresinol. In oat bran, the levels of secoisolariciresinol and matairesinol were measured at 238 and 1550 mg/kg, respectively, while in oatmeal, they were found to be 134 and 3 mg/kg, respectively [53]. In warm-blooded animals, lignans exhibit strong antioxidant properties and low oestrogenic activity, which contribute to their biological effects and health benefits. In mammals, lignans have been shown to provide protection against heart diseases and chemicals associated with breast and prostate cancer [54]. They also inhibit the growth of colon cancer cells and interfere with the progression of the cell cycle. Lignans in grains are primarily concentrated in the outer fibre-containing layers, so the milling of oats can significantly impact their lignan content.

Lignans are known to induce various bioactivities, including acting as phytoestrogens, similar to isoflavones and coumestans. Collectively, phytoestrogens are defined as plant-derived compounds that exert oestrogen-like effects [55]. Plant lignans themselves do not possess inherent oestrogenic activity but are converted by intestinal bacteria into more bioactive mammalian lignans, also known as enterolignans [56]. Upon ingestion, sugar moieties are hydrolysed, and it is the released aglycones that are metabolized by gut bacteria into enterolignans. Dietary phytoestrogens like lignans may also have weakly anti-oestrogenic properties.

Lignans exhibit antioxidant activity, which has been investigated in vitro for compounds such as secoisolariciresinol diglycoside and its mammalian lignans, enterodiol, and enterolactone. Their ability to scavenge hydroxyl and peroxyl radicals has been assessed in both lipid and aqueous models, including tests involving lipid oxidation, deoxyribose degradation by hydroxyl radicals to evaluate site-specific and non-site-specific scavenging activities, and a plasmid DNA-nicking assay. All three lignans showed effectiveness in reducing lipid peroxidation, but mammalian lignans were more efficient than secoisolariciresinol diglycoside in reducing deoxyribose oxidation and DNA strand breakage. These findings suggest structural and functional differences between the three lignans regarding antioxidant activity and highlight the potential health benefits of oat-derived lignans, positioning them as an excellent source for superfood and nutraceutical applications.

10.3.11 Flavonoids

Flavonoids are compounds characterized by two aromatic rings linked by a 3-carbon connection, and they encompass various subgroups such as anthocyanins, flavonols, flavones, and flavanones. In oats, flavonoids are evenly distributed in the pericarp (outer layer). Oats exhibit a notably wide range of flavanones, which are typically found in fruits and vegetables but are also present in cereals. While most grains contain only trace amounts of flavonoids, some oats contain measurable levels of catechin. The total flavonoid content in oat grains falls within the range of 754.16 to 1056.66 mg of quercetin equivalent (QE), while total flavonol content ranges from 663.75 to 697.5 mg QE [57]. Flavonoids are recognized for their various health-promoting properties, including antioxidant, anticancer, anti-allergy, anti-inflammatory, anti-carcinogenic, and gastro-protective effects [58]. The discoveries regarding oat-derived flavonoids highlight their potential health advantages, establishing them as a valuable source for superfood and nutraceutical applications.

10.4 CONCLUSION

Superfoods and nutraceuticals have gained popularity globally due to their perceived health benefits, offering a potential solution to address food insecurity. However, this trend raises environmental concerns, particularly regarding the intensified production methods required to meet the growing demand. These production changes can have profound effects on landscapes, diets, and carbon footprints. Achieving sustainable intensification in agriculture is crucial to address these challenges while also addressing climate change and other environmental issues. Science-based policies, including resource reduction, efficient water use, and long-term assessment of productivity and ecosystem services, are essential to support this transition. Regulation of superfoods and nutraceuticals is essential to provide consumers with accurate information about these products and establish minimum health claim requirements. Additionally, transparency and traceability in food supply chains can be improved through digitalization and technologies like the Internet of things, blockchain, and distributed ledger technologies to ensure food quality and safety.

Future research on superfoods should focus on human intervention studies to scientifically support their health benefits. Establishing a standardized definition for superfoods by food authorities can improve understanding and regulation. Oats, in particular, have shown promise in protecting against various diseases and supporting weight control. While more research is needed to understand their mechanisms of action, the link between whole oat grains and health holds potential for the development of nutritious oat-based foods.

Overall, enhancing production, reducing costs, and improving the bioavailability of nutrients and bioactive compounds in whole-grain-based products are key priorities for promoting health and addressing the rising prevalence of chronic diseases in affluent countries. Innovative manufacturing processes, equipment, and product standards are essential for achieving these goals and meeting consumer demand for healthy and nutritious foods.

REFERENCES

[1] M. Tomar et al., "Nutritional composition patterns and application of multivariate analysis to evaluate indigenous Pearl millet ((*Pennisetum glaucum* (L.) R. Br.) germplasm," *J. Food Compos. Anal.*, vol. 103, p. 104086, 2021, doi: 10.1016/j.jfca.2021.104086.

[2] D. Šamec and B. Urlić, "Salopek-Sondi, Kale (Brassica oleracea var. acephala) as a superfood: Review of the scientific evidence behind the statement," *Crit. Rev. Food Sci. Nutr.*, vol. 59, pp. 2411–2422, 2019, doi: 10.1080/10408398.2018.1454400.

[3] M. Tomar et al., "Interactome of millet-based food matrices: A review," Food Chem., vol. 385, p. 132636, 2022, doi: 10.1016/j.foodchem.2022.132636.

[4] D. Granato, F. J. Barba, D. Bursać Kovačević, J. M. Lorenzo, A. G. Cruz and P. Putnik, "Functional foods: Product development, technological trends, efficacy testing, and safety," *Annu. Rev. Food Sci. Technol.*, vol. 11, pp. 93–118, 2020, doi: 10.1146/annurev-food-032519-051708.

[5] S. Rodgers, "Minimally processed functional foods: Technological and operational pathways," *J. Food Sci.*, vol. 81, pp. R2309–R2319, 2016, doi: 10.1111/1750-3841.13422.

[6] K.D. Hall, "From dearth to excess: The rise of obesity in an ultra-processed food system," *Philos. Trans. R. Soc. B: Biol. Sci.*, vol. 378, p. 20220214, 2023, doi: 10.1098/rstb.2022.0214.

[7] J. Melo and C. Quintas, "Minimally processed fruits as vehicles for foodborne pathogens," *AIMS Microbiol.*, vol. 9, pp. 1–19, 2023, doi: 10.3934/microbiol.2023001.

[8] S. Sharma et al., "Vegetable microgreens: The gleam of next generation super foods, their genetic enhancement, health benefits and processing approaches," *Food Res. J.*, vol. 155, p. 111038, 2022, doi: 10.1016/j.foodres.2022.111038.

[9] M. Margallo Blanco, J. Laso Cortabitarte, A. Fernández Ríos and R. Aldaco García, "Superfoods: A super impact on health and the environment?," *Curr. Opin. Environ. Sci. Heal.*, vol. 31, p. 100410, 2023, doi: 10.1016/j.coesh.2022.100410.

[10] Ž. Pećanin and T. Vukasović, "Factors influencing consumer purchase behaviour when buying superfoods," *Mednarodno Inovativno Poslovanje = J. Innov. Bus. Manag.*, vol. 14, pp. 1–12, 2022, doi: 10.32015/JIBM.2022.14.1.4.

[11] A. Fernández-Ríos et al., "A critical review of superfoods from a holistic nutritional and environmental approach," *J. Clean. Prod.*, vol. 379, p. 134491, 2022, doi: 10.1016/j.jclepro.2022.134491.

[12] C. MacGregor, A. Petersen and C. Parker, "Promoting a healthier, younger you: The media marketing of anti-ageing superfoods," *J. Consum. Cult.*, vol. 21, pp. 164–179, 2021, doi: 10.1177/1469540518773825.

[13] S.L. DeFelice, "The nutraceutical revolution: Its impact on food industry R&D," *Trends Food Sci. Technol.*, vol. 6, pp. 59–61, 1995, doi: 10.1016/S0924-2244(00)88944-X.

[14] A. Santini et al., "Nutraceuticals: Opening the debate for a regulatory framework," *Br. J. Clin. Pharmacol.*, vol. 84, pp. 659–672, 2018, doi: 10.1111/bcp.13496.

[15] G. Picone, C. Mengucci and F. Capozzi, "The NMR added value to the green foodomics perspective: Advances by machine learning to the holistic view on food and nutrition," *Magn. Reson. Chem.*, vol. 60, pp. 590–596, 2022, doi: 10.1002/mrc.5257.

[16] E. Gupta and P. Mishra, "Functional food with some health benefits, so called superfood: A review," *Curr. Nutr. Food Sci.*, vol. 17, pp. 144–166, 2021, doi: 10.2174/157340 1316999200717171048.

[17] J. C. Espín, M. T. García-Conesa and F. A. Tomás-Barberán, "Nutraceuticals: Facts and fiction," *Phytochemistry*, vol. 68, pp. 2986–3008, 2007, doi: 10.1016/j. phytochem.2007.09.014.

[18] K. Gul, A. K. Singh and R. Jabeen, "Nutraceuticals and functional foods: The foods for the future world," *Crit. Rev. Food Sci. Nutr.*, vol. 56, pp. 2617–2627, 2016, doi: 10.1080/10408398.2014.903384.

[19] M. Saka, B. Özkaya and İ. Saka, "The effect of bread-making methods on functional and quality characteristics of oat bran blended bread," *Int. J. Gastron. Food Sci.*, vol. 26, p. 100439, 2021, doi: 10.1016/j.ijgfs.2021.100439.

[20] M. Rabie Abd El-Rahman, "Effect of dry and germinated oat on hypercholesterolemic rats," *Egypt. J. Nutr.*, vol. 38, pp. 44–66, 2023, doi: 10.21608/enj.2023.233786.1011.

[21] A. Mackie, "The role of food structure in gastric-emptying rate, absorption and metabolism," *Proc. Nutr. Soc.*, pp. 1–7, 2023, doi: 10.1017/S0029665123003609.

[22] M. Rawat et al., "A comprehensive review on nutraceutical potential of underutilized cereals and cereal-based products," *J. Agric. Food Res.*, vol. 12, p. 100619, 2023, doi: 10.1016/j.jafr.2023.100619.

[23] H. Rafique et al., "Dietary-nutraceutical properties of oat protein and peptides," *Front. Nutr.*, vol. 9, 2022. Accessed: Sept. 23, 2023. [Online]. Available: www.frontiersin.org/articles/10.3389/fnut.2022.950400

[24] M. Kumar et al., "Cottonseed feedstock as a source of plant-based protein and bioactive peptides: Evidence based on biofunctionalities and industrial applications," *Food Hydrocoll.*, vol. 131, p. 107776, 2022, doi: 10.1016/j.foodhyd.2022.107776.

[25] M. Kumar et al., "Advances in the plant protein extraction: Mechanism and recommendations," *Food Hydrocoll.*, vol. 115, p. 106595, 2021, doi: 10.1016/j.foodhyd.2021.106595.

[26] M. Kumar et al., "Functional characterization of plant-based protein to determine its quality for food applications," *Food Hydrocoll.*, p. 106986, 2021, doi: 10.1016/j. foodhyd.2021.106986.

[27] M. Kumar et al., "Cottonseed: A sustainable contributor to global protein require-ments," *Trends Food Sci. Technol.*, vol. 111, pp. 100–113, 2021, doi: 10.1016/j.tifs.2021.02.058.

[28] M. Kumar et al., "Plant-based proteins and their multifaceted industrial applications," *LWT.*, vol. 154, p. 112620, 2022, doi: 10.1016/j.lwt.2021.112620.

[29] T.J. Ashaolu and I. Suttikhana, "Plant-based bioactive peptides: A review of their relevant production strategies, in vivo bioactivities, action mechanisms and bioaccessibility," *Int. J. Food Sci. Technol.*, vol. 58, pp. 2228–2235, 2023, doi: 10.1111/ijfs.16384.

[30] V. Ashokkumar et al., "Technological advances in the production of carotenoids and their applications– A critical review," *Bioresour. Technol.*, vol. 367, p. 128215, 2023, doi: 10.1016/j.biortech.2022.128215.

[31] X. Zhao, K. Liang and H. Zhu, "Carotenoids in cereals and related foodstuffs: A review of extraction and analysis methods," *Food Rev. Int.*, vol. 39, 2023, pp. 4513–4528, doi: 10.1080/87559129.2022.2027438.

[32] I. G. Loskutov and E. K. Khlestkina, "Wheat, barley, and oat breeding for health benefit components in grain," *Plants.*, vol. 10, 2021, p. 86, doi: 10.3390/plants10010086.

[33] P. Crupi, M. F. Faienza, M. Y. Naeem, F. Corbo, M. L. Clodoveo and M. Muraglia, "Overview of the potential beneficial effects of carotenoids on consumer health and well-being," *Antioxidants.*, vol. 12, p. 1069, 2023, doi: 10.3390/antiox12051069.

[34] S.K. Steffensen et al., "Bioactive small molecules in commercially available cereal food: Benzoxazinoids," *J. Food Compos. Anal.*, vol. 64, pp. 213–222, 2017, doi: 10.1016/j.jfca.2017.10.001.

[35] K.B. Adhikari et al., "Benzoxazinoids: Cereal phytochemicals with putative therapeutic and health-protecting properties," *Mol. Nutr. Food Res.*, vol. 59, 2015, pp. 1324–1338, doi: 10.1002/mnfr.201400717.

[36] M. Tomar et al., "Development of NIR spectroscopy based prediction models for nutritional profiling of pearl millet (*Pennisetum glaucum* (L.)) R.Br: A chemometrics approach," *LWT.*, vol. 149, 2021, p. 111813, doi: 10.1016/j.lwt.2021.111813.

[37] A. P. M. Bloot, D. L. Kalschne, J. A. S. Amaral, I. J. Baraldi and C. Canan, "A review of phytic acid sources, obtention, and applications," *Food Rev. Int.*, vol. 39, pp. 73–92, 2023, doi: 10.1080/87559129.2021.1906697.

[38] Y. Zhang, Y. Li, X. Ren, X. Zhang, Z. Wu and L. Liu, "The positive correlation of anti-oxidant activity and prebiotic effect about oat phenolic compounds," *Food Chem.*, 402, p. 134231, 2023, doi: 10.1016/j.foodchem.2022.134231.

[39] A. Poonia, D. S. Phogat, Versha, S. Nagar, P. Sharma and V. Kumar, "Biochemical assessment of oat genotypes revealed variability in grain quality with nutrition and crop improvement implications," *Food Chem.*, vol. 377, p. 131982, 2022, doi: 10.1016/j.foodchem.2021.131982.

[40] M. Kumar, M. Tomar, S. Punia, R. Amarowicz and C. Kaur, "Evaluation of cellulolytic enzyme-assisted microwave extraction of punica granatum peel phenolics and anti-oxidant activity," *Plant Foods Hum. Nutr.*, vol. 75, pp. 614–620, 2020, doi: 10.1007/s11130-020-00859-3.

[41] P. Van Hung, "Phenolic compounds of cereals and their antioxidant capacity," *Crit. Rev. Food Sci. Nutr.*, vol. 56, pp. 25–35, 2016, doi: 10.1080/10408398.2012.708909.

[42] A. Purushothaman, P. Jishnu Gopal and D. Janardanan, "Mechanistic insights on the radical scavenging activity of oat avenanthramides," *J. Phys. Org. Chem.*, vol. 35, p. e4391, 2022, doi: 10.1002/poc.4391.

[43] M. Kumar et al., "Guava (Psidium guajava L.) leaves: Nutritional composition, phyto-chemical profile, and health-promoting bioactivities," *Foods.*, vol. 10, p. 752, 2021, doi: 10.3390/foods10040752.

[44] D.M. Peterson, "Oat antioxidants," *J. Cereal Sci.*, vol. 33, pp. 115–129, 2001, doi: 10.1006/jcrs.2000.0349.

[45] X. Li, L. Zhou, Y. Yu, J. Zhang, J. Wang and B. Sun, "The potential functions and mechanisms of oat on cancer prevention: A review," *J. Agric. Food Chem.*, vol. 70, pp. 14588–14599, 2022, doi: 10.1021/acs.jafc.2c06518.

[46] D.P. Belobrajdic, H. Brook, P. Orchard, G. James-Martin and W. Stonehouse, "Australian mushroom β-glucan content and in vitro bile-acid binding capacity compared to oats," *Proc. Nutr. Soc.*, vol. 82, p. E93, 2023, doi: 10.1017/S0029665123001027.

[47] S. Fan et al., "Metabolomics reveals the effects of Lactiplantibacillus plantarum dy-1 fermentation on the lipid-lowering capacity of barley β-glucans in an in vitro model of gut-liver axis," *Int. J. Biol. Macromol.*, 2023, p. 126861, doi: 10.1016/j.ijbiomac.2023.126861.

[48] R. Ranasinghe, M. Mathai and A. Zulli, "Revisiting the therapeutic potential of tocotrienol," *BioFactors.*, vol. 48, pp. 813–856, 2022, doi: 10.1002/biof.1873.

[49] Z. Khan, S. Ahmed, Marya, H. Ullah and H. Khan, "Vitamin E (tocopherols and tocotrienols) (natural-occurring antioxidant; bright and dark side)," in *Antioxidants Effects in Health*, S. M. Nabavi and A. S. Silva, Eds. Elsevier, 2022, pp. 547–560, doi: 10.1016/B978-0-12-819096-8.00066-5.

[50] S.P. Bangar and N. Kaushik, "Functional cereals: Functional components and benefits," in *Functional Cereals and Cereal Foods: Properties, Functionality and Applications*, S. Punia Bangar and A. Kumar Siroha, Eds. Cham, Germany: Springer International Publishing, 2022, pp. 3–25, doi: 10.1007/978-3-031-05611-6_1.

[51] S. S. Yadav, L. Kaur, P. Nath and N. Deep, "Bioactive compounds and phytonutrients from cereals," in *Plant-Based Bioactive Compounds and Food Ingredients (First Edition)*, Palm Bay, Florida: Apple Academic Press, 2023, pp. 1–51.

[52] M. Tomar, Reetu and S. S. Changan, "Potato vitamins," in *Potato: Nutrition and Food Security*, P. Raigond, B. Singh, S. Dutt and S. K. Chakrabarti, Eds. Singapore, Singapore: Springer, 2020, pp. 113–132, doi: 10.1007/978-981-15-7662-1_7.

[53] D. Ryan, M. Kendall and K. Robards, "Bioactivity of oats as it relates to cardiovascular disease," *Nutr. Res. Rev.*, vol. 20, pp. 147–162, 2007, doi: 10.1017/S0954422407782884.

[54] S. Soleymani, S. Habtemariam, R. Rahimi and S. M. Nabavi, "The what and who of dietary lignans in human health: Special focus on prooxidant and antioxidant effects," *Trends Food Sci. Technol.*, vol. 106, 2020, pp. 382–390, doi: 10.1016/j.tifs.2020.10.015.

[55] N.S. Plaha, S. Awasthi, A. Sharma and N. Kaushik, "Distribution, biosynthesis and therapeutic potential of lignans," *3 Biotech.*, vol. 12, p. 255, doi: 10.1007/s13205-022-03318-9.

[56] A. Mueed, M. Ibrahim, S. Shibli, P. Madjirebaye, Z. Deng and M. Jahangir, "The fate of flaxseed-lignans after oral administration: A comprehensive review on its bioavailability, pharmacokinetics, and food design strategies for optimal application," *Crit. Rev. Food Sci. Nutr.*, 2022, 1–19, doi: 10.1080/10408398.2022.2140643.

[57] M. S. Ibrahim, A. Ahmad, A. Sohail and M. J. Asad, "Nutritional and functional characterization of different oat (Avena sativa L.) cultivars," *Int. J. Food Prop.*, vol. 23, 2020, pp. 1373–1385, doi: 10.1080/10942912.2020.1806297.

[58] Z. Li et al., "Unique roles in health promotion of dietary flavonoids through gut microbiota regulation: Current understanding and future perspectives," *Food Chem.*, vol. 399, 2023, 133959, doi: 10.1016/j.foodchem.2022.133959.

Index

Note: Page numbers in *italics* indicate a figure and page numbers in **bold** indicate a table on the corresponding page.

T

terpenes, 105
TG2 antibodies (TG2-Abs), 196–197
thermal processing, 164, **165**
    extrusion, 169–171
    hot-air dry roasting, 168–169
    kilning, 172–173
    microwave, 166–167
    superheated steam treatment, 171–172
threshing, 28
tocols, 125, *126*, **127**, 126–127, 376
trading, 56–59
transformation techniques, 349–351

U

ultrasound treatment, 178–181
United States, 30–31
USDA Foreign Agricultural Service, 49

V

vitamins, 88–90, *90*, **91**, 377
    vitamin A, 88–89
    vitamin C, 89
    vitamin D, 89
    vitamin K, 89

W

water-holding capacity (WHC), 306–307
weeding, 22
wet extrusion, 171
wireworms (*Agriotes* spp.), 26

Y

yield
    improvements, 55–56
    and quality, 27